Feeding Dogs

Dry or Raw?
The Science Behind the Debate

D1737964

Dr. Conor Brady

ISBN 978-1-9162340-0-0

Cover image credit: Merran Kavanagh of Mkaotearoa Photography.

Design and typesetting: Orla Kelly

Editing by Red Pen Edits

Published by Farrow Road Publishing

Dedicated to the four great women in my life – my mother Joan for fueling first my passion in the subject and then the work ethic that sustains me to this day; my most-adored dog Meg for showed me everything I was doing was wrong; my ever-patient wife Elaine, my enabler, I could not have done it without your love and support; and finally to my daughter Holly – never stop asking questions.

About the Author

After college, I spent 5 years in guide dogs as a pup supervisor and guide dog trainer. Fourteen years ago while I was working in Guide Dogs Australia, the true powers of raw feeding came to light. Since then, bar a couple of years as a producer myself, I have been a full-time writer, speaker and dedicated advocate for natural canine food and health (available at my website www.dogsfirst.ie). As a dog lover and keen researcher, the subject fascinates and consumes me, providing me with near bottomless rabbit holes that demand exploration. I live with my wife and daughter in Wicklow, Ireland, and am proud father to a slightly odd blue roan cocker called Dudley. What he lacks in brains and finesse he makes up with single-minded determination, although that statement is equally true for the both of us.

Conor Brady, PhD

Contents

Introduction

Everything was fine until I moved to Perth, Western Australia. Before that I was a dog trainer in the disability sector, happily pursuing a lifelong ambition of working full time with dogs, something I truly loved. Then, while working in Australia in 2009, two things came to my attention which forced me back to the office. Back to the laptop, back to research and long, dog-less days spent trawling through veterinary libraries and journals. It felt like no sooner had I started my career, then it was all over.

Before I get to these two events, a little background is needed. For as long as I can remember, I have been obsessed with dogs, much like you, I'm sure. There are seven of us in our family but each of our family dogs, four in total since the very day I was born, has been profoundly attached to me. Not inexplicable. In their eyes I provided everything they needed. It was my job to feed and walk them.

More than that, though, I lavished attention on them. They went everywhere with me, whether I wanted their company or not. There are countless stories of my first dog, Prince, escaping the garden to sit outside my school all day – ears erect, head cocked, patiently waiting for me. If I'd go in one supermarket door but out another, he'd wait outside the entrance all day and sometimes into the night before we found him.

There was the time my Dad's friend hid behind a wall to scare me. As I passed the wall, he jumped out and gave me a terrible shock. I cried out, which pleased him. But what he hadn't anticipated was my little ginger bodyguard, Prince. He came hurtling up and actually did the stereotypical rip-the-seat-of-the-pants bite on him. The sight of him running around the yard shouting and flapping his arms with my dog hanging off his butt made my scare worthwhile. I guess the strongest bonds are forged on these fearless acts of devotion. God, I loved that dog.

Suffice it to say, the time my parents spent driving an hour to the animal shelter and waiting in the car for their teenage son to emerge every Saturday morning for 3 years was apparently worth it. I went on to feed my interest in animals, obtaining a degree in zoology and ultimately leaving college with a PhD in Animal Behaviour, investigating the effect of nutrition on both the behaviour and digestive morphology of mammals.

In 2006, upon leaving college, I was accepted into Irish Guide Dogs and schooled as a dog trainer. For me, this was the dream achieved. My role as guide dog trainer and ultimately, pup supervisor, guaranteed me total puppy immersion from 9 to 5 – a job second to none for canine enthusiasts.

Pup supervisors have to visit each of their 40 pups twice a month during their first year, train the owners as well as the pups and keep tabs on their general development. From a behavioural point of view, it was a fascinating opportunity to watch the pups mature. I took detailed notes on all aspects of their life, both mental and physical. I documented the changes that could occur from the smallest tweaks to their environment. Few people out there today have such access to animals *in vivo*, that is to say, non-caged, non-laboratory animals that are out and about in their natural surroundings but at the same time under relatively strict control, certainly dietary control. There was a steep learning curve.

I left Irish Guide Dogs in 2009 and set off for Perth, Western Australia, to help establish a pup training program, was walking dogs in the sunshine was marginally more attractive than walking them in the lashing rain at home. It was while I was in Perth that the two life-altering realisations came to me, one in the dog world and one in my own, which ultimately forced me back underground into the lonely, gloomy realms of laborious research.

The first realisation occurred while I was doing some work on the side, as most trainers do. I began to notice that an exceedingly high number of Perth dogs received long-term doses of very serious medications: steroids, non-steroidal anti-inflammatory drugs (NSAIDs), antibiotics and antihistamines. For the large part, these dogs were suffering recurring skin and gut conditions. These medications were potent tablets, powerful injections, creams and eardrops. In fact, of the 18 dogs that I began to see regularly, a whopping seven received long-term steroids or NSAIDs. Seven of 18 dogs! Can you imagine a random sample of 18 kids in a school?

And they weren't attending one rogue vet in Perth. This was a casually accepted epidemic of sick dogs or more commonly (but incorrectly) termed allergy dogs' — hot spots; flaring skin conditions; itchy, sore feet; weeping eyes; mucky ears; almost always accompanied with some form of recurring diarrhoea, poor condition or weight loss. All the pills and potions used at this point were, in essence, an attempt to relieve the dog's symptoms. When the symptoms disappeared, the drugs were hailed a success. When their effects wore off, more drugs were administered, and so on.

I was uncomfortable with this, having seen the effects of these immune-suppressing drugs during my time with Guide Dogs. Steroids and NSAIDs are an incredible development in medicine. Steroids can shut down various parts of the immune system, immediately ridding you of the symptoms resulting from an immune system that is working overtime, such as rashes, itching and swelling. NSAIDs, don't so much work on the immune system itself but inhibit the production of prostaglandins, which represent the chemicals that promote inflammation. For many sick people, including transplant patients and anyone suffering with an auto-immune disease (where the immune system goes awry and begins to attack the body), these drugs are absolute lifesavers.

However, as the saying goes with some of the more impressive drugs, 'the bigger the front, the bigger the back', meaning the more amazing the results, the greater the potential for side effects. In the case of steroids or NSAIDs, excluding the fact that they prevent your immune system from doing its job correctly, their dark side involves a heavy impact on various organs, namely, the liver and kidneys. They are known to negatively affect joint integrity by weakening connectivity over time. They disrupt how your body deals with fat so your weight can balloon, compounding the issue. Then there is behaviour. It's unfair to ask anything complicated of a working dog on steroids. They appear a little tetchy, lack focus – although perhaps what we are seeing is the side effects of the underlying illness. Whatever the reason, it makes steroids a wholly unsuitable drug for long-term use, particularly in younger animals.

More to the point, drugs like steroids, NSAID's and pain relief do not provide the patient with a cure; unlike antibiotics, which do work to kill an infection, they are not designed to remedy the underlying issue. They merely serve to mask the symptoms, a short-term bandage to reduce your discomfort, giving you time to think and act. Break your ankle? Take a painkiller with an anti-inflammatory agent and let the bone re-set. Have a heart attack? Take these drugs, but to avoid a recurrence, you need to eat right, lose weight, de-stress and exercise.

As opposed to fighting strange symptoms, such as a funny rash or constantly upset gut, they often serve as a form of smoke detector; alerting us to a bigger issue lurking beneath. It's like putting a fresh plaster on gangrene each week, if you do not tackle the underlying cause, the issue is likely to continue to boil away under the surface. Symptoms will remerge, often growing to affect other systems and materialising in an increasing array of forms. Over time the plaster gets bigger and bigger and has to be changed more regularly. More and more medications are required until eventually either the underlying disease kills you or your exhausted immune system permits something else to do it.

This is the modern way of things. Since the accidental discovery of penicillin a hundred years ago (from a simple fungus), our health system has turned wholeheartedly toward chemistry. The average medical practitioner's approach to health is now, 'When the symptoms pop up, we have great pills here to get rid of them'. We see a similar approach applied particularly to patients with cancer.

The survival rate of cancer is much improved these days, but we seem to be ignoring the fact that cancer rates continue to soar in the general population. Today, incredibly 1-in-2 of us may be affected by it. With diabetes and heart disease showing similar trends, we are very clearly looking through the wrong end of the telescope.

Did you know we used to pay doctors to keep us healthy? Makes sense, doesn't it? Now it seems we pay them only when we're sick. But why would you keep paying a mechanic for an un-fixed car? Strange knocking sound from your engine? Here, pop these earmuffs on! Funny smell? Here's a peg for your nose! Spurred on by vast profits from multinational drug companies, health care has now become sick care. And all the while we ignore the fact that prescription drugs dished out by doctors are now the second biggest killer in the United States.

The true route to health care is not disease *treatment* but disease *avoidance*. Should you be unlucky enough to get a disease, you must find the *cause* of the symptoms you are experiencing — known as the aetiology of disease.

This point alone is perhaps the crux of this entire book.

I wanted to know the aetiology of the disease affecting my Perth dogs but it's exactly where things always seem to get a bit murky. Everyone had an answer. Unfortunately, all the answers were different. For dogs, Perth, apparently, is the allergy capital of the world. The offending antigens (substances that cause a negative reaction in your body) were suspected to be a wide range of things — from the grass and carpets they lie on, to the air they breathe, the food they eat, the dust mites they nibble, the fleas in the sand and, somewhat bizarrely for meat-eaters, the beef and chicken in their diets.

As everyone knows, everything in Australia is dangerous! So, it's hardly surprising that there is a whole host of potential allergens that bother dogs. From the top ten most poisonous spiders and snakes in the world to the man-eating sharks in the water and the deadly weather, we can now add vicious pollen and fleas.

In this way, recurring skin and gut conditions have become the casually accepted norm for many Perth dogs today, an irritating part of daily life in a converted desert. But I wasn't convinced. It simply didn't add up. Not only were humans not affected to anywhere near the same degree, but I was seeing dogs overreacting, sometimes quite violently, to the likes of a fleabite. Two even suffered mange outbreaks, something I hadn't seen in a dog since my shelter days and then only in the worst cases. Mange (certainly *Demodex* mange, the more common and less harmful cousin of *Sarcoptes* mange) can only get hold of very sick, stressed or weakened animals. The mite that causes mange is, invariably, on and off them throughout their lives. Just like fleas, these critters are normally kept in check by a healthy, in-balance body and robust immune system. For a well-cared for dog, mange should be no more common than scurvy for a well-fed human. So, if a dog presents with mange, the focus of a more holistic-minded vet would not be simply on the mites or fleas running rampant on the dog, but essentially what is wrong with this dog *under the hood*. Why couldn't his immune system keep these baddies at bay? Is he sick? Is he stressed? Or is an insidious disease lurking in the background, sapping his reserves? But these well-pampered Perth dogs did not appear to have any of these conditions. They were young, robust, well-fed and well-cared for pets.

Apart from the fact that these dogs were clearly distressed, something we would all find upsetting, I was vexed by the absolute lack of veterinary explanation that followed all their expensive and invasive tests. The affected dog owners would hand me over a lengthy report with an apologetic 'I dunno' expression, like it might be something they could be doing wrong.

The reports were always the same. Either a vague reference was made to an unexplained, recurring mystery allergy, such as atopic dermatitis, which means a skin disorder with no known cause. Or it would be accompanied by a dizzying list of potential allergens, always including mundane challenges like pollen and dust mites. As if these Perth dogs were some of the weakest animals in the world.

Whatever the cause, the solution was always the same – some incredibly scientific and exorbitantly priced pet food and a barrage of expensive, powerful, synthetic drugs to keep the dog's *symptoms* in check, often administered monthly.

This bothered me considerably. Of course, there was a *cause*, we just hadn't identified it yet. And I couldn't stop thinking about it.

The second thing that happened to me in Perth occurred around the same time as all the above was going on. It led to my own personal eureka moment. Perhaps not on par with the importance of Sir Isaac Newton's, but for me it was certainly akin to discovering gravity as it changed the course of my career and my life forever. It was when my wife began to complain about my snoring. Now this was a new grumbling for me to deal with. I was horrified when the other occupants of the house, who actually lived some distance down the hall, verified it, in spite of us being separated by a spare room, bathroom and linen cupboard. Rather than give the houseowners time to ponder their new life with a hippopotamus, I took action and started asking around for some advice. Having exhausted some of the more popular ideas and remedies, I found myself standing at the door of a holistic, food nutritionist person.

Now for anyone who knew me, this was an event. Having been immersed in science for years in college, my stance on *heebie-jeebie* medicine was clear. I didn't like it. The countless stories of their failures under scientific scrutiny were enough for me to label the whole lot of holistic and homeopathic practitioners, water diviners, psychics and astrologists, as crackpots – refugees from the 1960s eking out a living from gloomy tents in carnivals.

The very ordinarily dressed lady sat me down in her ordinarily decorated office in front of a machine that, to my surprise, was already familiar to most of us. Unlike the more uncomfortable pinprick test under the skin, used to test the body's reaction to various proteins, the Vega Test is a quick, noninvasive technique (that I'm still unsure about).

Essentially, you sit there holding two little rods. It uses a harmless current to detect the body's reaction to various food groups. She was going to test over 200 foods, so we got to chatting and it quickly became apparent that this lady knew her stuff. She was a scientist. She had the same degree as me, was going on to obtain a master's degree in nutrition, then to work as a nutritionist in a hospital before specialising in food allergies full-time. I began to relax and answer her questions.

When does this occur? Have you any other symptoms? What did you eat prior to your issues developing? How are your movements? FLINCH! I'm Irish. We are positively averse to talking seriously about anything concerning reproductive organs or bottoms. And all the while, her cute little machine made perpetual chirping noises, which I took to be good.

Once she established that my snoring was worse after poker nights and parties, she quickly diagnosed me as possibly gluten-sensitive, at which point her machine dutifully gave a rather over-the-top electronic wail, which I took to be bad.

INTRODUCTION

And bad it was. Testing out her diagnosis, we verified that my snoring (and blocked nose, waxy ears and headaches) was, indeed, much worse after poker night. This was due largely to my beer consumption. Like all the nice things, beer is of course, wheat-based (as is bread, cakes, biscuits, pizza, muffins, batter, crackers and anything else tasty in the average person's life). I was distraught. We had had some good times, wheat and me. I hadn't realised how friendly we'd become or how hard it would be to say goodbye.

Dietary sensitivity is a very new realm of science, only really gaining popularity in the last two decades. Like all new sciences, it is initially causing a lot of confusion. At best, there's scorn, such as the general perception in social media, 'Ah, sure, everyone's wheat intolerant now!' Or worse, there's cynicism about its effects – even its existence is regularly scoffed at by totally unversed, medical professionals. The problem is that food sensitivity is a very, very sneaky little issue. When viewed from the outside, it has many different symptoms ranging from mild to severe, and without further testing, your doctor is hard pushed to come up with a diagnosis.

Added to this, doctors have no way of finding out exactly what you had been eating a week previously, nor could you recall it reliably. In this way, many gluten intolerants (up to 30% of Europeans believe it or not) never even realise they are in the gang. Off they go, not-so-happily about life, suffering regular bouts of undiagnosed inflammatory disease — from gastrointestinal upset, headaches, acne, asthma and mood swings to poor joint formation and arthritis, resulting from its consumption. Incredibly, those with coeliac disease, where the effects of gluten are far more dramatic and even life-threatening, wait an average of 10 years before a diagnosis is made.

Which symptoms you express is down to your genetic makeup. When I eat gluten, I get mucus and inflammation, particularly in the nasal area. A few hours later I'm rattling the panes with my death snore, sucking the whole world in on itself like a black hole. We are still together, my wife and I, by the way. While I'm a sub-par night breather, I'm told I'm an above-average cook.

I was 30 before I was diagnosed as gluten intolerant. This was something that was unheard when I was growing up. If something like food intolerance had been mentioned, you would be frowned upon in that typically Irish way we have for dealing with unusual happenings. Like people wearing sunglasses, it was something to be suspicious of and derided, maybe prayed over, but certainly not investigated. Everyone had simply ignored my stuffed nose over the years. I was the snotty kid with the tissue attached to his hand, as was my father and likely his father (or mother) before him.

You'd often hear my mother saying, 'We didn't have allergies when we were growing up, you just got a slap in the head and were told to eat your lunch!' She said this as she plonked her delicious, warm, gluten-tastic scones in front of me. In fairness, this was something she said for most issues identified in the last 50 years, but I'm only just coming to realise how much truth there is to that statement. Back then, food sensitivity and a whole host of other health issues, including asthma, diabetes and childhood cancers, were significantly rarer in the general population. We now know they were less prevalent, allowing for increased awareness and diagnosis in the present day. This alone is fascinating. Why are all these chronic conditions increasing year after year?

So Mum, I'm not soft or weird. I'm a grown man with sensitivities, which result in me getting the sniffles.

Ok, at this point you are possibly thinking, where is this guy going with all this? A perfectly reasonable question, considering you have just forked out some hard-earned cash on another of what is a growing line of canine nutrition books and so far, all you've heard about is my holidays, sleeping habits and at times, fraught relationships with my wife and mother. Here it is, the eureka moment, if you haven't already come to it yourself.

After banging my head against the veterinary wall for a few months and getting no closer to a solution for all the sickness I was seeing in the dogs around me, I had the beginnings of an idea. If 30% of European humans are still unable to deal with gluten effectively, and we are pretty good at breaking down plant matter, then how well do carnivorous dogs fare? After all, these days, gluten-laden wheat is the mainstay of their diet, approximately 50 - 60% of it, in fact. Plus, all my sick dogs were eating it. How did dogs develop systems that were better able to cope with all the gluten, than me?

This seemed like an obvious enough question when you consider that the ability to digest plant matter, certainly wheat gluten, decreases as you move from herbivore to omnivore to carnivore. You will learn that dogs diverged from wolves around 30,000 years ago, depending on who you talk to. Wolves have been out-and-out carnivores for at least 5 million years, normally consuming a diet of almost all animal matter. So, if it takes a lot of time and many thousands of generations to develop a system that can cope with a new food group, how are today's dogs coping with this transition to incorporating a wheat gluten diet in only five decades?

The answer is, we don't really know. This is understandable to a point because gluten intolerance is still a very new issue in humans, really only a few decades old. But I like to know things! Equipped with my research background and my access to pups, I started reading everything produced by the leaders in the field at the time. Both were Australian vets as it happens, Ian Billinghurst (author of *Give a Dog a Bone*) and Tom Lonsdale (*Raw Meaty Bones*).

Now partly versed, I began conducting a few tests. First, I changed three of my absolute worst, most steroid-dependent dogs to an all-natural, cereal-free, raw meat and bone diet. The trial dogs were one Golden Labrador, one Cocker Spaniel and one absolute nutter of a Labradoodle. They were from different breeders and all suffered recurring skin rash, with two also suffering continuous stomach upset.

In the 5 months before the changeover, these three dogs had racked up a costly 19 veterinary visits specifically for their ailments. There were multiple diagnoses, multiple causes and multiple uses of medicine. I alerted the overseeing vets to what I was doing and said I'd come back with results, one way or the other.

Within days I knew it was working. The dogs instantly stopped itching. Their skin cooled. Their poos were suddenly nice and firm and didn't stink. They drank less and urinated less. Two weeks into the change, their hair started to grow back on bald spots. Very soon, the dogs were off their steroids, apparently allergy-free. Four weeks later, they looked incredible with softer coats, better muscle tone and a new focus, now back in training. Four months after the change, all the dogs were positively thriving. One pup returned to the vet for a skin care follow-up. Without using a single drug, their issues had expediently been resolved – which the best vets in Perth couldn't manage.

The results of this simple test were pretty astounding to me, these being the worst cases I could get my hands on and my head started racing. Was this just the removal of wheat or was there perhaps a whole lot more going on here that I didn't know about. For a researcher, this is like hitting a thick vein of gold? How far does this go? But it was only the lack of veterinary interest that had taken me to the position I'm in today. Interest is perhaps the wrong word, but they certainly didn't join me in my jitterbug in their corridor. This for me, as someone who has always been naturally inquisitive, something that has been honed and greatly accentuated by 8 years in college studying science, was completely unacceptable. 'You, sir, are a trained scientist! Here I am presenting the results of a little trial that had gotten your worst cases off recurring drug use and into full recovery and you don't bat an eyelid?' No follow-up investigation of their own. No questions. They simply refused to believe me.

It's fair to say I was very put out by it. Within 3 months of my little Australian food trial, I had quit my dream job with Guide Dogs and reluctantly but determinedly reentered the research world full-time, ending up 10 years later with the book you are about to read.

While I was writing this book, between the research and dozens of interviews, I have embarked on a number of enterprises, mostly in an effort to keep the money coming in to meet the mortgage. As most of you know, making a living in the pet world without ripping people off can be very tricky. I began writing in-depth articles for my website *www.dogsfirst.ie* which proudly had 250,000 readers a month by the start of 2019. I took my canine nutritional seminar 'What Do Dogs Eat?' on the road.

In 2011, I created *Gráw Dog Food* – the word stems from the Irish for love, *grá (*pronounced *graw).* That was 3 years of my life I will never get back. It was terribly hard work, most certainly because I did most of it by myself for the first year. In 2013, I had a bit of luck with it on the TV show "Dragons' Den" and nearly half a million Irish people were introduced to Dr. Conor Brady and the world's finest raw dog food. It was the boost I badly needed, and the business took off.

However, with an increase in demand came an increase in issues. Making money from good dog food is difficult. You need to get paid for the better ingredients you use; to achieve that takes very solid business acumen – a field where I was sorely lacking. Soon my costs overran my abilities and I was forced to accept that my strengths were less product manufacturing and more examining the research that surrounds it. That is what I have been trained to do and being seen as a pet food manufacturer was not working out for the message I was trying to put out. So just a few years after I had started, I left pet food manufacturing behind. But I have learned so much. Besides something close to a degree in business, the experience gave me an irreplaceable insight into the meat chain, and indeed, pet food manufacturing as a whole. I befriended a number of competitors, some dry manufacturers, mostly raw, and was often permitted in to see how things were done. Some were ok, most were…less so. As they say about sausages, once you see it being made, you rarely want to eat them afterward. I have had the luxury of examining the pet food industry from both sides of the divide.

Since then, I have been full-time researching, writing and lecturing on canine nutrition and the pet food world as a whole. In that regard, the result of my efforts can be summed up as follows: once you peek behind the curtain, it becomes apparent that what you have been watching is possibly one of the greatest orchestrated money-making shows on earth today, one where you pay with your money and your pet pays with his health. This should come as no surprise. The UK dog food industry is worth £1.1b per year, the same size as their entire music industry; a market that doubles when you include cats and treats. With so much money at stake, most pet owners have been duped into feeding overpriced junk foods of the poorest quality. The industry is little more than a profitable dumping ground for the world's food waste, and you are paying top dollar for the pleasure of feeding it to your best friend. With little by way of regulation to protect them, all the indicators are now screaming that chronic illness in pets is at an all-time high. It has never been more important for you, your pet's guardian, to get informed on the subject that matters most to their health, well-being and longevity.

This book is an amalgamation of the available literature on the subject of canine nutrition. It studies the nutritional cause of many canine diseases we take as the norm today. It is a factual account of the colossal importance of good nutrition and it is written in the hope that it will be of assistance to both veterinarian, and dog owner alike.

In the following chapters I attempt to present a strong, scientific argument for a vast array of topics, covering a large selection of health issues. In the first section, I tackle the age-old argument concerning whether the dog is a carnivore or omnivore. This is the most important consideration as to how we might feed the animal once in our care. The second section concerns the many issues with dry pet food as a food source for the dog. The third is an analysis of how things have gotten so bad, in particular, the role of manufacturer pseudoscience in our corporate-funded veterinary sector. The final section concerns what and how you might feed your dog properly.

I try to support all my points with independent, peer-reviewed studies. While doing so, I try to filter out the industry-produced nonsense which is no small feat. Trawling through studies in this manner is laborious work. It takes a little skill, a lot of patience and often the determination of a Jack Russell at a ridiculously large branch. Sometimes though, when a relevant point is found in the dank pages of a 1970 *Nature Journal*, conducted by a now largely forgotten Japanese scientist, it provides you with that little eureka moment and makes the labour worthwhile. This book is a collection of those sorts of studies.

In an effort to paint as broad a picture as possible, I have touched on a great variety of topics, few of which I pretend to be a great specialist of. I have done my best to do justice to each section. Any additions or, indeed, corrections a true specialist may have, thereafter, ideally with attached references, will be very gratefully received with the intention of revisiting the text in the future. Please send these corrections to me directly at www.dogsfirst.ie. I sincerely hope you enjoy reading this book as much as I suffered putting it together.

Warning: This book may contain some tests on laboratory dogs that were sacrificed—none of which I was ever, or will ever be, involved in. However, as the worst of these sorts of experiments wind down, we can glean some useful information.

SECTION ONE

Carnivore or Omnivore?

CHAPTER 1

What Is an Omnivore?

With adequate nutrition being one of the most important factors in the health and longevity of an animal, it may come with some surprise that there is currently great confusion concerning one of the most fundamental questions in canine nutrition. What does the dog eat normally, left to his own devices? If we assume that none of us thinks the dog is a herbivore (i.e. an animal that derives its nutrition from plant matter only), is the domestic dog a carnivore (i.e. an animal that derives its nutrition from the flesh of other animals) or is he perhaps an omnivore (i.e. an animal that derives nutrition from both meat and plants)? Can you imagine a modern zoo housing an animal and not knowing the answer to that question? So, let's tackle it first.

There are a number of physiological and behavioural adaptations that occur in animals to facilitate the exploitation of a particular dietary niche, most of them concerning how they obtain and process food. Largely based on these adaptations, mammals are split into the three broad feeding styles – carnivores, herbivores or omnivores.

In general, carnivores such as big cats are equipped with typically pointy, jagged teeth that pierce and tear flesh. These teeth are set in jaws that hinge open and closed only. There is no sideways movement. This adaptation results from a need to grab and hold the prey. Any sideways movement would reduce bite force and allow it to shake free. Also, there is less need to chew large lumps of meat as they are quickly swallowed down a wide gullet. This easily digested meat meal rapidly dissolves in the low-acidity stomach, which is around pH 1–1.5, akin to battery acid. The carnivore's digestive system is short and fast. It consists of a small stomach in relation to their body size, with short intestines that are only three to four times the length of the body. Their whole system is designed to consume and digest meat meals quickly.

Compare this body plan with that of an omnivore. Plant fibre is tough and hard to break down. First, it requires plenty of mastication. This is best achieved with a flat dental arcade set in a jaw that allows some sideways grinding movement for the slow grinding down of fibrous plant material. Picture the blunt back teeth of humans. This material digests better in the slightly higher stomach acidity of around pH 2.5 (which is considered ten times less acidic than pH 1.5). This meal must then pass through the intestinal tract slowly, leaving time for the 1.5 kg of specialised anaerobic microflora housed in the gut to break down the tough plant cell walls and allow access to the goodies inside. Hence, animals that consume a diet high in plant material have a much longer intestinal tract – between 6 and 16 times the length of the body, depending on how much plant food and what type are generally included.

Herbivores on the other hand, consume only plant material. Often the most nutritionally poor and hardest to digest diet of the three, herbivores generally must consume huge amounts in order to get their nutrient hit. Hence, they are often larger in size with cavernous foreguts. In some herbivores, this foregut is divided in four, where the coarse meal can be brought up again for a second chew. Their long intestinal tracts, often more than 20 times the length of their bodies, are full of dead ends to further slow the passage of the digesta, giving the bacteria more time to do their work.

But it's not as simple as carnivore or omnivore. Within these groups there is a dizzying array of specialisations. If you are a zookeeper in charge of a group of animals, it is not enough to know that your particular herbivore requires *plant matter*. Which plants? Grass? Fruit? Vegetables? Roots? Leaves? And which type?

Take the family *Cervidae* (deer), a collection of 62 herbivorous species, each with their own feeding style. There are those that choose a grazing lifestyle, munching all year-round largely on a diet of grass. While nutritionally very poor, their dinner is readily available. But they must consume large amounts of grass to hit their daily nutritional targets, so these deer are usually larger species, with flat muzzles and typically large digestive systems.

Then there are those deer that opt for a more browsing lifestyle, carefully selecting the choicest bits of each plant, young leaves and fruit. This is a nutritionally superior diet, certainly easier to digest, but it requires more work to find. So, this lifestyle favours a smaller body size, with smaller gut capacity and a pointier face to get in between troublesome branches.

If you are a deer farmer and did not do your research, feeding one herbivorous deer species like another would greatly affect their long-term prospects. If a grazing-type animal with a slower system is fed a high-protein diet of fruits and shoots, it will naturally hold on to this easily digested meal for too long. This disturbs the microflora balance and increases gas production to bloat levels, among other unpleasant factors. In the same way, if you were to feed a browsing-type herbivore a cow's diet of poor, fibrous grass, it would not retain the food long enough to extract the necessary nutrients. It would die of malnutrition – if the rotten matter accumulating in its digestive system didn't kill it first.

Then there are sex differences, the reproductive stages and seasonal variations to consider. Knowing exactly what species of deer you have and what exactly they consume year-round when left to their own devices, is *modus operandi* for zookeepers and animal husbandry worldwide.

You won't be surprised to hear that carnivores are just as complicated as herbivores. Take the group *Carnivora*, for example, to which the dog belongs. Consisting of over 260 different species, many in this category are far from carnivorous, despite what their name may suggest. Cats obviously are. However, pandas today are almost totally herbivorous. They will include the occasional raw fish or grub in their diet in times of low forage availability, but this is rare. After all, few others can process bamboo.

To make matters worse, there are different types of carnivores. A strict carnivore is often termed an obligate carnivore. That is a mammal that *only* consumes other animals every day of its life, as opposed to a facultative carnivore that is vaguely defined as needing *mostly* meat, which of course is getting into omnivore territory.

But in terms of broad definitions, omnivore take the biscuit. This category contains the greatest myriad of feeding types. It includes animals that spend 90% of their lives eating meat, compared to those that take it on occasion, often simply if it is abundant and easy to catch. Every omnivore is different, eating only certain animals, certain plants, at certain times, many of which are endemic to their habitat.

For example, take the common red (European) fox whose diet consists of 70% animal matter, which is closer to a carnivorous way of life than herbivorous. Compare this to American black bears that consume meat 25% of the time, the rest being made up of fruit, berries and roots. Being told that both of these animals are omnivores doesn't help all that much. Of course, you can feed one like the other, at least on a short-term basis. However, over time this is not expected to work out for them. Nutritional deficiencies and excesses would creep in and the animals would suffer chronically in a myriad of ways.

The question then becomes, if not a meat-eater and actually an 'omnivore', where on this broad scale of omnivory does the domestic dog lie? Are plants really on the menu? If so, how much and of what?

There are a number of tools available to a zoologist when attempting to decipher the answer to this question. There is ancestry, evolution, anatomy, internal physiology, stomach and faecal analysis and, though highly debatable, taste tests. Assuming we all know the answer to the question, 'Which would your dog prefer, a sausage or a brussels sprout?', we can exclude the latter from our investigation. We know our dogs love meat. We make their toys look like bones. We flavour their dry food stuffs with meat protein. They drool ridiculously when meat is taken from the cooker and stare at us so pathetically that we can't even enjoy eating our own dinner. How much of it do they *need*, though? That is the question.

TAKE-HOME POINTS

- ✓ Carnivores have pointed teeth, hinged jaws and short, fast, acidic digestive tracts that are between three and four times their body length.

- ✓ Omnivores generally have blunt back teeth, jaws allowing sideways movement, less acidic guts that are 6 - 16 times the length of their body, all of which are modifications to enhance the digestion of plant forage.

- ✓ However, the carnivore, omnivore or herbivore descriptors are not sufficient to understand what the optimal nutrition might be for an animal's day-to-day diet. Within each of the descriptions is an enormous array of diverse, entirely unique feeding styles.

- ✓ The true extent of the wrong diet takes time to materialise.

- ✓ To work out the optimal diet of the dog, we must dig deeper by looking at the pattern of evolution, the diet studies and their digestive biology.

CHAPTER 2

Ancestry

The diet habits of the Wolf, the Dingo and the Dingo Hybrid

In 1997,[1] 162 different samples of wolf DNA were taken from 27 populations in Europe, Asia and North America. These were compared with DNA samples from 140 individual dogs from 67 breeds worldwide. It was concluded that all wolves you see today (37 species of them) diverged from a grey wolf-type ancestor (*Canis lupus*) between 76,000 and 135,000 years ago.

What is less clear is when domestic dogs (*Canis lupus familaris*) made their appearance. Genome sequencing indicates that dog is not a direct descendant of the extant (living) grey wolf but these are sister taxa which share a common ancestor from a ghost population of wolves that went extinct at the end of the Late Pleistocene,[2] giving us an age range of 12,000 to 120,000 years. More recent genetic work reveals it was likely in the last 20,000 to 40,000 years.[3] It's thought humans were relatively central to the process but when exactly we teamed up is also up for discussion. In 1978, the remains of a dog buried with a human in Palestine put the earliest domesticated dog at around 12,000 years ago.[4] This held until 1987, when analysis of the lower bone of a dog found in the grave of a 50-year-old man and 25-year-old woman, at a burial site in Bonn-Oberkassel, Germany, came up with 14,000 years ago.[5] Recently all this has been blown out of the water by two major finds. In 2008, reexamination of fossil material excavated from Goyet Cave in Belgium in the late 19th century identified that this was actually a 31,700-year-old proto-dog, a large and powerful animal that ate horse and large bovids.[6] The author explains that this is the proto-dog painted on the walls of the ancient Chauvet Cave in France. Recently this has been topped by Russian scientists, who in 2010 identified the remains of a 33,000-year-old 'incipient dog' (to come into being) in the Altai Mountains of southern Siberia.[7]

Some authors make a strong case for a single, Asian domestication[8,9] while others campaign for a Middle Eastern domestication.[10] The majority of authors, however, believe their domestication was not an isolated event, but rather a common practice of humans.[11,12]

What we do know is that beginning somewhere around 30,000 years ago, dogs and humans began sharing the same space. It is assumed the earliest wolf ancestors began helping themselves to our kill scraps, food waste and faeces. These 'less frightened' wolves may have then been fed and eventually utilised in hunts by some early wolf-admirers. A decreasing body size for handling purposes and general affinity toward humans would have been favoured by these early domesticators. While small pockets of selection and domestication began from this point forward, the earliest definitive records we have of humans and dogs coupling up in earnest is a shallow grave containing a man, a woman and a puppy, dating back to the Palaeolithic era some 14,000 years ago. By 5,000 years ago we had hunting dogs, guard dogs, scent hounds and terriers for ratting.

At any rate, the exact dates matter little to this discussion. The dog and grey wolf descended from a single ancestor around 100,000 years ago. And that ancestor has been an out-and-out meat-eater for at least the last 5 million years.[13-15] Outside of small bits ingested for medicinal purposes, though possibly also for nutrition, it appears plant matter is not on the menu for the grey wolf to any great degree. A large review of 26 diet studies published in the *British Journal of Nutrition*, involving 31,276 wolf scat and stomach analyses, revealed little to no vegetative matter being consumed, though in one or two, plant matter could be as high as – 2–3%, consisting of berries, nuts and other fruit.[16] From this, the authors noted that the selected protein/fat/carbohydrate profile of wolves was 54%, 45%, 1%, respectively, by energy contribution.

The 2–3% plant matter inclusion is an interesting and still debated topic, in that we are still unsure how much of this is self-selected and how much arises from the stomach contents of smaller prey. We do know the grey wolves of Yellowstone National Park include a small amount of plant material, largely fruit, in their diet in the summer months[17] (something we will return to in Chapter 3), but few are suggesting the grey wolf is anything but the total carnivore, much like the other 37 subspecies of wolf we see descended from it today.[15]

One myth you commonly find perpetuated online is that wolves gorge on the stomach contents of their prey. Numerous sources indicate this is absolutely not true.[17-24] In his book *Raw Meaty Bones Promote Health*, Lonsdale (2001) draws our attention to the often mentioned but never referenced suggestion that wolves consume the stomach contents of their prey. Lonsdale highlights that, except where the prey is so small as to render it unavoidable, nothing could be further from the truth.

> ...the only part [of the prey] *consistently ignored* is the stomach and its contents.
> **Kerwood Wolf Education Center, Canada *cited in* Lonsdale, (2001)**

David Mech and his research team are considered the world's authority on wolves. Their 2003 book *Wolves: Behavior, Ecology, and Conservation*[13] is a compilation of 350 collective years of research, experiments and careful field observations. These quotes are taken from Chapter 4, *The Wolf as a Carnivore*. I have italicised relevant words for emphasis.

> ...to grow and maintain their own bodies, wolves need to ingest all the major parts of their herbivorous prey, *except* the plants in the digestive system...

> ...the large rumen is usually punctured during removal and its contents spilled. The vegetation in the intestinal tract is of *no interest* to the wolves, but the stomach lining and intestinal wall are consumed...

Wolves appear to be total carnivores and there is little evidence suggesting otherwise. Apart from the occasional piece of plant material taken largely in self-medication, or the stomach contents of the smallest prey (birds, rodents, juveniles), wolves do not include plant material as normal nutrition. You would actually have to go back around 5 million years, back to when the coyote and the grey wolf diverged, to find a canid in the dog's family tree with truly omnivorous tendencies. African wild dogs (also called painted dogs) are seen to be quite omnivorous on occasion. However, this animal diverged from the wolf line even earlier than coyotes, closer to 6 million years ago; hence, they do not get the *Canis* classification but *Lycaon pictus*.

To be clear, these guys diverged around the time man was climbing down from the trees. Any comparisons of the domestic dog to the African wild dog is the equivalent of us studying the diet of chimpanzees to understand the best way to feed our children. In the same way, some researchers have highlighted the omnivorous habits of the maned wolf as an example of the omnivorous tendencies of 'some wolves'. However, the maned wolf (*Chrysocyon brachyurus*) isn't actually a wolf, he's more of a fox, though he's not that either. He went his own way 7 or 8 million years ago, along with the South American foxes.[1] So those, too, must be excluded from the conversation. Sadly, you will find many examples online of these animals being held aloft in conversations concerning the diet habits of the domestic dog.

While the domestic dog is his own species today, and deservedly so, the similarities that remain between the domestic dog and the wolf are as undeniable as they are obvious. From form to behaviour, common dogs have deviated relatively little from the wolf blueprint and given the time and space seem to revert quickly back to form.

Andrei Poyarkov of the Severtsov Institute of Ecology and Evolution in southwest Moscow is a leading researcher of these dogs. A specialist in wolves, Poyarkov has dedicated 30 years to studying the stray dogs of the Moscow underground and surrounding area. Among a number of interesting findings, he maintains that their appearance and behaviour have changed even during the relatively short time he's been studying them, and certainly over the last 200 years of their existence. These dogs have evolved (or reverted, so to speak) into a group of animals that 'all look similar to one another' and appear to be 'somewhere between dogs and wolves.' They have developed the thicker fur, wedge-shaped heads, almond eyes, long tails and erect ears of wolves.[25]

The Moscow dogs' apparent return to a more wolf-like form reminds us that dogs are not long removed from their wolf ancestors. But before we start making crude comparisons of the domestic dog to his cousin the wolf, as many are tempted to do, we must remember that dogs have not been wolves for 30,000 years or more. They are very different animals today. While direct descendants, they shouldn't be compared to them in anything but the loosest sense – certainly not while there are far more appropriate comparisons to be made, such as with the dog's brother, the dingo.

Most of us are familiar with the Australian dingo (*Canis dingo*). These are the rust red coloured wild dogs emblematic of the Australian outback. With this beautiful canid, we can make two very important points concerning canine nutrition as a whole. But first, some background is essential before we get to one of the most important canine nutrition studies to date.

Much like his wolf cousin, the dingo is unquestionably a meat-eating carnivore.[15,26-28] What is interesting about this canid is that in the land of marsupials, it was always assumed the dingo was Australia's only native mammal, a direct descendant of domestic dogs that accompanied Asian travellers landing in Australia around 3,500–4,000 years ago (the earliest dingo fossil found in Australia being 3,500 years old).[15,27,29] In that time, they have evolved to suit their niche. This hypothesis was particularly alluring as the dingo is the perfect colour for the iron-rich red soils of the Australian outback. But now, thanks to DNA and archaeological analyses, there is general agreement that the dingo's ancestor is likely to have originated in Asia – likely China – before spreading to Southeast Asia between 5,000 and 12,000 years ago.[30,31] This has since been narrowed down by archaeologists Fillios and Tacon (2016)[31] to the dingo possibly arriving with the seafaring Tolean people from the island of Sulawesi. The DNA folk counter by offering evidence suggesting they may have simply walked themselves across in two waves, some 8,000 years BP,[32] likely aided by a now-submerged land bridge that existed between Papua New Guinea and Australia at the time.

So, it seems the dingo is not Australian after all. However, this is not the only bit of controversy surrounding the dingo of late. Now folk are furiously debating whether it is even a *dog*. This will surely come as a surprise to most of us. While the exact point of divergence cannot be pinpointed, few are disagreeing the dingo and domestic dog share a common ancestor in the not so distant past,[32] with current theory suggesting the dingo is highly similar at the genetic level with both the Papua New Guinea Singing Dog and the African Basenji. The singing dog is very similar in appearance to the dingo and both currently fall under the same classification *Canis lupus dingo*. Incidentally, with a diet of middle-sized marsupials, rodents, birds and some fruits when available,[33,34] the wild singing dog of Papua New Guinea appears to be as much the carnivore as his dingo brother. In their summer newsletter, the Zoological Association of America[35] note that they thrive on lean raw meat diets, as does the dingo.

The problem the dingo is having is its scientific classification as a dog. Being classified as a dog permits it to be hunted, trapped and killed by farmers who believe dingoes to be a threat to their livestock. This is a concern as most Aussies love their dingoes and, as you are soon to discover, there are not as many dingoes around as was once thought. For this reason, in the last decade there has been a flurry of research and heated debate in an attempt to reclassify the dingo as a separate species, giving them and the domestic dog a little more taxonomical space and more protection as a result. So, the question becomes: in the 4,000 years he has been roaming the outback and adapting to his new dietary niche, has the dingo evolved enough characteristics to be properly classified as his own species?

The dingo certainly has clearly evolved some unique features compared to the domestic dog. These include rotating wrists and being virtually double jointed (tree climbers), as well as having far more impressive set of teeth. However, these physical characteristics alone are not enough.[36] The really important detail is whether the dingo was ever a domesticated animal in the first place. If it was, it would instantly demote the dingo to a *feral* dog, one that has returned to the wild following domestication. Feral animals are permitted to be hunted at will. This is very different to being a *wild* dog – an animal that was never domesticated such as the African wild dog – an animal, it has to be assumed, that has more rights.

For the dingo, it comes down to an analysis of their behaviour and DNA. It's fair to say dingoes are typically aloof and wary of humans. While revered by Aboriginal people, and allowing for the occasional friendship, dingoes have never been domesticated by them. They were not even used to much extent in hunting.[37] Hence, they remain difficult to train; even when raised by us, they lack much body language, such as facial expressions, to which we humans have now become so accustomed to in the canids sitting on our couch. And yet, dingoes make a lot more eye contact with humans than wolves.[38] In fact, they can follow social cues from humans better than wolves, which, as these authors conclude, may show dingoes shared an early domestication history with dogs.[39]

On the DNA front, it was recently discovered that domestic dogs have more copies of the gene (ranging from three or four to 32 more copies) necessary to produce the enzyme involved in starch digestion (pancreatic α-amylase 2B, or simply, AMY2B,[40] compared to dingoes or wolves that have only two.[30] This, it appears, is a rare glimpse of evolution in action. Ultra-carnivorous animals that live on protein and fat do not require a lot of amylase, enough to help with the digestion of a handful of berries taken in summer and the glycogen stored liver of their prey. In contrast, dogs have been living with agricultural people for thousands of years. During this time, it is expected they would have encountered more carbohydrates in their diet, encouraging some adaption over time.

Like eye contact and the ability to pick up social cues, multiple copies of this gene simply wouldn't have evolved in the domestic dog without some prior need. It was this difference in the number of AMY2B genes between the domestic dog and the dingo (and the similarity of the dingo to the wolf) that was held up by some authors as evidence the dingo is of wolf lineage and not a subspecies of the domestic dog.[32]

But again, there are holes. The Siberian Husky has only three or four copies of the AMY2B gene,[30] likely a result of their evolution alongside hunter – gatherers in the Arctic, but few would doubt the Husky is a fully signed-up member of the domestic dog family. While he may look like a wolf, the Husky is no more wolf than an English bulldog. Nor are huskies the only domestic dog lacking a great expansion of this gene. Reiter *et al.* (2016)[41] investigated this further in breeds known to have evolved on either starch-rich diets (Pekingese and Shar Pei) or low-starch, seafood-rich diets (both the Akita and Shiba Inu of Japan, the Siberian Husky and Alaskan Malamute). They found dogs with historically high-starch diets had a higher number of these genes compared to the dogs on low-starch diets. As the Pekingese, Shar Pei and Shiba Inu breeds are each no more than 2,000 years old, this shows how relatively quick minor genetic steps can be taken within a species to exploit a feeding niche. Nor is it just dogs. Great variation in the AMY gene is also evident between and even within human populations where populations with more copies historically consume more starch.[42] In fact, it appears unrelated mammals living in different habitats and eating different types of food have similar numbers of amylase gene copies if they have the same level of starch in their diet.[43] It's a fascinating insight that Darwin would have killed to have understood at the time.

Furthermore, if a few thousand years is enough to bring about these genetic variations among the dog breeds previously described, it could be that all of these things, from the ability to digest starch to human aloofness and physical alterations of the body, could be as much explained by a *loss* at the genetic level instead of having *never developed* the trait in the first place. Much like our practically useless and now shrinking appendix and little fingers – in nature, if you don't use it, you lose it (this is why the Simpson's characters have four fingers, it was Matt Groening's apparent nod to evolution). The recent explosion of genomic data is now revealing that gene loss has been crucial to the divergence of animal phyla across the planet. While gene appearance occurs naturally with genetic drift (this is the normal fluctuation of genes in a population from mutation or chance disappearance as individuals die or do not reproduce), the same applies to gene loss. Today, gene loss is increasingly viewed as a major adaptive and evolutionary force, a response to abrupt environmental challenges. Gene loss is now implicated in adaptations such as colour changes in flowers to attract new pollinators, to enable insects to colonise different habitats and exploit different environmental conditions.[44] Supporting this, Inchley *et al.* (2016)[42] detected 'multiple secondary losses of...AMY2A [pancreatic amylase] and associated low copy number of

AMY1 [salivary amylase] in northeast Siberian populations [of humans] whose diet has been low in starch content'.

Previous authors hypothesise that the limited expansion of the AMY2B genes in ancient breeds, such as the Dingo and Siberian Husky, suggests that these breeds arose alongside hunter–gatherers rather than agriculturists.[30] However, if gene loss was at play, that is not a given. This matter would be put to bed once we see how expanded this gene is in the Papua New Guinea Singing Dog.

For now, the most recent genetic evidence reveals that the dog and the dingo are not at all a separate species.[32,36,45] It is why a dingo–dog hybrid is so fertile – unrelated animals do not produce fertile offspring. In fact, it is largely because of dog interbreeding that pure dingo populations are on the endangered list. Once European dogs arrived in Australia, during the 18th century,[27] domestic dogs began to freely interbreed with their 3,500-year-old ancestors so frequently to the extent that feral non-dingoes (hybrids and feral domestic dogs) now outnumber the pure dingo by a considerable degree. According to Steve Davidson of *Ecosystem Magazine* (2004), studies show the dog population of southeast Australia and along the East Coast to consist of roughly 90% dingo hybrids. Researchers using skull structure have noted a decline in *pure* dingoes in the south east of Australia from 49% in the 1960s to 17% in the 1980s.[28] The number of feral dogs and hybrids may now be so great that pure populations of dingo may no longer exist. There are estimated to be little more than 10,000 genetically pure dingoes left. Dingo expert, Dr. Ricky Spencer of the University of Western Sydney, predicts that Australia's native canine may effectively go extinct within the next 20 years.

> Nowhere on the east coast of Australia can you find a dingo population that isn't at least fifty per cent, and in some cases eighty percent, domestic dog.
>
> **Ricky to the *Australian Geographic*, 2011**

In comparison, a review of dog–wolf hybridisation reveals it is so uncommon that it is not an important conservation concern 'even in small, endangered wolf populations near human settlements'.[46]

Ironically, it is feral domestic dogs and the dingo hybrids they produce that are more aggressive toward livestock than dingoes themselves.[27] But convincing Australian farmers of this fact appears to be as difficult as teaching Irish and UK farmers that exterminating badgers will not rectify the potential for TB in their cattle left grazing outside.

> Overwhelming current evidence from archaeology and genomics indicates that the Dingo is of recent origin in Australia and shares immediate ancestry with other domestic dogs as evidenced by patterns of genetic and morphological variation… we are strongly sympathetic to arguments about the historical, ecological, cultural, or other significance of the Dingo, but these are issues that will have to be considered outside of the more narrow scope of taxonomy and nomenclature.
>
> **Jackson *et al.*, 2019**[36]

While we continue to debate such asinine details, conservationists will continue to be hamstrung when trying to protect yet another beautiful animal from the undue pressures wrought by what is surely the world's most ignorant animal. Luckily, wildlife managers are all too aware of the plight of the dingo. Thus, when they are employed to cull roaming dogs they are employed by farmers to cull roaming dogs to protect livestock or by conservation groups to protect the last few remaining true dingo populations from inbreeding, they go to great lengths to remove only feral domestic dogs and anything they deem to be a hybrid near the protected areas. This is something they have been doing for many years.

Ethics aside, this has given rise to one of the world's largest bodies of data on what dogs might eat when left to their own devices in the wild. Using the results of numerous published works, Fleming *et al.* (2001)[27] gathered impressive and unprecedented 13,000 stomach samples of largely dingo hybrids and feral domestic dogs over 30 years, spanning the six different climatic regions of the Australian continent. It is today the largest dietary study of any single canid that I can source. They found animal protein comprised 97% of their diet (mammals making up the greater part at 72%, mainly rabbits and kangaroo, with birds, insects, fish, crabs, frogs and reptiles making up another 25%). Like the grey wolves, vegetation made up just 3% of all these samples. This plant contribution in the rain forest-dwelling wild dogs consisted largely of seeds from the stomach contents of small birds which would be too small to be shaken free. Just like their cousin, the wolf, the dingo does not consume the rumen contents of their larger prey. Based on their findings, Fleming *et al.* (2001)[27] classified Australian feral dogs, a group consisting largely of domestic dogs and dingo-cross domestic dog hybrids, as *specialist carnivores*.

TAKE-HOME POINTS

✓ Dogs evolved, likely more than once, from a grey wolf-type ancestor 20–40,000 years ago. Immediately or very soon thereafter, they started sharing the same space with humans.

✓ Wolves are true carnivores, rarely averaging more than 3% vegetation in the diet.

✓ Wolves do not usually eat the stomach contents of large prey.

✓ Canids, such as the African wild dog, maned wolf and coyote, have not been related to the domestic dog for more than 5 million years.

✓ The dingo was once a domestic dog, arriving in Australia some 4–8,000 years ago. He is also a true carnivore, consuming no more than 3% plant matter.

✓ The more copies of the AMY gene for amylase production a mammal has, the more carbohydrates they are thought to have included in their diet. The dingo has only two copies of the AMY2B gene for carbohydrate digestion. Domestic dogs have 3–32 more copies, depending on their historic association with farmers and exposure to carbohydrates. Siberian Huskies and Akitas have the least number of copies of this gene.

✓ One of the largest canid diet analysis in existence is of feral dogs and dingo hybrids in Australia. Using some 13,000 stomach samples, researchers found these animals to be specialist carnivores, averaging no more than 3% vegetation in the diet.

Chapter Two References

1   Vilà, C., Savolainen, P., Maldonado, J.E. *et al.* (1997). Multiple and ancient origins of the domestic dog. Science, 276(5319): 1687–1689

2   Wozencraft, W.C. (2005). Order Carnivora. In Wilson, D.E.; Reeder, D.M (eds.). *Mammal Species of the World: A Taxonomic and Geographic Reference* (3rd ed.). Johns Hopkins University Press. pp. 575–577

3   Irving-Pease, E.K.; Ryan, H., Jamieson, A. *et al.* (2018). Paleogenomics of animal domestication. In Lindqvist, C.; Rajora, O. (eds.). Paleogenomics: Genome-Scale Analysis of Ancient DNA. Cham: Springer

4   Davis, S.J.M. and Valla, F.R. (1978). Evidence for domestication of the dog 12,000 years ago in the Natufian of Palestine. Nature, 276: 608–610

5   Benecke, N. (1987). Studies on early dog remains from Northern Europe. Journal of Archaeological Science, 14: 31–49

6   Mark, D. (2011). *How the dog became the dog: from wolves to our best friends*. New York: Penguin

7   Ovodov, N.D., Crockford, S.J., Kuzmin, Y.V. *et al.* (2011). A 33,000-year-old incipient dog from the Altai Mountains of Siberia: Evidence of the earliest domestication disrupted by the last glacial maximum. PLoS One, 6(7): e22821

8   Savolainen, P., Zhang, Y.P., Luo, J. *et al.* (2002). Genetic evidence for an east Asian origin of domestic dogs. Science, 298: 1610–1613

9   Pang, J.F., Kluetsch, C., Zou, X.J. *et al.* (2009). mtDNA data indicate a single origin for dogs south of Yangtze River less than 16,300 years ago, from numerous wolves. Molecular Biology and Evolution, 12: 2849–2864

10 VonHoldt, B., Pollinger, J.P., Lohmueller, K.E. *et al.* (2010). Genome-wide SNP and haplotype analyses reveal a rich history underlying dog domestication. Nature, 464(7290): 898–902

11 Honeycutt, R.L. (2010). Unravelling the mysteries of dog evolution. Biomedical Central Biology, 8:20

12 Bradshaw, J. (2011). *Dog Sense*. New York: Basic Books

13 Mech L.D. and Boitani L. (Eds) (2003). *Wolves: behavior, ecology, and conservation*. Chicago: University of Chicago Press

14 Peterson, R.O. and Ciucci, P. (2003). The Wolf As A Carnivore. In L. D. Mech and L. Boitani (Eds). *Wolves: behavior, ecology, and conservation*. pp123–124. Chicago: University of Chicago Press.

15 Sillero-Zubiri, C., Hoffmann, M. and MacDonald, D.W. (2004). *Canids: foxes, wolves, jackals and dogs. Status survey and conservation action plan*. Gland, Switzerland: IUCN

16 Bosch, G., Hagen-Plantinga, E.A. and Hendriks, W.H. (2015). Dietary nutrient profiles of wild wolves: insights for optimal dog nutrition? British Journal of Nutrition (2015), 113:S40–S54

17 Stahler, D.R., Smith, D.W. and Guernsey, D.S. (2006). Foraging And Feeding Ecology Of The Gray Wolf (*Canis lupus)*: Lessons from Yellowstone National Park, Wyoming, USA. The Journal of Nutrition, 136(7): 1923S–1926S

18 Mech, L.D. (1970). *The wolf: the ecology and behaviour of an endangered species*. New York: Doubleday

19 Peterson, R.O. (1977). *Wolf ecology and prey relationships on isle royale*. PhD Thesis, Purdue University, West Lafayette

20 Potvin, F., Jolicoeur, H. and Huot, J. (1988) Wolf diet and prey selectivity during two periods for deer in Quebec: Decline versus expansion. Canadian Journal of Zoology, 66: 1274–1279

21 Fuller, T.K. (1989) Population dynamics of wolves in North-Central Minnesota. Wildlife Monographs, 105: 1–41

22   Peterson, R.O. and Ciucci, P. (2003). *The wolf as a carnivore*. In Mech, L D and Boitani, L (Eds). *Wolves: Behavior, Ecology, And Conservation*, p104-111. Chicago, IL: University of Chicago Press.

23   Wilmers, C.C., Crabtree, R.L., Smith, D.W.*et al.* (2003). Trophic facilitation by introduced top predators: grey wolf subsidies to scavengers in Yellowstone National Park. Journal of Animal Ecology, 72: 909–916

24   Bump, J.K., Peterson, R.O. and Vucetich, J.A. (2009). Wolves modulate soil nutrient heterogeneity and foliar nitrogen by configuring the distribution of ungulate carcasses. Ecology, 90: 3159–3167

25   Sternthal, S. (2010). *Moscow's stray dogs*. Financial Times. Published online. April 30th, www.ft.com

26   Gill, J., Hoffmannowa, H. and Piekarz, R. (1964). Studies on digestive physiology in the wolf, dingo, and jackal. II. Digestive ability of the pancreas, duodenum and salivary glands and size of the alimentary tract and weight of internal organs. Acta Physiologica, 15(1): 137–148

27   Fleming, F., Corbett, L., Harden, R. and Thomson, P. (2001). Managing the impacts of dingoes and other wild dogs. Canberra, Australia: National Heritage Trust, Bureau of Rural Sciences.

28   Corbett, L. (2004). *Dingo*. In Canids: Foxes, Wolves, Jackals and Dogs. International Union for Conservation of Nature and Natural Resources. Publisher IUCN, Gland, Switzerland

29   Milham, P. and Thompson, P. (1976). Relative antiquity of human occupation and extinct fauna at Madura Cave, southeastern Western Australia. Mankind, 10: 175–180

30   Freedman, A.H., Gronau, I., Schweizer, R.M. *et al.* (2014). Genome Sequencing Highlights the Dynamic Early History of Dogs. PLOS Genetics 10(8): e1004631

31   Fillios, M. and Tacon, P. (2016). Who let the dogs in? A review of the recent genetic evidence for the introduction of the dingo to Australia and implications for the movement of people. Journal of Archaeological Science: Reports, 364

32   Cairns, K.M., Brown, S.K., Sacks, B.N. *et al.* (2017). Conservation implications for dingoes from the maternal and paternal genome: Multiple populations, dog introgression, and demography. Ecology and Evolution, 7(22): 9787–9807

33   Koler-Matznick, J., Lehr Brisbin Jr, I., Feinstein, M. and Bulmer, S. (2003). An updated description of the New Guinea Singing Dog (*Canis hallstromi*), Troughton 1957. Journal of Zoology, London. 261(2): 109–118

34   Koler-Matznick, J., Lehr Brisbin Jr., Yates, I. *et al.* (2007). The New Guinea singing dog: its status and scientific importance. The Journal of the Australian Mammal Society. 29(1): 47–56

35   Ehrlich, D. (2011). Singers singing – Hear the cry of the New Guinea Singing Dog. Zoological Association of America Newsletter and Journal. 5(2): 111–128

36   Jackson, S.M., Fleming, P.J.S., Eldridge, M.D.B *et al.* (2019). The dogma of dingoes — taxonomic status of the dingo: A reply to Smith *et al.* Zootaxa, 4564(1)

37   Smith, B.P. and Litchfield, C.A. (2009). A review of the relationship between indigenous Australians, Dingoes (*Canis dingo*) and Domestic Dogs (*Canis familiaris*). Anthrozoös, 2: 111–128

38   Johnston, A.M., Turrina, C., Watson, Arrea, A.L. *et al.* (2017). Uncovering the origins of dog–human eye contact: dingoes establish eye contact more than wolves, but less than dogs. Animal Behaviour, 133: 123–129

39   Smith, B.P. and Litchfield, C.A. (2010). Dingoes (*Canis dingo*) can use human social cues to locate hidden food. Animal Cognition, 13: 367–376

40   Axelsson, E., Ratnakumar, A., Arendt, M.L *et al.* (2013). The genomic signature of dog domestication reveals adaptation to a starch-rich diet. Nature, 495(7441): 360–364

41   Reiter, T., Jagoda, E., and Capellini, T.D. (2016). Dietary variation and evolution of gene copy number among dog breeds. PLoS ONE 11(2): e0148899

42   Inchley, C.E., Larbey, C.D.A., Shwan, N.A. *et al.* (2016). Selective sweep on human amylase genes postdates the split with Neanderthals. Scientific Reports, (6): 37198

43   Pajic, P., Pavlidis, P., Dean, K. *et al.* (2019). Independent amylase gene copy number bursts correlate with dietary preferences in mammals. eLife, 8: e44628

44   Albalat, R. and Cañestro, C. (2016). Evolution by gene loss. Nature Reviews Genetics, 17(7): 379-391

45   Fan, Z., Silva, P., Gronau, I. *et al.* (2016). Worldwide patterns of genomic variation and admixture in Grey Wolves. Genome Research, 26(2): 163–173

46   Vilà, C. and Wayne, R.K. (1999). Hybridization between Wolves and Dogs. Conservation Biology, 13(1): 195–198

Diet Selection by Feral and Free-Ranging Domestic Dogs

1. The hunting ability of the domestic dog

Since moving in with humans, changes have necessarily occurred in the dog that facilitate us both living and working together. Behaviour was most likely the first thing to change, as aggression toward humans would never do. Thousands of years ago our ancestors would have naturally chosen proto-dogs that were less wary, less aggressive and more affectionate toward humans. Wary proto-dogs would have steered clear of camps and not contributed to the gene pool. Over time, canine behaviour would have adapted to take advantage of what they must have perceived as human walking/talking vending machines. One crucial strength was their ability to read and interpret our body language. One group of researchers[1] found that when it comes to locating hidden food, wolves raised by humans do not show a capability to read human, communicative skills, whereas domestic dog puppies only a few weeks old, even those that have had little human contact, absolutely do.

The next thing to change was how they look. Since the advent of farming we have been selecting smaller, more docile dogs.[2] In order to avoid starving, at the very least grey wolves require 1 kilo of fresh meat per day,[3] while early proto-dogs would have been roaming most of the time, topping up their fat stores. Over the last 30,000 years domestication and constant slim, but readily accessible, pickings from around humans would have favoured a smaller size in proto-dogs. Meggitt

(1965)[4] found tame dingoes living with Aboriginals to be smaller than their wild brothers, which the author notes was due to poorer nutrition. In this way over time, there evolved a smaller, less aggressive animal in the domestic dog.

It's also important to note that free-ranging domestic dogs no longer organise in structured, finely tuned hunting packs but rather loose groups, commonly called social or feeding units[5, 6,7] ranging in size from two to ten.[8]

Couple a decrease in size, aggression and pack organisation with a decrease in parental teaching and exposure to prey, the latter two being absolutely crucial for the development of hunting efficiency in wolf pups,[9] then we begin to see that the domestic dog is a very different type of canid to his wolf cousin today. For one thing, dogs have little impact on larger wildlife such as cattle or moose, which require serious, organised hunting.[5,10-12] While isolated incidences of both feral and free-ranging dogs attacking large prey do of course exist, including cattle[13] and black buck,[14] these are the exceptions. In contrast to the findings of Fleming et al. on Australian wild dogs, in some cases authors looking for livestock predation by feral dogs didn't document one instance of live predation over periods as long as 5 years.[15,16] Although it is accepted that years of feral and dingo hybridisation and access to prey may be clouding the waters here. These authors reported numerous, short, apparently uncoordinated and certainly unsuccessful hunting chases during which the feral dogs were constantly barking. Although they may not actually be killed, this harassment can take a heavy toll on these larger species, resulting in increased stress and energy loss[17] as well as decreasing the breeding success of native ungulate species.[18]

Large prey is generally consumed as carcass. Aided by large noses and colossal olfactory centres that take up almost 25% of their brain, dogs are highly efficient scavengers of carcass, finding an incredible 67% of the available carcass in their area.[19] In fact, dogs appear to outcompete vultures where the two exist together.[11,20]

However, although larger animals may be off the menu, this should not be confused with a decrease in predatory instinct. A strong prey–drive is alive and well in the dog,[7, 8] it has just been shifted to smaller prey. At the larger end of their kill range are sheep, of which dogs are well known to take terrible advantage. Ask any farmer. I have seen the aftermath of some of these frenzies and it can be absolutely horrific. Kill rate aside, the actual death offered by a canid to larger, exhausted prey can seem cruel in the extreme. Unlike muscular big cats that tend to go for the neck, killing the animal quickly, dogs and wolves lack the front-end power to easily inflict that killer blow. Dogs are more long-distance running machines than ambush killer. They are the marathon runner compared to the 100 metres sprinter and are built accordingly. Dogs prefer to stalk and harass the animal, often for hours or even days (in the case of the wolf), until it collapses with exhaustion. Much like hyenas, hungry dogs have been known to begin feeding from the hindquarters of the animal while it is still very much alive. If they are not hungry, they can bite indiscriminately, frenzied, until the animal lies still.

Larger ungulates aside, any prey smaller than a sheep is in very real danger when dogs are around. Populations of marine iguanas and turtles in the Galapagos, capybaras in Venezuela, nonflying birds such as kiwi in New Zealand and numerous species of frogs worldwide have suffered drastically from dog predation.[8,21-23] Manor and Saltz (2004)[24] found that free-roaming dogs predated heavily on gazelle kids. Gazelle numbers, however, responded positively and quickly to dog culling. One German Shepherd bitch was known to have killed 500 of a 900-strong population of kiwis in *one* single feeding frenzy before she was shot dead.[25] Such formidable hunters are they, that their mere presence in an area deters other prey animals such as squirrels, rabbits and even deer,[17] as well as rival carnivores such as wolves, bobcats and foxes[17, 26, 27, 28] from using an area, even when those dogs are on a lead.[29]

Left to their own devices, where they are readily and easily available, dogs are shown to largely pursue a diet of small animals including rodents, birds, rabbits, insects, lizards and frogs, as well as smaller ungulates such as sheep, white tail deer and gazelle kids.[5,8,11,23,24,30-36] The rest of the time they spend scavenging carcass and faeces. Indeed, some studies show that in Zimbabwe, faeces can account for 20% of a dog's diet.[11] The authors note that it is a symptom of their protein deficient diet.

Dogs are tough to narrow down to a single mode of feeding. They are so adaptive and opportunistic that they are best described as scavenging carnivores rather than true hunters,[37] happily switching between prey when abundance makes it easy to do so. While they may not be the biggest, in areas where top carnivores have been removed, feral and free-roaming dogs are often the top predators of many habitats.[38]

All that said, some of the authors above,[5,8,11,12,35] noted some domestic dog populations consuming various amounts of plant material, some as much as 50% of their diet. There is a crucial, all-too-often overlooked reason for this disparity.

2. The Difference Between Feral and Free-Roaming Dogs

People constantly point out to me the small studies of village dogs, as proof that the domestic dog takes vegetation as part of its *normal* diet. There is a lot in this statement, so bear with me while I tease it out a bit.

There are too few studies conducted to date on the diet of dogs. No study yet exists of feral or free-ranging domestic dogs on a scale that is comparable to that of the 13,000 samples of domestic dog-dingo hybrids in Australia.[39] And, while we have a small handful of studies to work with, sadly their results appear to differ greatly.

Butler *et al* (2004)[11] studied the stomach contents of free-ranging village dogs in Zimbabwe and concluded that they were 'scavengers of human waste and carcass.' While their human families sometimes fed them porridge, the authors noted that when *left to their own devices,* the village dogs consumed '97% animal matter', coincidentally the *exact* same amount of animal matter as the dingo-dog hybrid in the study by Fleming *et al.* (2001)[39].

Campos *et al.* (2007),[35] using field observation together with scat analysis of free-ranging dogs in suburban and rural Brazil, agree closely with these findings. Dogs here consumed an almost all-meat diet consisting of 82% mammals and invertebrates with the rest made up of a mix of birds, frogs, human faeces and small amounts of plant matter.

Much like their ancestors, the diet of the feral dog is looking quite carnivorous so far. This explains why geneticists tracking wolves regularly struggle to tell both scats apart.[13]

But not all studies agree. Using only field observation, Scott and Causey (1973)[5]concluded that feral dogs in Alabama consumed 'small mammals, garbage and some vegetable material'. Gipson (1983)[40] too, using observation only, noted the principal food of feral dogs in Alaska was small mammals, snowshoe hares, scavenged moose and bison and some garbage. Incidentally, this author noted a mother and her pups foraging out of the den at −45°C (−49°F)! A third observational study by Boitani and Ciucci (1995)[8] echoed findings of previous studies, with Italian feral dogs consuming a diet of small mammals and some vegetable material.

Some plant material is beginning to creep in now.

When analysing diet studies, there are a number of factors that must be controlled and allowed for. The first is the sampling method. There are essentially three ways to study the diet of an animal: observation (using a telescope from afar) and scat [droppings] and stomach content analyses. Which method you use can greatly affect your results.

In terms of diet analysis, field observation could be viewed as the least reliable form of data as it is the one most prone to error. Field observation involves a researcher setting predetermined study intervals, such as every minute, and taking a note of what the animal appears to be consuming at that point. This method can rarely take account of what is specifically chosen from the ground nor, most importantly, *how much* is consumed – both details are crucial to the overview of why the dog was nosing around there in the first place. For example, a fox feeding in a vegetable patch could lead to a conclusion that foxes eat vegetables, when he is actually after the slugs lurking underneath. Via observation alone, wolves teasing the fatty lining from the exposed gut of their prey could give rise to the incorrect conclusion that wolves consume the stomach contents of their prey, which we now know does not occur. In this way, observations, even by the most qualified and diligent scientists, are highly prone to error.

A human dump is a scavenger's takeaway. Most free-roaming dogs are found in and around them. Our dumps have *always* been the attraction. They are probably the reason dogs started hanging around us in the first place. In dumps there are meat leftovers, insects and grubs, rodents, small birds with their eggs and good old faeces for those who wish to indulge, and God knows, dogs do. Coprophagy, the act of poo-eating, is unfortunately a very natural thing for dogs. As noted above by Butler *et al*, the village dogs in Zimbabwe consumed nearly 20% human faeces. This act is probably due to the relatively high protein and possible vitamin content of faeces which are produced by gut microflora in the back passage of omnivores and herbivores. Polar bears are notoriously fond of scavenging in human dumps, and nobody would argue that they are anything but total meat-eaters.

Scat (droppings) analysis is a better method for evaluating diet but it, too, has its share of issues. Fragments can be hard to identify. More importantly, harder to digest items tend to get overrepresented in the results. For example, if you eat meat and cabbage, then the cabbage plant fibres would make up the bulk of the stool, the meat being almost fully digested. This residue plant matter is often over-represented in animals that consume both.

The most accurate method by far is analysis of the stomach contents. For the large part, this unfortunately requires the animal to be sacrificed. Hence, although considered as the gold standard of diet studies, stomach content analysis is conducted less often, usually in conjunction with population control measures.

Apart from the sampling method, there is another vital factor confusing the whole affair, and that is human influence, or more aptly, the dog's experience while young.

Truly feral or wild domestic dogs are those that have never had and positively avoid human contact. Free-roaming village dogs are free to forage during the day but return to their human families at night for food handouts. While these anatomically and taxonomically identical animals differ only in a generation or two of wild breeding, some differences do exist between them. For instance, in their study of the social biology of free-roaming domestic dogs and feral dogs, Bekoff (1989)[6] concluded that free-roaming domestic dogs were less social than expected, while feral dogs characteristically had reverted to operating in functional packs, much like their ancestors.

Free-roaming village dogs naturally are found in poorer areas of the world, where roaming laws are lax. On returning to their families in the evening, these dogs are observed to rely heavily on human handouts.[11,12] As meat protein is of significantly higher value in these economically poorer regions, village dogs tend to be offered a high amount of plant material. In central India they existed 'largely on human-derived handouts' such as millet bread, corn and peanuts[41] or in Zimbabwe, *sadza* (porridge). In some dogs human handouts made up to 50% of the food they consumed.

It's interesting to note that when these same dogs were left to their own devices, they tended to follow an all-carnivorous way of life.

> ...although they are fed regularly by their owners they are given little high-quality protein... they fed on animal matter to top up their failing protein levels...
>
> **Butler *et al* 2004**[11]

All this highlights an interesting quirk in dogs that is often overlooked when authors analyse the feeding habits of dogs. As part of his research for *The Dynamics of Behaviour Development*, Kuo (1967)[42] hand-reared 100 chow pups from birth to 6 months of age on one of three diets. One group was fed nothing but soybeans. The second was fed an all-vegetable material diet. The third was fed a mix of meat and vegetables. What he found was that those dogs reared on a single-protein diet such as soybeans would eat no novel foods presented to them later in life. Those reared on the vegetarian diet would eat no animal protein. Those reared on the meat and vegetarian diet would eat any new food. What Kuo amply demonstrated is that dogs seem to fixate their food preferences early in life, likely during the *imprinting period* (the first 5 months of life, a period long known by trainers to be crucial to their social, and mental development). It is likely a key feature to many scavenging carnivores, if not humans too.

In his book, *The Domestic Dog: Its Evolution, Behaviour, and Interactions with People*, Serpell (1995)[43] highlights the importance of this human factor in diet selection by dogs. Serpell reared a variety of small-breed dogs – poodles, dachshunds, Yorkshire Terriers and Cavalier King Charles Spaniels, on specific diets, until 2 years of age. One diet was a 'limited flavour experience' in the form of a nutritionally complete puppy food. Two others provided a variety of prepared and fresh foods. The author found that those fed a variety of flavours showed an immediate preference for novel foods, but the flavour-restricted groups preferred their usual food. In short, variety while young reduces pickiness in dogs.

Serpell notes that while some food preferences in dogs are genetically mediated, such as for sweet and salt, the behavioural processes involved in food selection are modified in response to the experience gained in life. Amniotic fluid and mother's milk are flavoured with foods eaten by the mother. Then food is regurgitated and presented whole by parents. In this way, animals that experience flavours early in life will link these to 'safe food sources'.[43] From here the animal develops a food selection strategy based on those experiences, selecting foods that are not only available but nutritious (no matter to what degree) and, most importantly, safe.

This process likely begins in the womb. *In utero* exposure to apple solution in rats results in an increased preference for that flavour later in life.[44] The same applies to odours. Exposure of pregnant female rats to citral (tasteless lemon scent) resulted in their pups selecting nipples that had been scented with citral.[45] These authors go on to show that rats restricted to a single flavour choose that flavour subsequently. Whereas those provided with a variety of flavours early on will more readily consume a novel one.

This goes some way to explaining why many domestic cats have been documented eating plant items. Village cats in South East Asia have a staple diet, consisting of rice flavoured with wok scrapings containing vegetables and sometimes fish bones; they will select similar items in garbage dumps.[46] However, their wild counterparts absolutely do not to any degree (see reviews by Doherty *et al.* [2015][47] who accumulated the results of 49 studies spanning six climatic regions, and Bonnaud *et al.* [2011][48] who used 72 studies of island cats).

It may even, and I'm going out on a limb here, explain why some grey wolf packs might very occasionally gorge on fruit items such as berries when available when most of the species possibly do not. I have seen the scat images – it appears as if nothing else but berries was eaten the previous meal. However, it is hard to discern if this is a *normal* practice for grey wolf populations. As we discussed in Chapter 2, a large review of some 26 wolf diet studies published in the *British Journal of Nutrition*, involving 31,276 wolf scat and stomach analyses, revealed 'a negligible amount of vegetative matter' being consumed.[49] Only in one or two studies was plant matter as high as 2–3%. This would seem strange with fruit being so easily available to the wolf in the summer months. It suggests that fruit 'gorging' is not a common or at least not the regular practice of wolves. Here's the rub – as we learn how important it is for our landscapes to have some apex predators about to keep the herbivores down, wolf re-introductions, are becoming more commonplace these days. However, a previous history of being fed by humans who had their own opinions on how these wolves should be fed may inadvertently muddy the waters for generations to come.

In such dietary studies, the free-roaming village dogs were fed plant scraps by their carers from a young age. In fact, their mothers were fed the same material, so they were likely primed to select it since before they were born.

This also explains why vegetarians believe their dogs *love* vegetables. It is a strange quirk of dogs that we can target them to eat pretty much any material, meat, vegetables or dry food. However, it says nothing of its *long-term* suitability to that animal. In fact, if we use longevity as a measure of fitness, then it would appear that when vets aren't involved, it's not working out too well for them. Boitani and Ciucci (1995)[8] found only 2% of Italian free-roaming and feral domestic dog populations living in a dump made it to 1 year of age.[50] Most free-roaming dogs die of malnutrition, in combination with predation, diseases, parasites and exposure.[51]

This is another crucial point. Plant food is far more abundant and accessible to animals when compared to meat, which is harder to find and certainly harder to catch. If we assume food availability is the most important factor in malnutrition, then it follows that if plant food is on the menu for dogs in any major way, then these free-roaming dogs would happily turn to it to sustain them (crops, plants, fruit and vegetables, garbage scraps), as true omnivores might do. But that doesn't seem to happen. Van't Woudt (1990)[51] suggests it is only 'where not subject to predation and where native or introduced prey is adequate' that they can survive to form truly feral populations.

All studies of canine diet from this point forward must take note of this crucial fact. Studies of pet, free-roaming or village dogs that have been fed by humans cannot be extrapolated to reflect the *normal* diet of the species as a whole.

3. Grass eating by dogs and hunger

We have all seen our dogs chewing on a grass stem now and again. *Canis lupus* species are notorious for self-medication.[52] In a survey of 1,571 dogs, 79% were documented to eat grass at least monthly.[53] However, this behaviour says no more about the dog's normal diet than it does in cats or wolves who are also known to indulge.[54-56] It is surely a natural solution to a variety of health issues, mostly concerning the digestive tract, but what exactly still eludes us. One reason may be that dogs seek fresh chlorophyll from young rye grass stems to aid the digestion process. Other stems induce vomiting or diarrhoea depending on the perceived need.[57] Indigestible, fibrous stems may even be an age-old strategy of reducing gut parasitic load. We're not quite sure which. As early as 1944, the famous wolf biologist Murie reported seeing parasitic worms in wolf scats alongside recently consumed grass.[58] More recently, wild chimpanzees have been found to eat leaves from a variety of plants that pass through the intestinal tract undigested, purging the intestinal tract of nematodes.[59] However, we recently tested the scat of 20 avid grass-eaters and found only one housed gut worms (*pers. comm.*). Indeed, in the aforementioned survey only 9% of the plant-eating dogs appeared ill prior to eating grass and only 22% regularly vomited afterward, the great majority appeared normal. A final interesting finding of the survey was that young dogs tended to eat more grass than older dogs. It may be that young animals, with their developing immunity, are much more affected by parasites. However, we do know dogs learn *over time* to associate certain foods with its physiological consequences. Thus, while they are born with an inherent knowledge of *what* to select, it is likely they are unsure exactly *when*, something that would be developed with time and *in utero* exposure to medicinal foods.

Never underestimate a dog's innate ability to heal himself. Indeed, this is the whole basis of Zoopharmacognosy, whereby various healing foods and herbs are offered to sick dogs. The patient, with their supreme olfactory system, is free to choose what they perceive they might need or walk away. Caroline Ingraham, the founder of the discipline, is incredible. Please check out her work. In Section 4, you will see we apply some of her principles when feeding dogs ourselves.

Of course, the occasional piece of grass taken by your dog is not a reason to include huge amounts of plant material in the dog's diet. Hippos and, indeed, cows will chew the bones of other animals for calcium. Red deer and sheep on the Scottish island of Rum have been known to eat the heads and legs of live seabird chicks to get the minerals they need to grow their antlers and horns.[60] We consider these occasional feeding quirks as medicinal and, thus, more rare than habitual.

Then there is hunger. Deep-chested dogs are permanently hungry.[61] Take Labradors, for example. Originating in the cold straits of Labrador in Northern Canada, they were bred to put on fat quickly to enable them to retrieve game from icy waters. In this, they are aided by webbed feet and an oar-like tail. Genetically predisposed to gorge large amounts of food, labs, like many other breeds, can distend their stomachs, an adaptation of scavenging carnivores who are not quite sure when the next meal will be. It means they can eat 10% of their body weight in one sitting – that's 3kg of food for the average lab! Instead, you pour 300 g of rapidly digested dry kibble into his bowl. A starving dog will be less choosy.

TAKE-HOME POINTS

- ✓ Compared to wolves, dogs are smaller, less aggressive and lack pack-hunting ability. They are still highly efficient predators; only today their prey is now smaller.

- ✓ Typical food items included by the dog are rodents, birds, rabbits, insects, lizards, frogs, and smaller ungulates, such as white tail deer, sheep and gazelle kids, should they be readily available and accessible. Larger prey, such as cattle, are normally consumed in carcass form which makes up approximately 25% of their diet. Faeces is also on the menu. This is the diet of an opportunistic hunter or scavenging carnivore.

- ✓ Dogs and cats establish lifelong taste preferences based on experiences while young. Humans can interfere with this process by feeding inappropriate items during the imprinting period (and explains why cats might 'love vegetables', something feral cats most certainly do not). This sullies the diet data and all diet works using previously dry-fed dogs and cats.

- ✓ Studies of village dogs indicate the more vegetation in their diet, the more likely they are affected by the fact they were fed leftover plant matter when young by their families and on returning home after a day roaming.

- ✓ Free-roaming dogs follow an almost completely carnivorous way of life when roaming during the day.

- ✓ Truly feral dogs consume significantly less plant matter when left to their own devices and given adequate access to prey, but we have very little dietary data on this group.

- ✓ Most carnivorous mammals consume some plant matter, often on a medicinal basis. It may act as a digestif, induce vomiting, help to remove parasites. For others it may be nutritional.

Chapter Three References

1   Hare, B., Brown, M. Williamson, C. *et al*. (2002). The Domestication of Social Cognition in Dogs. Science, 298(5598): 1634–1636

2   Wayne, R.K. vonHoldt, B.M. (2012). Evolutionary genomics of dog domestication. Mammalian Genometrics, 23(1-2): 3–18

3   Mech L.D. and Boitani L. (2003). *Wolves: Behavior, Ecology, and Conservation*. University of Chicago Press

4   Meggitt, M. J. (1965). The association between Australian Aborigines and dingoes. In A. Leeds and A. Vayada (Eds.), Man, culture and animals: The role of animals in human ecological adjustments. Washington, DC: American Association for the Advancement of Science pp7-26

5   Scott, M.D. and Causey, K. (1973). Ecology of feral dogs in Alabama. Journal of Wildlife Management, 37: 253–265

6   Daniels, T.J. and Bekoff, M. (1989). Population and social biology of free-ranging dogs, *Canis familiaris*. Journal of Mammology, 70: 754–762

7   Bradshaw, J. (2011). *Dog sense*. New York: Basic Books

8   Boitani, L. and Ciucci, P. (1995). Comparative social ecology of feral dogs and wolves. Ethology Ecology and Evolution, 7(1): 49–72

9   Mech, L.D. (1970). *The wolf: The ecology and behaviour of an endangered species*. New York: Doubleday

10   Sweeney, J.R., Marchinton, R.L. and Sweeney, J.M. (1971). Responses of radio monitored white-tailed deer chased by hunting dogs. Journal of Wildlife Management, 35: 707–716

11   Butler J.R.A., du Toit, J.T., Bingham, J. (2004). Free-ranging domestic dogs *Canis familiaris* as predators and prey in rural Zimbabwe: Threats of competition and disease to large wild carnivores. Biological Conservation 115: 369–378

12   Vanak, A.T. and Gompper, M.E. (2009b). Dogs (*Canis familiaris)* as carnivores: their role and function in intraguild competition. Mammalian Review, 39(4): 265–283

13   Echegaray, J. and Vilà, C. (2010). Non-invasive monitoring of wolves at the edge of their distribution and the cost of their conservation. Animal Conservation, 13: 157–161

14   Jhala, Y.V. and Giles, R.H. (1991). The status and conservation of the wolf in Gujarat and Rajasthan, India. Conservation Biology 5: 476–483

15   Scott, M.D. and Causey, (1973). Ecology of feral dogs in Alabama. Journal of Wildlife Management, 37: 253–265

16   Nesbitt, W.H. (1975). *Ecology of a feral dog pack on a wildlife refuge*. In The wild canids. New York: Van Nostrand Reinhold. M. W. Fox (Ed.), p391–395

17   Lenth, B., Knight, R., Brennan, M.E. (2008). The effects of dogs on wildlife communities. Natural Areas Journal 28: 218–227

18   Gingold, G., Yom-Tov, Y., Kronfeld-Schor, N. *et al* (2009). Effect of guard dogs on behavior and reproduction of gazelles in cattle enclosures on the Golan Heights. Animal Conservation, 12:155–162

19   Butler J.R.A. and du Toit, J.T. (2002). Diet of free-ranging domestic dogs *Canis familiaris* in rural Zimbabwe: Implications for wild scavengers on the periphery of wildlife reserves. Animal Conservation, 5: 29–37

20   Prakash, V., Pain, D.J., Cunningham, A.A. *et al.* (2003). Catastrophic collapse of Indian White-backed *Gyps bengalensis* and Long-billed Q vulture populations. Biological Conservation, 109: 381–390

21   Iverson, J.B. (1978). The impact of feral cats and dogs on populations of the West Indian rock iguana, Cyclura carinata. Biological Conservation, 14: 63–73

22   Kruuk, H. and Snell, H. (1981). Prey selection by feral dogs from a population of marine iguanas *Amblyrhynchus cristatus*. Journal of Applied Ecology, 18: 197–204

23   Galetti, M. and Sazima, I. (2006). Impact of feral dogs in an urban Atlantic forest fragment in southeastern Brazil. Nature and Conservation, 4(1): 146–155

24   Manor, R. and Saltz, D. (2004). The impact of free-roaming dogs on gazelle kid/female ratio in a fragmented area. Biological Conservation, 119(2): 231–236.

25   Taborsky, M. (1988). Kiwis and dog predation: observations in Waitangi State Forest. Notornis, 35: 197-202

26   Sillero-Zubiri, C. and Gotelli, D. (1995). Spatial organization in the Ethiopian wolf *Canis simensis* - large pack and small stable home ranges. Journal of Zoology, 237: 65–81

27   Mitchell, B.D. and Banks, P.B. (2005). Do wild dogs exclude foxes? Evidence for competition from dietary and spatial overlap. Australian Ecology, 30: 581–591

28   Lacerda, A.C.R., Tomas, W.M. and Marinho-Filho, J. (2009). Domestic dogs as an edge effect in the Brasília National Park, Brazil: Interactions with native mammals. Animal Conservation, 12: 477–487

29   Banks, P.B. and Bryant, J.V. (2007). Four-legged friend or foe? Dog walking displaces native birds from natural areas. Biology Letters, 3: 611–613

30   Lowry, D.A. and McArthur, K.L. (1978). Domestic dogs as predators on deer. Wildlife Society Bulletin, 6: 38–39

31   Gipson, S. (1983). *Evaluation and control implications of behaviour of feral dogs in interior Alaska Vertebrate Pest Control and Management Materials: Fourth Symposium*. ASTM Special Technical Publication 817, p285–294. West Conshohocken, PA

32   Miller, J.E. and Leopold, B.D. (1992). *Population influences: Predators*. in Dickinson, J.G. (Ed.). The Wild Turkey: Biology and Management, p119–128. Stackpole.PA

33   Bouvier, M. and Arthur, C.P. (1995). *Protection et indemnisation des degats d'xours aux troupeaux domestiques dans les Pyrenees occidentales: Fonctionnement, importance economique et role dans la protection de l'ours*. In Bourliere F, Barre V, Camerra JJ, Herrenschmidt V, Moutou F, Serveen C, Stuart S, Saint Girons MC, eds. Proceedings on the Management and Restoration of Small and Relictual Bear Populations, p510–521. Museum of Natural History

34   Pierce, R.J. and Sporle, W. (1997). Causes of Kiwi Mortality in Northland. Conservation Advisory Science Notes no. 169. Department of Conservation, Wellington, New Zealand

35   Campos, C.B., Esteves, C.F., Ferraz, K. M. *et al* (2007). Diet of free-ranging cats and dogs in a suburban and rural environment, south-eastern Brazil. Journal of Zoology, 273(1): 14–20

36   Young, J.K., Olson, K.A., Reading, R.P. *et al* (2011). Is Wildlife Going to the Dogs? Impacts of Feral and Free-roaming Dogs on Wildlife Populations. BioScience 61(2): 125–132

37   Macdonald, D.W. and Carr, G.M. (1995). *Variation in dog society: between resource dispersion and social flux*. In: Serpell J, editor. *The domestic dog: its evolution, behaviour and interactions with people*. Cambridge: Cambridge University Press; 1995. p. 199–216

38   Prugh, L.R., Stoner, C.J., Epps, C.W. *et al* (2009). The rise of the mesopredator. BioScience, 59: 779–791

39   Fleming, F., Corbett, L., Harden, R. *et al* (2001). Managing the impacts of dingoes and other wild dogs. Canberra, Australia: National Heritage Trust, Bureau of Rural Sciences

40   Gipson, S. (1983). Evaluation and control implications of behaviour of feral dogs in interior Alaska. Vertebrate Pest Control and Management Materials: Fourth Symposium. ASTM Special Technical Publication 817, pp. 285–294. West Conshohocken, PA: ASTM

41   Vanak, A.T. and Gompper, M.E. (2009a). Dietary niche separation between sympatric free-ranging domestic dogs and Indian foxes in Central India. Journal of Mammalogy, 90(5): 1058–1065

42   Kuo, Z.Y. (1967). *The dynamics of behaviour development: An epigenetic view*. New York: Random House.

43   Serpell, J. (1995). The domestic dog: Its evolution, behaviour, and interactions with people. Cambridge, UK: Cambridge University Press

44   Smotherman, W.P. (1982). In utero chemosensory experience alters taster preferences and corticosterone responsiveness. Behavioural and Neural Biology, 36: 61–68

45   Pedersen, P.E. and Blass, E.M. (1982). Prenatal and postnatal determinants of the 1st suckling episode in albino rats. Developmental Psychobiology, 15: 349–355

46   Von Goldschmidt-Rotschild, B. and Lüps, P. (1976). Untersuchungen zur Nährungs-Ökologie verwilderter Hauskatzen im Kanton Bern (Schweiz). Revue Suisse Zoological, 83: 723–735 (in German, cited in Van't Woudt 1990)

47   Doherty, T.S., Davis, R.A., van Etten, E., *et al*. (2015). A continental-scale analysis of feral cat diet in Australia. Journal of BioGeography, 42(5): 964–975

48   Bonnaud, E, Medina, F.M., Vidal, E., *et al*. (2011). The diet of feral cats on islands: a review and a call for more studies. Biological Invasions, 13(3): 581–603

49   Bosch, G., Hagen-Plantinga, E.A. and Hendriks, W.H. (2015). Dietary nutrient profiles of wild wolves: insights for optimal dog nutrition? British Journal of Nutrition (2015), 113, S40–S54

50   Boitani, L., Francisci, F., Ciucci, P. *et al* (1995). Population biology and ecology of feral dogs in central Italy. In J. A. Serpell (Ed.), The domestic dog: Its evolution, behaviour, and interactions with people. Cambridge, UK: Cambridge University Press, pp. 217–244

51   Van't Woudt, B.D. (1990). Roaming, stray and feral domestic cats and dogs as wildlife problems. Vertebrate Pest Conference Proceedings collection. Lincoln, NE: University of Nebraska

52   Wynn, S. (2006). *Veterinary herbal medicine*. New York: Mosby

53   Chieko Suedaa, K.L., Hart. B.L. and Davis Cliff, K. (2008). Characterisation of plant eating in dogs. Applied Animal Behaviour Science, 111(1–2): 120–132

54   Robinette, W.L., Gashwiler, J.S. and Morris, O.W. (1959). Food habits of the cougar in Utah and Nevada. Journal of Wildlife Management, 23:261–273

55   Andersone Z, Ozolins J. Food habits of wolves Canis lupus in Latvia. Acta Theriologic, 49:357–367

56   Stahler, D.R., Smith, D.W. and Guernsey, D.S. (2006). Foraging and Feeding Ecology of the Gray Wolf (*Canis lupus*): Lessons from Yellowstone National Park, Wyoming, USA. The Journal of Nutrition, 136(7): 1923S–1926S

57   Trainys, K.V. (2001). Dogs eat grass: what, when, why and how much? Veterinarija Ir Zootechnika, 16 (38).

58   Murie A. (1944). The wolves of Mount McKinley. Fauna of the National Parks, No. 5. Washington, DC: US Government Printing Office. (Reprinted by University of Washington Press 1985.)

59   Huffman M.A. and Caton J.M. 2001. Self-induced increase of gut motility and the control of parasitic infections in wild chimpanzees. International Journal of Primatology, 22: 329–346

60   Furness, R.W. (1988). Predation on ground-nesting seabirds by island populations of red deer *Cervus elaphus* and sheep *Ovis*. Journal of Zoology, 216(3): 565–573

61   Hand, M.S., Thatcher, C.D., Remillard, R.F. *et al* (1998). *Small animal clinical nutrition* (4th ed.). Topeka, KS: Mark Morris Associates

Digestive Anatomy and Physiology of the Domestic Dog

Dogs have differed in size and shape from their wolf cousins for more than 30,000 years. Five thousand years ago we had hunting dogs, guard dogs, scent hounds and terriers for ratting. Lap dogs appeared around 2,000 years ago.[1] Only in the last 150 years has breeding really exploded and produced many of the 339 breeds of dog 'evident today (numbers dependent on who you talk to).'The question is, has anything changed on the inside of the dog, over the last 30,000 years of evolution: which might support the more omnivorous way of life that the majority of Western dogs are being forced to live?

The short answer is no, it hasn't. All the physiology experts agree that dogs have the internal anatomy and physiology of a carnivore.[2-6]

Head

Look at a dog's mouth. Does that look like a plant-eater to you?! Dogs have the dentition of a meat-eating carnivore.[2,6-8] As opposed to large, flat molars for grinding plant material, dogs have pointed jagged teeth for nipping, piercing, tearing and shredding flesh.[9] Their huge bite force, coupled with large, reinforced carnassial molars which slide past each other, aids the cutting and chopping of flesh and bone alike. Unlike omnivores, dogs have no sideways movement of the jaw to grind down fibrous plant forage. Dog's chomp and swallow large chunks. As scavenging carnivores, dogs tend to eat quickly before bigger meat-eaters get a chance to move them on. In this way, aided by large quantities of saliva and a wide, keratinised throat,[7] they can gulp down large lumps of meat and bone.

Unlike herbivores and true omnivores, dogs have no amylase in their saliva.[3,5,10] This is telling. Amylase aids in the breakdown of plant carbohydrate. Carnivores do not have salivary amylase as they do not consume plant material to any large degree. Any carbohydrates consumed by these animals are broken down via enzymes released by the pancreas and the villi of the intestines.

Like all scavenging carnivores, dogs have various lysozymes in their saliva. They dissolve bacteria cell walls, rather like an in-built, antibacterial oral disinfectant. Lysing means that the lysozyme attaches itself to the cell wall of the bacteria and weakens it until the point where the cell wall ruptures, and the bacterium dies. On top of this, their saliva contains the enzymes peroxidase, lactoferrin, defensins, cystatins and the antibody IgA, which are all antibacterial. It also contains thrombospondin, an anti-viral, as well as protease inhibitors and nitrates that break down into nitric oxide on contact with skin, inhibiting bacterial growth.[11-15] Hart and Powell (1990)[16] found canine saliva highly effective at destroying *Escherichia coli* and *Streptococcus canis,* among other baddies. This would help protect the dog when consuming raw meat from not-so-fresh carcasses or digging up meaty bones buried days previously, but also, on return to the pack, to not spread disease when allogrooming.

In this way, a dog's kiss is relatively sterile, certainly cleaner than yours. It's why they show such interest in that cut on your leg. They tentatively lick it, to clean it. There are numerous examples historically of cultures using a dog's saliva for its curative powers.[17] The French have a saying *Langue de chien, langue de médecin*, meaning 'A dog's tongue is a doctor's tongue.' And for many years the French Foreign Legion had them around for this very reason. In Latin there is a quote *Lingua canis dum lingit vulnus curat* or 'A dog's tongue, licking a wound, heals it' which appears in *The Aberdeen Bestiary*, a 13th century English illuminated manuscript.

That said, don't snog the dog. These aren't my words. This is the very sound advice of Ngaage *et al.* (1999)[18] who documented a case of infective endocarditis due to *Capnocytophaga canimorsus* in a 63-year-old man who made a habit of 'snogging his dog'. Honestly, you don't want that! It's a common bacteria in and around a dog's mouth in 60-86% of dogs,[19,20] though it rarely makes it into a human's blood stream. Should you be unfortunate enough to pick it up, normally through a bite, you could be in trouble. Of 484 affected patients suffering various degrees of sepsis, septic shock, gangrene, meningitis and endocarditis, 26% died.[21]

The taste system of a dog is also adapted to carnivory. The presence of both amino acid and nucleotide sensitive receptors indicates a specialised taste system geared to detect compounds found only in raw flesh and carrion,[7,22] one that is very different to that of rats, humans and omnivores in general.[22] Dogs have salt-specific taste buds, which tends to reflect a predominantly carnivorous diet in which the food is salt-balanced.[7] This results in the dog having both a smell[23,24] and taste,[25,26] preference for meat over all other food sources. Bhadra *et al.* (2016)[27] offered free-range dogs a choice of dry kibble pet food, plain bread or plain bread soaked in chicken broth. They found that the dogs would consistently choose the bread that smells of meat above all else, which the authors state demonstrated that dogs 'have retained a clear preference for meat, which is manifested by their choice of anything that smells of meat, irrespective of the actual nutrient content. They like meat.'

Also note their eye position, which is forward, on the front of their skull. This is to enable focus on prey animals. Herbivorous animals have eyes set to the sides of their skulls to watch for attacks.[28] Have you ever waggled a sausage at a hungry dog? They stare, transfixed. They want to and will devour it. Compare this to waggling some grass at a horse. There isn't quite the same reaction.

Gut

Dogs have highly elastic, highly acidic stomachs, with undeveloped caecum and the short, fast intestinal tracts of a carnivore.[3-5]

The dog's gut is highly acidic. During digestion it can reach $< pH1.0$, equivalent to car battery acid. It can remain at that level for 5 hours, if need be.[29-31] Youngberg *et al.* (1985)[30] found the average gastric pH of (dry-fed) dogs was pH 1.5, becoming steadily more alkaline as it prepares to empty into the duodenum.

While fasting, dogs and humans actually have a very similar gastric pH, averaging 1.5 and 1.7, respectively. Following stimulation (food), the gastric acid secretion rates in dogs greatly exceeds that of humans. A human's stomach can rise to pH 5, while a dog's does not get above pH 2.[32]

Acidity aside, during digestion dogs hold on to the ingested meal longer and pulverise it more. Meyer *et al.* (1979, 1981)[33,34] measured the stomach-emptying rate of a liver and steak meal in both dogs and humans and discovered, somewhat surprisingly considering their overall rapid throughput time, that dogs retained food in their stomachs far longer than humans. Once emptied, however, transit time in the small intestines is far more rapid in dogs than in humans,[35] as you would expect in a carnivore. Also, Schemann and Ehrlein (1986)[36] note that a dog's gut contracts on average 5.2 times per minute when digesting, while a human's only 3 times per minute. The dog is literally pulverising the meal in order to decrease digestion and throughput time.

This level of acidity is ideal for the enzyme pepsin, released by the stomach to get to work on the protein in the meal. Couple this with a longer processing time and greater mechanical compression, and the dog's stomach is a meat-and-bone digesting machine. Fresh meat and bone meal are shown to rapidly break down into chyme (goo) within an hour.[37]

A low pH has another vital benefit in that it is highly effective at killing bacteria, particularly normally pathogenic bacteria like certain *Salmonella* spp., *Clostridia*, *Campylobacter* and *Escherichia coli*, a vital adaptation for a scavenging carnivore that thrives on carcass. We see this in Griffon vultures, who have evolved a very acidic gastric environment of pH between 1.0 and 2.0, which authors note helps to minimise infection by pathogens from rotten meat.[38]

Post digestion, the stomach will abruptly change to neutral, presumably to neutralise the corrosive acid before it hits the duodenum and intestines, which are both less equipped to withstand the corrosive power of a pH 1.5 acid broth. Authors note that once in the intestines, the pH of the food bolus in dogs gradually rises to a near neutral pH 6.0, via the large intestine where it remains for defecation.[29,31]

Total intestinal tract length is a good indicator of feeding ability, with carnivores having shorter tracts and herbivores having the longest. The total gut length of the dog is approximately 3.5 to 4.1 times their body length.[39] The longest reliable length I can find for a dog's intestinal tract is in a Turkish study of seven Turkish shepherd dogs (Karabash, a large-breed), which had intestinal tracts five times the length of the body.[40] For this study Yildiz *et al.*[40] measured intestinal tracts of canine cadavers used in student classes. However, measurements of an intestinal tract should only be conducted on very fresh samples, as the intestinal tract significantly lengthens by roughly 20% after the death of the animal[41] due to a relaxation of collagen fibres. Serpell (1995)[7] found intestinal tracts of dogs to be 4.1 times the length of the body which would "equate to the value reported in the study by Yildiz *et al.* (2006)[40] value above, allowing for 20% distention. Gill *et al.* (1964)[39] measured the intestinal tracts of wolves, feral dogs and dingoes while still fresh in the field and found their intestinal tract length to be comparable–grey wolves 3.0 to 4.2 times body length, domestic dogs 3.5 to 4.1 times body length, dingoes 4.1 times the length of the body. This is the intestinal length you would expect of a carnivore.[7]

The dog's intestines are host to a simple, limited number of gut microflora[42] with bacterial numbers rarely exceeding 10^4 to 10^5 per millilitre. The low numbers are due to the very low acidity of the environment, but also to the rapid throughput of the digesta. It prevents colonisation by non-adherent bacteria and pathogenic microorganisms.

The dominant bacteria in the canine gut, include *Bacteroides*, *Clostridium*, *Lactobacillus*, *Bifidobacterium* and *Enterobacteriaceae*, which are species adapted to meat digestion.[43] However, no two dogs are the same. Davis *et al.* (1977)[44] found that housed dogs, fed the same food for years, have marked differences in their microflora.

The acidity of the dog's gut, coupled with undeveloped caecum, a rapid passage of digesta through the intestines and a microflora ill-equipped for plant fibre digestion, means the dog's system is totally unprepared for the digestion of raw plant material.

In this way dogs still have virtually the same internal anatomy and physiology as wolves, which is why they are often used as models for wolves in physiological studies.[45]

Digestive Physiology

We know that dogs have zero need for plant carbohydrate in their diet. They make their own glucose from protein and fat in a process called gluconeogenesis (*gluco-neo-genesis*), a process that, in dogs, is constantly switched on.[3,5,10,46]

> *Canis lupus* sub-species do not consume plant carbohydrate by means of nutrition.
>
> **Sillero-Zubiri *et al.*, 2004**[47]

> Dogs have no requirement for plant carbohydrate
> **Association of American Feed Control Officials (AAFCO), 2016**[48]

> There appears to be no requirement for carbohydrate [in dogs] provided enough protein is given.
>
> **National Research Council (NRC), 2006**[5]

Compared to say true omnivores, dogs are poorly equipped to gather and process plant matter. Their hinged jaw and jagged, carnassial teeth allow no sideways movement for flat dental surfaces for grinding tough plant forage. They have no salivary amylase. Their taste receptors are geared for a meat diet. Their quick, highly acidic gut and undeveloped caecum is ill-adapted to plant fibre digestion. For all these reasons, all the independent anatomy and physiology experts agree that the dog today is best geared for a carnivorous way of life.

...carnivores such as dogs and cats...

Akers and Denbow, 2008[6]

...dogs are carnivores...

NRC, 2006[5]

...dogs have the internal anatomy and physiology of a carnivore...

Feldhamer, 2003[3]

Now, this is no great revelation. It is clear that in just a few thousand years dog breeds have, to varying degrees, taken some minor evolutionary steps toward, plant carbohydrate digestion – certainly at the genetic level when compared to the dingo or wolf. However, the major changes in anatomy and physiology that would be required for a once meat-eating animal to thrive on the largely plant-based diet now endorsed by the veterinary community seem not (yet) to have evolved. Such a seismic shift in dietary practice would surely take far longer – hundreds of thousands, if not millions of years (and deaths). Dogs have only been around for 30,000 years, or so.

But we altered everything else about domestic dogs, I hear you cry! Absolutely, while this is most certainly true of external phenotypes, including body size, ear and tail carriage, muzzle shape, coat form and many behaviours, it doesn't hold for dietary preference. At no point could it be argued that humans made a conscious effort to breed dogs according to their internal digestive dynamics. Dogs have been living in close proximity to humans off and on for 30,000 years. Initially, free-roaming proto-dogs would, for the very large part, have chosen their own partners. Where hunter–gatherers carried out selective breeding, it was likely to have been first for correct behaviour (don't eat me) and later for size. Lacking bin charges, it's highly unlikely they cherished the dog's ability to consume their leftovers. Furthermore, any family pets would have been free-to-roam and thus mate, day and night. In this way, the haphazard and sporadic domestications of dogs from 30,000 to 200 years ago, when breeding really picked up, have not altered the gut anatomy or feeding style of this species.

This simple fact is evident in red setters today. Largely accepted to be the coeliacs of the dog family (more on that later), at no point has a Red Setter breeder attempted to breed the condition out by selecting only those setters that can digest wheat safely, at least not to this author's knowledge. It's fair to say that, should inherited disease be a measure of fitness, breeders seem to be making dogs less fit, not more. Why else would mongrels be cheaper to insure?

But the evidence previously discussed above concerning the increased starch-digesting ability of some breeds of domestic dogs should not be overlooked.[49-52] Dogs clearly have more copies of the AMY2B carbohydrate-digesting gene than wolves. First noted by Axelsson *et al.* (2013),[50] these authors further showed that the dogs in their sample had small changes in specific genes that allow for the breakdown of maltose into glucose, another key starch digestion step, as well as in genes allowing for the body to make use of this glucose.

In addition, the liver and pancreas of the dog produce hepatic glucokinase (GCK), an enzyme used to digest sugar.[53] True carnivores, such as domestic cats and indeed all other true carnivores such as owls, dolphins and trout, do not.

This all results in dogs being better able to utilise sugar than cats. A glucose tolerance test is a laboratory test to check how well your body breaks down sugar. Schermerhorn (2013)[53] notes how intravenous glucose tolerance tests, where glucose is injected into the bloodstream and monitored for how quickly it is utilised by the animal, revealed a delayed glucose clearance after 90 minutes in cats. This compared with about 40–60 minutes in dogs – humans are 30–40 minutes.

> In these carnivorous species, hepatic GCK is replaced by hexokinase I, an adaptation that enables the cat to function normally during periods of fasting. It is part of the adaptive genetics of the cat, which places the cat in a physiological "pre-diabetic state". This is not pathological; it is what the cat requires, so long as its diet remains carnivorous.
>
> **Billinghurst,** *personal comment,* **2018**[54]

Nor are these the only omnivorous tricks performed by the dog. Authors note that dogs appear to be able to convert carotene (derived from plant material such as carrots) to vitamin A, although they appear extremely poor at it.[5] While the exact conversion rate for dogs is unknown, we humans can only convert one-twelfth of the available carotene we eat to vitamin A,[55] and only about one-third of that one-twelfth is actually absorbed into the body. Then again, perhaps that is all we need. Dogs can also convert some tryptophan (an amino acid) to niacin (vitamin B$_3$), cysteine (an amino acid) to taurine (another amino acid) and linoleate (a salt form of linoleic acid) to arachidonate (polyunsaturated omega-6 fatty acid). While we are unsure whether many wolves have this ability, we know these are things the likes of the ultra-carnivorous cat cannot do. These may be an adaptation to facilitate the dogs more scavenging lifestyle. While cats want it fresh, it's more a matter of best-before-not-bad-after for our humble hero. The dog is happy to exploit less desirable options such as carcass, garbage and faeces. In a body conducting literally thousands of carnivorous processes each minute, the three processes above might facilitate the dog's move to a more scavenging lifestyle. As the nutrient content of food diminishes rapidly over time, being able to produce some vitamins and proteins from more readily available material might have its advantages. Some information on polar bears or vultures here would be very useful.

It is metabolic quirks such as these that result in cats being defined as obligate or *true* carnivores, while dogs get the vaguer *facultative* carnivore definition. Sadly, where there is vagary, there are people screaming obscenities at each other on social media forums. The difference in the two definitions is that obligate carnivores *need* meat to thrive. Whereas facultative carnivores, while still very, very carnivorous in their daily routine, can make use of other plant-based bits and pieces when necessary. Of course, the words 'can take some plant material if needs be' sounds ominously like an omnivore. For this reason, I urge caution with the use of all these terms. Again, being told an animal is either a facultative carnivore or omnivore does little to help a novice zookeeper feed it adequately over the course of the year.

The fact remains, these minor physiological quirks have not (yet) seemed to affect what dogs tend to eat *when left to their own devices.*

In fact, a review of the dog's ancestry, foraging habits and now digestive machinery and physiology, all indicate that the modern dog is a formidable, often devastating predator of smaller prey animals. Free of human influence, they pursue an almost all-meat diet.

Thus, if we are concerned with optimum health in our dogs, the basics of animal husbandry dictate that we are required to feed them as close to their natural, biologically appropriate diet as possible. In the case of the domestic dog, that would be a diet consisting of a very large amount of fresh animal matter.

With this in mind, you would be forgiven for wondering what the effects of feeding dogs ultra-high-carbohydrate diets long term might be?

TAKE-HOME POINTS

✓ Dogs have the dentition of a carnivore. Their jaws can exert immense bite force useful only for catching and crunching prey. Their jaws allow no sideways movement.

✓ They have no amylase in their saliva for digesting plant carbohydrates.

✓ With various lysozymes in their saliva, the dog's lick is virtually anti-bacterial (but don't snog the dog!).

✓ Their taste system is adapted to meat. Studies show they have retained a clear taste-preference for meat.

✓ Dogs have highly elastic, highly acidic stomachs, undeveloped caecum and the short, fast intestinal tracts of a carnivore. Their gut tract lengths are around 3.5–4.1 times the length of their body.

✓ Dogs have zero physiological need at any stage for plant carbohydrate in their diet.

✓ Dogs do have some omnivorous leanings, including more copies of the AMY2B gene than dingoes or wolves. Also, unlike so many true carnivores, they can produce hepatic glucokinase. These two traits result in dogs being better at utilising carbohydrates than cats.

✓ Other potentially omnivorous physiological traits include the conversion of carotene to vitamin A, tryptophan to niacin, cysteine to taurine and linoleate to arachidonate. Taken together, this indicates some plant material has been consumed in the past.

Chapter Four References

1   Bradshaw, J. (2011). *Dog sense*. New York: Basic Books

2   Stevens, C.E. and Hume, I.D. (1995). *Comparative physiology of the vertebrate digestive system* (2nd ed.). New York: Cambridge University Press

3   Feldhamer, G.A. (2003). *Mammology: Adaptation, diversity, and ecology*, 2nd Ed. New York: McGraw-Hill

4   O'Reece, W. (2004). *Dukes' physiology of domestic animals* (12th ed.). Ithaca, NY: Comstock Publishing

5   National Research Council (NRC) (2006). *Nutrient requirement of dogs and cats*. Washington, DC: National Academies Press

6   Akers, R.M. and Denbow, D.M. (2008). *Anatomy and physiology of domestic animals*. Oxford: Blackwell

7   Serpell, J. (1995). *The domestic dog: Its evolution, behaviour, and interactions with people*. Cambridge, UK: Cambridge University Press

8   Bradshaw, J.W.S. (2006). The Evolutionary Basis for the Feeding Behavior of Domestic Dogs (*Canis familiaris*) and Cats (*Felis catus*). Journal of Nutrition 2006, 136(7): 1927S–1931S

9   Coppinger, R. and Coppinger, L. (2001). *Dogs: A new understanding of canine origin, behavior, and evolution*. Chicago, IL: University of Chicago Press

10   Pasquini, C., Spurgeon, T. and Pasquini, S. (1989). *Anatomy of domestic animals: Systemic and regional approach* (10th ed.). Pilot Point, TX: Sudz Publishing

11   Benecke, N. (1987). Studies on early dog remains from Northern Europe. Journal of Archaeological Science, 14: 31–49

12   Ashcroft, G.S., Lei, K. and Jin, W. (2000). Secretory leukocyte protease inhibitor mediates non-redundant functions necessary for normal wound healing. Natural Medicine, 6(10): 1147–1153

13   Baron, S., Singh, I., Chopra, A. *et al.* (2000). Innate antiviral defenses in body fluids and tissues. Antiviral Research, 48(2): 71–89

14   Abiko, Y., Nishimura, M. and Kaku, T. (2003). Defensins in saliva and the salivary glands. Medical Electron Microscopy, 36(4): 247–252

15   Ihalin, R., Loimaranta, V. and Tenovuo, J. (2006). Origin, structure, and biological activities of peroxidases in human saliva. Archives of Biochemistry and Biophysics, 445(2): 261–268

16   Hart, B.L. and Powell, K.L. (1990). Antibacterial properties of saliva: Role in maternal periparturient grooming and in licking wounds. Physiology and Behaviour, 48(3): 383–386.

17   Hatfield, G. (2004). Encyclopedia of folk medicine: Old World and New World traditions. Santa Barbara, CA: ABC-CLIO

18   Ngaage, D.L., Kotidis, K.N., Sandoe, J.A.T. *et al.* (1999). Do not snog the dog: infective endocarditis due to *Capnocytophaga canimorsus*. European Journal of Cardiothoracic Surgery, 16: 362–363

19   Mally, M., Paroz, C,. Shin, H. *et al.* (2009). Prevalence of *Capnocytophaga canimorsus* in dogs and occurrence of potential virulence factors. Microbes and Infection, 11(4): 509-514

20 Suzuki, M., Kimura, M., Imaoka, K. and Yamada, A. (2010). Prevalence of *Capnocytophaga canimorsus* and *Capnocytophaga cynodegmi* in dogs and cats determined by using a newly established species-specific PCR. Veterinary Microbiology, 144(1-2): 172-176

21 Butler, T. (2015). *Capnocytophaga canimorsus*: an emerging cause of sepsis, meningitis, and post-splenectomy infection after dog bites. European Journal Clinical Microbiology of Infectious Disease, 34(7): 1271–1280

22 Boudreau, J.C. (1989). *Neurophysiology and stimulus chemistry of mammalian taste systems.* In: Teranishi R, Buttery RG, Shahadi F, editors. Flavor chemistry trends and developments, p122-137. American Chemical Society Symposium Series no 67; Washington, DC: American Chemical Society

23 Houpt, K.A., Hintz, H.F. and Shepherd, P. (1978). The role of olfaction in canine food preferences Chemical Senses, 3(3): 281–290

24 Beaver, B.V., Fischer, M. and Atkinson, C.E. (1992). Determination of favorite components of garbage by dogs. Applied Animal Behaviour Science, 34(1–2): 129–136

25 Kitchell, R.L. (1972). Dogs know what they like. Friskies Research Digest 8: 1-42

26 Houpt, K.A. and Smith, S.L. (1981). Taste preferences and their relation to obesity in dogs and cats. Canandian Veterinary Journal, 22(4): 77–81

27 Bhadra, A., Debottam, B., Manabi, P. *et al.* (2016). The meat of the matter: A thumb rule for scavenging dogs? Ethology Ecology & Evolution, 28(4): 427–440

28 Schultz, K.R. (1998). *Natural nutrition for dogs and cats*. Carlsbad, CA: Hay House

29 Itoh, Z., Honda, R., Aizawa, I.. (1980). Diurnal pH changes in duodenum of conscious dogs. American Journal of Physiology, 238(2): 91–96

30 Youngberg, C.A., Wlodyga, J., Schmaltz, S. *et al.* (1985). Radiotelemetric determination of gastrointestinal pH in four healthy beagles. American Journal of Veterinary Research, 46(7): 1516–1521

31 Sagawa, K., Li, F., Liese, R. *et al.* (2009). Fed and fasted gastric pH and gastric residence time in conscious beagle dogs. Journal of Pharmacological Science, 98(7): 2494-2500

32 Kararli, T.T (1995). Comparison of the gastrointestinal anatomy, physiology and biochemistry of humans and commonly used laboratory animals. Biopharmaceuticals and Drug Disposition, 16: 351–380

33 Meyer, J.H., Thomson, J.B. and Cohen, B. (1979). Sieving a solid food by the normal and ulcer-operated canine stomach. Gastroenterology 76: 804–813

34 Meyer, J.H., Ohashi, D.J., Jehn, D. *et al.* (1981). Size of liver particles emptied from the human stomach. Gastroenterology, 80:1489–1496

35 Youngberg, C.A. (1984). *Radiotelemetric Determination of GI pH in Man and Dog.* M.Sc. Thesis, University of Michigan, Ann Arbor, 1984

36 Schemann, M. and Ehrlein, H.J. (1986). Postprandial patterns of canine jejunal motility and transit of luminal content. Gastroenterology, 90(4): 991–1000

37 Lonsdale, T. (2001). *Raw meaty bones promote health*. Wenatchee, WA: Dogwise Publishing

38 Houston, D.C. and Cooper, J.E. (1975) The digestive tract of the white back griffon vulture and its role in disease transmission among wild ungulates. Journal of Wildlife Diseases, 11: 306–313

39   Gill, J., Hoffmannowa, H. and Piekarz, R. (1964). Studies on digestive physiology in the wolf, dingo, and jackal. II. Digestive ability of the pancreas, duodenum and salivary glands and size of the alimentary tract and weight of internal organs. Acta Physiologica, 15(1): 137–148

40   Yildiz, H., Arslan, K., Corfikun, H. *et al.* (2006). A geometric modeling of dog intestine. Turkish Journal of Veterinary Animal Science, 30: 483–488

41   Hounnou, G., Destrieux, C., Desmé, J. *et al.* (2002). Anatomical study of the length of the human intestine. Surgical and Radiologic Anatomy, 24(5): 290–294

42   Kearns, R.J., Hayek, M.G. and Sunvold, G.D. (1998). *Microbial changes in aged dogs. Recent Advances in Canine and Feline nutrition.* Vol. II. 1998 Iams International Nutrition Symposium Proceedings. 337–351

43   Suchodolski, J.S. (2005). *Assessment of the canine intestinal microflora using molecular methods and serum markers.* PhD Thesis. Texas A&M University

44   Davis, C.P., Cleven, D., Balish, E. *et al.* (1977). Bacterial association in the gastrointestinal tract of beagle dogs. Applied Environmental Microbiology, 34: 194-206

45   Mech L.D. and Boitani L. (Eds) (2003). *Wolves: Behavior, Ecology, and Conservation.* Chicago: University of Chicago Press

46   Hand, M.S., Thatcher, C.D., Remillard, R.L. *et al.* (2010). *Small Animal Clinical Nutrition*, 5th Edition. Published by The Mark Morris Institute, Kansas, U.S

47   Sillero-Zubiri, C., Hoffmann, M. and MacDonald, D.W. (2004). *Canids: Foxes, wolves, jackals and dogs. Status survey and conservation action plan.* Gland, Switzerland: IUCN.

48   AAFCO (Association of American Feed Control Officials) 2016. Official Publication. Available at AAFCO.org

49   Yang, R. and Newgard, C.B. (2004). *Balancing hepatic glucose disposal and production.* In: Matschinsky FM, Magnuson MA, editors. Glucokinase and Glycemic Disease: From Basics to Novel Therapeutics. Front Diabetes (Belfiore F, editor), 16: 379–397

50   Axelsson, E., Ratnakumar, A., Arendt, M.L. *et al.* (2013). The genomic signature of dog domestication reveals adaptation to a starch-rich diet. Nature, 495(7441): 360–364

51   Freedman, A.H., Gronau, I., Schweizer, R.M, *et al.* (2014). Genome Sequencing Highlights the Dynamic Early History of Dogs. PLOS Genetics 10(8): e1004631

52   Reiter, T., Jagoda, E., and Capellini, T.D. (2016). Dietary Variation and Evolution of Gene Copy Number among Dog Breeds. PLoS ONE 11(2): e0148899

53   Schermerhorn, T. (2013). Normal Glucose Metabolism in Carnivores Overlaps with Diabetes Pathology in Non-Carnivores. Front Endocrinol (Lausanne), 4: 188

54   Billinghurst, I. (1993). *Give your dog a bone.* Self-published.

55   Tang, G. (2010). Bioconversion of dietary provitamin A carotenoids to vitamin A in humans. American Journal of Clinical Nutrition, 91(5): 1468S–1473S

SECTION TWO

Issues with Kibble

CHAPTER 5

Introduction to Dry Pet Food

As the vast majority of western dogs today are consuming dry, cereal-based pet foods, and as it appears to be the only food promoted by the majority of our vets, this section is going to investigate it as a suitable food source for dogs.

Dry pet meal as we know it was likely invented by James Spratt sometime in the 1850s. The young electrician from Cincinnati went to London with his lightning rod business. While there, he saw the crew of a ship feeding leftover ship's biscuits to dogs. Cheap, easy to make and with a long shelf life, Spratt had stumbled on a gold mine. Very soon he had taken his idea back to New York and made himself a lot of money-making biscuit meal for dogs.

From this humble start, the pet food business was born. By the 1880s, a Massachusetts veterinary surgeon called A.C. Daniels, first thought of manufacturing Medicated Dog Bread. In 1908, The F.H. Bennet Biscuit Company tweaked the concept and began making various bone-shaped biscuits. In 1931, Nabisco (The National Biscuit Company) bought Bennet's product and renamed it *Milkbones*. They put 3,000 salespeople on the road. Their job? To make *Milkbones* the new national standard in dog food and a regular in the weekly grocery shop.

The first canned dog food appeared in 1922, called *Ken-L-Ration*. Made of horsemeat, of which there was a lot around, it was a big hit with pet owners, thanks largely to being advertised during the popular *Adventures of Rin Tin Tin* radio show. The ads brought canned dog food to the forefront of dog and cat nutrition. In fact, by the 1930s the Chappel Brothers, makers of *Ken-L-Ration*, had absorbed all available horsemeat and had to get into the horsemeat business themselves, resulting in the slaughter of more than 50,000 horses a year by the end of the 1930s, for dog food alone. Before World War II, it was estimated that canned dog food made up 90% of the dog food market. With the advent of war, there was suddenly less metal and meat about the place, and canned dog food became almost impossible to produce.

In 1950, the market quickly shifted to a new product manufactured by Ralston Purina Company using a new automatic process called extrusion cooking. In essence, a mix of cereal, meat, plant ingredients, supplements and chemical ingredients are added to a giant hopper. This mix is fed into a high pressure vat and cooked at approximately 121°C for 30 minutes, when it is extruded (forced through a small die) to form the required shape, then chopped into kibble pieces, baked dry and bagged. Purina's Dog Chow was born. This post-war invention, born of necessity, remains a regular on supermarket shelves to the present day.

By the 1960s the Pet Food Institute, the mouthpiece of the pet food industry, began a campaign to get pet–parents to only feed their dogs dry pet food. They started funding reports concerning the 'dangers' of table scraps for pets. To quote the chair for the Manufacturers Committee of the National Pet Association 'our biggest competitor is still table scraps'.[1] Together with the post-war economy boom, dry pet food rapidly became the wise choice for health-conscious consumers.

The concept of 'complete' was introduced in the 1970s. These were specialty diets for working dogs. Some health issues, including obesity, arrived 10 years later. By the 1990s we had veterinary-prescribed diets. These increasingly focused on breed-specific foods, varying ages and an increasing array of health conditions and reproductive stages. The rapid expansion of this specialisation process continues to this day.

In 2015, 68% of Americans were dry feeding only, compared to 90% in France, 78% in China and 56% in Great Britain.[2]

At the lower end of the quality scale of dry food are *economy brands*. These products are usually the cheapest and as they are perceived to be based on the lowest-quality ingredients, possibly offer the least in terms of nutrition and digestibility. Economy brands are rarely termed '*complete*' or '*balanced*'.

The next level up is termed *mainstream* or *supermarket brands*, and these are thought to represent better value for money. Often termed 'complete and balanced', many adhere to the criteria set by the AAFCO (Association of American Feed Control Officials, more on this group later), which is hoped to ensure adequate 'life-feeding'.

Then there is *premium* dry food. These products are most likely to be sold by pet shops and vets. They are always termed 'nutritionally complete', claiming to contain higher-quality ingredients with better palatability and digestibility. Authors noted that dogs fed dry food designated as premium appeared less distressed and agitated over an 8 week period.[3] They are significantly more expensive.

Super premium products are assumed to be the best. They are certainly the most expensive. They are always 'complete' and when sold by vets, they can often carry terms such as 'prescribed'. However, as we will discover later, this word indicates the product contains a restricted drug of importance to health, which is most certainly not the case. Prescribed pet food remains a hotly debated topic today. These products are more often than not breed and health issue-specific, focusing on different stages of life, including performance diets, growth diets and weight-control diets.

However, it's important to note here that the words '*economy*' and '*super premium*' are not defined by the industry. While the latter often claim to have optimum nutritional quality and higher digestibility, there are no set principles by which products can earn the loftier title. In fact, Krogdahl *et al.* (2004)[4] set out to explore if there were any differences whatsoever between the nutrient digestibility of both lower-(cheapest) and higher-quality (more expensive) commercial dry foods sold by vets. They found no difference in the dietary level of nutrients. Nor did they find any difference in the digestibility of those nutrients between the types. Furthermore, the protein and amino acid content and digestibility were similar between the two types. There were no discernible differences between them whatsoever. This suggests the only real difference between 'lower' and 'higher' quality dry foods is their price tag and marketing budgets.

Within the *premium* and *super premium* classifications, there are a great many varieties of foods. Still, the most popular and dominating veterinary recommendations remain cereal-based dry food (usually based on wheat or corn). However, of late, and in response to the market's demand for more 'natural' products,[5] grain-free pet food (which is more likely to be using pea, potato or tapioca as fillers) and much meatier ranges which replace their carbohydrate filler with more meat (which can make up 80% of the product and hence are often coined 80:20s, a ratio that is supposed to better represent how the dog would feed in the wild) have entered the market.

As well as better ingredients, many pet owners are now seeking to avoid the high-temperature cooking step in the hope that more of the nutritional value of the mix will be preserved. In response, less harsh processing techniques were developed to meet market demands including cold-pressed and freeze or air-dried pet food. By increasing processing pressure, 'cold-pressed' dry foods claim to employ lower temperatures of 40–70°C during manufacturing. However, when questioned, I have yet to meet a cold-pressed food manufacturer who does not subject the mix to a blast of high heat, which they call an antimicrobial step (though others might call it cooking). When it comes to sterilising your mix, you have two choices – use heat or use chemical antimicrobials to kill the pathogenic bacteria meat can contain. Clients buying the more expensive products are usually trying to avoid these chemical preservatives, so the heat step becomes something of a necessity.

Still, these less-heat-treated products continue their advance on the market. In fact, the more expensive freeze-dried pet food alone accounted for $182 million of the US pet food market in 2015, up from $75 million in 2012.[6]

For our analysis, we will be focusing on dry, premium and super premium, cereal-based diets, as these remain the products most recommended, promoted and sold by vets worldwide today.

TAKE-HOME POINTS

✓ Dry pet food is said to vary in quality from *economy* to *super premium*. However, studies can detect no nutritional differences whatsoever between the two types of food.

✓ As cereal-based pet food remains the food of choice by the world's vets, we focus on it in this section.

Chapter Five References

1 Anreder, S. S. (1962). *The pet industry is growing by leaps and bounds*. Barron's National Business and Financial Weekly. January 29th, p3,8,10,12–13

2 Lange, M. (2017). *Pet Food Trends Shaping the World*. Pet Food Industry Leadership Conference, 2017

3 Case, L.P., Carey, D.P., Hirakawa, D.A. *et al.* (2000). *Canine and feline nutrition: A resource for companion animal professionals* (2nd ed.). New York: Mosby

4 Krogdahl, A., Ahlstrøm, Ø. and Skrede, A. (2004). Nutrient digestibility of commercial dog foods using mink as a model. American Journal of Nutrition, 134: 2141S–2144S

5 Lummis, D. (2012). *Natural, organic and eco-friendly pet products in the U.S.*. Packaged Facts, Rockville, MD

6 Lange, M. (2017). *Pet Food Trends Shaping the World*. Pet Food Industry Leadership Conference, 2017

CHAPTER 6

Carbohydrates

The Science Supporting the Use of Carbohydrates in Dogs

Dogs do not require any carbohydrates whatsoever in their diet.[1-3] As the previous section highlighted, they happily make their own energy from protein and fat. Studies of beagle pups fed carbohydrate-free diets all exhibited normal blood glucose concentrations, growth rates and weight gain over time.[4,5] Despite this, the pet food industry is now feeding them more than 50% carbohydrates every meal of their lives. We know carnivorous dogs and cats are capable of utilising much of these carbohydrates. Equipped with the ability to produce maltase, sucrose and lactase from the pancreas, they are at least enzymatically able to digest carbohydrates.[6] If carbohydrates are presented to them correctly in their cooked form, they can digest up to 84% of them,[7] which is equivalent to what we can do. In fact, studies show dogs can almost fully digest cooked starch in dry extruded pet food diets, above 99%.[8]

In this way, manufacturers of these high carbohydrate products are correct when they proclaim that carbohydrates, while not *essential* for dogs, *may* provide an excellent source of energy to dogs. This is true, they absolutely can. Nobody is disputing that.

> When ranked with other major ingredients that supply protein and fat, carbohydrates are generally considered the least important and are often regarded as the "filler ingredient". To the contrary, carbohydrates do not just provide "bulk" in the diet. Instead they provide an excellent source of metabolisable energy for dogs.
> **Murray and Sunvold, 2003, Research and Development Division of Mars/Eukanuba**
> **www.eukanuba.co.uk/en/professionals/ articles/carbohydrates-for-dogs**

Many things are *excellent* sources of energy. Doughnuts are one example. Mars bars another. It seems more relevant to ask if they are *suitable*. We know dogs do not require carbohydrates in their diet which is why, in taste trials funded by the cereal-based dry food manufacturers themselves, the dog appears disinclined to obtain its energy needs from carbohydrates. Hewson-Hughes *et al.* (2013)[9] conducted an interesting study for The Waltham Centre for Pet Nutrition, the science and marketing arm of Mars Pet Food. The authors highlight that many types of predators (vertebrate and invertebrate) appear to regulate their intake of foods to balance the gain of macro-nutrients, and that failure to do so can result in fitness penalties for the animal. To examine this effect in dogs, they used a range of dry and canned cereal-based pet food products. In essence, they were trying to find the average level of carbohydrates, fat and protein a dog might include in its diet when given the freedom to choose from a range of specially formulated diets presented. The diets offered differed in their fat, protein and carbohydrate concentrations. It was found that dogs chose approximately 30% of their metabolisable energy (ME) from protein, 63% from fat and only 7% from carbohydrate, or 1:2 protein to fat, on an ME basis. This figure was apparently similar across breeds.

However, a ratio of 1:2 protein to fat on an ME basis cannot be expected to be the average fat content for a normal dog. We know the average protein to fat ratio on an ME basis for wolves is closer to 1:1 (54:45)[10] and wolves are expected to have a fattier diet than the average dog. Wolves are big game hunters and proportional body fat content of mammals increases with size.[11] The dog is a smaller animal, an opportunistic hunter of smaller prey.

If we estimate 1g of fat offers twice the amount of ME than protein (1g of carbohydrates produces approximately 4 kilocalories, as does 1g of protein, whereas 1g of fat produces approximately 9 kilocalories), then this 1:2 ME ration equates to very roughly 1:1 protein to fat, on a dry matter (DM) basis, which I think we all agree is an easier way to view things. One of the fattiest meals the dog is going to find in the wild appears to be a rat, which is around 2:1 protein to fat DM[11,12], while the fat content of mice is seen to vary widely from 3.7:1 protein and fat at birth to 2.4:1 by adulthood.[11] Insects average 3:1 protein to fat DM[12]. A rabbit ranges from 3:1[12] to 4 or 5:1[11] protein to fat DM. Toads are 4:1 protein to fat while green frogs are a lean 7:1 protein to fat DM.[11,12] However, crucially, many of the animals used for these previous figures are from farmed stock, used for feeding to zoo animals, so we might expect their up-and-running wild counterparts to be considerably leaner. Indeed, the protein to fat contents of wild rodents and birds only begin at 7:1[13] on a DM basis.

This means, if we take the average protein to fat ratio of a rabbit (4:1), the domestic dog might normally have a protein to fat ME ratio of something like 2:1.

The problem with the work by Hewson-Hughes *et al.* is likely twofold. The first is diet formulation and the second is time. The authors used a range of ultra-processed food products that consisted of ground rice, wheat flour, poultry meal, corn gluten (the indigestible husks of corn leftover from human food processing) and beef tallow. Over just 7 days, dogs were given three diets simultaneously – one was high in carbohydrates (rice and wheat flour), the other higher in protein (meat meal) and the third high in fat (beef tallow). Section 1 showed us that dogs have a taste and smell preference for meat and will choose it over all other forms of foods offered, and the fresher the better. Meat meal arrives at the factory from rendering plants as a grey powder and is considered an extremely poor standard of meat protein, if it is even recognisable as such by the animal. When this is coupled with the assumption that fat must be a very sought-after energy source for carnivores, it comes as no surprise that the dogs in this short study were initially choosing meals higher in beef tallow.

When Roberts *et al.* (2018)[14] repeated the study (again using previously dry-fed dogs) but this time using real food ingredients including raw lamb loin fat, green tripe, venison (mechanically deboned) and corn (maize), they found that overall fat and carbohydrate portions of the diet significantly declined from 6,382 to 917 kcals per day and from 553 to 214 kcals, respectively, over the course of their 10-day trial. Protein consumption remained relatively even (dropping from 4,786 to 4,156 kcals per day). The authors explain the fat decrease as a 'feast or famine' mentality in dogs, where higher fat diets might be consumed initially but this drops over time in favour of a more moderate protein to fat ratio. This time ME ratio was closer to 4:5.

In light of the actual protein to fat contents of their prey, this still seems a little high, particularly as we know it is at this ME ratio that hard-working sled dogs perform best[15] and they have a far greater demand of fat than the average dog. Is it that dogs are simply hard wired to be gluttons for meat fat? This area requires more work.

Further highlighting the inadequacies of using dry diets and indeed dry-fed animals in such trials, Hewson-Hughes *et al.* (2011a)[16] had actually conducted this experiment first using dry-fed cats. Feeding them a variety of Mars pet care products, they found cats included in their diets substantially more protein and less fat than dogs (52:36:12, protein, fat and carbohydrates, respectively)! But of greater interest here is that their cats appeared to be choosing more carbohydrates in their diets than feral cats (52:36:12 versus 52:46:2, protein, fat and carbohydrates, where the average carbohydrate content of small prey is 1.7%).[17] Truly wild domestic cats clearly do not consume carbohydrates as part of their normal diet. Clearly, food trials using previously dry-fed carnivores that were offered a range of unnatural, cereal-based mixes say very little about what these animals might require *normally* in their diet.

The fact remains, if carbohydrates were truly an *excellent* or even suitable source of energy for a meat–eater, don't you think they would feed carbohydrates to sled dogs, animals that have some of the toughest, most demanding and energy-sapping jobs in the animal kingdom? But, more often than not, sled dogs are not fed carbohydrates.[18-20] In fact, Kronfeld, a giant of the field, later went on to run his sled dogs on three different diets – one group was fed a high-carbohydrate diet, the other a medium carbohydrate and the third zero carbohydrates. No adverse effects were observed in dogs fed the zero-carbohydrate diet.[15] On the contrary, dogs on this diet maintained higher serum concentrations of albumin, calcium, magnesium and free fatty acids during the racing season. They also exhibited the greatest increases in red cell count, haemoglobin concentration and packed cell volume during training (all of which would increase their fitness). The authors concluded that a carbohydrate-free diet 'appeared to confer advantages for prolonged strenuous running in terms of certain metabolic responses to training'.

To support their stance that the high cereal/carb content of Mars Iams can provide a suitable source of ME for dogs, Murray and Sunvold (2003)[21] used 20 references. Only three of these had anything at all to do with dogs and only one of these had anything to do with carbohydrate digestion. It was a study of blood sugar/insulin response in three groups of dogs fed dry, soft-moist and canned pet food. The assessment period lasted 5 days. Murray and Sunvold's own feeding trial, analysing blood sugar and insulin response in groups of dogs fed various grains, lasted 2 weeks. They concluded that the choice of starch would influence the glucose and insulin response in dogs after a meal. Fair enough. It absolutely does, as we will see later. It is the authors' conclusions, however, that are of particular interest:

> Iams' carbohydrate research has shown that some products are best formulated using a combination of carbohydrate sources to fit the special nutritional requirements of your dog during specific life stages and lifestyles...

As the authors offer no supportive long-term studies to back up this statement, we remain unsure what these 'specific life stages and lifestyles' that require a specific carbohydrate content may be as, again, carnivorous dogs *require* zero plant carbohydrates in their diet at any stage of their life.

One life-stage this end of the industry seems particularly focused on is gestating and lactating bitches. Any time the 'need' for carbohydrates by dogs is discussed, the study by Romsos *et al.* (1981)[7] often pops up.[22-24] This study compared two groups of dry-fed, pregnant beagle bitches. Group A was fed a diet consisting of 26% ME from protein (beef kidney), 44% from carbohydrate and 30% from fat. Group B also received 26% ME from protein, but with zero carbohydrates, substituting them instead with even more fat, ultimately equating to 74% ME of the diet. If we assume the ideal protein to fat ME ratio for the dog is approximately 2:1, then it's fair to say a protein to fat ME ratio of 1:3 would be considered a very high fat diet for this animal.

The authors found that the Group B dogs (zero-carb/high-fat) displayed elevated levels of free fatty acids. Also, while the two groups gave birth to the same number of pups, only 63% of Group B's pups were alive at birth and only 35% of these survived to 3 days. As this is not normal, we could assume this, too, is related to the fat content. While litter size was unaffected, rat pups, born of mothers fed a high fat diet, had significantly higher mortality over the first 3 days of life.[7]

The high-fat fed bitches also exhibited ketosis.[25] This is when the body doesn't have enough blood sugar to conduct normal business and turns to the body's fat stores for energy. In this instance, the authors note that a higher protein intake may have helped dogs by providing additional glycogenic precursors (the building blocks necessary for dogs to perform gluconeogenesis properly). In other words, had they balanced the protein-fat content to a more biologically appropriate level, these struggling mothers would have been able to conduct gluconeogenesis as normal, preventing ketosis.

From their feeding trial, the authors concluded:

> The demonstration that consumption of a low carbohydrate diet by bitches during gestation severely reduced survival of their pups was the most pronounced finding of this study...

I feel it might have been more accurate to write, 'the demonstration that consumption of a *very high-fat* diet by bitches during gestation severely reduced survival of their pups'. In the past, a high fat diet such as this (7 g of lean meat, 10 g of lard, per kg of body weight) induced liver disease in dogs over a relatively short space of time.[26]

But it is the last line of their abstract that is the most astounding (italics added by me for effect):

> We conclude that pregnant bitches *require* dietary carbohydrate for optimal reproductive performance…

While some carbohydrates or, better still, protein, in this instance would have been very beneficial to these dogs to reduce the fat content, for this study to be used as evidence by the industry that a carnivorous dog might *normally* benefit from some carbohydrates in their diet is pretty audacious.

During the course of this entire section, and indeed the next, you will be hearing a lot about two large collections of studies that form the backbone of veterinary opinion on canine (and feline) nutrition. The first is the SACN (*Small Animal Clinical Nutrition*), edited by Hand *et al.* (2010)[27] and now in its 5th edition. The SACN is a colossal work of more than 1,300 pages (not including references) and is used extensively by vets worldwide to inform on all matters of canine and feline nutrition. The second is the US National Research Council's *Nutrient Requirement of Cats and Dogs* (NRC 2006).

In its section entitled "Canine Carbohydrate Requirements" (itself a misnomer as carbohydrates are not required by dogs at any stage of their life, that we yet know of), the SACN has but three short paragraphs taking up half a page. They cite just four references. Each is entirely focused on the use of carbohydrates in gestating and lactating bitches. The first is the Romsos *et al.* (1981)[7] work discussed previously. The second, conducted for the Waltham Symposium (Mars Inc.), found that pregnant bitches that were fed a higher protein and starch-free diet performed as well as those on starch-containing diets.[28] The third was again a study of the viability of pups born to mothers on varying protein rations and found that dogs need 'at least 33% of ME from protein'.[29] The fourth and last study mentioned in this section was the NRC (2006), which apparently states 'foetal abnormalities, embryonic reabsorption, ketosis, and reduced milk production are other possible adverse effects of providing inadequate carbohydrate during gestation and lactation'. When you go to the relevant section in the NRC (2006, Carbohydrates and Fibre, subsection "Effects on Reproductive Performance") you find they, too, are referring to the study by Romsos *et al.* (1981)[7] study.

The SACN's concluding paragraph states the following (italics added by me for effect):

> Overall, a minimum of 23% carbohydrate is recommended in foods for gestating and lactating bitches. *Excess starch in the food typically does not cause health problems in dogs.* Dry, extruded dog foods typically contain 30 to 60% carbohydrates, mostly starch, *and cause no adverse effects.*
>
> **Hand *et al.,* 2010**[27]

In the face of a raging canine obesity and diabetes epidemic, the SACN (the canine nutrition bible for our vets today) does not use a single study in support of the statement that a diet containing more than 50% carbohydrates does not cause adverse health effects in dogs.

The very next section in the SACN is titled "Feline Carbohydrate Requirements" correctly refers to cats as strict carnivores and yet 'starch levels found in commercial cat foods, up to 35% of the food's DM, are well tolerated'. Sadly, no references are used to support this rather crucial statement of fact.

Dr. Stefanie Handl (vet. med. Dipl. ECVCN), editor-in-chief of the journal *Veterinary Medicine Austria* (a journal sponsored by Mars Royal Canin, as of 2016), but writing in 2014 for *Veterinary Focus* (a journal owned by Mars Inc.), states the following (italics added by me for effect):

> The idea that gluten and cereals, in general, are damaging to dogs and cats is another *popular rumour with no scientific basis*. One can assume that *many domestic dogs received lots of grain-based products* (e.g., bread, dog biscuits) before the introduction of commercial dry diets. *Current research suggests that dogs have genetically adapted to carbohydrate foods* throughout their evolution...

This is a very common statement by the industry, and it is factually incorrect. Studies of sled dogs revealed that dogs maintained on high-carbohydrate diets suffered more injury than those on a high-protein feed.[30] High-starch diets stimulate the formation of struvite crystals in cats,[30] while high-protein diets can rectify the issue.[31] Studies show that reducing carbohydrates in the diet prevents tumour growth in dogs.[32]

This is before we flip the statement to ask Dr. Handl on what 'scientific basis' is she advocating a diet of 50–60% carbohydrates for a meat-eater? Has she a *single* long-term study to indicate that high-carbohydrate diets are safe for carnivorous dogs when compared to a higher-protein or, dare we hope, a more natural diet? No, she hasn't, as this study does not exist. If it did, the industry would deploy it repeatedly. She has taken it on faith – with no scientific basis whatsoever.

Dr. Handl goes on to say, 'one can assume that many domestic dogs received lots of grain-based products (e.g. bread, dog biscuits) before the introduction of commercial dry diets'. We can *assume* this statement is largely true. Dogs have surely received some amount of carbohydrates in their daily fare from humans in the past but how much and what these free-to-roam dogs spent the rest of their days eating is unknown. Was it enough to force a major evolutionary shift in the animal? Free-foraging diet and anatomy studies suggest not. Until we know more, Dr. Handl here is merely stating her unreferenced opinion.

Eventually, Dr. Handl makes a referenced point, stating 'current research suggests that dogs have genetically adapted to carbohydrate foods throughout their evolution', which she supports by using the work of Axelsson *et al.* (2013)[33] that found many breeds of dogs have multiple copies of the AMY2B gene for carbohydrate digestion.

First, this is a very liberal use of the word 'throughout'. Humans have only been farming in earnest for some 8,000 years. Before that, we can only assume that dogs were out and out meat-eaters, suggesting dogs have only been adapting to carbohydrates for less than 25% of their 30,000-year evolution from wolves. In fact, an analysis of three ancient dog remains from Germany, dated somewhere between 4,700 and 7,000 YBP, showed no increase in the AMY2B gene copy number although agriculture was thriving in the region at the time, very much questioning the role of agriculture in dog domestication up to even that point.[34]

As we learned from our analysis of the dingo, it appears the domestic breeds that evolved alongside farmers have taken some minor steps toward carbohydrate digestion at the gene level. They certainly have higher activities of these enzymes compared to domestic cats.[24,35] This, along with a small number of other omnivorous-leaning physiological quirks, would not have arisen if some minor plant matter inclusions were not on the menu to some degree for dogs in the past. However, to use this handful of genes (in a body using thousands of genes every minute for digestion) as the sole scientific basis for your ultra-high carbohydrate argument for every dog on the planet, above all other modes of feeding, is lax in the extreme.

There is no better rebuke to this position than that of Doug Knueven who once stated to Dr. Jean Dodds:

> To say that because dogs can digest some starch better than a wolf proves that they can thrive on a high-starch diet long-term is like asserting that because people can process ethanol and glucose, we should thrive on a diet of 50% rum and cookies!

There is no evidence to suggest high-carbohydrate diets offer much by way of benefit to meat-eaters and still, despite their own food trials clearly demonstrating that carnivorous dogs repeatedly opt for protein and fat over carbohydrates,[17] manufacturers of such diets continue to drive the cereal-based pet food message. Even worse, the practice continues with the full support of our evidenced-based veterinary sector despite there being no works of any value suggesting it's particularly safe for dogs long-term. Let's take a look at the possible repercussions of that decision.

The Canine Obesity Epidemic

Why Humans Get Fat

To understand a little about the effects of carbohydrate consumption by the dog, we must first begin with what we know of humans. What?! But we just heard dogs are carnivores, not omnivores, I hear you cry! Yes, while this is true, the fact remains that because cereal-based, dry food promoters have never provided us with a single long-term study of normal dogs fed such diets compared to those fed a more normal diet significantly lower in carbohydrates, we need to look elsewhere for a bit of inspiration to start the ball rolling.

We know that dogs share many physiological and metabolic attributes associated with the digestion and metabolism of humans. This results because we share an extensive parallel genomic evolution, particularly genes governing digestion, metabolism and numerous neurological processes and diseases including cancer.[36] They react in the same way as we do to many foods and chemicals, making them a suitable test subject for questions on human disease, nutrition and translational medicine.[37] It's why we, despicably, test all our new food chemicals and pharmaceuticals on them. The causes of many nutritional illnesses in humans, such as rickets and pellagra, were discovered by denying many thousands of beagles' certain vitamins and nutrients at the cost of their lives. In particular, we have known for 20 years that dogs respond in the same way physiologically to sugar as humans, with both carbohydrate amount and type dictating their glycaemic response[38-40] and it is exactly this process we are about to discuss.

The world has a terrible obesity problem and it is destroying our health. The body mass index (BMI) is a measure of body fat based on an individual's weight in relation to his or her height and age. In general, a person with a BMI of 25–29.9 is considered overweight, while a person with a BMI of over 30 is considered clinically obese. Let's start with the United States, so far, the most obese nation in the known universe. In 2010, the Centers for Disease Control and Prevention reported that 66% of American adults were overweight (*National Obesity Trends*, 2010). By 2018, 40% of their adults were obese,[41] meaning significantly more were obese than overweight. And the toll on the sufferer and economy is staggering. In 2011 an estimated 186,000 Americans died as a result of their excess BMI.[42] Medical costs associated with obesity are now topping $200 billion, 20% of the US annual health care spent.[43] And, of course, it's not just the United States. Statistics from WorldObesity.org, working with *The Lancet*, tells us that in the United Kingdom, 27% of both males and females were obese as of 2015. In Australia, it is around 28%, and in Ireland it is 24%. And we are all getting fatter, putting on an average of 10% more fat every decade.[44]

We all know by now the effect of this excess body fat on our physical health– from cardiovascular disease, diabetes, cancer and a range of associated inflammatory diseases, is utterly disastrous. As for a cause, very few world bodies are in doubt. The Pan American Health Organization (PAHO) and the World Health Organization (WHO), in a joint effort, state:

> The most striking change in food systems of high-income countries, and now of low- and middle-income countries, is displacement of dietary patterns based on meals and dishes prepared from unprocessed or minimally processed foods by those that are increasingly based on ultra-processed food and drink products. The result is diets with excessive energy density, high in free sugars and unhealthy fats and salt, and low in dietary fibre that increase the risk of obesity and other diet-related noncommunicable diseases. The proportion of ultra-processed products in food supplies can be seen as a measure of overall population diet quality.

PAHO 2015[45]

We are getting fatter because we have moved away from eating real, whole, unprocessed food items to processed foods. Professor Carlos Monteiro from the University of Sao Paulo in Brazil knows more about the dangers of ultra-processed food consumption than most. His research was the basis of a recent special edition of *Publish Health Nutrition* on ultra-processed food.[46] Using more than 45 large-scale studies and incorporating hard data on millions of people across the globe, the study found that approximately half of Irish, German and UK shopping baskets (45%, 46% and 51%, respectively) contain ultra-processed foods. The report concludes with deep concern, the association between ultra-processed food and poor health, in particular its certain links to obesity and diabetes, cancer and poor health in general.

> Highly processed foods are calorie dense but not filling…[they] contain, besides salts, sugars, oils and fats, substances such as additives that imitate the taste and texture of foods prepared from scratch… future generations will look at today's food consumption in the same way we view sending children up chimneys...
>
> **Monteiro *et al.* 2017**[47]

While heart disease used to make all the headlines (it is still the number one killer in both the European Union and the United States), the link between obesity and cancer is now abundantly clear. The World Cancer Research Fund is a collection of dozens of world leaders in cancer research. They have now published three colossal 'state of the union' reports, beginning in 1997, 2007 and now 2017, the most recent titled *Body Fatness and Weight Gain and the Risk of Cancer*. They investigate the effects of diet and being overweight on the incidence of cancer in the general population. Their findings are equally as clear and bleak as the findings of Monteiro's team.There is strong evidence that greater body fatness leads to a greater incidence of practically every cancer you can think of – colorectal cancer, endometrial cancer, gallbladder cancer, kidney cancer, liver cancer, cancers of the mouth, pharynx, and larynx, oesophageal cancer, ovarian cancer, pancreatic cancer, prostate cancer, postmenopausal breast cancer and stomach cancer – where the fatter you are, the more at risk of those diseases you become.

So, being overweight is extremely bad for your health. But before we get into *why* exactly processed foods make us fat, we must first highlight that obesity is a complex disease. Until recently, the dominant theory for our rapidly expanding waistlines was simply a matter of calories. Ultra-processed foods are higher in calories. You are eating too many calories. Eat less, move more, right? Now we know it's not as simple as that. Many factors affect how fat you will be including your genes (well, not your genes *per se)*, this is not a genetic issue, it's increasing far too rapidly for that, but *epi*genetically, which means simply that obese people can pass on the fat genes 'switched on' to their children, making them far more likely to be fat when they grow up.[48] Your gut flora, too, plays a role. Obese people have a predictable gut flora although while people debate which came first – is it obesity that changes the gut flora or is it a disrupted gut flora that leads to increased obesity? To investigate this, a fascinating study published in *Science* took the gut flora from an obese mouse and inserted it into his lean twin that promptly became fat.[49] *When* you eat IS PIVOTAL (in 2017 Jeffrey C. Hall, Michael Rosbash and Michael W Young received the Nobel Prize for physiology or medicine for their work in circadian rhythm. While the implications were vast, what is important here is what time of day you eat will affect how you process and store that food (with eating in the morning and after sundown being the biggest offenders) as well as *when you don't* eat (intermittent periods of fasting will result in weight loss, even if the fasting group consumes the same level of calories as another.[50] Then there is physical and mental health, stress and of course, your level of physical activity, to name but a few more. But of all culprits, absolutely nothing affects your waistline as much as *what* you eat.

As the overly simplistic 'calories in, calories out' hypothesis falls by the wayside, this is a good time to highlight the difference between scientific *hypothesis* and scientific *theory*.

A *scientific hypothesis* is little more than an educated guess as to what might be going on. It remains to be formally tested. It is not yet supported by the literature. The hypothesis is then put to the test, often repeatedly from a variety of angles and by a number of different scientific authors who each set out to accept or reject the hypothesis. If it stands up to scientific scrutiny better than any other competing hypothesis out there, then the hypothesis is confirmed to be possibly true and gradually makes its way into the more factual realm of *scientific theory*.

There are times however, when a hypothesis can seem so plausible and hang around for so long that it morphs into scientific theory. That is, until someone thinks to actually put it to the test. At this point, it's not uncommon for popular dogma to be found utterly wrong down the line. For instance, for the longest time we believed the earth was flat. The suggestion we are all walking around a globe is still today too much for many to comprehend. There was a time when putting lead in petrol was a good idea. It stopped our engines knocking. For decades, as the physical and mental health of the public plummeted, the industry-lead hypothesis that this was a perfectly safe thing to do remained untested, unproven and very far from scientific theory. Too many decades later, a number of tests soon utterly refuted this hypothesis. The scientific theory now is it that micro particles of lead in the air can accumulate in our bodies where they have a disastrous effect on particularly the nervous systems of our unborn. Today, we continue to inject highly inflammatory nanoparticles of aluminum into children, particles that we know are capable of passing through the mammalian blood-brain barrier,[51] in the full *belief* the practice is entirely unrelated to the shocking rise of childhood neurodevelopmental disabilities in the general population. However, that belief is very far from scientific theory. It is a hypothesis that today remains virtually untested.

We have all the famine evidence we need to show you can starve the weight off someone easily enough and, conversely, people who consume far too many calories on a daily basis are going to put on weight. The problem over the last few decades is that nobody thought to look much further than this. Because when we do, we realise the 'calories in, calories out' hypothesis is rejected on a number of fronts.

First, simply stating we have an obesity epidemic because people are suddenly consuming too many calories is nonsense. Humans have always enjoyed eating but to suggest that everyone was absolutely nailing their calorific intake in the first 70 years of the 1900s is ridiculous, constantly factoring in their exercise levels, that extra hour in bed, the little bit more they ate after a hard day's work, the fact they burned a few more calories when the temperature dropped while they were working outside, those few drinks on a Friday night, where the calories from just two glasses of wine (160 kcal) would result in several extra pounds of body fat a year, where suddenly in the 1970s, 60% of Westerners entirely lost the run of themselves, turning into greedy, lazy idiots, seems a bit hard to swallow.

According to Taubes, simply saying it's about calories is about as elucidating as saying you get richer by making more money than you spend. We are lacking the how and the why. Better authors than me have already adequately laid out the scientific evidence in this regard, including Fung (*The Obesity Code*), Taubes (*Good Calories, Bad Calories* and later *The Case Against Sugar*) and in the case of dogs, Schulof (*Dogs, Dog Food and Dogma*), all of whom I now lean on to explain the obesity epidemic in the following pages.

As the name of Taubes's most recent book implicates, it's not so much about calories *per se*, but how they are delivered to the body. In this respect, most of us are now becoming aware of just how disastrous our addiction to sugar is to our health. We have always loved sugar and through the centuries the sugar content of our diet has been very slowly increasing. However, it wasn't until 'fat' was incriminated for making us fat in the 1970s (made sense right? Only it was completely wrong, as you are about to find out), that low-fat-and-thus-high-sugar processed foods began to rapidly expand our waistlines. Never mind being more addictive than cocaine, it certainly seems to be more destructive to the nation. A colossal systematic review by the WHO found that the intake of sugar is an important determinant of body weight in people[52] and this, in turn, is the road to both our diabetes[53,54] and cancer[55,56] epidemics. On the back of such evidence, the WHO revised its sugar recommendation on March 5, 2015. They now recommend, at most, 25–50 g of sugar per day to avoid obesity, diabetes and tooth decay.

But we're not listening. Today, the Western world is eating a staggering amount of sugar, the most refined carbohydrate of them all. Americans are consuming 126 g of sugar per day (that's 46 kg a year). Germany and Netherlands are next in line with 103 g while Ireland and the UK consumed 97 g and 93 g per day, respectively.[57] The only good news is this is likely our ceiling for sugar consumption, thanks to various market trends, health initiatives, artificial sweeteners and an increasing array of sugar alternatives now on the market.

What many people are still failing to grasp, however, is that it is not just refined sugar we are concerned about here. But to understand a little more, we first need a quick lesson in the different types of carbohydrates out there.

Carbohydrates are sourced from plants and there are three different types – simple sugars, complex carbohydrates and indigestible plant fibre. Simple sugars, as their name suggests, are the ready-to-go carbohydrates. They comprise single or double sugar units (monosaccharides or disaccharides), require little to no digestion and are quickly assimilated into the body. They are an instant source of energy and are found in such items as table sugar, fruit juices and honey.

Complex carbohydrates (called polysaccharides, meaning many sugar units joined together) are the starchy bit in cereals, potatoes, rice and vegetables, such as peas and carrots. They take slightly longer to break down than simple sugars, requiring a few extra steps, but once that's done, they may be utilised as energy by the body.

The carbohydrate digestion process looks something like this: when a human eats soluble complex carbohydrates such as a starch-filled potato, digestion begins in the mouth thanks to the presence of amylase in our saliva which is an enzyme that can break down carbohydrate into single units. The partially digested mix then makes its way down to the stomach, which pulverises the acid mix into chyme, a liquid form suitable for passing into the intestines. No digestion occurs in the stomach due to the acidic environment. Once the mix passes to the first part of the intestine, known as the duodenum, the pancreas now kicks in and releases lots of amylase to finish the digestive process. Now broken down into simple single units, your starchy meal is absorbed readily through the gut wall and into the bloodstream. The liver then converts these sugar units into glucose for use by the cells of the body. Surplus-to-demand glucose gets stored in the liver as glycogen or, with the help of insulin, converted into fatty acids and stored as fat in adipose tissue for later deployment or periods of self-loathing.

It's important to reiterate here that whether you eat simple sugars (sugar, honey, fruit juice) or complex carbohydrates (wheat, rice, bread), they both end up as sugar for use by the body. It's just that complex carbohydrates take a little longer to digest and this makes all the difference to your body, as you will soon learn.

The third plant carbohydrate is structural, commonly known as fibre. There are a few types of plant fibre but they can be lumped into two groups depending on whether they dissolve in water (soluble fibre) or not (insoluble fibre). Both types are entirely resistant to enzymatic digestion by mammals. It all passes through the small intestines undigested and arrives in the colon relatively unscathed. It is here the differences kick in. Unlike indigestible plant fibre, our gut flora loves soluble plant fibres such as inulin, oligofructose and fructooligosaccharide (FOS). They are premium bacteria food or, far more commonly, prebiotics (*before-life*). In perfect symbiosis, we provide our beneficial bacteria with food, they ferment it, multiply and then we digest them, in turn, harvesting many benefical nutrients and by-products. But this is not the only difference between the two. Both fibres regulate the flow of digesta through the intestines but in apparently opposite manners. They can be summed up as follows:

(i)   **Soluble fibre.** Dissolves in water to form a gel-like material in the intestines. These are the pectins, gums and mucilages that are commonly found in plant items such as oats, legumes (peas, beans, lentils), seeds (think chia), fruits and vegetables. Soluble fibre swells in the intestines; as such, it slows the passage of digesta, much to the delight of our gut flora that have more time to act (aided by our longer, slower intestinal tracts and dead ends such as the caecum). Soluble fibre not only increases the feeling of satiety we get after a meal but also it alleviates the symptoms of diarrhoea.

(i)   **Insoluble fibre.** Does not dissolve in water. Examples include cellulose in the outside of food items such as the husks of grains, wheat and corn or the skin of tomatoes. This fibre passes straight through the system undigested to the large intestines where it acts like a sponge, sucking in water via osmosis from the large intestines, increasing stool bulk. In this way, insoluble fibre is great for constipation, promoting the movement of material through the digestive system, maintaining bowel health (but bad for patients with diarrhoea).

By slowing the rate of digesta, soluble fibre encourages a more gradual percolation of sugar into the bloodstream and this, in turn, lowers blood glucose levels. This is pivotal to the obesity epidemic we are witnessing in both humans and pets, so it is crucial we now get more familiar with the details.

The speed at which a food item releases its energy has become a science in its own right. In the 1980s the Glycaemic Index (GI), a measure of the effects of a food's carbohydrate on our blood sugar levels, was born. Those carbohydrates that break down quickly during digestion and release glucose rapidly into the bloodstream (such as pasta) have a high GI, while those that break down more slowly, releasing glucose more gradually into the bloodstream (such as porridge), have a low GI. You can now find the GI online at www.glycemicindex.com where you can search practically any food item you can think of.

The problem with the GI is that it doesn't tell you how *much* carbohydrate is in a particular food, just how quickly it hits the blood compared to something else. For instance, watermelon has a high GI ranking of 72. Using only the GI, you may be reluctant to eat it, fearing a rapid rise in glucose, but in fact, a serving of watermelon has only about 6 g of carbohydrates. Glycaemic load (GL) combines both the quality and quantity of carbohydrate in one simple value. It's the best way to predict a food's impact on our blood glucose readings. GL alerts us to the fact that a lower GI isn't everything. It might tempt you to choose brown bread over white but bear in mind that their GLs are almost comparable. Just two slices of bread made with whole-wheat flour can raise blood sugar higher than six teaspoons of table sugar – higher than many candy bars.[58] Similarly, peas and sweet potatoes (both boiled) have a similar GI of 51 and 46, respectively. Low-ish, which is ok. However, the GL in peas is only a quarter of that in sweet potatoes. So, a serving of peas gives a lot less punch to your blood sugar.

Focusing on more relevant foodstuffs, the Glycaemic Index shows us that cooked cereals like wheat, barley, corn and oats have low to medium GL values.

However, they have a medium GL load of 15–17. (GL values of 0–10 are low, GL values of >10 are moderate, GL of >20 are high.)

We cook these grains to break down the fibre and enable access to the goodies inside. The knock-on effect is that when the fibre is broken down, the food delivers its large sugar payload far quicker. In other words, whole cereals such as wheat, corn and barley don't remain 'complex' for very long. When cooked, cereals and grains pack a very big punch. In this way, it is the high GLs of cereals such as wheat and corn that make them an unsuitable, long-term food choice for us humans. A fantastic work by Bertoia *et al.* (2015)[59] highlights this. They tracked the fruit and vegetable consumption of 133,468 American men and women from 1986 to 2010 (makes you feel really lazy, doesn't it?) and found, quite simply, that people who ate items with a higher GL, such as corn and potatoes, put on more weight.

This implies if skinny is what you're after, you need to keep up your intake of fibre-containing foods. You should choose low/medium GL whole grains (with fibre) over higher GL processed flours (without fibre), eat them in whole, unprocessed (fibre-removed) form insofar as possible and reduce your intake of simple, refined carbohydrates such as sugar, fruit juices, cake and pop to effectively nil.

But it's not just obesity, diabetes and cancer you need to worry about. By spiking blood sugar, you prompt the body to produce pro-inflammatory chemicals called cytokines, increasing inflammation in the body, and this can worsen the symptoms of inflammatory heart disease,[60] joint inflammation,[61] and is strongly linked to depression.[62] By contrast, whole grains and fibre have been reported to play a protective role in the aetiology and management of the chronic diseases previously mentioned. [60,63-67]

For all these reasons, excess sugar in the blood is bad news and the body knows it. It wants to get rid of it from the blood as soon as you consume it. Enter insulin. When beta glands in the pancreas note a rise in blood sugar, insulin is released from the islets of Langerhans. Insulin is a hormone that 'shuttles' all the glucose out of the bloodstream and into the fat stores. But that's not all it does. Insulin is what's known as an anabolic hormone, meaning it is responsible for cell growth. In terms of obesity, diabetes and cancer, now we have our master villain.

> We don't get fat because we over eat, we over eat because we're getting fat.
>
> **Taubes, *Why We Get Fat*[68]**

Hats off to Taubes – it's a hell of a line. Unfortunately, to understand the obesity epidemic in people and dogs, you need to wrap your head around it! So, let's start with a more obvious example. Wade *et al.* (1972)[69] examined the relationship between the sex hormones, weight and appetite in rats. After removing the ovaries from a group of rats, they found that they began to eat more and quickly became obese. At first, this seems to support the 'calories in, calories out' hypothesis – removing the gonads turned them into gluttons, they ate more and got fat. Pretty simple. However, it was Wade's second experiment that forces you to reassess. To avoid the effect of gluttony this time, Wade put his female rats on a strict post-surgery diet. This way, even if they wanted to, they couldn't consume more calories than they were consuming pre-surgery. It simply wasn't available to them. Despite being on the *same number* of calories, the rats managed to get just as fat, just as quickly. Want to know how they did it? They became more sedentary. Despite having the same opportunities to do so, the rats decided to move as little as possible between meals. It's like their bodies were *determined* to get fat. People that stick to the 'calorie in, calorie out' theory might at this point push and say removing the ovaries made these rats lazy, so they burned fewer calories, etc. But if that was the case, wouldn't the rats be gluttons and be lazy at the same time? They only got lazy when option A 'eat more food' was removed from them.

In this way, removing the sex hormones doesn't necessarily make you lazy but it might make you fat. This is likely why neutered dogs are more likely to be overweight.[70]

No matter what way you cut it, those de-sexed rats were going to get fat. The path was set. Something is governing the process and that something is hormones, in this case the sex hormones (in particular oestrogen). By disrupting the normal hormonal regulation of the fat stores (removing the ovaries), Wade *et al.* put their rats on the train to Fatville–a train, it seems, they weren't able to get off (incidentally, the same effect is seen in male rats by removing testosterone but it's not as prominent as it is in females).

> Gluttony and sloth are effects of the *drive* to get fatter.
> **Taubes, *Why We Get Fat*[68]**

Nowhere are the effects of sex hormones more evident than in the 10 year old prepubescent boy. We know he's about to undergo some impressive growth over the next couple of years. Will he eat more during this time? Absolutely. But he's not growing because he's eating more, he's eating more because he's growing.

It's not his food consumption resulting in growth, it's the other way around. The cause and effect are reversed. Are boys that age lazy? You betcha. But they're not growing because they're lazy, they're lazy because they are growing. The hormones gave the order to grow and the rest of the body gets to work.

While we are focusing on the effect of hormones on body height and size, it's the very same with the fat stores. Insulin regulates blood sugar by signalling for the liver, muscle and fat cells to take in glucose as fuel from the blood (generally obesity is not the creation of new fat cells, it is the fat cells you have swelling in size). But insulin has one more dirty trick up its sleeve – the blocking of leptin in the brain.[71]

Do you know what the largest endocrine (hormone-producing) mass in the body is? Surprisingly, it's body fat. The fat cells produce the hormone leptin. When you eat a big meal and the fat cells are full to their normal levels, they produce leptin which tells your brain (the hypothalamus) they have enough, to stop eating and start doing other stuff. You would think the more body fat you have, the more leptin would be coursing around your blood and the more your brain would listen to it. But that's not the case. For nearly 20 years, scientists such as Dr. Robert Lustig, Professor of Paediatrics in the Division of Endocrinology at the University of California, San Francisco, suspected leptin resistance was at the centre of the obesity conundrum[72] and recently his team have unlocked the answer.

Take the following example, nicely explained by Lustig himself in his YouTube interview, *The Skinny on Obesity (Ep. 3): Hunger and Hormones–A Vicious Cycle.* He explains that when you inject insulin into a patient with diabetes their blood sugar drops accordingly. Let's say it goes from 250 mg/dl to a more appropriate and safer, 100 mg/dl. But where did all that blood sugar go? Insulin directed it into the fat cells for storage. That's its job. In this way, insulin *drives* weight gain.

Now imagine for a moment taking a healthy, active person that consumes 2,500 kcal per day from a great diet, going about life all lean and lovely with their relatively balanced 'calorie in, calorie out' type lifestyle, and injecting them with a certain amount of insulin each day. As long as everything else is kept the same, the added insulin will shunt say 500 kcal into the fat stores. No ifs, no buts, no debate – that's what it does. You inject that insulin and you will gain 50 g of body fat, give or take.

But this now means, if nothing else changes, you have a body that wants to burn 2,500 kcal each day but now only has 2,000 kcal available as the insulin shunted 500 kcal of it into the fat stores and out of use. So, what did Wade's mice do when the extra calories weren't available? They slowed down to conserve power. Next thing you know, you are slightly less mobile, a bit more sluggish, less inclined to exercise, maybe sitting on the couch more, watching a movie, taking a nap. Most of all, you will soon be hungry. With today's access to food, you will naturally increase your intake. All in a bid to recoup the 500 kcal you shuttled away with the insulin shot.

Now, instead of eating 2,500 kcal per day, you will take in 3,000 kcal per day to compensate. But you're still injecting with insulin. So, what happens? The insulin will now take 600 kcal of the 3,000–kcal consumed and shunt it into the fat stores. On and on. A vicious, ever-increasing spiral of obesity and insulin need in the soon-to-be person with Type 2 diabetes.

Imagine going to the doctor at this point, begging for help – 'doc, what do I do?' The answer? 'You're greedy. Eat less, move more…' Which is true! You ARE eating too much, and you are not moving enough but not because you *chose* to be. It's because you *have to* be. You have been biochemically driven to laziness by injecting with insulin each day.

Makes sense, right? At this point you may be wondering what this has to do with the obesity epidemic. We're not injecting insulin every day, which is true, we're not. But what we are doing is consuming huge daily doses of refined carbohydrates and sugar and it is making our bodies produce more and more insulin, constantly driving the process forward.

A final rhetorical question: Why doesn't the leptin produced by my fat stores tell my brain to stop? Because insulin won't let it. Insulin blocks the leptin receptors in the brain,[72] keeping you perpetually hungry.

In this way, the higher GL in the foods you consume the more glucose in your blood, the more glucose in your blood; the more insulin will be present; the more insulin present, the more fat you store and the hungrier you get.

For now, we know one of the only ways to get off this train is to consume low GL foods. And what food has the lowest GL values as it doesn't contain any carbohydrates whatsoever?

Meat.

Obesity and Diabetes in Dogs

How much carbohydrate a human might normally include in their diet is up for debate. A colossal diet study tracked the eating habits of more than 135,000 adults over 7 years. These included high-income, medium-income and low-income nations, resulting in two papers, published in *The Lancet*.[73,74] The authors found that keeping carbohydrate content down was a good thing. People eating high quantities of carbohydrates (more than 70% of their diet) had a nearly 30% higher risk of dying during the study, than people eating a lower carb diet. They further noted that eating lower GL foods such as vegetables and legumes lower your risk of dying prematurely. If you were to push for a guiding figure, we omnivorous humans are advised by the likes of Harvard nutrition, to include no more than 30% complex carbohydrates in our diet. Ideally, this would be in the form of whole grains, vegetables and a little fruit, although this figure undoubtedly varies widely between populations and fluctuating needs. Today the vast majority of Western dogs are fed a high-carbohydrate, ultra-processed dry food, with cereals such as wheat and corn making up around 50–60% of their diet.

As it's not stated on the label, it's not immediately clear to consumers how much cereal/carbohydrate is in pet food. Here's how to work it out.

Here are the ingredients of one of the best-selling, super premium brands of veterinary-prescribed, dry foods for Labradors on the UK market:

> Chicken, Ground Corn, Ground Sorghum, Ground Whole Grain Wheat, Chicken By-Product Meal, Soybean Meal, Corn Gluten Meal, Animal Fat (preserved with mixed tocopherols), Brewers Rice, Chicken Liver Flavor…

These ingredients are included in order of weight. The fact that chicken is the number one ingredient is appealing to the consumer and desirable for the carnivorous dog. However, the next three ingredients are cereal.

It's important to note here that the chicken portion is included as fresh, meaning *with* water (chicken is, let's say, 70% water), while the cereal components are included dry, which usually means a water content of 10% or less. Food chemists get very upset about this as it does not compare like with like. To make meaningful comparisons of nutrient levels between products/ingredients, they should be expressed on a *dry-weight basis*, i.e. with the water removed. Had this been done, the first meat ingredient would have become very significantly lighter. Consequently, it would be much further down the ingredient list.

Imagine, for example, the manufacturer decides to include 100 g of fresh-weight chicken, 98 g of dry corn, 95 g of dry sorghum and 90 g of dry wheat, in the above mix. Fresh-weight chicken breast, 100 g, contains 70% water. Thus, in 100g of fresh chicken breast, you only have around 30g of dried chicken.

If we look at this list again on a dry-weight basis, it might contain 30–40 g of dried meat (dried meat actually has 10% water, remember) and 283 g of dry cereal. Not so meaty now, is it?

Author's note:

Please remember the dry-weight phenomenon when comparing dry and canned dog food. A kilo of canned dog food might give its protein content as 10%. This does not sound like a lot compared to the 20% in dry dog food. But the canned food contains roughly 75% moisture. If you remove this water from the product, you are left with 25% DM. To determine the amount of protein on the new DM basis, simply divide the reported amount of protein (in this case, 10%) by the total amount of dry matter (25%) and multiply the result by 100. This gives you a DM protein content of 40%, which is now a lot better than the dry food, on a dry basis. By removing the water, you even the playing field. This is why food chemists only work on a DM basis.

This clever loading of individually listed, dry cereal ingredients is just one of the many tricks employed by the industry to convince the consumer they are picking up a meaty feast for their pet. Another is that manufacturers do not state the actual carbohydrate content in their products. As Section 3 will show you, they are not required. While such a thing would never be permitted in human food production, you're in pet food world now, where everything is upside down and nothing is quite as it seems. So, pet owners have to do a little math. If you are told that your product contains (per 100 gms) say 20 g of protein, 15 g of fat, 10 g of moisture and 5% ash and fibre, then you simply add these values and subtract from 100 g, leaving you with 50 g of high GL carbohydrate.

We know dogs require zero carbohydrates whatsoever in their diet.[1-3] As the previous section highlighted, they happily make their own energy from protein and fat. That's why, unlike what you would expect in say humans, studies of beagle pups fed carbohydrate-free diets all exhibited, over time, normal blood glucose concentrations, growth rates and weight gain.[4,5] Despite this, the pet food industry is now feeding them 50–60% carbohydrates in the form of wheat, corn and rice, every meal of their life. This is perhaps twice the amount recommended for nearly-plant-eating humans. And we are advised to avoid eating such high GL options.

We know that our excess consumption of refined carbohydrates with the resulting insulin payload is driving our obesity epidemic. Plus, once you get on this train, you won't be getting off it until you change your diet to unprocessed, low GL food items. We know that despite having zero physiological requirement for carbohydrates, dogs can both digest and utilise them perfectly when presented correctly and, indeed, they respond in the same way physiologically to sugar as humans.[38,39,40] The question clearly is not *can* they use all these carbohydrates for energy but, as we saw with the sled dogs, the real question is whether this sort of diet is suitable or even safe for dogs *long-term*. Without a retrospective analysis to guide us, all we can do is look at the figures…and hang our heads.

As in humans, obesity in dogs is soaring. Approximately 21% of the UK dog population was obese in the 1980s.[75] By 2017, the most recent review of the situation revealed that while 65% of UK dogs were, at least, overweight (body condition scores of 6/9 to 9/9), a shocking 37% of UK juvenile dogs were obese.[76] In the United States, during 2006–2011 alone, overweight and obesity in dogs rose by 37% and in cats by more than 90%.[77]

Unfortunately for our pets, they share many of the same issues that come with human obesity.[77] The range of orthopaedic diseases includes osteoarthritis and ruptured cruciate, as well as skeletal disease and hip dysplasia, but also, urinary disorders, reproductive disorders and the other usuals, including diabetes, cardiorespiratory disease, neoplasia (mammary tumours, transitional cell carcinoma), dermatological diseases and anaesthetic complications.[70,79-83] Banfield Hospital, with access to the health records of over 2 million dogs and 430,000 cats from 800 vet hospitals across 43 states in the US, produces a report called *The State of Pet Health*. In 2012, Banfield found that 61% of dogs with hypothyroidism were overweight and 40% had arthritis.

Then there is diabetes. The link between obesity and diabetes in humans is certainly established but the exact details remain a little fuzzy. Too much carbs/sugar in the diet is not a direct causal factor of diabetes, at least not in humans, but excess body fat clearly is, and excess carbohydrates clearly cause that. Obesity plays such a central role in the development of diabetes in humans, that since the turn of the century, the term 'diabesity' has been used in health circles.[84] Studies now verify the link at least in cats.[85,86]

Diabetes is characterised by high blood sugar. There are two types: Type I diabetes means you have an autoimmune condition. The body attacks the cells (Islets of Langerhans) that make insulin. Type II comes about as either your body doesn't make enough insulin or your insulin doesn't work properly. This is known as insulin resistance.

As in humans, the most common form of diabetes in cats is Type II diabetes whereas, the most common form of diabetes in dogs is Type I. Whatever the exact trigger for this immune response in dogs, we know their rates of diabetes are increasing at an alarming pace, tripling in the last 30 years[87-89] Banfield (2016)[90], using data from over 2.5 million US dogs, revealed that canine diabetes has increased by 80% since 2006. For this reason, while there may well be a genetic basis to the condition, as with cancer, it appears environmental factors are chiefly at play. Something is causing this disease in dogs that goes far beyond breeding. Thankfully, with the development of modern veterinary medicine, fatality rates have decreased from 37% to 5%.[88] Bitches and smaller breeds are most at risk of diabetes[89] with Samoyeds, Tibetan Terriers and Cairn Terriers among the more susceptible.[91]

Whatever the exact cause, the dietary advice for both types of diabetes remains the same. Reduce the carbohydrate assault. A higher protein (and thus lower carbohydrate) diet and/or increasing dietary fibre (as it slows the rate of digesta and thus carbohydrate absorption) aids glycaemic control in both diabetic dogs and cats.[88,89,92-94] High-protein diets maximise the metabolic rate, improve satiety and prevent lean muscle mass loss in, at least, the diabetic cat.[95] In fact, Kirk (2006)[96] shows low-carbohydrate food improves the odds of achieving diabetic remission in cats by fourfold.

Few are in disagreement. Lori Wise, a highly qualified vet with special interests in diabetes mellitus, agrees with this dietary advice. In a piece for *Veterinary News Magazine* (March 1, 2012), she states:

> …we know now that low-carbohydrate diets are more advantageous for diabetic cats, and the weight-control diets happen to be high carbohydrate diets…

And yet Wise concludes her piece with…

> …the jury is out, and I don't think we have strong evidence to say that all cats need to be on low-carbohydrate diets.

This baffles me. Despite having zero evidence to show that a normal, healthy and very carnivorous cat actually benefits from *any* carbohydrates whatsoever in their diet and cats with diseases such as obesity and diabetes clearly doing better the less carbs you feed them, this vet is happy to promote highly processed, obesity-inducing diets for cats containing 50–60% carbohydrates, at least until someone can produce a study that explicitly states she should try not feeding cats carbohydrates in the first place.

Obesity and diabetes are terrible, chronic diseases that will lay waste to their health, well-being and emotional state. It will shorten their lives and cause you significant stress in the process. The tragic irony of it is that we, their guardians, are causing it by feeding them the wrong food. Sadly, owners appear completely unaware of this. In a survey of 1,104 American pet owners, 356 (32%) reported that their pets were overweight or obese but, incredibly, only three people considered this obesity a health concern.[97] The remainder are very wrong. Part of the problem is that nobody dies of obesity, they die of its effects – heart disease, diabetes and cancer– all of which account for the very vast majority of early death across the Western world. Sadly, it seems like the public aren't the only ones with very clouded judgment when it comes to obesity.

Light Dog Food

While it should now seem entirely plausible that a dry, high-carb, ultra-processed food stuff might at least be a *potential* risk factor in the dramatic surge of obesity and diabetes in the canine population, as they are in humans, our vets stubbornly refuse to entertain the notion. Despite all the evidence to the contrary, ultra-processed, *light* dry food remains the veterinary diet of choice to resolve the canine obesity epidemic. Almost identical to the food the dog got fat on, light pet food is still desperately high in carbohydrate but this time it now has a magic component – a greater amount of indigestible plant fibre.

As of 2017, the most popular, vet-recommended light dry food for large adult dogs in the United Kingdom still contains corn as its primary ingredient. This results in a rapidly digested carbohydrate content of at least 50%, only this time it contains 12.5% fibre, in comparison to their normal adult dog foods that are less than 2% fibre.

The first six ingredients of this product are corn (a totally unnecessary high GL punch to the gut), poultry meal, cellulose (virtually indigestible plant fibre), soybean meal (a large indigestible component), maize gluten (virtually indigestible rubbery pulp left over after corn processing) and beet pulp (a practically indigestible source of fibre). The final four ingredients here offer protein to the mix but little of it is bioavailable to the dog. Thus, in a move reminiscent of catwalk models filling up on paper tissue days before a show in order to shed those final few grams, a high indigestible component of the diet is used to reduce the overall calorie load of the meal. To ensure calorie restriction, these high-carb, high-fibre diets are then coupled with a slightly reduced recommended daily allowance. Slaves to the 'calories in, calories out' notion, 'light', 'weight management' or 'metabolic' dry food remains the very *best* way to diet a dog, in the opinion of the very vast majority of vets today. And unfortunately for obese dogs worldwide, these diets *do* have supportive studies to back them up. In-house feed trials, conducted by pet food manufacturers on caged dogs, support the notion that dogs maintained on these light diets can and do lose weight over time.[98]

Let's think on that for a moment. Consider the average Labrador on a cereal-based diet. This dog was engineered to put on weight to keep him from freezing in the frigid waters of Labrador, Canada. He can distend his stomach, meaning he can eat 10% of his body weight. This means a 30-kg lab wants to eat up to 3 kg in a sitting. Instead, you feed him 300 g of carb-rich, rapidly digested crackers for breakfast which he quickly turns to blood sugar. The body responds by flooding the system with insulin, which in turn, encourages the body to store fat. Blood sugar levels fall and as the hypothalamus is not getting the leptin message, your dog gets hungry soon after his meal. This is why weight-loss programs in dogs, based on food restriction, increases begging and scavenging behaviour.[99] Starving, you might feed him some more in sympathy, if he does not find it himself. Worse still, hunger can fuel aggression which ranges from a dog resource–guarding his own bowl or a meaty bone from an unsuspecting toddler. Either way, over time, a dog in this situation is going to gain weight, particularly if they are neutered.

Nor is this the only problem with *light* dry foods. The indigestible fibre ingredients described, including soybean meal, corn gluten meal and beet pulp, all account for some of the protein in the mix; only little of this protein is actually available to the dog (more on this later). Further, this added fibre can affect the dog's ability to absorb the necessary nutrients. Burkholder and Bauer (1998)[100] found dogs on reduced energy intake dry diets had a suboptimal intake of essential nutrients, especially protein. They documented considerable net losses of trace elements in dogs fed diets containing increased amounts of hard-to-digest carbohydrates and crude fibre, most notably a depression of zinc and iron absorption in the small intestines.[101] Ko and Fascetti (2016)[102] found that when dietary fibres such as rice bran (the leftovers from rice processing), cellulose and beet pulp (leftovers from beet processing), are included in complete dry food mixes, it results in taurine deficiencies in dogs, with beet pulp being the worst offender, a potential risk factor for Dilated Cardiomyopathy DCM in dogs, something to which we will return later.

> As if more reasons were needed to show that dry diets play no role in weight loss, cats allowed to feed *ad libitum* on a 40% hydrated diet, compared to a dry diet with 12% moisture, resulted in the former eating less (77g/d $\pm$ 10.8 vs. 86g/d $\pm$ 18.4, P < 0.05). These cats gained less body weight increased (312g/d $\pm$ 95.9 vs. 368g/d $\pm$ 120.7; P = 0.28) and significantly increased their activity levels.
>
> **Cameron *et al.*, 2011**[103]

Common sense at this point would tell us that it might be time to drop all the carbohydrates and increase the protein for this animal. Authors note that protein has a greater satiating effect in dogs, evidenced by reduced voluntary intake. This has the potential to lead to greater compliance in weight-loss programs.[99] A multitude of studies clearly demonstrate that dry-fed dogs receiving higher protein diets (>100 g crude protein/1,000 kcal ME) achieved not only greater weight loss in obese dogs but maintained their lean body mass during the process, with the higher the protein/carb ratio the better.[104-108] The same applies to cats[109] and humans.[110] Lean body mass is the proportion of your muscle to your overall body weight, and retention of it during dieting is crucial as it is one of the primary drivers of basal energy metabolism. Hence, loss of lean muscle tissue during a weight-loss regime will contribute to weight gain, as well as decreasing immune competence and increasing susceptibility to stresses, such as infection and injury.[111]

One of the most convincing works in this regard is Diez *et al.* (2002).[106] They took a number of obese beagles and divided them into two groups, one was placed on a high-protein dry diet (48% protein, 5% fat), whereas the other received a conventional weight-loss dry diet. They fed each dog whatever it took to induce weight loss at the rate of 2% per week. Once the dogs reached their target weights, Diez *et al.* assessed how they got there. The first thing they noted was that the dogs eating the higher protein diets actually consumed *more* calories (76% of maintenance requirements versus 68% on the weight-loss food). Second, while both groups lost the same amount of weight, the high protein group lost on average 13% more body fat compared to their brethren on the weight-loss foods. Nestlé Purina repeated this study 3 years later, this time in cats, substituting corn for protein-rich ingredients.[108] They had similar results, where both groups lost similar amounts of weight in the same time. The only difference was that the cats on the higher protein diet lost more fat and less lean muscle mass than the higher carbohydrate group.

Bierer and Bui (2004)[112] took this one step further. With a similar format as in the work by Diez *et al*, Bierer and Bui calorie restricted two groups of beagles, one on a high-protein formulation, the other on a low-protein (high-carb) formulation. They found that the dogs on the high-protein diet lost nearly *six times* the amount of body fat as their high-carb brethren.

Their current approach ensures overweight dogs – protein-eating machines that require zero carbohydrates in their diet – continue to consume obscenely high levels of carbohydrates. The insulin effect will continue, as will their hunger. Assured that science is on their side, should a client present to a vet with an overweight pet, the blame is shifted to the owner. This product is clinically proven to work, so *you* must have been doing it wrong. *You* made him fat by feeding him *too much* of the high-carb diet. *You* are simply loving him to death.

> You love your dog, and you want to provide him with the best nutrition to keep him in top shape. But when it comes to portion size or the number of snacks you share per day, you're not really sure whether you're giving him too much…
> **"Risks of Over-Feeding Your Dog", Hill's Pet Food Website, 2019**
> **https://www.hillspet.com/dog-care/nutrition-feeding/overfeeding-**
> **your-dog**

Irrespective of whether you think the dog is a carnivore or omnivore, a dry, high-carbohydrate *light* pet food is contrary to all scientific theory on the subject of obesity. It is, however, highly profitable, as many of the ingredients in this new light food are nothing more than fibrous waste left over from food processing. If anything highlights how grossly ill prepared our vets are to appropriately advise on the role of proper nutrition in the health of our pets, it is their backing of such an approach to canine obesity.

Sadly, this is not the only potential problem with increasing plant fibre to such a degree in the dogs' diet.

Bloat with Torsion in Dogs

Few diseases require more immediate attention in dogs than bloat with torsion, or gastro dilation and volvulus (GDV). It is a shocking, agonising end for a dog that is sadly far too common in deep-chested breeds. Lately, the thinking on this condition has moved on and, in my opinion, diet should now be very much top of the agenda.

Gastric dilation (bloat) is a filling of the stomach with gas and/or liquid, which can be uncomfortable. It's a common enough issue in both humans and dogs. In humans, it can occur for a variety of reasons but one of the most common is the consumption of foods you find hard to digest. Fibrous foods are a stand out food example here. Milk being ingested by people who are lactose intolerant is another. In both cases, large amounts of undigested matter make it into the large intestines, much to the delight of certain groups of bacteria that live there but usually in smaller numbers. A common by-product of these industrious microbes is gas which builds up, normally resulting in a fart or two. So far, so relieving.

GDV, is a progression of the bloat condition in dogs. It involves the stomach (and spleen, as they're attached) flipping or twisting between 90 degrees and 360 degrees. This seals both the entrance and exit to the stomach. Neither fluid nor gas from the digestive process can enter or leave the chamber. If allowed to progress, gas can build up. If swelling continues, the pain is immense and death can happen quickly. Fatality is the end result for on average 33% of cases, with a range of 15 to 60% of cases.[113,114]

Symptoms initially include a dog standing motionless, reluctant to sit down, or he may be having trouble getting comfortable, doing a lot of stretching with his front legs, head down, bum in the air. You might hear a lot of gurgling coming from his rock hard stomach. An examination may reveal the abdomen is hard, with a hollow 'thump' when gently tapped. He may not be in pain at this point. If allowed to progress, the dog might get extremely restless with excessive panting, excessive salivation, and unsuccessful attempts to vomit or defecate. In the final stages of this disease, the stomach area *may* appear swollen and distended, the dog will be breathing rapidly, have pale-coloured gums and tongue. The dog will finally collapse from shock. It's important to note that while bloat often leads to GDV in dogs, GDV does not always arise from bloat. A survey of 1,165 Great Dane owners revealed 12.8% of owners (149) experienced GDV in their dogs but less than half noticed any bloating whatsoever.[115]

If you think your dog is suffering from bloat or, worse still, GDV, you must take him to the vet **immediately**. Ring them in advance to prepare them. If a vet is beyond your reach, you need to get one on the phone as you may have to perform a procedure yourself at home to release the gas to save his life. It involves a sharp knife.

It's concerning that such a terrifying infliction is relatively common in the general canine population. It is the cause of death for 2.5% of the UK's pure-bred dogs (n=15,881, 165 breeds represented).[116] However, some breeds are significantly more affected than others. We know that GDV is a major risk for larger, deep-chested dogs such as Great Dane, German Shepherd, Bloodhound, Red setter, Weimaraner, St. Bernard, etc.[117,118] The chest cavity is deep and narrow, where the greater the depth to width ratio, the more prone they are to GDV.[114,119] As such, it comes as no surprise that Glickman *et al.* (2000)[120] found that being related to a GDV sufferer increases their risk by 63%, suggesting a genetic basis. The effect is particularly significant for first-degree relatives (parent, sibling, or offspring). [113,120,121]

Other risk factors include age, where advancing age, certainly from 5 years of age, increases their likelihood of a GDV strike by 20% each year[122-125] and body weight. Lean, deep-chested dogs are potentially at greater risk.[113,126] The hypothesis goes that some extra abdominal fat would reduce the amount of internal space available, working to keep the stomach somewhat in place. Supporting this, Uhrikova *et al.* (2015)[127] found intact males were at greater risk of GDV (neutered dogs are more likely to be overweight) while the number of spayed females with GDV was significantly lower than expected.

So now we have our at-risk dog – deep-chested, possibly lean, where age and being related to a sufferer increase the risk. But crucially – this concerns a dog's predisposition to GDV, not bloat *per se*. After all, the majority of dogs with this shape do not experience GDV. To put it another way, your dog's physical shape may load the gun but it is the bloat that pulls the trigger. The question is: why are their stomachs filling with gas?

It was commonly thought that it was aerophagia causing bloat in dogs, a particular concern for deep-chested, and thus, at-risk-of-torsion breeds. However, when Van Kruiningen *et al.* (2013)[128] examined the stomach gas of 10 dogs admitted to an emergency clinic for GDV surgery, they found the CO_2 composition of the gas was between 13% and 20%. As the CO_2 concentration of the atmosphere is less than 1%, the authors concluded that the gas is far more likely to be coming *up* from the intestinal tract, similar to the fermentative bloat that occurs in cattle, in other words, the gas produced by busy microbes in the intestines.

This explains why authors can find no validation for some of the more popular, but yet-to-be-verified, hypotheses for GDV in dogs including the speed of eating[129] and bowl height (this was originally and only found by Glickman *et al.* 2000a[125] but it was later revealed giant dogs are more likely to be offered high feed stations assumedly to help long-necked breeds get to their meal – correlation not causation), both of which were thought to affect air intake in the dog. Similarly, allowing dogs to rest after a meal does not affect the risk of GDV. Authors find no link between the timing, duration or intensity of GDV, whether before or after exercise.[124,125] Supporting this further, anecdotally speaking, I polled more than 100 owners of dogs that suffered a torsion episode and learned that in excess of 80% of episodes happen more than an hour after a meal, just when we expect the stomach to begin emptying into the intestines.

We all know eating a meal containing a lot of plant fibre (beans, lentils, raw vegetables) produces excess gas. You are feeding and encouraging the multiplication of a certain group of bacteria, and a by-product of their activity is bacteria farts which build gas inside the system. When Manichanh *et al.* (2013)[130] wanted to test the effect of their 'flatulogenic diet' on healthy human patients, they based it on a greater intake of more fibrous items including whole grains, beans and soya, as well as a variety of fibrous fruit and vegetables, including good old cruciferous vegetables (brussels sprouts, cauliflower, broccoli, cabbage). Hullar *et al.* (2018)[131] studied the faecal biome of Great Danes that suffered GDV and found the patients had a significantly more diverse faecal microbiome than healthy control dogs. In particular, dogs with GDV showed a greater number of *Firmicutes* and *Actinobacteria* and a significantly lower abundance of *Bacteroidetes*. As the gut biome is intricately linked to how our immune system fires, Hullar *et al.* concluded there may be an immunogenicity to GDV in dogs, one that is kicked off by a gut microbiome imbalance (or *dysbiosis*).

While the actual spark for GDV may still elude us, it seems we are now honing in on the most aggravating factor for bloat gas in dogs – dietary ingredients that encourage the growth of bacterial communities that, in turn, increase gas in the system.

Numerous authors have highlighted the role of kibble in bloating.[132-134] To prevent a first episode of GDV, their advice is to avoid feeding exclusively dry, cereal-based and specifically soy protein-based commercial dog foods, until more is known.

> The widespread practice of extruding dry dog food began in 1957. An epidemic of GDV in dogs was reported in the United States from 1965 to 1995.
>
> **Raghavan *et al.*, 2006**[135]

> During the past 30 years there has been a 1,500 percent increase in the incidence of bloat, and this has coincided with the increased feeding of dry dog foods. There is a much lower incidence of bloat in susceptible breeds in Australia and New Zealand. Feeding practices in these countries have been found to be less dependent on dry foods.
>
> **Bell, 2013**[136]

In fact, simply decreasing the amount of dry food fed to your dog lowers their risk of GDV. Glickman *et al.* (1997)[126] found that the addition of table foods or canned foods to the predominantly dry food diet of large- and giant-breed dogs resulted in a 59% and 28% decreased risk of GDV, respectively. Other authors note adding fish or eggs may decrease the risk.[124,137]

That is not to say raw-fed dogs do not suffer bloat with torsion. It appears they can but to what degree and under what circumstances is unknown. But that they can is enough to suggest that simply raw-feeding (whatever your definition of that may be) is not a suitable protector from this horrible disease, certainly not if that raw diet contains a preponderance of ingredients known to fuel the problem.

Of all ingredients, those high in plant fibre, specifically *soluble* fibre, are at the top of the list of suspects as soluble fibre is consumed by gut bacteria. We know the more of this we have in a mix, the more gas is produced. Excess gas is surely something we want to avoid in dogs prone to bloat. However, nobody has ever concerned themselves with the amount of soluble fibre in their pet food products.

Section 1 suggests wild dogs eat as little as 3% plant matter when left to their own devices. If we take the average crude fibre value for this plant matter as 10%, this would be the equivalent of perhaps 0.3% crude plant fibre. Dry pet foods start at around 2% *crude* fibre and range upward from there. However, the 'crude fibre' measure pertains only to the amount of indigestible fibre in the mix. It is the stuff resilient to chemical digestion in the laboratory and bacterial digestion in your intestines. This is why it's so good for constipation in humans and dogs. While both types of fibre greatly slow the passage of digesta through the intestines, once indigestible fibre hits the colon undigested, it draws in water to the stool passively by osmosis. Now it speeds things up.

Total dietary fibre (TDF) is a far more accurate type of fibre analysis as it includes the soluble fibre content. This measure is required for human food products. However, as TDF is considerably more expensive than crude fibre measurement, it is not employed by pet food manufacturers.

To give you an idea of the potential *soluble* fibre content of typical ingredients used in pet food, a 100 g of sweet corn has a CF content of around 8 g (although this depends on the species). However, it has a TDF content of more than double that at 17.2 g. If we look at the UK's most popular 'light' dry food, its *crude fibre* content is 12.5%. The first six ingredients are corn, poultry meal, cellulose (indigestible plant fibre), soybean meal (high in soluble fibre), maize gluten (high in indigestible plant fibre) and beet pulp (high in soluble fibre). With these sorts of ingredients making up perhaps three quarters of the mix, we have to assume the insoluble fibre content of this meal is at least the same amount of soluble fibre again. This product now becomes at least 25% TDF. A 400-g meal of this would provide 100 g of plant fibre to your dog. The inevitable result is that this slow-to-digest meal will move slowly through the dog's normally rapid system. This alone is a potential threat to GDV in dogs. Studies show plant fibre ingredients greatly delay canine gastric emptying time.[138] Authors note delayed gastric emptying may cause chronic gastric distention, stretching the hepatogastric ligament.[139,140] That aside, delayed transit coupled with large amounts of soluble plant fibre will fuel the growth of the wrong bacteria and, inevitably, gas buildup.

The only author to examine the link between dietary ingredients and bloat is Raghavan *et al.* (2006).[135] Using dry dog food label information, they checked whether the risk of GDV increases with an increasing amount of cereal ingredients such as wheat, corn or soy (and a decreasing number of animal-protein ingredients) used in the food. Soy is high in difficult-to-digest oligosaccharides, making them notorious for flatulence in humans and dogs alike[141]. Raghavan *et al.* detected no link between cereal–usage and GDV in the 85 cases analysed. However, only six dogs were consuming a pet food with soy in the first four ingredients, making the test beyond irrelevant. They did find something with corn where the presence of one corn-based ingredient or two among the first four label ingredients increased the risk of GDV. However, the trend was not quite statistically significant (P=0.11).

Unfortunately, the authors only tested the first four ingredients of the pet foods consumed and made no effort to determine the fibre contents of the food. This means the risk posed by fibrous filler ingredients further down the list such as beet pulp, corn gluten and soybean meal was not assessed. As little as 1–2% of ingredients such as cellulose and beet pulp can have a dramatic biological effect in dogs, radically altering not only the gut flora but also stool quality.[142,143]

In my opinion, considering the small sample size used, more work is urgently required here. If we accept GDV has increased 1,500% in US dogs since the early 80s, an issue these authors attribute to the increased use of dry food, it's worth noting that around this time, and due to matters of cost, corn began to become a dominant ingredient in pet food production. The reason was twofold. First, demand for corn as a human and agri–animal food source rose. Chemical advancements in its cultivation soon resulted in corn replacing wheat as the most affordable cereal crop to American food producers. The difference was further increased when the Chinese and Indian wheat belts became the world's largest producer of cheap wheat. Perhaps it's a coincidence but, coupled with the increased usage of indigestible plant-fibre filler ingredients in pet food, it sure isn't helping matters.

There is another issue with feeding dogs large amounts of fibre and that is a heavier stomach weight (excluding the contents), expressed as a percentage of body weight, risks stretching the hepatogastric ligament of dogs, resulting in the flip that turns bloat from uncomfortable to life threatening in deep-chested dogs.

Part of my doctorate involved weighing the stomach and intestinal tracts of herbivores through the seasons. On top of diet analysis, we wanted to see if there was a significant difference in gut weight during this time. As expected, we found gut weights were lighter in summer and heavier in winter. This was not a novel finding. As the fibre content of forage increases toward winter, the more fibrous meal demands more mechanical effort from the gut to break it down. As the gut is essentially a muscle, a well-worked gut is known to get larger and heavier.

The same effect is seen in dogs. Plant fibre requires more work of the dog's digestive tract. As previously described, it initially delays gastric emptying time. From there, it disrupts the pulsing of the intestines. In dogs, the normal pattern of duodenojejunal (where the duodenum, the first short segment of the intestines meets the small intestines) contractions following a meal consists of bursts of 4–10 rhythmic contractions per burst. When wheat bran or cellulose were added, the contractions not only increased (12–15 contractions per burst) but there was also a delay during burst of anywhere from 4–15 minutes.[144] In contrast, when guar gum was added, contractions occurred continuously at a rate of 7-8 per minute, but their amplitude was one-half of that seen with the other fibres. In other words, the type of fibre fed to a dog greatly increases the mechanical labour on the intestinal tract. And all this shows how quickly it passes through. Bueno *et al.* (1981)[144] measured the effect of wheat bran and cellulose on the jejunal (small intestine) transit time in dogs. Just 30 g of wheat bran per dog increased the jejunal transit time by 28% but the indigestible cellulose caused a 900% increase in transit time, resulting in an over 50% reduction in the flow of digesta. This gives bacteria therein more time to digest the soluble plant fibre meal, fueling gas production. Moreover, the greater work rate increases the weight of the dog's stomach. The stomachs of healthy dogs fed dry food once daily for a year were larger and heavier (as a percentage of body weight) than the stomachs of healthy dogs fed meat-and-bone.[139]

At least in deer, their gut weight (as a %/body weight) reduces in the summer months. In dogs fed nothing but high fibre food, gut weight stays heavy, constantly working on the fibrous meal, consistently straining the hepatogastric ligament. That takes a toll over time and with increasing age is a risk factor for GDV in dogs.

The high plant fibre content of dry food fits all the hypotheses for this dreadful and all too common condition of deep-chested dogs. The risk factors so far established for GDV in dogs are as follows:

- A large volume of food at once (more undigested plant fibre reaches the intestines at once).

- Delayed gastric emptying time (plant fibre delays canine gastric emptying time).

- Resting doesn't help as most attacks happen an hour after a meal (when the fibre meal enters the intestines).

- Bacterial fermentation (indigestible fibre slows the passage of digesta, giving bacteria more time to work on the high soluble fibre content of the meal).

- Increased weight of the stomach may cause flip (fibre increases the workload of the digestive tract).

It is for this reason, until more is known about the exact dietary cause of GDV in dogs, I implore vets to reconsider their use of dry, cereal-based pet food products high in plant fibre, if just in deep-chested breeds.

Pancreatitis in Dogs

Pancreatitis is a terrible disease and one of the most painful you can endure. In short, pancreatitis is inflammation of the pancreas. It can occur as a result of a poor diet, drug abuse, an infection or an injury. If, as a result, the pancreas starts to malfunction, digestive juices leak out into the surrounding tissue and the body begins to digest itself, causing agony to the sufferer. This is a terribly debilitating infliction that you need to take very seriously. By the time the dogs show outward signs of discomfort, you can be quite sure they are in a great deal of internal pain.

Pancreatitis can be either acute or chronic. Acute pancreatitis is a sudden, dramatic and crippling, painful infliction. Abnormal pancreatic function causes the release of digestive enzymes into the pancreas tissue and surrounding organs. Called necrotising pancreatitis, self-digestion begins to occur. Without rapid veterinary intervention and aggressive treatment, your dog is unlikely to survive.

Chronic pancreatitis takes time to develop and is thus more likely to occur in animals of 2 years and older. It is characterised by an inflammation of the pancreas that does not subside. It results in an inability of the afflicted pancreas to secrete digestive enzymes or hormones. Symptoms will not appear until 85–90% of the dog's pancreas has shut down.[145] Fewer enzymes mean that less fat and protein are digested. These undigested fatty acids in the gut give the diarrhoea a yellowy-grey and oily nature, typical of the disease. In the initial stages, symptoms are not as severe as acute pancreatitis. These are associated with the lack of digestion, including weight loss, poor hair coat quality, flatulence, increased appetite and coprophagy (poo-eating, likely as a result of nutrient deficiency) and diarrhoea.

In humans the pancreatitis is usually acute. It is one of the most frequent gastrointestinal causes of hospital admission in the United States.[146] It resulted in 275,000 hospitalisations in 2009, affecting around 1:1,400 US citizens. In the majority (approximately 70%) of these cases, alcohol was thought to play a significant role with troubled gallbladders and drug abuse was thought to explain much of the remainder.

In dogs, it is usually chronic pancreatitis that we see. The exact prevalence of the disease in the population is difficult to determine because most chronic canine (and feline) pancreatitis slips under the radar.[147] However, clinical features of samples taken randomly, post-mortem, indicate that pancreatitis in dogs and cats occurs at epidemic proportions. In a study of the 200 samples it was found that 34% of dogs were suffering chronic pancreatitis at the time of death.[148] In another study, of 73 apparently normal dogs presented for postmortem examination, 64% of pancreata displayed evidence of chronic pancreatitis.[149] These figures are mirrored in our cats. An examination of 115 feline pancreata from healthy and sick cats revealed pancreatitis in 67% of cases, including 45% of apparently healthy cats.[150-153]

So, what can possibly be causing all this in dogs? In their review entitled *Chronic Pancreatitis in Dogs and Cats*, Panagiotis *et al.* (2008),[147] highlight how little is known about the aetiology of pancreatitis in these species. Genetics is thought to play a role in some forms of pancreatic issues, such as exocrine pancreatic insufficiency (EPI), where individuals are genetically unable to secrete certain pancreatic enzymes, unrelated to inflammation of the organ). German Shepherds can constitute up to two-thirds of cases reporting with EPI,[154] with rough collies, Yorkshire and Silky Terriers, Dachshunds, Miniature Poodles and Cocker Spaniels also noted to be at risk (all breeds that have gone through tight genetic bottlenecks). However, the more common form of pancreatitis is the result of inflammation of the pancreas and here genetics is thought to play significantly less of a role. It cannot explain the shocking amount of pancreatitis we see in cats, where pedigree inbreeding is far less of an issue.

Genetics aside and with booze and drug abuse out of the equation, we must look for another common factor for the rate of this disease in dogs and cats. The very next place to look is diet.

Hyperlipidaemia (excess fat in the blood), characterised by elevated plasma triacylglycerol concentrations, is one of accepted causes of acute pancreatitis or recurring bouts of acute pancreatitis in humans.[155] It is thought to account for 7% of cases, making it the most common cause of the disease after gall stones and alcohol.[156] In fact, the presence of excess fat is how your vet typically diagnoses the condition in your dog. A pancreas in trouble does not digest fat very well. One of the (later) signs of pancreatitis in dogs is yellowy, greasy stools. Hence, one way to detect the possible signs of pancreatitis is to measure the amount of triglycerides (fat) in the blood. Another way is to test for canine pancreas-specific lipase, the enzyme secreted by the pancreas to digest fat. A stressed pancreas is assumed to produce much more of it, something a simple blood test in a fasted dog would reveal.

So concerned are our vets for fat that when discussing a possible cause of the issue, the line 'it can be something as simple as that bit of fat off your steak' is often trotted out. And it makes perfect sense. If there is too much fat in the blood, then surely you have been eating too much of it. Only that statement is not only entirely unsupported by literature but, as we have since learned from the obesity epidemic, very likely to be absolutely false. Of course, dogs should be able to eat a big lump of fatty meat now and again, that's what they are designed to do. As you will learn, they are more adept at utilising fat than we are. Remember *fat* was blamed initially for the obesity epidemic. We thought initially getting fat was from eating too much fat. It made sense, only it was entirely wrong. Fat actually switches *off* our hunger. It ironically paved the way for us moving to more low-fat (and thus increasingly higher sugar) options. Now the obesity trap has slammed shut. We have become a race of gelatinous, sugar junkies and our hormones will ensure it stays that way for quite some time.

To understand a little more about this, we need to first discuss the three different energy pathways (again, for the sake of flow, please forgive me while I grossly simplify here). You may remember that your body runs on Adenosine Tri-Phosphate (ATP). That's adenosine with three phosphates on the end. Energy is created when one of these phosphates is broken off (to form Adenosine diphosphate). This energy production reaction occurs in one of three ways. The first is the ATP-PC system, which is essentially your body using all the ATP it has stored ready to go in the mitochondria. As nothing is required by the body, this system is typically rapid but short lasting. In gym terms, it can produce lots of power but only for a very short duration, perhaps 12 seconds of maximal effort. Think of it as the *favoured* pathway of your 100-m sprinter, for instance.

The second system is known as the glycolytic system. This system runs on glycogen stored in the muscles and liver, which you create after consuming carbohydrates and, to a lesser degree, protein. In gym terms, this pathway provides for you moderate power of moderate duration, perhaps 30 seconds. If you work too hard and push the glycolytic system beyond this, fast glycolysis results in an increase in pyruvic acid and subsequently lactic acid production. This builds up in your muscles, rapidly increasing muscle fatigue and decreasing your power (this is you 'hitting the wall'). Your other option here (long-distance runners) is slow, controlled glycolysis where, given time, pyruvic acid is instead converted to acetyl coenzyme A and fed through the Krebs cycle (part of the third system below), producing ATP and delaying fatigue.

The third system is known as the fatty acid oxidation system. This is essentially three systems (of which the Krebs cycle is part of it). For now, all we need to note is that instead of blood glucose, it uses stored fat (lipolysis) to fuel the ATP conversion. In gym terms, it offers the least power but the greatest duration. It is why top marathon runners (and long-pursuit animals such as wolves) are all bordering skeletal.

Many of us are now familiar with keto diet. This is a process where followers exclude all carbohydrates from the diet. Without blood glucose, the body is forced into a permanent state of ketosis (this is the term used to describe the fat stores being broken down to produce energy, a by-product of which is ketones). First made popular by the Atkins diet, the very first benefit you can expect from this approach is weight loss but also any diseases associated with being overweight, such as diabetes and cancer. However, as being fat is inflammatory to the body, studies show that reducing body fat via keto diets have also proven beneficial to patients suffering inflammatory issues such as Alzheimer's, Parkinson's and brain issues.

One of the most interesting academics studying this phenomenon of high-fat diets, weight loss and performance is Professor Timothy Noakes. Noakes is a long-distance runner of some renown and it is essentially upon his advice back in the 1980s, after running out of gas too early in the 1980 Comrades race, forcing him to walk the last 6 miles, that lead to us all carb-loading before a race. He summarised his thoughts on the matter in his extremely successful book *The Lore of Running*. In essence, the idea was that as the glycolytic system runs on glycogen, the more you have stored before a race, the more you push back the 'wall' effect that often kicks in around 20 miles. This is where all stored sugar has been depleted and the body switches to burning fat to keep you going. However, this energy system lacks the power of glycolytic system. The inevitable result is slowing down just as you need to push. The idea sounds right, and it is why runners today are seen to guzzle energy drinks during a race, all in an effort to avoid running out of power. However, he has recently made a commendable U-turn and admitted that his advice of carb–loading the long-distance running athlete was not correct and that it's actually all about fat. He now advises to keep buying his book but to throw that chapter in the garbage! His advice is now a low-carb high-fat (LCHF) diet for everyone, from the average joe, to the obese to the ultra-athlete. His supporting piece on the matter, "Evidence that supports the prescription of low-carb high-fat diets: a narrative review", published in the *British Journal of Sports Medicine*, is an eye-opener.[157] It cites numerous studies and ample clinical evidence that LCHF diets consistently improve all markers of cardiovascular risk, lowering elevated blood glucose, insulin, triglyceride, ApoB and saturated fat concentrations, reducing small dense LDL (bad cholesterol) particle numbers, glycated haemoglobin (HbA1c) levels, blood pressure and body weight while increasing low HDL cholesterol concentrations (good cholesterol) and reversing non-alcoholic fatty liver disease NAFLD. They state that a reduction in insulin is obviously beneficial from a weight perspective, in that in terms of weight loss LCHF diets consistently outperform any other variation of nutrients in this manner, but that a lot of it may simply be, in part, due to reduced hunger which leads the patient to consume less calories throughout the day.

It's worth noting that his efforts to push the LCHF diet regime has met some rebuke, as all diets do and should. When Noakes, a South African, began to promote his new message, the Health Professions Council of South Africa (HPCSA) (which governs the medical professions in South Africa) charged Noakes with violating medical ethics by giving such poor advice, calling it 'disgraceful conduct'. They tried to take his license and the matter went to court. He was successful in his defence. The HPCSA appealed the decision and lost again. His science was found to be sound. Noakes sees the whole affair as an orchestrated conspiracy, a result of big pharma and the food industry corrupting the medical profession 'in order to sell more carb-rich foods and diabetes medications'.

> I think the goal is to shut me up and humiliate me, like how they used to lock people in stocks in medieval England.
>
> **Prof. Noakes to Gifford, 2016**[158]

Now to the role of carbohydrates in pancreatitis. It happens that the more carbohydrates you consume, the less likely you are to use the fatty acid oxidation system. In humans, the ingestion of high-carbohydrate diets for a long period of time decreases fatty acid oxidation by decreasing the rate of fatty acid entry into the mitochondria.[159] This means, rather paradoxically, the more carbohydrates you consume, the less fat is consumed by the mitochondria and the net result is an *elevation* of plasma triacylglycerol (blood fat). In other words, it is a high-carb diet that raises your blood fat. Authors note that when the content of dietary carbohydrate is elevated above 55% of ME, blood triglycerides rise.[160] It even has a catchy name too – carbohydrate-induced hypertriglyceridemia.

Studies show this is very much what's happening in dry-fed dogs. Raw-meat-and-bone fed dogs (very low-carb diet) exhibited reduced blood triglycerides when compared to dogs fed a dry, cereal-based diet.[161] In fact, Dr. Mark Roberts is a leading authority on the role of dietary fat in dogs, particularly in relation to sporting dogs. His latest work (in print) seeks to dispel the mythological role of dietary fat in causing pancreatitis in dogs. He found that dogs' pancreas were not working harder on high-fat diets by any measure available to them. Using 20 dogs that were fed regular diets and then alternatively fed high-carb or high-fat diets, then he measured blood fat, lipase and stool quality. Roberts found blood triglycerides were not higher in the high-fat diets, as expected by conventional veterinary medicine, but actually lower than dogs on high-carb diets. The pancreas does not produce more lipase under a high-fat challenge but the same as a high-carb diet. Even stool quality is better in the high-fat fed dogs. Thus, by all measures, increasing dietary fat failed to induce the parameters linked to pancreatitis in dogs which conventional veterinary medicine says it does.

In short, if blood fat is an accepted cause of pancreatitis and we know high-carb diets increase blood fat, perhaps they should ease off the carbohydrates in dogs.

It gets worse for dry-fed dogs suffering pancreatitis on their high-carb meals. Once it sets in, pancreatitis will result in a vitamin E deficiency.[162] vitamin E is primarily an antioxidant, mopping up excess fats in the system. As the failing organ struggles to break down fat in the diet, more vitamin E is required to clean up the excess fat. But vitamin E is notoriously unstable. And in dry pet foods, after just 6 months' storage, it is proven to reduce by 30%.[163] With vitamin E in short supply, a vicious cycle may begin. And as this is what dry-fed dogs receive in the way of fresh nutrients, a vicious circle begins.

As fat builds in the blood of dogs consuming high-carb diets, the body screams for more lipase to get the fat out of the blood and the pancreas complies. Measure the dog for lipase at this point and the values will be worryingly high. What do conventional vets recommend now? Low-fat (and thus higher-carb) diets. It is at this near-breaking point that, one more load of fat might push the system over the pancreatic cliff. In a perfect straw-camel's-back scenario, it's not the final piece of straw but the heavy load already in place. Of course, the carnivore's pancreas should have been able to cope with that bit of fat, as meat-eater dogs are better as its digestion than we are (later). Sadly, it is at this low moment that modern vets tend to blame the owner for a dietary indiscretion, when it was far more likely that the vets' own poor dietary advice put the dog on the table in the first place.

In this way, in all but the midst of an acute bout of pancreatitis, where scientists such as Roberts suggest lower fat (and zero carbohydrates) is the order of the day, for chronic pancreatitis that plagues so many cats and dogs today, a lower fat diet is less likely to be the advice. In fact, due to their deflammatory properties, therapeutic doses of omega-3 fatty acids (perhaps 700 mg of combined EPA and DHA per 10 kg of dog, according to the ACVN), will help alleviate some of the more painful symptoms of pancreatitis by decreasing the inflammation and possibly help avoid its occurence in the future.

Carbohydrates and Cancer

In a paper titled "The Role of Carbohydrates in the Health of Dogs", nicely tying the word carbohydrates in with the word health, Rankovic et al. (2019)[164] state:

> Obesity, diabetes mellitus, cancer, adverse food reactions and gastrointestinal diseases are common medical concerns for dogs. Diet, and carbohydrates in particular, plays an important role in the treatment of these conditions.
>
> **Rankovic et al., (2019)[164]**

This is an incredible statement and one the authors do little to support in the eight pages that follow, beyond the now typical overreliance on dogs *can* digest carbohydrates and fibre *can* play a role in weight loss. To understand the level of scientific evidence and reasoning currently being employed by the industry in defence of feeding carnivores a high-carbohydrate diet, this article is a very good place to start. But of all those diseases they mention, to suggest carbohydrates play an 'important role' in treating dogs with cancer is perhaps the most unforgiveable of all.

Dogs are more likely to die of cancer than any other animal on the planet. While cancer is rife in humans, only 500/100,000 Americans are diagnosed with cancer each year. Compare this to 5,300/100,000 dogs.[165] That's quite a statistic when you consider they lack the ability to light their own cigarettes. Sadly, when looking through the literature for the potential role of improper nutrition in this scandal, there is a great big hole where the really useful studies should be, in particular, the role of high-dose carbohydrates in the whole affair.

It happens that dogs provide an ideal solution to filling the gap in models of natural disease and translational medicine in humans,[166] particularly cancer. Many cancers are shared between humans and dogs, including sarcoma (osteosarcoma, soft tissue sarcoma, histiocytic sarcoma, hemangiosarcoma), haematological malignancies (lymphoma, leukaemia), bladder cancer, intracranial neoplasms (meningioma, glioma) and melanoma.[167] In fact, when viewed under a microscope, it is impossible to distinguish between a tumour from a human and a dog. Bone cancers, lymphomas and even bladder cancer in dogs are molecularly identical to cancers in people. Moreover, their cancer responds to treatments in similar ways. In this way, dogs are excellent models for how cancer develops in humans.[36,167,168] However, it stands to reason that the opposite must apply too. For this reason, we will be leaning on nutritive lessons learned in human cancer development.

While genetics today absorb the lion's share of cancer research budgets, it may come as a surprise to learn that we can only attribute 5–10% of all cancer cases in humans to genetic defects at birth.[169] Cancer arising from genetic flaws are called inherited cancers or germline mutations. In dogs, we would say inbred lines, such as the Rottweiler or Boxer, are *predisposed* to certain inherited cancers. However, more than 90% of cancers are sporadic, the result of genetic defects acquired, during the life of the animal, from environment and lifestyle.[169] This means you can avoid its occurrence.

In terms of cancer, you will now hear people saying that genetics loads the gun and environmental factors pull the trigger. The most common environmental factors negatively affecting humans are tobacco, ultraviolet radiation, age and now, poor nutrition. In respect of the latter, a new realm of science has popped up termed nutrigenomics. This is the study of the effects of certain nutrients to up- or downregulate an individual's gene expression, essentially turning things on or off. Diet plays a very significant role here, with poor-quality fats, too much red meat (particularly processed meats), too much salt and too much sugar/carbohydrates listed among the most common protagonists in human cancers today.[170]

Tumours are total carb junkies. In fairness, all cells need sugar to operate, but cancer cells use glucose at 10-20 times the rate of normal cells.[171,172] Their high sugar-uptake is the primary way we can look for them, using a method called a positron emission tomography and computed tomography (PET-CT) scan. PET scans use radioactively labelled glucose to detect sugar-hungry tumour cells. When patients drink the sugar water, the cancer cells preferentially take up this liquid and they light up. This helps physicians see where the cancer is, to evaluate the extent of the disease to deduce which treatments to use and check if those treatments are working. In fact, all the way back in 1931, Otto Warburg won the Nobel Prize for his discovery that cancer cells have a different energy metabolism to healthy cells, most notably, a greater rate of glycolysis (the process of converting glucose to energy) compared with normal cells.

In this way, cancer loves a high-sugar diet, but the relationship goes deeper than that. Macrophage-mediated programmed cell removal PrCR, or phagocytosis for short, plays an essential role in tumour surveillance and elimination. These are the 'seek, engulf and destroy' cells of the immune system. We've known since 1971 that just 100 g of sugar via sucrose, honey or orange juice significantly reduces the effectiveness of phagocytosis in humans for up to 5 hours.[173,174] If you're a cancer cell thinking of getting up into mischief, this is most welcome.

And it gets worse. As more and more sugar is consumed, cell resistance to insulin builds, meaning more and more insulin is released into the blood. Insulin is a powerful stimulant of cell growth, as it drives fuel into the cell. Cancer cells have 10–20 times the insulin receptors of normal cells[168,169] This enables them to gorge on glucose and in this way, excess sugar leading to obesity and high blood insulin is an important factor in cancer.[175] In this way, too much sugar leading to excess insulin is now firmly linked to the development of cancer of the breast, ovaries, pancreas, biliary tract, lung, gallbladder, stomach and colorectal cancer in humans[176-184]

Tavani *et al.* (2006)[185] studied 2,569 women with breast cancer and 2,588 females without. They found a direct association between breast cancer risk and sugar consumption, a result of an increase in insulin and insulin growth factors. Unsurprisingly, the advice for humans with mammary tumours is to reduce the carbohydrate/sugar content of their diet to effectively nil.

Mammary cancer is the most common form of cancer in dogs by a considerable degree.[167] Of more than 3,000 tumour biopsy specimens received from local veterinarians in the Municipality of Genoa, between 1985 and 2002, mammary cancer accounted for 70% of the female samples.[186] Mammary gland tumours share common features between dogs and humans with authors noting that dogs make excellent models for the development, prognosis and treatment of breast cancer in humans.[167,168] We know dogs maintained on even a relatively low-starch, dry diet (23% starch) exhibit significant increases in blood insulin.[187,188] Dogs fed a low (10%) and moderate (32%) starch diet show a near doubling in plasma insulin release (190 versus 360 pmol/L plasma insulin). Most cereal-based dry foods contain almost twice as much starch as this. This might lead us to suspect that carbohydrates also play a role in the development of this cancer in dogs.

Whatever the cause, studies show that dogs with cancer have reduced tumour growth on diets containing fewer carbohydrates.[31]

The problem is it's complicated to firmly establish whether cancer rates in dogs are increasing due to diet alone, as so many other environmental factors can potentially be muddying the waters. The Veterinary Cancer Society tells us that cancer will play a role in nearly half of canine deaths today with older dogs significantly more likely to get it. This is somewhat as you would expect following a life of high carbohydrate, ultra-processed food products and not to mention the copious amounts of chemical parasite control and annual boosters.

One of the most confounding factors is the effect of various gene pool bottlenecks that so many breeds have passed through. For example, the breeds most affected by cancer include the Boxer, Bernese Mountain Dog, Saint Bernard, Wolfhound, Leonberger, Rottweiler, Staffordshire Bull Terrier, Vizsla, Irish Water Spaniel and Giant Schnauzer.[168] Here, genetics is surely at play. Giant dogs, for instance, the Bernese, St. Bernard, Wolfhound and Leonberger, have each arisen from a handful of individuals, following war and hard economic times. Boxers, Vizslas, Irish Water Spaniels and Giant Schnauzers too, have been reduced to a handful of individuals in the past. The breed most susceptible to cancer is the poor old Golden Retriever. Astoundingly, the Golden Retriever Club of America National Health Survey revealed that an incredible 60% of American Golden Retrievers would suffer cancer[189] compared to 40% of European Golden Retrievers. The worldwide average for UK dogs, as of 2010, is 27% of purebred dogs.[190]

Most certainly, until more is known, if you are the owner of a dog breed at risk of cancer, the best diet is one entirely free of carbohydrates. Should your dog develop cancer, a suitable canine nutritionist will recommend a fresh, species-appropriate diet. This diet will be based on very fatty meat inclusions, fat being the one energy source cancer cannot utilise. This is the keto diet humans are now embarking on. It ensures the body is using ketones from fat, something dogs are known to be remarkably adept at,[191] reducing blood sugars way down, starving the tumour of what it needs to grow. But, please, do not take another step without first holding the hand of a good vet, who is adequately versed in fresh nutrition. You will know you're in safe hands if those hands are not holding out a high-carb diet for your cancer-stricken pet. Or simply check out www.ketopetsanctuary.com. They are possibly the world leaders in the field and, in return for helping you, you donate to their cause, which is rescuing cancer dogs with no hope from pounds. Win-win.

TAKE-HOME POINTS

✓ While they can digest them, at no stage do dogs require carbohydrates in their diet.

✓ Food trials conducted by dry pet food companies show us that, given the choice, dry-fed dogs will consume largely protein and fat with very little carbohydrates for energy (30%, 63% and 7% of their daily MEneeds, respectively). This equates to a protein/fat ME ratio of 1:2.

✓ Mars feed trials revealed that dogs are disinclined to use carbohydrates for energy. Given the option, they will choose higher fat diets initially and choose leaner products over time, possibly in line with a 'feast or famine' mentality.

✓ When ad libitum feed trials are repeated using real ingredients, the protein to fat ME ration becomes a leaner 4:5.

✓ We expect dogs to have evolved upon a very lean diet. If we take a rabbit as the average dog meal, that would be a protein/fat ratio of 4:1, on a DM basis (2:1 on an ME basis), with wild prey expected to be much leaner than rabbit again.

✓ The industry claims carbohydrates are an *excellent* source of energy. Sled dogs perform better without them.

✓ There is no scientific evidence that suggests feeding dogs carbohydrates over the long term is safe. The only scientific evidence offered by a leading veterinary canine nutrition manual in support of feeding dogs high carbohydrate diets was four, old, short studies (over days to weeks) in reproducing bitches, some of which have highly questionable conclusions.

✓ Sled dogs on higher carbohydrate diets have more injuries. High-starch diets stimulate the formation of struvite crystals in cats, while high-protein diets can rectify the issue. Studies show that reducing carbohydrates in the diet prevents tumour growth in dogs.

✓ We have a raging obesity epidemic in humans and in dogs. In humans it's because of high calorie, unfulfilling, high GL, ultra-processed foods. In dogs, we are assured they have nothing to do with it, that we are simply feeding them *too much*.

✓ Dogs share many physiological and metabolic attributes associated with digestion and metabolism in humans, and they respond in the same way physiologically to sugar, so the two can be used interchangeably in the obesity debate.

✓ Obesity is terrible for your health, increasing your risk of diabetes, cancer and inflammatory diseases.

✓ Rapidly digested, calorie dense ultra-processed foods are directly implicated in the human obesity epidemic.

✓ The 'calories-in, calories-out' hypothesis no longer holds. While the cause of obesity is multifaceted, there is nothing more important than *what* you eat.

✓ In relation to obesity, the problem is a blood sugar spike and the subsequent flood of insulin.

✓ The GI is just a measure of how quick a food releases its energy. More accurately here, GL estimates how much a food will raise an individual's blood glucose level after eating it. After sugar in its various forms, rapidly digested carbohydrates such as cooked cereals (corn, wheat, rice) are among the worst offenders.

✓ We overeat (or get lazy) in the hormonal drive to get fat: insulin regulates blood sugar by signalling to the liver, muscle and fat cells to take in glucose. Unfortunately, it also blocks leptin (produced by the fat cells) in the brain, a hormone that normally tells the body you are full.

✓ Obesity in a nut shell: higher GL foods increase the more glycogen you have in the blood, the more blood sugar, the more insulin will be released and the more insulin you have, the more you store fat, and the hungrier you get.

✓ Meat is the lowest GL food you can eat.

✓ Studies suggest carb-based *light* dry food is not the answer to the canine obesity epidemic. As it is still high in carbohydrates, the large part of the diet is still rapidly digested. The higher indigestible-fibre content likely explains the suboptimal intake of nutrients by dogs on such diets, particularly protein.

✓ Studies show higher protein diets (with water) facilitate greater weight loss in pets, retaining lean body mass.

✓ Bloat with torsion is a frightening, often deadly and all too common infliction of pet dogs today. However, while your dog's physical shape may load the gun, it is bloat that pulls the trigger. The question is: why are their stomachs filling with gas?

✓ Studies show bloat is not aerophagia (air in from the mouth) but fermentation gas coming up from the intestines.

✓ Authors suspect it is something in dry food. Studies show using less dry foods reduces the risk of GDV in dogs, as does selecting dry foods with more meat in them.

✓ The chief suspects for GDV in dogs are the fibrous plant fillers used so liberally by the dry pet food industry.

✓ There is no evidence resting before or after a meal helps.

✓ Studies show bloat gas is not a result of aerophagia (air in from the mouth) but fermentation gas from the intestines. Hence, there is no established link between speed of eating or high feed stations.

✓ Numerous authors link the increased incidence of bloat to dry feeding. Studies show feeding less dry food reduces the risk of GDV in dogs, as does adding more real, meat-based ingredients such as fish or eggs.

✓ The chief dietary ingredient suspect for GDV in dogs is plant fibre. Both soluble and insoluble fibre slows the passage of digesta through the intestines. Soluble fibre then is then digested by bacteria, resulting in gas production.

✓ Ingredients such as corn but also beet pulp, and soybean meal are high in both soluble and insoluble fibre.

✓ The fibre content you see on a pet food label is crude fibre. That is the indigestible (insoluble) fibre content. Total dietary fibre is a measure of both digestible (soluble) and indigestible fibre. It is more accurate and appropriate but it is expensive, so it is not offered by pet food manufacturers.

✓ Higher fibre diets require more manual contractions of the gut, increasing gut weight. Higher gut weights are a risk factor for GDV in dogs.

✓ Until we know more, it is advised to feed at-risk breeds less plant fibre.

✓ Chronic pancreatitis in dogs is most likely explained by poor diet. The veterinary industry believes hyperlipidaemia (excess fat in the blood) is caused by eating fat. It's not. This belief results in the advice that even the 'fat off your steak' can cause the disease. This is incorrect. Your dog should be able to cope with that bit of fat.

✓ Chronic pancreatitis in dogs is likely caused by a diet high in carbohydrates. It causes your body to run on sugar, using the glycolytic energy system and not the fatty-acid oxidation system. The result is the more carbohydrates that are consumed, the more fatty acids build in the blood.

✓ The lack of vitamin E in ultra-processed pet food and the need of it in dogs with pancreatitis is likely an exaggerating factor for pancreatitis in dogs.

✓ Only 5–10% of all human cancer cases are linked to genetic defects at birth.

✓ Tumours are carbohydrate junkies. They use glucose 10–20 times more than normal cells.

✓ Tumours also have a great number of insulin receptors, as insulin is the growth hormone.

✓ Diets high in carbohydrates mean blood full of sugar and insulin.

✓ The advice for human cancer patients is reduce carbohydrate content immediately.

✓ As in humans, carbohydrates are shown to spike canine blood insulin.

✓ Studies show dogs have reduced tumour growth on lower carbohydrate foods.

✓ Despite their potential for harm, particularly in a meat eater, Association of American Feed Control Officials continues to leave carbs and sugar out as requirements for ultra-processed pet food labels. Manufacturers are free to use as much as they like.

Chapter Six References

1   Sillero-Zubiri, C., Hoffmann, M. and MacDonald, D.W. (2004). *Canids: Foxes, wolves, jackals and dogs. Status survey and conservation action plan*. Gland, Switzerland: IUCN

2   National Research Council (NRC) (2006). *Nutrient requirement of dogs and cats*. Washington, DC: National Academies Press

3   American Association of Feed Control Officials (AAFCO, 2008). *Dog and Cat Food Nutrient Profiles*. Official Publication

4   Belo, P.S., Romsos, D.R. and Leveille, G.A. (1976). Influence of Diet on Glucose Tolerance, on the Rate of Glucose Utilization and on Gluconeogenic Enzyme Activities in the Dog. The Journal of Nutrition, 106(10): 1465–1474

5   Romsos, D.R., Belo, P.S., Bennink, M.R. *et al.* (1976). Effects of Dietary Carbohydrate, Fat and Protein on Growth, Body Composition and Blood Metabolite Levels in the Dog. The Journal of Nutrition, 106(10): 1452–1464

6   Hore, P. and Messer, M. (1968). Studies on disaccharidase activities of the small intestine of the domestic cat and other carnivorous mammals. Comparative Biochemistry and Physiology, 24:717–725

7   Romsos, D.H., Palmer, H.J., Muiruri, K.L. and Bennink, M.R. (1981). Influence of a low carbohydrate diet on performance of pregnant and lactating dogs. Journal of Nutrition, 111: 678–689

8   Murray, S.M., Flickinger, A.E., Patil, A.R. *et al.* (2001). *In vitro* fermentation characteristics of native and processed cereal grains and potato starch using ileal chyme from dogs. Journal of Animal Science, 79: 435–444

9   Hewson-Hughes, A.K., Hewson-Hughesa, V.L., Colyera, A. *et al.* (2013). Geometric analysis of macronutrient selection in breeds of the domestic dog, *Canis lupus familiaris*. Behavioral Ecology, 24(1): 293–304

10   Bosch, G., Hagen-Plantinga, E.A. and Hendriks, W.H. (2015). Dietary nutrient profiles of wild wolves: insights for optimal dog nutrition? British Journal of Nutrition, 113: S40–S54

11   Dierenfeld, E.S., Alcorn, H.L. and Jacobsen, K.L. (2002). *Nutrient Composition of Whole Vertebrate Prey (Excluding Fish) Fed in Zoos*. U.S. Department of Agriculture. Available at www.researchgate.net

12   Plantinga, E.A., Bosch, G. and Hendriks, W.H. (2011). Estimation of the dietary nutrient profile of free-roaming feral cats: possible implications for nutrition of domestic cats. British Journal of Nutrition, 106(S112): 35–48

13   McWilliams, S. (2013). Non-destructive techniques to assess body composition of birds: A review and validation study. Journal of Ornithology, 154(3): 597–618

14   Roberts, M.T., Bermingham, E.N., Cave, N. J. *et al.* (2018). Macronutrient intake of dogs, self-selecting diets varying in composition offered *ad libitum*. Journal of Animal Physiology and Animal Nutrition, 102(2): 568–575

15 Kronfeld, D.S., Hammel, E.P., Ramberg, C.F. Jr. *et al.* (1977). Hematological and metabolic responses to training in racing sled dogs fed diets containing medium, low or zero carbohydrate. American Journal of Clinical Nutrition, 30: 419–430

16 Hewson-Hughes, A.K., Gilham, M.S., Upton, S. *et al.* (2011a). The effect of dietary starch level on postprandial glucose and insulin concentrations in cats and dogs. British Journal of Nutrition, 106(1): S105–9.

17 Hewson-Hughes, A.K., Hewson-Hughes, V.L., Colyer, A. *et al.* (2013). Geometric analysis of macronutrient selection in breeds of the domestic dog, *Canis lupus familiaris*. Behavioral Ecology, 24(1): 293–304

18 Kronfeld, D.S. (1973). Diet and the performance of racing sled dogs. Journal of the American Veterinary Medical Association, 162(6): 470–473

19 Hinchcliff, K.W., Reinhart, G.A., Burr, J.R. *et al.* (1997). Metabolizable energy intake and sustained energy expenditure of Alaskan sled dogs during heavy exertion in the cold. American Journal of Veterinary Research, 58(12): 1457–1462

20 Loftus, J.P, Yazwinski, M., Milizio, J.G. *et al.* (2014). Energy requirements for racing endurance sled dogs. Journal of Nutritional Science, 3: e34

21 Murray, S.M., Sunvold, G.D. (2003). *Carbohydrates for Dogs. Carbohydrate puzzle: what's in it for my dog?* Presented at the Iams Breeder' Symposium, 2002–2003 Edition

22 Baker, D.H. and Czarnecki-Maulden, G.L. (1991). Comparative Nutrition of Cats and Dogs. Annual Review, 11: 239–263

23 Longland, A.C, Theodorou, M.K. and Burger, I.H. (2000). *The nutrition of companion animals.* In M. K. Theodorou and J. France (Eds.), Feeding systems and feed evaluation models. Wallingford, UK: CABI.

24 Prothero, J. (1995). Bone and fat as a function of bodyweight in adult mammals. Comparitive Biochemistry and Physiology, 111: 633–639

25 Blaza, S.E., Booles, D. and Burger, I.H. (1989). *Is carbohydrate essential for pregnancy and lactation in dogs?* Nutrition of the Dog and Cat. Waltham Symposium No. 7. Cambridge University Press, Cambridge, pp229–242

26 Lindsay, S., Entenman, C. and Chaikoff, I.L. (1948). Pancreatitis accompanying hepatic disease in dogs fed a high fat, low protein diet. Archives of Pathology, 45: 635–638

27 Hand, M.S., Thatcher, C.D., Remillard, R.L. *et al.* (2010). *Small Animal Clinical Nutrition*, 5th Edition. Topeka, KS: The Mark Morris Institute, Kansas, U.S.

28 Kienzle, E., Meyer, H. and Lohrie H. (1985). Influence of carbohydrate free rations with various protein/energy relationships on foetal development, viability of newborn puppies and milk composition. Advances in Animal Physiology and Animal Nutrition, 16: 78–99

29 Reynolds, A.J., Taylor, C.R., Hoppler, H. *et al.* (1996). *The effect of diet on sled dog performance, oxidative capacity, skeletal muscle microstucture, and muscle glycogen metabolism.* In: Carey, D.P., Norton, S.A., Bolser, S.M., eds. Recent Advances in Canine and Feline Nutritional Research: Proceedings of the 1996 Iams International Nutrition Symposium. Wilmington, OH: Orange Frazer Press, p181–198

30 Funaba, M., Uchiyama, A., Takahashi, K. *et al.*(2004). Evaluation of effects of dietary carbohydrate on formation of struvite crystals in urine and macromineral balance in clinically normal cats. American Journal of Veterinary Research, 65(2):138–142

31 Ogilvie, G.K. (1998). Interventional nutrition for the cancer patient. Clinical Techniques in Small Animal Practice, 13(4): 224–231

32 Kienzle E (1993) Carbohydrate metabolism of the cat. 1. Activity of amylase in the gastrointestinal tract of the cat. Journal of Animal Physiology and Animal Nutrition, 69: 92–101

33 Axelsson, E., Ratnakumar, A., Arendt, M.L. *et al.* (2013). The genomic signature of dog domestication reveals adaptation to a starch-rich diet. Nature, 495: 360–364

34 Botigué, L.R., Shiya, S., Scheu, A. *et al.* (2017). Ancient European dog genomes reveal continuity since the Early Neolithic. Nature Communications. 8: 16082

35 Washizu, T., Tanaka, A., Sako, T. *et al.* (1999) Comparison of the activities of enzymes related to glycolysis and gluconeogenesis in the liver of dogs and cats. Research in Veterinary Science, 67: 205–206

36 Wang, G.D., Zhai, W., Yang, H.C. *et al.* (2013). The genomics of selection in dogs and the parallel evolution between dogs and humans. Nature Communications, 4(1860)

37 Day, M.J. (2005). The canine model of dietary hypersensitivity. Journal of the Nutrition Society, 64: 458–464

38 Nguyen, P., Dumon, H., Biourge, V. *et al.* (1998). Glycemic and insulinemic responses after ingestion of commercial foods in healthy dogs: Influence of food composition. Journal of Nutrition, 128:2654S–2658S

39 Carciofi, A.C., Takakura, F.S., de-Oliveira, L.D. *et al.* (2008). Effects of six carbohydrate sources on dog diet digestibility and post-prandial glucose and insulin response. Journal of Animal Physiology and Animal Nutrition (Berlin), 92(3): 326–336

40 Elliott, K.F., Rand, J.S., Fleeman, L.M. *et al.* (2012). A diet lower in digestible carbohydrate results in lower postprandial glucose concentrations compared with a traditional canine diabetes diet and an adult maintenance diet in healthy dogs. Research in Veterinary Science, 93: 288–295

41 Hales, C.M. Margaret D., Carroll, D. *et al.* (2017). *Prevalence of Obesity Among Adults and Youth: United States, 2015–2016.* NCHS Data Brief #288

42 Preston, S.H., Vierboom, Y.C. and Stokes, A. (2018). *The role of obesity in exceptionally slow US mortality improvement.* Proceedings of the National Academy of Sciences

43 Spieker, E.A. and Pyzocha, N. (2016). *Economic Impact of Obesity.* Primary Care: Clinics in Office Practice. 43(1): 83–95

44 Flegal, K.M., Carroll, M.D., Ogden, C.L. *et al.* (2002). Prevalence and trends in obesity among US adults, 1999-2000. The Journal of the American Medical Association, 288: 1723–1727

45 PAHO (2015). Ultra-processed food and drink products in Latin America: Trends, impact on obesity, policy implications. Published on the Pan American Health Organisation website, www.paho.org

46   Kelly, B. and Jacoby, E. (2018). Special issue on ultra-processed foods. Public Health Nutrition, 21(1)

47   Monteiro, C., Moubarac, J., Levy, R. *et al.* (2017). Household availability of ultra-processed foods and obesity in nineteen European countries. Public Health Nutrition, 1–9

48   Lopomo, A., Burgio, E. and Migliore, L. (2016). Epigenetics of Obesity. Progress in Molecular Biology and Translational Science, 140: 151–184

49   Ridaura, V.K., Faith, J.J., Rey, F.E. *et al.* (2013). Gut microbiota from twins discordant for obesity modulate metabolism in mice. Science, 341:1079–U1049

50   Ravussin, E., Beyl, R.A., Poggiogalle, E. *et al.* (2019). Early Time-Restricted Feeding Reduces Appetite and Increases Fat Oxidation But Does Not Affect Energy Expenditure in Humans. Obesity, 27: 1244–1254

51   Khan, Z., Combadière, C., Authier, F.J. (2013). Slow CCL2-dependent translocation of biopersistent particles from muscle to brain. BMC Medicine, 4(11): 99

52   Te Morenga, L., Mallard, S. and Mann, J. (2013). Dietary sugars and body weight: systematic review and meta-analyses of randomised controlled trials and cohort studies. The British Medical Journal, 346(7492)

53   Malik, V.S., Schulze, M.B., Hu, F.B. *et al.* (2006). Intake of sugar-sweetened beverages and weight gain: a systematic review. American Journal of Clinical Nutrition, 84: 274–288

54   Malik, V.S., Popkin, B.M., Bray, G.A. *et al.* (2010). Sugar-sweetened beverages and risk of metabolic syndrome and type 2 diabetes: a meta-analysis. Diabetes Care, 33(11): 2477–2483

55   Cust, A.E., Slimani, N., Kaaks, R. *et al.* (2007). Dietary carbohydrates, glycemic index, glycemic load, and endometrial cancer risk within the European Prospective Investigation into Cancer and Nutrition cohort. American Journal of Epidemiology, 166: 912–923

56   Drake, I., Sonestedt, E., Gullberg, B. *et al.* (2012). Dietary intakes of carbohydrates in relation to prostate cancer risk: a prospective study in the Malmö diet and cancer cohort. American Journal of Clinical Nutrition, 96: 1409–1418

57   Ferdman, A. (2015). *Where people around the world eat the most sugar and fat.* Washington Post. Available at www.washingtonpost.com

58   Mullin, G.E. and Swift, C.M. (2011). *The Inside Tract: Your Good Gut Guide to Great Digestive Health.* Rodale PA

59   Bertoia, M.L, Mukamal, K.J., Cahill, L.E. *et al.* (2015). Changes in Intake of Fruits and Vegetables and Weight Change in United States Men and Women Followed for Up to 24 Years: Analysis from Three Prospective Cohort Studies. PLOS Medicine 13(1): e1001956

60   Ye, E.Q., Chacko, S.A., Chou, E.L. *et al.* (2012). Greater whole-grain intake is associated with lower risk of type 2 diabetes, cardiovascular disease, and weight gain. Journal of Nutrition, 142: 1304–1313

61   Yang, H., Costenbader, K.H., Gao, X. *et al.* (2014). Sugar-sweetened soda consumption and risk of developing rheumatoid arthritis in women. American Journal of Clinical Nutrition, 100(3): 959–967

62 Knüppel, A., Shipley, M.J., Llewellyn, C.H. *et al.* (2017). Sugar intake from sweet food and beverages, common mental disorder and depression: prospective findings from the Whitehall II study. Scientific Reports, 7(6287)

63 Liu, S., Willett, W.C., Manson, J.A.E. *et al.* (2003). Relation between changes in intakes of dietary fiber and grain products and changes in weight and development of obesity among middle-aged women. American Journal of Clinical Nutrition, 78:920–927

64 Koh-Banerjee, P., Franz, M., Sampson, L. *et al.* (2004). Changes in whole-grain, bran, and cereal fiber consumption in relation to 8-y weight gain among men. American Journal of Clinical Nutrition, 80: 1237–1245

65 De Munter, J.S.L., Hu, F.B., Spiegelman, D. *et al.* (2007). Whole grain, bran, and germ intake and risk of type 2 diabetes: a prospective cohort study and systematic review. PLOS Medicine, 4: e261

66 Aune, D., Chan, D., Greenwood, D. *et al.* (2012). Dietary fiber and breast cancer risk: a systematic review and meta-analysis of prospective studies. Annals of Oncology, 23: 1394–1402

67 Post, R.E., Mainous, A.G., King, D.E. *et al.* (2012). Dietary fiber for the treatment of type 2 diabetes mellitus: a meta-analysis. Journal of the American Board of Family Medicine, 25: 16–23

68 Taubes, G. (2011). *Why we get fat: and what to do about it.* Anchor

69 Wade, G.N. (1972). Gonadal hormones and behavioral regulation of body weight. Physiology and Behaviour, 8(3): 523–34

70 Lund, E.M., Armstrong, J.P., Kirk, C.A. *et al.* (2006). Prevalence and risk factors for obesity in adult dogs from private US veterinary practices. Journal of Applied Research Veterinary Medicine, 4(2): 177–186.

71 Kellerer, M., Lammers, R., Fritsche, A. *et al.* (2001). Insulin inhibits leptin receptor signalling in HEK293 cells at the level of janus kinase-2: a potential mechanism for hyperinsulinaemia-associated leptin resistance. Diabetologia, 44(9): 1125–32

72 Lustig, R.H., Sen, S., Soberman, J.E. *et al.* (2004). Obesity, leptin resistance, and the effects of insulin reduction. International Journal of Obesity, 28: 1344–1348

73 Dehghan, M., Mente, A., Zhang, X. *et al.* (2017). Associations of fats and carbohydrate intake with cardiovascular disease and mortality in 18 countries from five continents (PURE): a prospective cohort study. The Lancet, 390(10107): 2050–2062

74 Miller, V., Mente, A., Dehghan, M. *et al.* (2017). Fruit, vegetable, and legume intake, and cardiovascular disease and deaths in 18 countries (PURE): a prospective cohort study. The Lancet, 390(10107): 2037–2049

75 Edney, A.T.B. and Smith, P.M. (1986). Study of obesity in dogs visiting veterinary practices in the United Kingdom. Veterinary Record, 118: 391–396

76 German, A.J., Woods, G.R.T., Holden, S.L. *et al.* (2018). Small animal health: Dangerous trends in pet obesity. Veterinary Record, 182(1): 25

77 Mars Banfield (2012). *State of Pet Health 2012 Report.* Banfield Pet Hospital Publication. Available at www.banfield.com

78 Ostoa, M. and Lutza, T.A. (2015). Translational value of animal models of obesity—Focus on dogs and cats. European Journal of Pharmacology, 759(15): 240–252

79 Kasstrom, H. (1975). Nutrition, weight gain and development of hip dysplasia. Acta Radiologica, 334: S135–179

80 Kealy, R.D., Olsson, S.E., Monti, K.L. et al. (1992). Effects of limited food consumption on the incidence of hip dysplasia. Journal of the American Veterinary Medical Association, 201: 857–863

81 German, A.J. (2006). The growing problem of obesity in dogs and cats. Journal of Nutrition, 136: 1940S–1946S

82 Fascetti, A.J. and Delaney, S.J. (2012). Applied Veterinary Clinical Nutrition. John Wiley and Sons. Chapter 10. Nutritional Management of Orthopaedic Diseases by Herman Hazelwinkel

83 Lim, H.Y., Im, K.S., Kim, N.H. et al. (2015). Effects of Obesity and Obesity-Related Molecules on Canine Mammary Gland Tumors. Veterinary Pathology, 52: 1045–1051

84 Golay, A. and Ybarra, J. (2005). Link between obesity and type 2 diabetes. Best Practice Research Clinical Endocrinology Metabolism, 19(4): 649–663

85 Bloom, C.A. and Rand, J. (2014). Feline diabetes mellitus: clinical use of long-acting glargine and detemir. Journal of Feline Medical Surgery, 16(3): 205–215

86 Sparkes, A.H., Cannon, M., Church, D. et al. (2015). ISFM consensus guidelines on the practical management of diabetes mellitus in cats. Journal of Feline Medical Surgery, 17(3): 235–250

87 Hoenig, M. (2002). Comparative aspects of diabetes mellitus in dogs and cats. Molecular and Cellular Endocrinology, 197(1–2): 221–229

88 Guptill, L., Glickman, L. and Glickman, N. (2003). Time Trends and Risk Factors for Diabetes Mellitus in Dogs: Analysis of Veterinary Medical Data Base Records (1970–1999). The Veterinary Journal, 165(3): 240–247

89 Fleeman, L. and Rand, J. (2005). Beyond insulin therapy: Achieving optimal control in diabetic dogs. Brisbane, Australia: Centre for Companion Animal Health, University of Queensland

90 Banfield (2016). State of pet health report. Published online https://www.banfield.com/banfield/media/pdf/downloads/soph/banfield-state-of-pet-health-report-2016.pdf

91 Catchpole, B., Ristic, J.M., Fleeman, L.M. and Davison, L.J. (2005). Canine diabetes mellitus: Can old dogs teach us new tricks? Diabetologia, 48(10): 1948–1956

92 Kimmel, S.E., Michel, K.E., Hess, R.S. et al. (2000). Effects of insoluble and soluble dietary fiber on glycemic control in dogs with naturally occurring insulin-dependent diabetes mellitus. Journal of the American Veterinary Medical Association, 216(7):

93 Graham, P.A, Maskell, E., Rawlings, J.M. et al. (2002). Influence of a high fibre diet on glycaemic control and quality of life in dogs with diabetes mellitus. Journal of Small Animal Practice, 43(2): 67–73

94 Bennett N., Greco, D.S., Peterson, M.E. *et al.* (2006). Comparison of a low carbohydrate-low fiber diet and a moderate carbohydrate-high fiber diet in the management of feline diabetes mellitus. Journal of Feline Medical Surgery, 2006 Apr;8(2):73–84.

95 Zoran, D.L. and Rand, J.S. (2013) The role of diet in the prevention and management of feline diabetes. Veterinary Clinical North American Small Animal Practice, 43(2): 233–243

96 Kirk, C.A. (2006). Feline diabetes mellitus: low carbohydrates versus high fiber? Veterinary Clinics of North America and Small Anim Practices, 36(6):1297–1306

97 Freeman, L.M., Abood, S.K., Fascetti, A.J. *et al.* (2006). Disease prevalence among dogs and cats in the United States and Australia and proportions of dogs and cats that receive therapeutic diets or dietary supplements. Journal of American Veterinary Medical Association, 229(4): 531–534

98 Hahn, K.A. and Meyer H. (2013). Evidence-based nutrition for obesity management and weight gain prevention. Hill's Global Symposium on Obesity, pp26–28

99 Weber, M., Bissot, T., Servet, E. *et al.* (2007). A High-Protein, High-Fiber Diet Designed for Weight Loss Improves Satiety in Dogs. Journal of Veterinary Internal Medicine, 21(6): 1203–1208

100 Burkholder, W. J. and Bauer, J. E. (1998) Foods and techniques for managing obesity in companion animals. Journal of American Veterinary Medical Association, 212: 658–662.

101 Zentek J. (1995). Observations on the apparent digestibility of copper, iron, zinc and magnesium in dogs. Deutsche tierarztliche Wochenschrift, 102(8): 310–315.

102 Ko, K.S. and Fascetti, A.J. (2016). Dietary beet pulp decreases taurine status in dogs fed low protein diet. Journal of Animal Science and Technology, 58: 29

103 Cameron, K.M., Morris, P.J., Hackett, R. M. *et al.* (2011). The effects of increasing water content to reduce the energy density of the diet on body mass changes following caloric restriction in domestic cats. Journal of Animal Physiology and Animal Nutrition, 95(3): 399–408

104 Hannah, S.S. and Laflamme, D.P. (1998). Increased dietary protein spares lean body mass during weight loss in dogs. Journal of Veterinary International Medicine, 12: 224

105 Hannah, S. (1999). Role of dietary protein in weight management. Compendium on Continuing Education for the Practicing Veterinarian, 21: 32–33

106 Diez, M., Nguyen, P., Jeusette, I, *et al.* (2002). Weight loss in obese dogs: Evaluation of a high-protein, low-carbohydrate diet. Journal of Nutrition, 132: 1685S–1687S

107 Blanchard, G., Nguyen, P., Gayet, C. *et al.* (2004). Rapid weight loss with a high-protein low-energy diet allows the recovery of ideal body composition and insulin sensitivity in obese dogs. Journal of Nutrition, 134: 2148S–2150S

108 German, A.J., Holden, S.L., Bissot, T. *et al.* (2010). A high protein high fibre diet improves weight loss in obese dogs. Veterinary Journal, 183: 294–297

109 Laflamme, D.P. and Hannah, S.S. (2005). Increased dietary protein promotes fat loss and reduces loss of lean body mass during weight loss in cats. International Journal of Applied Research in Veterinary Medicine, 3(2): 62–68

110   Wadden, T.A., Stunkard, A.J., Brownell, K.D. *et al.* (1985). A comparison of two very-low-calorie diets: Protein-sparing-modified fast versus protein-formula liquid diet. American Journal of Clinical Nutrition, 41: 533–539

111   Young, V.R. and Marchini, J.S. (1990). Mechanisms and nutritional significance of metabolic responses to altered intakes of protein and amino acids, with reference to nutritional adaptation in humans. American Journal of Clinical Nutrition, 51: 270–289

112   Bierer, T.L. and Bui, L.M. (2004). High-protein low-carbohydrate diets enhance weight loss in dogs. The Journal of Nutrition, 134(8): 2087S–2089S

113   Raghavan, M., Glickman, N., McCabe, G. *et al.* (2004). Diet-related risk factors for gastric dilatation-volvulus in dogs of high-risk breeds. Journal of American Animal Hospital Association, 40(3): 192–203

114   Glickman, L.T., Glickman, N.W., Pérez, C.M. *et al.* (1994). Analysis of risk factors for gastric dilatation and dilatation-volvulus in dogs. Journal of the American Veterinary Medical Association, 204: 1465–1471

115   Neill (2015). *Australian Great Dane Health and Lifestyle Survey*. Available at www.australiangreatdanehealthsurvey.com

116   Evans, K.M. and Adams, V.J. (2010). Mortality and morbidity due to gastric dilatation-volvulus syndrome in pedigree dogs in the UK. J Small Anim Pract 51:376–381

117   Brockman, D.J., Washabau, R.J. and Drobatz, K.J. (1995). Canine gastric dilatation/volvulus syndrome in a veterinary critical care unit: 295 cases (1986–1992). Journal of the American Veterinary Medical Association, 207: 460–464

118   Evans, K.M. and Adams, V.J. (2010). Mortality and morbidity due to gastric dilatation-volvulus syndrome in pedigree dogs in the UK. Journal of Small Animal Practice, 51: 376–381

119   Schaible, R.H., Ziech, J., Glickman, N.W. *et al.* (1997). Predisposition to gastric dilatation-volvulus in relation to genetics of thoracic conformation in Irish setters. Journal of the American Animal Hospital Association, 33:n379–383

120   Glickman, L.T., Glickman, N.W., Schellenberg, D.B. *et al.* (2000). Non-dietary risk factors for gastric dilatation-volvulus in large and giant breed dogs. Journal of the American Veterinary Medical Association, 217(10): 1492–1499

121   Schellenberg, D., Yi, Q., Glickman, N.W. *et al.* (1998). Influence of thoracic conformation and genetics on the risk of gastric dilatation-volvulus in Irish setters. Journal of the American Animal Hospital Association, 34: 64–73

122   Glickman, L.T., Glickman, N.W., Schellenberg, D.B. *et al.* (2000b). Incidence of and breed-related risk factors for gastric dilatation-volvulus in dogs. Journal of the American Animal Hospital Association, 216: 40–45

123   Theyse, L.F., van de Brom, W.E. and van Sluijs, F.J. (1998). Small size of food particles and age as risk factors for gastric dilatation volvulus in Great Danes. Veterinary Record, 143: 48–50

124   Elwood, C.M. (1998). Risk factors for gastric dilatation in Irish setter dogs. Journal of Small Animal Practice, 39: 185–190

125 Glickman, L.T., Glickman, N.W., Schellenberg, D.B. *et al.* (2000a). Non-dietary risk factors for gastric dilatation-volvulus in large and giant breed dogs. Journal of the American Veterinary Medical Association, 217(10): 1492–1499

126 Glickman, L.T., Glickman, N.W., Schellenberg, D.B. *et al.* (1997). Multiple risk factors for the gastric dilatation-volvulus syndrome in dogs: a practitioner/ owner case-control study. Journal of the American Animal Hospital Association, 33: 197–204

127 Uhrikova, I., Machackova, K. Rauserova-Lexmaulova, L. *et al.* (2015). Risk factors for gastric dilatation and volvulus in central Europe: an internet survey. Veterinarni Medicina, 60(10): 578–587

128 Van Kruiningen, H.J., Gargamelli, C., Havier, J. (2013). Stomach Gas Analyses in Canine Acute Gastric Dilatation with Volvulus. Journal of Veterinary Internal Medicine, 27(5): 1260–1261

129 Buckley, L.A. (2016). Are dogs that eat quickly more likely to develop a gastric dilatation (+/- Volvulus) than dogs that eat slowly? Veterinary Evidence, 1(4): Knowledge summaries

130 Manichanh, C., Eck, A., Varela, E. *et al.* (2014). Anal gas evacuation and colonic microbiota in patients with flatulence: Effect of diet. Gut, 63(3): 401–408

131 Hullar, M.J.H., Lampe, J.W., and Harkey, M.A. (2018). The canine gut microbiome is associated with higher risk of gastric dilatation-volvulus and high risk genetic variants of the immune system. PLoS One, 13(6): e0197686.

132 Van Kruiningen, H.J., Gregoire, K. and Meuten, D.J. (1974). Acute gastric dilatation: a review of comparative aspects, by species, and a study in dogs and monkeys. Journal of the American Animal Hospital Association, 10: 294–324

133 Kronfeld, D. (1979). Common questions about the nutrition of dogs and cats. Compendium on Continuing Education for the Practising Veterinarian, 1: 33–42

134 Morgan, R.V. (1982). Acute gastric dilatation-volvulus syndrome. Compendium on Continuing Education for the Practising Veterinarian, 4: 677–682

135 Raghavan, M., Glickman, N.W. and Glickman, L.T. (2006). The effect of ingredients in dry dog foods on the risk of gastric dilatation–volvulus in dogs. Journal of the American Animal Hospital Association, 42: 28–36

136 Bell, J.S. (2013). Inherited and Predisposing Factors in the Development of Gastric Dilatation Volvulus in Dogs. Topics in Companion Animal Medicine, 29(3): 60-63

137 Pipan, M., Brown, D.C., Battaglia, C.L. *et al.* (2012). An Internet-based survey of risk factors for surgical gastric dilatation-volvulus in dogs. Journal of American Veterinary Medicine Association, 240: 1456–1462

138 Russell, J. and Bass, P. (1985). Canine gastric emptying of fiber meals: influence of meal viscosity and antroduodenal motility Gastrointestinal and Liver Physiology, 249(6): G662–G667

139 Van Kruiningen, H.J., Wojan, L.D., Stake, P.E. *et al.* (1987). The influence of diet and feeding frequency on gastric function in the dog. Journal of American Animal Hospital Association, 23: 145–153

140 Hall, J.A., Willer, R.L., Seim, H.B. *et al.* (1995). Gross and histologic evaluation of hepatogastric ligaments in clinically normal dogs and dogs with gastric dilatation-volvulus. American Journal of Veterinary Research, 56(12): 1611–1614

141 Yamka, R.M., Harmon, D.L., Schoenherr, W.D. *et al.* (2006). In vivo measurement of flatulence and nutrient digestibility in dogs fed poultry by-product meal, conventional soybean meal, and low-oligosaccharide low-phytate soybean meal. American Journal of Veterinary Research, 67: 88–94

142 Russel, T.J. (1998). *The effect of natural source of non-digestible oligosaccharides on the fecal microflora of the dog and effects on digestion.* St. Joseph, Mo. Friskies R&D Center

143 Howard, M.D., Kerley, M.S., Sunvold, G.D. *et al.* (2000). Source of dietary fiber fed to dogs affects nitrogen and energy metabolism and intestinal microflora populations. Nutrition Research, 20(10): 1473–1484

144 Bueno, L., Praddaude, F., Fioramonti, J. *et al.* (1981). Effect of dietary fiber on gastrointestinal motility and jejunal transit time in dogs. Gastroenterology, 80(4): 701–707.

145 Ettinger, S., Feldman, J. and Edward, C. (1995). *Textbook of veterinary internal medicine* (4th ed.). Philadelphia, PA: Saunders

146 Yadav, D. and Lowenfels, A.B. (2013). The Epidemiology of Pancreatitis and Pancreatic Cancer. Gastroenterology, 144(6): 1252–1261

147 Panagiotis, X.G., Suchodolski, J.S. and Steiner, J.M. (2008). *Chronic pancreatitis in dogs and cats.* College Station, TX: Department of Small Animal Clinical Sciences, Texas A&M University

148 Watson, P.J., Roulois, A.J., Scase, T. *et al.* (2007). Prevalence and breed distribution of chronic pancreatitis at post-mortem examination in first-opinion dogs. Journal of Small Animal Practice, 48(11): 609–618

149 Newman, S. J. and Woosley, K. (2004). Localization of pancreatic inflammation and necrosis in dogs. Journal of Veterinary Internal Medicine, 18: 488–493

150 Owens, J.M., Drazner, F.H. and Gilbertson, S.R. (1975). Pancreatic disease in the cat. Journal of the American Animal Hospital Association, 11: 83–89

151 Macy, D.W. (1989). Feline pancreatitis. In R. W. Kirk (Ed.), Current veterinary therapy: Small animal practice. Philadelphia, PA: Saunders, pp893–896

152 Steiner, J.M. and Williams, D.A. (1997). Feline pancreatitis. Compendium on the Continuing Education of Veterinary Practitioners, 19: 590–603

153 De Cock, H.E.V., Forman, M.A. and Farver, B. (2007). Prevalence and histopathologic characteristics of pancreatitis in cats. Veterinary Pathology, 44: 39–49

154 Kim, J., Jung, D., Kang, B. *et al.* (2005). Canine exocrine pancreatic insufficiency treated with porcine pancreatic extract. Journal of Veterinary Science, 6(3): 263–266

155 The Expert Panel (1986). Report of the National Cholesterol Education program. Expert Panel on Detection, Evaluation, and Treatment of High Blood Cholesterol in Adults. Archives of Internal Medicine, 148: 36–69

156 Seales, C.E. and Ooi, T.C. (1992). Underrecognition of chylomicronemia as a cause of acute pancreatitis. Canadian Medical Association Journal, 147: 1806–1808

157 Noakes, T.D., and Windt, J. (2016). Evidence that supports the prescription of low-carbohydrate high-fat diets: a narrative review. British Journal of Sports Medicine, 51:133–139

158 Gifford, B. (2016). *The Silencing of Tim Noakes*. Published online Dec 8th https://www. outsideonline.com/2140271/silencing-low-carb-rebel

159 Mittendorfer, B. and Sidossis, L.S. (2001). Mechanism for the increase in plasma triacylglycerol concentrations after consumption of short-term, high-carbohydrate diets. The American Journal of Clinical Nutrition, 73(5): 892–899

160 Parks, E.J. (2001). Effect of Dietary Carbohydrate on Triglyceride Metabolism in Humans. The Journal of Nutrition, 131(10): 2772S–2774S

161 Algya, K.M., Cross, T.L., Leuck, K.N. *et al.* (2018). Apparent total-tract macronutrient digestibility, serum chemistry, urinalysis, and faecal characteristics, metabolites and microbiota of adult dogs fed extruded, mildly cooked, and raw diets. Journal of Animal Science, 96(9): 3670–3683

162 Kalvaria, I., Labadarios, D., Shephard, G.S. *et al.* (1986). Biochemical vitamin E deficiency in chronic pancreatitis. International Journal of Pancreatology, 1(2): 119–128

163 Hoffmann LaRoche, F.T. and Nutley, N.J. (1995). Paper presented at the Science and Technology Center, Hill's Pet Nutrition, Inc, Topeka, KS, on vitamin stability in canned and extruded pet food, 1995

164 Rankovic, A., Adolphe, J.L., and Verbrugghe, A. (2019). Role of carbohydrates in the health of dogs. Journal of American Veterinary Medical Association, 255(5):546–554

165 Schiffman, J.D. and Breen, M. (2015). Comparative oncology: what dogs and other species can teach us about humans with cancer. Philosophical Transactions of the Royal Society B: Biological Sciences, 370(1673): 20140231

166 Rowell, J.L, McCarthy, D.O. and Alvarez, C.E. (2011). Dog Models of Naturally Occurring Cancer. Trends in Molecular Medicine, 17(7): 380–388

167 Moe, L. (2001). Population-based incidence of mammary tumors in some dog breeds. Journal of Reproducitve Fertility Supplement, 57: 439–443

168 Dobson, J. (2012). Breed dispositions to cancer in pedigree dogs. ISRN Veterinary Medicine, 1–23

169 Anand, P., Kunnumakkara, A.B., Sundaram, C. *et al.* (2008). Cancer is a preventable disease that requires major lifestyle changes. Pharmacology Research, 25: 2097–2116

170 Stewart, B.W. and Wild, C.P. (2014). "Ch. 2: Cancer Etiology: Diet, obesity and physical activity". World Cancer Report 2014. World Health Organization, pp124–33

171 Bäck, K. (2011). Interaction between insulin and IGF-I receptors in insulin sensitive and insulin resistant human cells and tissues. Linköping University Medical Dissertations No.1268

172 Connealy, L.E. (2017). *The Cancer Revolution: A Groundbreaking Program to Reverse and Prevent Cancer*. Published by Da Capo Press

173 Sanchez, A., Reeser, J.L., Lau, H.S. *et al.* (1973). Role of sugars in human neutrophilic phagocytosis. The American Journal of Clinical Nutrition, 26(11): 1180–1184

174 Ringsdorf, W., Cheraskin, E. and Ramsay R. (1976). Sucrose, Neutrophilic Phagocytosis and Resistance to Disease, Dental Survey., 52(12): 46–48

175 Calle, E.E., Rodriguez, C., Walker-Thurmond, K. (2003). Overweight, obesity, and mortality from cancer in a prospectively studied cohort of U.S. adults. New England Journal of Medicine, 348: 1625–1638

176 Takahashi, E. (1982). Tohoku University School of Medicine, Wholistic Health Digest, Oct 1982, 41

177 Moerman, C. J., Bueno de Mesquita, H.B. and Runia, S. (1993). Dietary Sugar Intake in the Etiology of Biliary Tract Cancer. International Journal of Epidemiology, 2(2): 207–214

178 De Stefani, E. (1998). Dietary sugar and lung cancer: a case control study in Uruguay. Nutrition and Cancer, 31(2): 132–137

179 Cornee, J., Pobel, D., Riboli, E. *et al.* (1995). A Case-control study of gastric cancer and nutritional factors in Marseille, France. European Journal of Epidemiology, 11: 55–65

180 Dana-Farber Cancer Institute (2002). *Study Suggests A Possible Link Between High-Starch Diet And Pancreatic Cancer.* Science Daily, Sep 4. Published online www.sciencedaily.com

181 Michaud, D. (2002). Dietary Sugar, Glycemic Load, and Pancreatic Cancer Risk in a Prospective Study. Journal of National Cancer Institute, 94(17): 1293–1300

182 Larsson, S.C., Orsini, N., and Wolk, A. (2005). Diabetes mellitus and risk of colorectal cancer: a meta-analysis. Journal of the National Cancer Institute, 97: 1679–1687

183 Schernhammer, E.S., Hu, F.B., Giovannucci, E. (2005). Sugar-sweetened soft drink consumption and risk of pancreatic cancer in two prospective cohorts. Cancer Epidemiol Biomark Prevent; 14: 2098–2105

184 Lamkin, D.M., Spitz, D.R., Shahzad, M.M. *et al.* (2009). Glucose as a prognostic factor in ovarian carcinoma. Cancer, 115(5): 1021–1027

185 Tavani, A., Giordano, L., Gallus, S. *et al.* (2006). Consumption of sweet foods and breast cancer risk in Italy. Annals Oncology, 17(2): 341–350

186 Merlo, D.F., Rossi, L., Pellegrino, C. *et al.* (2008). Cancer Incidence in Pet Dogs: Findings of the Animal Tumor Registry of Genoa, Italy. Journal of Veterinary Internal Medicine, 22(4): 976–984

187 Hill, S.R., Rutherfurd-Markwick, K.J., Ravindran, G. *et al.* (2009). The effects of the proportions of dietary macronutrients on the digestibility, post-prandial endocrine responses and large intestinal fermentation of carbohydrate in working dogs. NewZealand Veterinary Journal, 57(6): 313–318

188 Hewson-Hughes, A.K., Gilham, M.S., Upton, S. *et al.* (2011). The effect of dietary starch level on postprandial glucose and insulin concentrations in cats and dogs. British Journal of Nutrition, 106(1): S105–109

189 Glickman, L., Glickman, N. and Thorpe, R. (1999). *The Golden Retriever Club of America National Health Survey 1998-1999.* Purdue University School of Veterinary Medicine

190 Adams, V.J., Evans, K.M., Sampson, J. *et al.* (2010). Methods and mortality results of a health survey of purebred dogs in the UK. Journal of Small Animal Practice, 51(10): 512–524

191 de Bruijne, J.J. and van den Brom, W.W. (1986). The effect of long-term fasting on ketone body metabolism in the dog. Comparative Biochemical Physiology, 83: 391–395

CHAPTER 7

Wheat Gluten

If you review any human nutrition book written in the last 10 years, you will be hard-pressed to find a reputable nutritionist who would recommend wheat in its current state to be included as the main ingredient in anyone's diet at any time. And you will not find a single, independent canine nutritionist recommending it for dogs. There are many reasons for this, including its high carbohydrate load, high phytic acid content, high gluten content and the presence of various worrying chemicals used in its production.

1. Phytic Acid

Found in nearly all cereals such as wheat, corn and barley, this chemical in very small quantities is quite beneficial to the body, having antioxidant properties. However, when phytic acid is included in every meal in larger dose, it can cause you problems. Phytic acid is entirely resistant to cooking. When present, it will happily bind to calcium, zinc, magnesium and iron, rendering them difficult or impossible to absorb. A study of iron absorption in cereal porridges by humans found a 12-fold increase in the absorption of iron when the phytic acid was removed from the food.[1] Other experimenters have examined the effect of phytic acid on depression-fighting zinc and magnesium.

Researchers provided two groups of people with bread: one containing phytates and one with the phytates removed. With the bread contained phytic acid, participants absorbed only 13% of its magnesium and 23% of its zinc. Without it, the figure was closer to 30% for both.[2,3] Calcium, zinc, magnesium and iron are all vital components of normal bone growth. This is just one of the reasons that a diet high in cereal grain is known to retard skeletal growth and induces both rickets and osteomalacia in humans.[1,4-10]

2. Chemical Content

Originally a simple grass, around 2 thousand years ago we began inadvertently selecting strains of wheat that were higher in gluten, and thus produced a better, tougher dough. Over the years, wheat has become so mutated it can no longer thrive in the wild without our chemical intervention. One such chemical is glyphosate, the active ingredients in Roundup. Made by Monsanto and used by casual gardeners and mega-agriculture alike, Roundup is the most popular weed killer in the world. A systemic herbicide and crop desiccant, it essentially allows wheat to grow quicker and bigger for longer periods increasing annual yields. Scientists have been warning us for years that it was very likely to be carcinogenic and that its presence in the flour we consume is a concern.[11] Unfortunately, like most chemicals produced by humans and introduced into the human food chain, it takes a lot of time, money and deaths to put the matter to bed. Recently school groundskeeper, Dewayne Johnson, successfully sued Monsanto for $289 million after his cancer diagnosis followed his exposure to Roundup. More than 5,000 similar lawsuits are waiting to be heard[12]–a figure that is sure to explode.

The risk of cancer aside, studies are now suggesting it is the glyphosate content in wheat that is driving many of the food sensitivity issues that often occur following the consumption of wheat by humans today.[13]

This is worrying for us but even more so for dogs. Studies show that dogs are eating more than their share of glyphosate. Zhao *et al.* (2018)[14] tested 18 companion animal feeds for the chemical's presence and concluded that the glyphosate pollution of companion animal feeds was 'likely to result in pet exposure that is 4-12 times higher than that of humans on a per kg basis'.

3. Gluten

Wheat is the number one ingredient in dog food. It happens that it is also the very worst, thanks largely to its carbohydrate load but also to the presence of wheat gluten. It absolutely must be removed from the diet of every dog and cat worldwide. While reading this section, please keep in mind whatever sick animal you may have or have had in the past. He is possibly the reason you picked up this book in the first place. The dog with constantly weepy eyes. The one with the recurring skin, ear or gut condition. The dog with chronic gut inflammation, constantly soft poos and possibly anal gland issues. A dog that you could never get to gain weight. One who never stopped scratching or nibbling his paws, no matter how many trips you took to the vet.

I can say with some confidence that his issue is likely to have begun on wheat-based dry food. You may have tried a number of dry foods since, but that was the start of it. But before we get into the effects of gluten sensitivity, we need to get the terminology correct as the word 'allergy' is being thrown around too often these days.

What Is the Difference Between a Food *Allergy* and a Food *Intolerance*?

When we think of a food allergy, we imagine the man on his hands and knees, coughing, spluttering, choking and projectile vomiting, minutes after accidentally consuming some peanuts. While this is not always the case, this is certainly a sign of a true allergy. It is a disorder of the immune system involving an inappropriate response to a food allergen. It can result in an exaggerated and often violent hypersensitive reaction. Crucially, allergy involves the antibody IgE. For now, you can think of IgE as the body's most effective arsenal, the Navy Seals of immune soldiers. IgE antibodies function mainly in the lungs, skin and mucous membranes of the eyes, nose, throat and gut. IgE coordinates the mast cells (a type of cell involved in the body's immune response) to release chemicals including histamine which causes the capillaries to become more permeable to the cells of the immune system. These cells rush via the blood through the capillaries into the affected tissue (usually the gut, the most likely entry, but also the skin or lungs) and proceed to attack and round up the perceived threat.

As with most actions of your immune system, you would never know this was even occurring except that the arrival of all this extra blood, immune-debris and by-products to the battle scene causes the area to swell. This results in the surrounding area becoming swollen or *inflamed*. Despite its intention to help you, it can have some very irritating side effects depending on where the battle is. If on the skin, it presents as an itchy, angry, red rash (eczema). Around the eyes, it takes the form of irritated and swollen, red eyelids (this can be annoying so when pollen is high, hay fever sufferers might take an *anti*histamine to prevent it from happening). Internally, it can result in or exasperate all sorts of issues, from those of the gut (irritable bowel, diarrhoea) to joint (stiffness). And these are just the tolerable symptoms of food allergy. For some, sadly, it gets much worse. The swelling can be so dramatic that airways are squeezed shut and blood pressure plummets, leaving the sufferer gasping for air and fighting for their life. This is anaphylactic shock. Without epinephrine to alleviate it, death can occur rapidly.

A food allergy, which can develop at any age and to foods you have encountered before, is said to send an American to the emergency room every 3 minutes. Each year 200,000 require emergency medical care for allergic reactions to food. Thankfully, true food allergy is rare in the general population. Between 1% and 3% of people and dogs are expected to suffer an IgE-associated food allergy today.[15,16]

Allergy is just one type of adverse food reaction. There are now a few different types defined in the literature. Here we are discussing the two most common – food *allergy* and a food *intolerance*. Until recently, it was thought a food intolerance reaction had nothing to do with the blood or immune system, that it was largely a *mechanical issue*, occurring exclusively *within* the digestive tract. However, there is now overwhelming evidence to suggest there is very much an immune pathogenesis to it, should it be allowed to persist.[17]

To recap, a food allergy is an inappropriate response to a substance in your body, one your body properly digested and absorbed, believing all was well until the proverbial poo hit the fan (or in this case, your underpants). In contrast, a food intolerance is your inability to mechanically break down that substance in the first place.

There are a number of reasons why you might suffer a food intolerance. It can result from a simple reaction to the chemical components of food – be they naturally occurring, such as in fish, or any one of the multitude of new chemical additives humans have come up with recently, such as the sulphites used to preserve dry fruit which we know can trigger asthma attacks in people. Infections from various parasites (food poisoning), viruses and mycotoxins, even a disruption of the gut flora balance, are all known to trigger food intolerances in some patients. However, it seems the most common cause of food intolerance is an inability to produce the enzymes necessary to break down certain proteins. These are called metabolic intolerances and include your wheat gluten or lactose intolerants. As it is mechanical in nature, unlike an allergy, small amounts of the food may be tolerated by the gut. If large enough amounts of the problem food are consumed often enough, there will be problems for the patient. The first is they upset the osmotic potential of the gut, drawing water into the digesta. This results in a looser stool and ultimately diarrhoea. When this occurs, valuable nutrition is lost, and if allowed to persist, can result in malnutrition through malabsorption in the individual. The second issue is an unbalancing of the gut microflora, known as gut dysbiosis, where the half-digested food encourages the growth of the wrong bacterial families in the gut. Allowed to bloom, the by-products of these feeding bacteria (which include short-chain fatty acids, methane, carbon dioxide and hydrogen) build up and give us bloating, flatulence and irritation of the gut membrane leading to a range of structural issues including irritable bowel syndrome (IBS) (for more on food intolerance, see Zopf *et al.*, 2009).[18]

Unlike a true food allergy, a food intolerance is far more common in the general population, affecting approximately 20% in the industrialised countries.[19] By far, the top two food culprits are wheat gluten (a protein) and milk lactose (a sugar). However, these are such accepted foodstuffs in society, so prominent in our diet and history, with so much industry, money and jobs behind them, that to even discuss problems with their consumption is still met with disbelief and often ridiculed by many.

Gluten Intolerance in Dogs

Since 1944, we have known that gluten is not the easiest protein for dogs. Wagner and Elvehjem (1944)[19] documented how doses of up to 40% gluten induce fits or 'canine hysteria' in beagles. It is suggested gluten plays a key role in protein-losing nephropathy in soft-coated wheaten terriers where administration of gluten resulted in a significant decrease in blood serum protein[20, 21] and it is IgE mediated.[22] Recently, gluten was found to play a role in the disorder in Border Terriers known as epileptoid cramping syndrome.[23] And yes, like us, being an issue of the genes, this food hypersensitivity is expected to be hereditary.[15]

We know dogs can struggle to safely digest gluten; the only unknown is to what degree. The top food allergens in dogs today are assumed to be beef, chicken and wheat gluten[24, 25] Compiling the available literature, Muller *et al.* (2016)[25] suggested the most common food allergen sources for dogs are beef (34%), chicken (17%), milk and dairy products (15%), lamb (15%) and wheat (14%). However, I suspect the true incidence of wheat gluten intolerance in dogs today is grossly under-reported by our veterinary community. To understand why, we must take a look at how gluten intolerance affects humans. For years, countless dogs have provided a suitable animal model for investigation of the immunopathogenesis of human dietary hypersensitivity,[15] and so it stands that the opposite will hold.

Gluten (from Latin *gluten*, meaning 'glue') is a protein commonly found in cereals. It is a strong, long-chained protein (like a necklace) that gives bread its tough, bouncy texture. It enables us to spread peanut butter on a thin slice of white bread. While less than 10% of the protein in wild wheat grass comprises of gluten, we have been unconsciously selecting for it since 400 AD. Gluten now consists up to 50% of the protein present in wheat today (it's particularly high in barley and rye).[26]

Gluten has many uses. First and foremost, it is used in the food sector where it is exploited for its binding, gluey properties in stretchy dough. It is also used in emulsifiers, gelling agents, film formation and as a stretch-ability agent in meat, sauces and soups. It's even central to many industrial-strength adhesives. As a result, it should come as no surprise that this protein is tough to digest.

An adverse reaction to gluten has been pursued with significant interest in the past 20 years.[27] You can be truly allergic to gluten although it is rare in the general populations of both humans and dogs (gluten allergy is thought to affect approximately 1% of the canine population.),[15,28-30] so we will leave the gluten allergy there for the moment.

A far more common reaction to gluten in humans is gluten intolerance, an inability of the sufferer at the genetic level to produce the enzymes necessary for the break of this tough protein. While gluten intolerance shot to prominence a couple of decades ago, spurring the growth of an entire industry, it's fair to say not everyone is on board with even its existence. In 2011, Biesiekierski *et al.* seemed to put the matter beyond all doubt when they recruited 34 people with IBS who were clinically proven to be free of celiac disease yet who had all previously benefited from a gluten-free diet, largely due to their exasperation with conventional medicine and movement to 'alternative health practitioners'. The 34 volunteers were all fed bread and muffins, half of which contained gluten and the other was gluten-free and acted as a placebo. Nearly 70% of the volunteers who ate the gluten reported pain, bloating, toilet problems and extreme tiredness. The authors concluded that 'gluten causes gastrointestinal symptoms in subjects without celiac disease'.

In short, and in line with classic intolerance, the pathology of gluten intolerance is half-digested gluten strands hanging around the gut, causing mechanical issues when water is drawn into the gut by osmosis as well as potentially gut dysbiosis, where the wrong bacteria are permitted to bloom. The result is a mixture of abdominal cramp, nausea, gas, intermittent diarrhoea, constipation and irritable bowel disease.[31,32]

Estimates on the incidence of gluten intolerance in the general population range from 15% to as high as 40%.[26,33,34] Braly and Hoggan (2002)[26] go some way to explaining this range of figures. Gluten intolerance, with its genetic basis, is strongly influenced by your ethnicity. Essentially, the longer your people have been eating it, the more likely you are to digest it safely. This is a great example of evolution at work, with all the digestively unfit individuals succumbing to gluten's health-sapping effects before getting a chance to contribute to the gene pool. Take African Americans, for example. In the 1600s, North Americans were abducting Africans from their homeland and using them as slaves to work on their farms. As if this wasn't bad enough, these slaves were faced with a major change in diet. African cereals such as sorghum and millet are gluten-free. Suddenly large amounts of gluten were introduced into their diet. Born without the ability to manufacture the necessary enzymes, problems ensued. As it takes time to develop the correct system, African Americans are still reeling today from the gluten insult, 40% are expected to be gluten intolerant.[26] As such, they are far more likely to develop diabetes, skin and nasal issues, than their White (more European) counterparts.[26] While the current rate of diabetes in the United States stands at 8.3% of the population, 18.7% of African Americans are thought to have the disease (US Department of Health and Human Services, National Institute of Diabetes and Digestive and Kidney Diseases). African Americans are more likely to suffer sleep-disordered breathing,[35] and asthma,[36] with African American children having an 80% higher prevalence of asthma than White American children.

The same biological and behavioural effects are visible in Aboriginal populations in Australia, who are ingesting gluten from bread and now beer, resulting in some alarming trends. In 1971, intestinal mucosal biopsies taken from 44 Aboriginal children showed an increased prevalence of abnormal mucosae (but only one coeliac) compared to Australian children of European descent. Six responded positively to a gluten-free diet.[37]

Now, think of carnivorous dogs. They are entirely ill adapted to plant digestion, lacking both the machinery and microflora to break down tougher plant matter. Wheat gluten is another level again in terms of digestive resilience. Surely, they are no better at it than omnivorous humans who have been eating it for hundreds of years? Logic dictates that as carnivores, only eating wheat in earnest for the last five or six decades, then they must fare worse, but by how much we don't know.

There is, however, another type of gluten intolerant out there, an unfortunate individual that has another two genetic defects which ultimately result in the ruination of the small intestines and individual's well-being. We call them coeliacs. To understand why so many dogs today seem to present with such a dizzying array of 'food allergies', we need to understand the pathogenesis of coeliac disease (CD), using humans as our guinea pigs.

CD in humans is receiving a lot of attention of late. It is a metabolic intolerance to gluten on steroids. It is in fact an autoimmune disorder where the body begins to attack itself (the gut, in particular). In sufferers with CD, inflammation in the small intestine area is stimulated by an enzyme known as tissue transglutaminase, unique to sufferers with CD. This enzyme results in large-scale, chronic inflammation of the gut in patients with CD and results in both villous (the finger-like projections in your gut that help you absorb nutrients) and gut membrane destruction. This occurs chiefly in the duodenum, which is the major absorptive segment of your intestines. Most of the B complex vitamins are absorbed here. As well as vitamin C, most water-soluble vitamins, macro-minerals such as calcium, iron and iodine, and micro-nutrients such as zinc, boron, manganese and magnesium. The damaged intestine is unable to perform its role effectively, ultimately resulting in malnutrition through malabsorption diseases. CD in children is frequently associated with a slower growth rate[38] while the blocking of vitamin B complex, vital in energy production and mental health, will sap energy levels and can seriously affect your mental health.

Now gluten comes in to make things a little worse for the coeliac patient. Zonulin is a protein that normally regulates the tight junctions of the gut cell membrane, dictating how easily substances pass through the intestinal wall. In coeliacs, it happens that gliadin (the alcohol fraction of gluten) stimulates the release of zonulin in the gut),[39,40] increasing intestinal permeability. Over time, this widening of the tight junctions results in small gaps in the intestinal barrier. Known as 'leaky gut', this is very bad news for the sufferer. It exposes the capillary-rich layers underneath (hence, blood may be apparent in the stool, common in approximately half of sufferers with CD).[34] But more importantly, now partially digested food and gluten proteins along with bacteria or toxins nearby can gain entry to the gut tissue and potentially the bloodstream. The body does not take this lightly because the blood leads to the body's nerve centres, the brain and heart. However, instead of the Navy Seal-type IgE antibodies, typically seen in true allergy, in sufferers with CD the 'milder' IgA and IgG antibodies are employed;[41, 42] hence, these antibodies are always the focus of tests for CD.

This process of leaky gut, the improper presentation of partially digested food molecules in the bloodstream and the body's immunological reaction to them, is the route to developing food allergens.[43] It is not normal for an animal to become hypersensitive (meaning it initiates an immune response to) to a large range of everyday food proteins. The immune cascade has tagged these various compounds as potential invaders. Once tagged, lasting pathogenic immune memory is established. The body will continue to react to these whole or partially digested proteins and sugars until you fix the leak.

Nor do the problems end there. With the flood gates open, the immune response can be so strong and constant that immune complexes build up quicker than the body can remove them. They clog the kidneys. They overrun the liver's ability to break them down. The body starts to stash these allergen-antibody complexes in various body tissues. These tissues do not accommodate their new guests too willingly and inflammation results. This contributes to a variety of health problems depending on where the complexes accumulate. For example, patients with CD are more prone to arthritis and diseases of the tendons, ligaments and bone,[44] but the list of potential affecting ailments is endless, effecting every system:

1. **Dermatological:** hives, dermatitis, psoriasis, eczema and other rashes

2. **Gastrointestinal:** vomiting, bloating, cramping, gas, nausea, diarrhoea (often with blood) and colic

3. **Respiratory:** sinusitis, runny noses and asthma

4. **Musculoskeletal:** aching joints, arthritis, osteoporosis, anaemia and general weakness

5. **Nervous:** mood disorders such as hyperactivity, depression, seizure, anxiety, poor concentration

And it gets worse for patients with CD. CD is present in patients with Type 1 diabetes 10 to 30 times more than the normal population.[45] Autoimmune disease, the third leading cause of mortality today,[46] is ten times more common in patients with CD than in the general population.[47] Vojdani *et al.* (2008)[42] linked CD to autoimmune endocrine disorders such as Addison's disease, auto-immune thyroid diseases, hypoparathyroidism and primary gonadal failure.

Then there's behaviour. Psycho-dietetics is a relatively new science. It is the study of the effects on behaviour of particles such as gluteomorphins (from the digestion of gluten) and casomorphins (from casein) entering the blood through a leaky gut. Gluteomorphins, as you may guess by their name, are morphine-derived compounds and, together with their cousins the casomorphins (from the incomplete breakdown of casein in milk), will wreak havoc on reaching the brain. These substances are known to result in and exacerbate a variety of disorders including epilepsy, autism, attention defect hyperactive disorder, bipolar disease, Multiple Sclerosis, Alzheimer's, Parkinson's and schizophrenia.[26,48-50] These molecules have a negative effect on attention, brain maturation, social interaction and learning in susceptible children. Symptoms are significantly reduced with a combined gluten-and-casein-free diet.[51-54] In fact, the absence of gluten and casein from a population is often characterised by a lack of these diseases. Braly and Hoggan (2002)[26] demonstrate how schizophrenia incidence decreased significantly during World War II in European populations suffering grain shortages.

Thus, CD can materialise in many forms. Known as the Great Imitator because of its insidious nature and broad spectrum of effects, we still know relatively little about CD, leading to misdiagnosis in the sufferer. It is estimated that less than 20% of sufferers with CD are ever diagnosed as such.[55] Those who are diagnosed wait, on average, more than 11 years for that diagnosis (Cranney *et al.*, 2007).[56] This is concerning. Rubio-Tapia *et al.* (2009)[57] conducted a 45-year follow-up study on undiagnosed coeliac disease sufferers and found a nearly fourfold increased risk of death.

In 2005, the *New England Journal of Medicine* claimed that 1 in 250 Americans suffered from CD; in 2006 the Mayo Clinic revised this figure to 1 in 122. Today, the figures rest somewhere between 1 and 50[41] and less than 1 in 100 (most CD websites). The number of known sufferers is almost certain to increase in the future in line with increasing awareness by medical practitioners.

While CD is common in humans, we have no idea of the incidence in dogs. We have not been looking to any real degree. We know red setters suffer it. Biopsies of intestinal segments of Irish setters suffered villus atrophy accompanied by increased intestinal permeability when exposed to gluten (the definition of CD). These dogs improved on a gluten-free diet and relapsed when given a subsequent gluten diet.[58-60]

What we do know is that the most common (at least the most obvious) symptoms of CD in humans are dermatological (hives, dermatitis, psoriasis, eczema and other rashes) and gastrointestinal (vomiting, bloating, cramping, gas, nausea, diarrhoea (often with blood) and colic). It happens that recurring skin conditions are among the most common reasons for your dog to visit the vet.[61] Gastrointestinal disease is the second biggest killer of dogs[62,63] after cancer. With more than 525,000 pets insured, Veterinary Pet Insurance (VPI) is America's largest insurance provider for pets. In 2008, VPI reported the most common reason for visiting the vet was ear infections, with skin conditions taking up the next two spots (skin 'allergies' and hot spots) and gut issues (gastritis and enteritis) occupying 4th and 5th positions. This range of maladies is remarkably consistent through the years and, indeed, across countries, and they are all potential symptoms of adverse food reactions (in case you're wondering). In America, the top five reasons for humans to visit their doctor are not so easily explained but they include skin conditions, joint problems, back issues, 'lipid metabolism' and upper respiratory issues.[64] Like my dogs in Australia, it seems we have an epidemic of chronically itchy dogs out there, dogs with hot, recurring skin rashes. Dogs nibbling their toes. Dogs with constant soft poos and often anal gland problems as a result. Dogs with IBD that you just cannot get to put the weight on (malnutrition through malabsorption). The inexplicably long list of potential allergens. All treated with drugs to tell an antagonised immune system to relax, drugs we know should not be part of a long-term health plan.

Considering how prevalent wheat is in their lives and the symptoms we are seeing in the general population – this is a field which urgently requires more attention. And if looking for a suitable breed to investigate after setters, I would put West Highland Terriers at the top of the list (with any small, white-coated breeds soon after). They always seem to present with a dizzying array of allergens which is a red flag for leaky gut. And they are notoriously tricky to get right. Until we know more, wheat should never be fed to these animals.

Owners commonly report that their dog's issues always appear to kick in all of a sudden, with owners saying they were fine one day and then scratching themselves raw the next. This is interesting because if this were a genetic inability to cope with the protein, we would be noticing issues in pups from a young age. However, we know 30–45% of the human population appears to have the CD-risk alleles and yet only 1% of the population ever develops the disease.[65] Therefore, there must be a trigger of CD, something that breaks the person's oral tolerance to gluten. Brown *et al.* (2018)[65] suggest a viral infection as a potential trigger for onset.

Are adverse food reactions the *only* cause of these stubborn issues sending so many dogs to the vets? Of course not, but they are most definitely the first (and easiest) place to look, with wheat being one of the chief offenders in a dog with a recurring skin, ear or gut condition. If you have a dog with one of these conditions, you should endeavour to remove *all* wheat from the diet. That means all processed pet foods, regardless of labels claiming to be wheat-free or single-protein. The issues with using these products to treat such food sensitivity are many. First, no human nutritionist would use a product that contains so many ingredients, particularly with so many chemicals not even making it to the label (later). Chemical additives used in dry foods are now shown to be second only to dietary protein in causing adverse food reactions in your dog.[66,67]

But more importantly is the issue of contamination. Ricci *et al.* (2013)[68]analysed twelve of the most popular single-protein and hypoallergenic, veterinary recommended dry foods for atopy and allergy and discovered that 10 of the 12 foods were contaminated with one or more potentially allergenic proteins or fats not listed on their labels, with wheat gluten being the chief offender. Nor is this sort of study a one-off for the single-protein pet food industry. Studies show they are constantly adulterated with proteins not on the label, even when they specifically state they do not contain that protein.[69-71] Dry food companies are simply not held to the same level of processing criteria as human gluten-free food manufacturers. It explains why these single-protein diets only work to cure gastrointestinal upset in dogs 50–60% of the time[72,73] and dogs on them will relapse.

We have known for years that a simple, homemade, single-protein diet (one that is based on the meat, organ and bone from one animal), one that focuses on healing the gut, is the best way to begin rectifying the issue. Termed an exclusion diet (the exact method is available at www.dogsfirst.ie), this has always been the method used by authors investigating food sensitivity in dogs to get a period of 'wellness' prior to rechallenge (Jeffers 1991 and 1996).[74,75]

> On the basis of these results, the commercial diet, skin testing and anti-IgE ELISA cannot replace an owner-prepared food elimination diet for food hypersensitivity testing in dogs.
>
> **Jeffers *et al.*, 1991**[74]

It's funny how modern vets *almost* know this to be the case. When a dog with recurring gut sickness presents itself, and all other avenues have been explored to no avail, sometimes a move to a homemade (and gluten-free) diet of something akin to boiled chicken and rice (not that this is recommended either) will be recommended. On this the dog often recovers. However, the diet is only employed while 'the right bag' of dry food is found. So close.

TAKE-HOME POINTS

✓ Phytic acid in wheat is entirely resistant to cooking, which binds vital nutrients from the diet.

✓ Glyphosphate is used in the production of wheat. The courts have now decided it is carcinogenic. The level of glycophosphate exposure in pets is likely 4–12 times higher than in humans.

✓ Wheat gluten is likely the most common food antigen in pets today.

✓ A food allergy is rare (1–3% of the dog population). It is the inappropriate response by the body to an everyday allergen. It is sudden, dramatic, very serious and involves the IgE antibody. It happens in the blood.

✓ A food intolerance is far more common. It is a mechanical issue in the gut. It happens for a number of reasons but is most commonly explained by an inability to produce the enzymes necessary to break down certain proteins. These are called metabolic intolerances. Half-digested compounds accumulating in the gut result in looser stool and/or gut dysbiosis (the wrong bacteria taking over) resulting in gut disruption and potentially, IBS.

✓ The two most common food intolerances in humans are to wheat gluten and milk lactose. At least 20–40% of humans suffer gluten intolerance. The longer a population has been consuming it, the better they are able to digest it.

✓ While dogs have been living on wheat-based diet for the last century, we know many dogs struggle to safely digest wheat gluten. It is one of the most common food allergens in dogs today; however, due to its insidious nature, its true prevalence is going grossly underreported today. It is simply not possible that a meat-eating carnivore, with a shorter digestive tract and inappropriate gut flora, would be better at digesting wheat than plant-eating humans who have been consuming it for thousands of years.

✓ CD is an autoimmune disorder whereby the ingestion of wheat gluten leads to chronic inflammation in the gut, malabsorption, gut barrier dysfunction with permeability (known as 'leaky gut') and immune system response. It results in a range of skin, gut, respiratory and behavioural issues. It is thought to affect 1-in-50 Americans today. Red Setters are known to suffer the disease.

> ✓ Single-protein and hypoallergenic dry foods are all known to be heavily contaminated with wheat gluten protein.
>
> ✓ A homemade exclusion diet based on a single protein has always been the advice to obtain a period of 'wellness' prior to food hypersensitivity testing in dogs. It remains the advice today.

Chapter Seven References

1 Hurrell, R.F., Reddy, M.B., Juillerat, M.A. *et al.* (2003). Degradation of phytic acid in cereal porridges improves iron absorption by human subjects. American Journal of Clinical Nutrition, 77: 1213–1219

2 Egli, I., Davidsson, L., Zeder, C. *et al.* (2004). Dephytinisation of a complementary food based on wheat and soy increases zinc, but not copper apparent absorption in adults. Journal of Nutrition, 134: 1077–1080

3 Bohn, T., Davidsson, L., Walczyk, T. *et al.* (2004). Phytic acid added to white-wheat bread inhibits fractional apparent magnesium absorption in humans. American Journal of Clinical Nutrition, 79(3):418–423

4 Weaver, C.M., Peacock, M. and Johnston Jr., C.C. (1999). Adolescent Nutrition in the Prevention of Postmenopausal Osteoporosis. The Journal of Clinical Endocrinology & Metabolism, 84(6): 1839–1843

5 Mann, J. and Truswell, S.A. (2002). Essentials of Human Nutrition, 2nd Ed. Editors Oxford University Press, UK

6 Forbes, R.M., Parker, H.M. and Erdman, J.W., Jr (1984). Effects of dietary phytate, calcium and magnesium levels on zinc bioavailability to rats. Journal of Nutrition, 114: 1421–1425.

7 Forbes, R.M, Parker, H.M. and Erdman Jr., J.W. (2012). Effects of Dietary Phytate, Calcium and Magnesium Levels on Zinc Bioavailability to Rats. Journal of Nutrition, 114(8): 1421–1425

8 Hellanda, S., Denstadlib, V., Wittena, P.E. *et al.* (2006). Hyper dense vertebrae and mineral content in Atlantic salmon (*Salmo salar* L.) fed diets with graded levels of phytic acid. Aquaculture, 261(2): 603–614

9 Ewer, R.F. (1973). *The carnivores*. London: Weidenfield and Nicolson Eds.

10 Nap, R.C. and Hazewinkel, H.A.W. (1994). Growth and skeletal development in the dog in relation to nutrition; a review. Veterinary Quarterly, 16(1): 50–59

11 Simonetti, E., Cartaud, G., Quinn, R. *et al.* (2015). Comparative Study on the Quantitative Determination of Glyphosate at Low Levels in Wheat Flour, Journal of AOAC International, 98(6): 1760–1768

12 Bellon, T. (2018). *Monsanto ordered to pay $289 million in world's first Roundup cancer trial*. Reuters. Published online, Aug 10th, available online www.reuters.com

13 Samsel, A. and Seneff, S. (2013). Glyphosate, pathways to modern diseases II: Celiac sprue and gluten intolerance. Interdisciplinary Toxicology, 6(4): 159–184

14 Zhao, J., Pacenka, S., Wu, J., *et al.* (2018). Detection of glyphosate residues in companion animal feeds. Environmental Pollution, 243(B): 1113–1118

15 Day, M.J. (2005). The canine model of dietary hypersensitivity. Journal of the Nutrition Society, 64: 458–464

16 Valenta, R., Hochwallner, H., Linhart, B. *et al.* (2015). Food Allergies: The Basics. Gastroenterology, 148(6): 1120–1131

17 Hadjivassiliou, M., Williamson, C.A. and Woodroofe, N. (2004). The immunology of gluten sensitivity: Beyond the gut. Trends in Immunology, 25: 578–582

18 Zopf, Y., Baenkler, H.W., Silbermann, A. *et al.* (2009). The differential diagnosis of food intolerance. Deutsches Arzteblatt International, 106(21): 359–370

19 Wagner J.R. and Elvehjem, C.A. (1944). A study of canine hysteria produced by feeding certain baked dog foods and wheat gluten flour. Journal of Nutrition, 28: 431–441.

20 Littman, M.P. and Giger, U. (1990). Familial protein-losing enteropathy (PLE) and/or protein-losing nephropathy (PLN) in soft-coated wheaten terriers (SCWT). Journal of Veterinary Internal Medicine, 4: 133–136

21 Littman, M.P., Dambach, D.M., Vaden, S. L. *et al.* (2000). Familial protein-losing enteropathy and protein-losing nephropathy in soft coated wheaten terriers: 222 cases (1983–1997). Journal of Veterinary Internal Medicine, 14: 68–80

22 Vaden, S.L., Hammerberg, B., Davenport, D.J. *et al.* (2000a). Food hypersensitivity reactions in Soft Coated Wheaten Terriers with protein-losing enteropathy or protein-losing nephropathy or both: gastroscopic food sensitivity testing, dietary provocation, and fecal immunoglobulin E. Journal of Veterinary Internal Medicine, 14(1): 60–70

23 Lowrie, M., Garden, O.A., Hadjivassiliou, M. *et al.* (2015). The Clinical and Serological Effect of a Gluten–Free Diet in Border Terriers with Epileptoid Cramping Syndrome. Journal of Veterinary Internal Medicine, 29(6): 1564–1568

24 Roudebush, P. (2013). Ingredients and foods associated with adverse reactions in dogs and cats. Veterinary Dermatology, 24: 293–294

25 Mueller, R.S., Olivry, T. and Prelaud, P. (2016). Critically appraised topic on adverse food reactions of companion animals (2): common food allergen sources in dogs and cats. BMC Veterinary Research, 12:9

26 Braly, J. and Hoggan, R. (2002). *Dangerous grains: Why gluten cereal grains may be hazardous to your health*. New York: Avery.

27 O'Bryan, V.T. and Kellermann, G.H. (2008). The immunology of immediate and delayed hypersensitivity reaction to gluten. European Journal of Inflammation, 6(1): 1–10

28   Loft, D.E., Marsh, M.N., Sandle G.I. *et al.* (1989). Studies of the intestinal lymphoid tissue, XII. Epithelial lymphocyte and mucosal responses to rectal gluten challenge in celiac sprue. Gastroenterology, 97: 29–37

29   Hall, E.J. and Batt, R.M. (1992). Dietary modulation of gluten sensitivity in a naturally occurring enteropathy of Irish setter dogs. Gut, 33: 198–205.

30   Hall, E.J., Carter, S.D., Barnes, A. *et al.* (1992) Immune responses to dietary antigens in gluten-sensitive enteropathy of Irish setters. Veterinary Science Research, 53: 293–299

31   Kajander, K. (2008). Pathophysiological factors of irritable bowel syndrome, and the effects of probiotic supplementation. Academic Dissertation. Faculty of Medicine, University of Helsinki. Published online, www.helsinki.fi

32   Ortolani, C. and Pastorello, E.A. (2006). Food allergies and food intolerances. Best Practice and Research: Clinical Gastroenterology, 20(3): 467–483

33   Sollid, L.M. and Lundin, K.E. (2001). Coeliac disease: An inappropriate immune response. Lancet, 358: S13

34   Fine, K.D. (1996). The prevalence of occult gastrointestinal bleeding in celiac sprue. New England Journal of Medicine, 334: 1163–1167

35   Redline, S., Tishler, P.V., Schluchter, M. *et al.* (1999). Risk factors for sleep-disordered breathing in children: Associations with obesity, race, and respiratory problems. American Journal of Respiratory and Critical Care Medicine, 159(5): 1527–1532

36   Wechsler, M.E., Szefler, S.J., Ortega, V.E. *et al.* (2019). Step-Up Therapy in Black Children and Adults with Poorly Controlled Asthma. New England Journal of Medicine, 381: 1227–1239

37   Walker-Smith, J.A. and Reye, R.D.K. (1971). Small intestinal morphology in Aboriginal children. Australian and New Zealand Journal of Medicine, 1(4): 377–384

38   Hernández, M., Argente J., Navarro, A. *et al.* (1992). Growth in Malnutrition Related to Gastrointestinal Diseases: Coeliac Disease. Hormonal Research in Paediatrics, 38(1)

39   Sander, G.R., Cummins, A.G., Henshall, T. *et al.* (2005). Rapid disruption of intestinal barrier function by gliadin involves altered expression of apical junctional proteins. FEBS Lett., 579(21): 4851–4855

40   de Punder, K. and Pruimboom, L. (2013). The Dietary Intake of Wheat and other Cereal Grains and Their Role in Inflammation. Nutrients, 5(3): 771–787

41   Korponay-Szabó, I.R., Dahlbom, I., Laurila, K. *et al.* (2003). Elevation of IgG antibodies against tissue transglutaminase as a diagnostic tool for coeliac disease in selective IgA deficiency. British Medical Journal, 52(11): 1567–1571

42   Vojdani, A., O'Bryan, T. and Kellermann, G.H. (2008). The immunology of immediate and delayed hypersenitivity reaction to gluten. European Journal of Inflammation, 6(1): 1–10

43   Perrier, C. and Corthésy, B. (2011). Gut permeability and food allergies. Clinical and Experimental Allergy, 41(1): 20–28

44   Atteno, M., Costa, L., Tortora, R. *et al.* (2013). The occurrence of lower limb enthesopathy in coeliac disease patients without clinical signs of articular involvement. Rheumatology, 52(5): 893–897

45   Funda D.P., Kaas, A., Bock, T. *et al.* (1999). Gluten-free diet prevents diabetes in NOD mice. Diabetes/Metabolism Research and Reviews, 15: 323–327

46   Arnson, Y., Amital, H. and Shoenfeld, Y. (2005). Vitamin D and autoimmunity: new aetiological and therapeutic considerations. Journal of Immunology, 175: 4119–4126

47   Alaedini, A., Okamoto, H., Briani, C. *et al.* (2007). Immune Cross-Reactivity in Celiac Disease: Anti-Gliadin Antibodies Bind to Neuronal Synapsin I. The Journal of Immunology, 178: 6590–6595

48   Dohan, F.C. (1980). Hypothesis: Genes and neuroactive peptides from food as cause of schizophrenia. Advances in Biochemical Psychopharmacology, 22: 535–548

49   Reichelt, K.L., Knivsberg, A.M., Lind, G. *et al.* (1991). Probable etiology and possible treatment of childhood autism. Brain Dysfunction, 4: 308–319

50   Kalaydjian, A.E., Eaton, W.N., Cascella, A. *et al.* (2005). The gluten connection: The association between schizophrenia and celiac disease. Acta Psychiatrica Scandinavica, 113(2): 82–90

51   Reichelt, K.L., Knivsberg, A.M. and Nodland, M. (1994). Nature and consequences of hyperpetiduria and bovine casomorphins found in autistic syndromes. Developmental Brain Dysfunction, 7: 71–85

52   Knivsberg, A.M., Reichelt, K.L., Nødland, M. *et al.* (1995). Autistic syndromes and diet: A follow-up study. Scandinavian Journal of Educational Research, 39(3): 222–236

53   White, J.F. (2003). Minireview: Intestinal pathophysiology in autism. Department of Physiology, Emory University, Atlanta, Georgia, Experimental Biology and Medicine, 228: 639–649

54   Millward, C., Ferriter, M., Calver, S. *et al.* (2007). Gluten-and casein-free diets for autistic spectrum disorder (Review). The Cochrane Library, available online, www.onlinelibrary.wiley.com

55   Lionetti, E., Gatti, S., Pulvirenti, A. *et al.* (2015). Celiac Disease From a Global Perspective. Best Practice and Research Clinical Gastroenterology, 29(3): 365–379

56   Cranney, A., Zarkadas, M., Graham, I.D. *et al.* (2007). The Canadian Celiac Health Survey. Digestive Diseases and Sciences, 52(4): 1087–1095

57   Rubio-Tapia, A., Kyle, R.A., Kaplan E.L. *et al.* (2009). Increased prevalence and mortality in undiagnosed celiac disease. Gastroenterology, 137(1): 88–93

58   Batt, V.R.M. and Hall, E.J. (1992). Gluten-sensitive enteropathy in the dog. Wiener Medizinische Wochenschrift, 79(8): 242–247

59   Daminet, S.C. (1996). Gluten-sensitive enteropathy in a family of Irish setters. Canadian Veterinary Journal, 37(12): 745–746

60 Pemberton, P.W., Lobley, R.W., *et al.* (1997). Gluten-sensitive enteropathy in Irish setter dogs: characterisation of jejunal microvillar membrane proteins by two-dimensional electrophoresis. Research in Veterinary Science, 62(2): 191–193

61 Hill, P.B., Lo, A., Eden, C.A. *et al.* (2006). Survey of the prevalence, diagnosis and treatment of dermatological conditions in small animals in general practice. Veterinary Record, 158, 533–539

62 Craig L.E. (2001). Cause of death in dogs according to breed: A necropsy survey of five breeds. Journal of the American Animal Hospital Association, 37: 438–443

63 Fleming, J.M., Creevy, K. E. and Promislow, D.E.L. (2011). Mortality in North American dogs from 1984 to 2004: An investigation into age, size and breed related causes of death. Journal of Veterinary Internal Medicine, 25: 187–198

64 St. Sauver, J.L., Warner, D.O., Yawn, B.P. *et al.* (2013). Why do patients visit their doctors? Assessing the most prevalent conditions in a defined US population. Mayo Clinical Proceedings, 88(1): 56–67

65 Brown, J.J., Jabri, B. and Dermody, T.S. (2018). A viral trigger for celiac disease. PLoS pathogens, 14(9): e1007181.

66 Roudebush, P. (1999). Hypoallergenic Diets for Dogs and Cats. In Kirk's Current Veterinary Therapy XIII, Bonagura, J.D. (ed.), W.B. Saunders Co., Philadelphia, 1999. p530-536

67 Kennis, R. (2006). Food allergies: Update of pathogenesis, diagnoses, and management. Veterinary Clinics of North America: Small Animal Practice, 36(1): 175–184

68 Ricci, R., Granato, A., Vascellari, M. *et al.* (2013). Identification of undeclared sources of animal origin in canine dry foods used in dietary elimination trials. Journal of Animal Physiology and Animal Nutrition, 97: 32–38

69 Raditic, D.M., Remillard, R.L. and Tater, K.C. (2011). ELISA testing for common food antigens in four dry dog foods used in dietary elimination trials. Journal of Animal Physiology and Animal Nutrition (Berlin), 95(1): 90–97

70 Willis-Mahn, C., Remillard, R. and Tater, K. (2014). ELISA testing for soy antigens in dry dog foods used in dietary elimination trials. Journal of American Animal Hospital Association, 50(6): 383–389

71 Horvath-Ungerboeck, C., Widmann, K. and Handl, S. (2017). Detection of DNA from undeclared animal species in commercial elimination diets for dogs using PCR. Veterinary Dermatology, 28(4):373–386

72 Allenspach, K., Culverwell, C., Chan, D. (2016). Long-term outcome in dogs with chronic enteropathies: 203 cases. Veterinary Record 178(15): 368

73 Volkmann, M., Steiner, J.M., Fosgate, G.T. *et al.* (2017). Chronic diarrhea in dogs – retrospective study in 136 cases. Journal of Veterinary Internal Medicine, 31: 1043–1055

74 Jeffers J.G., Shanley K.J. and Myer E.K. (1991). Diagnostic testing of dogs for food hypersensitivity. Journal of the American Veterinary Medical Association, 198: 245–250

75 Jeffers, J.G., Meyer, E.K. and Sosis, E.J. (1996). Responses of dogs with food allergies to single-ingredient dietary provocation. Journal of the American Veterinary Medical Association, 209: 608–611

CHAPTER 8

Protein

Proteins are the building blocks of life. They are the basis of all tissues – muscles, bones, tendons and ligaments. It is your hair, skin and fingernails. It is your joints, blood vessels and organs. Protein is vital to cellular regeneration, maintenance and repair, and for making hormones, enzymes and antibodies. It's hard to over-emphasize just how important good quality protein is to the body. In fact, the word protein comes from the Greek word *proteios*, meaning 'of prime importance'.

From a structural point of view, protein consists of individual building blocks called amino acids, strung together like a necklace. Animals can actually make some of their own amino acids and these are termed *nonessential* amino acids; in other words, they do not need to be consumed. The ones they can't make are called *essential* amino acids (EAAs), meaning they must be consumed daily to fulfil their needs. You can get your EAAs, by either eating other animals and using theirs (if you're a meat-eater), from plant tissues (if you're a plant-eater) or from both (if you're not picky!). Our hero is very much in the first category.

The most common food items selected by the dog appears to be small animals including rabbits, rodents, birds, frogs, carcass and perhaps a very small amount of plant matter. While the nutrient composition of smaller prey animals varies with species, season and living conditions, we have established that protein/fat ratio of small, whole prey animals such as rabbits is probably something around a lean 4:1, on a dry matter basis. In fact, few prey animals register below 60% protein, on a dry matter basis.[1,2] Millions of years on such a diet has resulted in dogs being particularly adept at meat digestion. They can digest 89% of chicken or turkey meal while humans can only digest 79% and a whopping 91% of fish compared to just 70% in humans.[3,4]

As protein is the mainstay of their diet, we might be forgiven for assuming protein is very important to them, as indeed it is to the rest of us. Cereal-based pet food manufacturers do not agree. Their stance, perpetuated by the veterinary industry, is too much protein can be potentially damaging to the dog. This we will call the 'too much protein' hypothesis. Due to its importance to the diet of the dog, we will now examine this hypothesis from every angle.

The New Low-Protein Norm for Dogs

To use the word 'complete' on your dry food, you must meet the minimum requirements of the Association of American Feed Control Officials (AAFCO 2016). The AAFCO set the standard for pet food manufacturers. They dictate the criteria manufacturers must adhere to before the word 'complete' can be used on the packet of pet food. On total crude protein, their requirement is 'complete foods must contain a *minimum* 18% protein for adult dogs and 22.5% for pups'. I have added the italics to draw attention to what is another crucial point in the book.

Both the Small Animal Clinical Nutrition (SACN)[5] and the National Research Council (NRC)[6] agree that the minimum protein requirement of dogs for normal growth is 225 g of protein per kilogram (22.5%) of dry food for pups aged 4–14 weeks, falling to 175 g per kg (17.5%) of dry food for older dogs. The Pet Food Industry magazine largely agrees (June 2000, p.38), stating large-breed puppies require a minimum of 21% protein.

For some reason, over time, these *minimum* guidelines have become an *optimum* for the industry to achieve. Check your dry food of choice. It's hard to get away from this one: your vet is recommending that a dry food with the *minimum* amount of protein is the *optimum* route to nutritional prowess in your dog.

If we accept dogs eat meat and meat consists largely of protein, then even the most cynical among us must raise an eyebrow at this new 18% protein (and 50-60% carbohydrate) norm for dogs. So, the likes of the SACN must have a good reason for this stance, right? Wellll…

To reach their conclusions on minimum protein requirements, arguably one of the most important decisions they can make in terms of feeding an animal the same meal every day of their developmental and adult life, the previous edition of the SACN[7] refers to just two studies to support their calculations, one by Romsos and Ferguson (1983)[8] and the other by Tôrres *et al.* (2003).[9] Both studies involved head-to-head comparisons of two very small groups of dogs fed ultra-processed, cereal-based dry foods. Both conclude the dog appears to choose 25-30% of his ME from protein with the remainder coming from largely fat and some carbohydrate. We have already highlighted the dogs potential desire to opt for ultra-processed mixes higher in animal fat, even more so when the other portions are cereal and meat meal. However, another possible flaw in these studies is the choice of protein in the diets. Romsos and Ferguson (1983)[8] supplied protein in the form of beef and soybean. Tôrres *et al.* (2003)[9] housed six beagles and tested six different diets over the course of a year to see which they preferred. However, instead of including beef as a protein source for their test dogs, they opted for casein and soybean protein in equal measure. It's clear that both these studies intended that particular food choice to bring results purely by protein content and not the *source* of the protein used.

It's fair to say soy for dogs has its critics. Daniel (2005) wrote a book titled *The Whole Soy Story: The Dark Side of America's Favorite Health Food*, which cites more than 170 epidemiological, clinical and laboratory studies that link processed soy to malnutrition, digestive problems, thyroid dysfunction, cognitive decline, reproductive disorders, heart disease and cancer in humans. When we know dogs will regulate their ingestion of foods based on their physiological consequences,[10] neither of these studies allowed for the fact that maybe dogs were trying to limit their ingestion of certain ingredients, such as soy. After all, phytoestrogens found in soy are known to have both beneficial and deleterious health effects on dogs.[11] These authors analysed the phytoestrogen content of 24 commercial dry foods that listed soy as an ingredient and found that all contained 'phytoestrogens in amounts that could have biological effects when ingested long-term'. Or maybe it wasn't the phytoestrogens. Perhaps it was the high levels of phytic acid in soy (known to cause growth issues in humans), the presence of trypsin inhibitors in soy (stunts growth), the fact that the processing of soy protein results in the formation of toxic lysinoalanine and highly carcinogenic nitrosamines, the fact that free glutamic acid (a potent neurotoxin) is formed during soy food processing, or even that soy foods are known to contain high levels of aluminium, which is toxic to the nervous system and the kidneys.

Whatever the reason, the results harvested from two feeding trials involving a handful of caged beagles fed a very unnatural, mostly plant-based food source, should be taken as anecdotal evidence at the very best, indicating a field where more could be done. They should certainly not be the basis for the long-term sustenance of every dog on the planet, certainly not those fed *real food*. For a manual that lauds itself as 'evidence-based nutrition,' it's slightly worrying that these results are not only included in support, but until very recently they appear to be the *sole basis* for the production of many millions of tonnes of extremely low-protein dry dog food each year.

In its latest edition, under the section titled "Protein Requirements of Dogs and Cats", the SACN[5] does not even refer to these two studies. Instead, it refers to just a single work regarding the protein requirements of the dog. The passage reads as follows (with italics added by me for effect):

> The absolute minimum dietary protein requirement can be estimated by feeding extremely high-quality protein or commonly used protein sources. If the estimate is based on feeding high-quality protein (e.g. lactalbumin), a growing dog requires approximately 18% DM protein and an adult dog 8% DM protein (NRC 2003).[6] AAFCO has established that canine foods containing commonly used protein ingredients should contain at least 22% DM protein for growth, and 18% DM protein for adult maintenance (AAFCO 2007). *It is important to note that AAFCO recommendations should be interpreted as daily allowances, not as absolute minimum requirements.*
>
> **Hand *et al.*, 2010[5]**

There is a lot in this. First, this is all from the most recent edition of the veterinary instruction manual on canine nutrition, on the total protein requirements of a dog. The book then moves on to cats, amino acids of special importance, protein deficiency, protein toxicity and protein sources. Preceding that paragraph was the definition of protein, its structure and metabolism, digestibility, usage, storage, excretion, the chemical analysis of protein and protein quality. But on the protein requirements of dogs, this 1,315-page behemoth affords the subject a single paragraph and just 18 pages on protein in total. Nowhere does it suggest a dog can or should satisfy his protein requirements with fresh meat.

Obviously, of most concern is their suggestion that adult dogs can maintain good health on just 8% protein in their diets and that by consequence the 'AAFCO recommendations should be interpreted as *daily allowances*, not as absolute minimum requirements', which AAFCO itself clearly states they are. This statement is supported by reference to the NRC's *Nutrient Requirement of Cats and Dogs*,[6] which itself uses five studies to support its stance. Four of these studies are each more than 50 years old and each involves just a handful of dogs. Most were but a few weeks long. Worst still, only 'nitrogen balance' was assessed in each dog at the end of trial – not health, not skin, bone or organ soundness, not behaviour, not reproductive ability or any other of the multitude of areas where adequate protein is central.

The final study was of protein restriction in just 17 beagles over 42 months. This time a fraction more information was gathered. They found that dogs maintained their body weight and blood chemistries during the period, although nearly all suffered a taurine deficiency (common in meat-eaters fed little to no meat), and one came down with dilated cardiomyopathy (DCM) and another had borderline DCM.

The quality of the evidence aside, we need to ask ourselves: why do both the SACN and the NRC focus purely on the *minimum* amount of protein we can feed a dog and not the optimum? To be fair, the NRC (2006) does conclude, '… the optimal concentrations for other variables and outcomes (e.g. optimal immune response, wound healing, health in old age) have to be evaluated before more specific recommendations can be made'. Strangely, this is yet to be done by the industry.

As opposed to beagles stuck in a cage eking out a wholly unnatural and sedentary existence, the normal way to test the effect of a protein-restricted diet is to put the protein-restricted animal under some form of stress, ideally outside the lab. When this is done, we see the true power of protein. Sled dogs were maintained at 16%, 24%, 32% and 40% of their calories from high-quality animal protein. The dogs fed the highest protein level maintained a larger plasma volume and red blood cell mass during strenuous training.[12] Moreover, all of the dogs consuming the low-protein diet had at least one injury during the racing season that resulted in it being removed from training for a minimum of one week. Those dogs consuming the highest amount of protein were injury free.

For now, I put it to you that the *minimum* amount of protein bears absolutely no relevance to the *optimum* health of a dog.

Why Meat Meal Is the Lowest Form of Protein on the Planet

Isn't it strange today that while most of us are growing increasingly concerned over the providence of our food, pet owners rarely spend a moment wondering where the ingredients in their pet food come from? It seems all we care about is that the correct *quantity* is consumed, as if knowing a product containing '18% protein' on the side was the normal route taken for optimal nutrition in our children. The whole notion that a correct quantity of food will sustain life was thought to have died out somewhere in the middle of the 19th century. Until then, people believed that all food contained a single sustaining nutritional substance, a universal element or Gia.[13] A kilo of meat or biscuits was deemed to have the same nutritional value as a kilo of fruit or vegetables. Happy days! All a person had to do was to eat enough biscuits each day and they'd be fine. It was only when enough sailors had died of scurvy that someone twigged this might not be the case.

To take this point further, if I were to offer you a dry food for your adult dog that I made myself and told you it was an enviable 22% animal protein, 17% fat and 50% carbohydrate, would you like the sound of it? Interestingly, for most vets, this is an ample description of a suitable canine diet. If you were to press me further regarding my new dry food, I might inform you beef meal was the number one ingredient. For most, that is all you will ever learn of the ingredients used. But what if you pressed me further, and I admitted that my dry food consisted of an old leather boot (protein), some used motor oil (fat) and a heap of used sawdust from a pig factory (carbohydrate), how quickly would you slip your wallet back in your pocket?

Like buying cheap burgers from a rat checker, we need to first find out exactly what we are trading our dollars for. Ingredients permitted by AAFCO (2008)[14] for use in pet food can make for a horrifying read. They include hair, dehydrated food waste, dehydrated garbage, dehydrated rumen contents, dried poultry waste and dried swine waste 'not containing less than 20% protein, 35% crude fibre or wood shavings or suitable bedding material, and not more than 20% ash'. Yummy!

The two most common forms of *meat* used are by-products and meat meals. Not all as bad as it sounds, by-products are by their very definition not classified as actual meat *per se*. By-products are everything but the meat from the carcass, including but not limited to organs such as the lungs, spleen, kidneys, liver, brain, ears, lips, tail, stomach and intestines freed of their contents as well as the blood, bone and fatty tissue of the animal. Each of these ingredients, bar the gut contents, is fine food for dogs when used in moderation, balance and in conjunction with a source of actual meat protein. Many, indeed, are positively vital. We will return to these in Section 4.

A more dubious form of *meat* used by the industry, however, is meat meal or, more correctly, meat and bone meal. Meat meal, which arrives to the pet food factory as a grey powder, is a profitable by-product of the rendering process. Think of a rendering vat like a giant pressure cooker, which stews up all the leftovers and waste of the meat industry under high temperature (121°C) and high pressure. The mix can consist of all sorts. The AAFCO (2008)[14], which set the rules for pet food quality, defines the animal debris permissible in pet food as 'the rendered product from mammal tissues, exclusive of any added blood, hair, hoof, horn, hide trimmings, manure, stomach and rumen contents except in such amounts as *may occur unavoidably* in good processing practices', leaving the door swinging widely open for 'less careful' producers, perhaps. Also permitted in the mix are spoiled animal carcasses, roadkill and garbage from the food industry.

Once this waste is adequately stewed, the fat floats to the top and is scraped off to make your soap and jellies. The protein portion, consisting of any meat and bone fragments and *other material,* sinks to the bottom as a lumpy grey goo. This is removed, dried under more temperature and pulverised into powder. Packaged in drums, it is now ready for transportation to animal feed companies.

Before we get into the nutritional qualities of such a product, we must first draw an important distinction between US and EU policy when it comes to their rendering plants, in particular, what they are permitted to handle, as it's fair to say the US system is a lot more porous.

The European Union was rattled by the bovine spongiform encephalopathy (BSE) crisis in the 1990s and since then has enforced tougher measures on rendering plants. For instance, EU rendering plants can only handle meat from slaughterhouses that has been passed fit for human consumption. The EU states:

> ...animal by-products derived from animals shown not to be fit for human consumption as a result of a health inspection should not enter the feed chain...
>
> **EU Regulation (EC) No. 1069/2009**

They are very specific about this, stating that animal by-products derived from animals not fit for human consumption should not enter the feed chain, be it pet or human. This immediately excludes 4D meat (dead, diseased, dying, disabled meat), roadkill, supermarket and restaurant waste and euthanised animals, including cats and dogs. This material must be sent for cremation and the waste from this industry is not permitted back into the food chain.

While US law dictates something similar to the EU stance, the problem is the Food and Drug Administration (FDA) and their various Departments of Agriculture are actively ignoring this law, at least when it comes to the pet food sector. So much so that the FDA has issued its own Compliance Policy (number 675.400), titled "Rendered Animal Feed Ingredients" (italics in the excerpt added by me). It reads:

No regulatory action will be considered for animal feed ingredients resulting from the ordinary rendering process of industry, *including those using animals which have died otherwise than by slaughter*, provided they are not otherwise in violation of the law.

For canned pet food, the FDA also has a policy (690.300), which states (italics added by me):

Pet food consisting of material from diseased animals or animals which have died otherwise than by slaughter, which is in violation of 402(a)(5) will not ordinarily be actionable, if it is not otherwise in violation of the law. *It will be considered fit for animal consumption.*

The basis for this law dodge is that the 'Center for Veterinary Medicine (CVM) is aware of no instances of disease or other hazard occurring' from this practice in a canned-food-packing house.

In this way, the American system leaves itself open for the inclusion of some very worrying ingredients, with dead pets being top of the list for actual pet owners. Described as 'quasi-cannibalism' by *The New York Times*,[15] six to seven million dogs and cats killed every year have been estimated to make their way into US rendering vats.

It gets worse. In the 1980s, a startling 40% of pets euthanised in large US cities were rendered for meat, bone meal and fat.[16] Martin (2008)[17] highlights that figures from the National Animal Control Association stated 13 million household pets are euthanised each year in the United States, 200 tonnes from Los Angeles each month – 200 tonnes! Of the 13 million pets, 30% are buried, 30% cremated and the rest, 5.2 million animals, are rendered. In a piece titled "How Dogs and Cats Get Recycled into Pet Food", Eckhouse (1990),[18] writing for the *San Francisco Chronicle*, quotes one rendering company estimating that it 'rendered somewhere between 10,000 and 30,000 pounds of dogs and cats a day out of a total of 250,000 to 500,000 pounds of cattle, poultry, butcher scrap and other materials.'

Nobody can tell the fate of the meat meal produced by the plants rendering cats and dogs. Hopefully, it was just fed to pigs and not back to our pets. The pet food companies will assure you they, of course, were never, ever, using meals containing dogs. But how they can say that is anyone's guess when, as of 2007, pet food companies were not DNA testing the meat meal flours arriving daily into their plants. A Pet Food Industry release in 2004, representing over 90%

of the pet food companies in the United States, assured readers that most of its clients did not use cat/dog by-products. However, its website is linked to the top five renderers in the country, two of which collect pets. Martin (1997)[17] points out that even if they decided to test meat meal coming in, not all meal supplied contains cats and dogs, and a lot of animal DNA is lost in cooking, certainly in the high-pressure, high-temperature cooking of extruded pet food. Thus, frequent and rigorous tests would be required. These would be expensive and time-consuming and are simply not conducted.

Not that Europe should rest on her laurels just yet. Just because we are not permitted does not necessarily mean it is not happening. After all, there is money at stake. Historically, very much like the United States, Ireland (and to a lesser degree the United Kingdom) slaughters a terrible number of dogs each year. Let's look at the ones we know about during our peak killing period, 2007 (things have significantly improved since the crash). In 2007, the Irish Greyhound Board (a semi-state body that is government-funded and in receipt of EU grants and subsidies such as the Farm Diversification Scheme, but thankfully open to the Freedom of Information Act as a result) bred 34,544 pups for racing, of which 20,916 were given identity cards making them 'eligible to qualify for racing' the following year.

Thus, 13,628 become 'unaccounted for' in a single year. While some will be picked up by the rehoming charities, it's difficult to get clear figures on the fate of all these dogs, largely as so much of the industry happens behind closed doors. Moreover, these figures are just from the government-funded kennels and do not include the privately run greyhound facilities. Then, any dogs that actually make it to the track have a 3-year shelf life at best, after which, unless used for breeding or picked up by the rescue agencies, they will be disposed of. This is where it can get even murkier. On May 21, 2009, *The Sun* newspaper exposed Larry Earle, owner of a knacker's yard (where horses are slaughtered) and a licensed meat-seller (meat from a knacker's yards is generally used in animal feed, be it pork or pet). Earle confessed to killing Irish greyhounds for €10 a go with a captive bolt gun. The piece did not elaborate if Larry, for the knockdown price of €10, was then adequately disposing of these greyhounds outside of his meat plant in the appropriate manner with the appropriate authorities (which would involve collecting all the dogs in a suitable refrigerated area and loading them into a truck each month, paying over the appropriate fee for their incineration, in a profitable manner, out of the €10 collected for each one). All we can do is hope that Larry's very cheap meat meal was not used by any Irish pet food manufacturers. And while we're all crossing our fingers, let's further hope that Larry is the only rogue meat producer in Europe, though the signs are not good.

In 2013, 13 separate EU countries were caught including horse and, worse still for Muslim and Jewish communities, pork meat in their beef burgers, it seems pretty unlikely that we know a fraction of what actually goes on, even in our own meat industry. Spurred on by the horsemeat scandal, in 2014, the British Food Standards Agency and the consumer watchdog Which? issued a joint report examining the meat content of British takeaway foods. During the course of their analysis, they found that lamb used in various kebab houses was routinely replaced with pork, beef, chicken, turkey and what could possibly be vermin or pets. Of 60 lamb dishes tested, they found 29 were 'suspect', 17 contained different meats, 7 contained no lamb at all and 5 had meat that could not be identified when compared to the meats they had on file. To be clear, on file they had all the usual meats, lamb, chicken, beef, pork, goat, fish, rabbit and some more worrying types, cat, dog, fox, badger, rodent. The agency was left hoping that the meat they were looking at was something 'not normally eaten in the United Kingdom'. Yum!

As for Asia, containing countries of mass populace, some of which actually eat dogs, others with often vast numbers of free-roaming dogs, I can only assume it has to be at least as poor as the United States. Not that it puts the market off in the slightest. The problem is that pet food producers do not get rewarded, financially or otherwise, for the quality of the meat meal they use in their mixes. Hence, the cheapest will always be the most attractive to producers. You would think the melamine scandal in 2007, which killed thousands and thousands of pets worldwide, (more on this later) would put manufacturers off using ingredients sourced from Asia for a spell. But since that very year there has been year-on-year growth in the importation of Chinese pet food into the United States market. The US Department of Agriculture figures which revealed that in 2007, the United States was importing 55 million pounds of dog and cat food from China. By 2011, this had risen to 85 million pounds ("FDA Investigates Animal Illnesses Linked to Jerky Pet Treats", published on the FDA website in 2012). So, whether the meal itself is imported or simply the finished product, there is a very high chance that millions of American pet food customers are feeding the remains of animals sourced from an Asian rendering plant.

A way to test for the possible presence of pets in pet food is to look for the chemical sodium pentobarbital (SPB). While occasionally SPB is used as both a sedative and sometimes slaughtering technique for larger animals (usually horses), this is the chemical most commonly used to euthanise small pets like cats and dogs. In 1998, the US FDA tested 90 different brands of dry dog food and 44 tested positive for SPB (almost 50%), a flagrant violation of federal law. In 2000, the agency again tested 60 brands of dry/kibble dog food and still 10 tested positive for pentobarbital.[19] Neither time did the FDA require the pet food companies to recall the product, loosely in line with the fact that policies 675.400 and 690.300 permit that sort of material to be included in pet food. Hence, 20 years on, they're all still at it. In 2017 and 2018 over 30 US brands of canned pet food were voluntarily recalled when SPB was identified in their products. It remains today the second most common cause of pet food recall, accounting for more than 30 million pounds of canned pet food recalled from 2012-2019.[20] It is yet to be the cause of a single recall of raw dog food (as of October 2019).

Pets eating pets aside, in 2018, ABC news in Australia did a great piece on how truly nasty the rendering industry can be. In their piece, they interviewed Dennis Pedretti, an employee of the Australian Tallows Producers who stated the following:

> Having been in the industry and seen what goes on, I can see why people are alarmed...we have sheep heads come through. They have a new tag. They go into the pit. There would be plastic, I mean butchers would be getting rid of their material and they don't care what they are putting in the bin, so it would be plastic, cans, all of those sorts of things you would see....
>
> A roller door goes up, a truck backs up, tips it in and tonnes of offal fall into the pit. It goes through an organ, it goes through a mincer. So it is ground up and crushed up and then goes through to the cooking process. So the ear tags with the heat effectively melt and then when it is going through the drying process effectively become a pinhead.
>
> The quantity that is going out is in containers, so 20-tonne containers and a lot of containers went out every day so it is a lot of product, a lot of containers, a lot of customers.

Pretty bad, but more was to come. When ABC news showed a photo of this meat waste and plastic mix to the owner of the operation, Dennis King, asking for comment. The conversation went like this:

> **Angelique Donnellan of ABC**: What do you see in those photos?
>
> **Dennis King**: I see little, hundreds of little pieces of ear tags or it could be blue gloves.
>
> **Angelique**: Is the plastic doing harm to pets?

Dennis: I don't believe so, no.

So, when it says *meat meal* in pet food, you and your pet food producer will never know for sure what is actually in there. A quick tip though, the least-worst type of meat meal is when it is labelled as *chicken meal* or *beef meal*. At least then you can hope it contains some form of chicken or beef debris. If it is simply labelled 'meat meal,' it means they can't even tell you what animal matter was in the mix.

With this sort of meat going in, it's probably lucky for dogs that cereal-based pet food manufacturers tend not to use a whole lot anyway. Take, for example, a cereal-based dry dog food that states on the front, 'with chicken'. They are only obliged to include 4% chicken meal in the product (AAFCO requirements). The rest of your dry food product, bar the 15% animal fat sourced from a rendering plant, is all plant-based carbohydrates and protein. Anything after that 4% inclusion rate is a bonus for your carnivorous pet. As cereal-based pet foods rarely list the percentage 'meat' in their products, they will not be rewarded for this little bonus, so I'll leave it to you to puzzle out the exact figure.

Quite clearly, meat meals are not used in pet food with your animal's nutritional needs at heart. I recommend avoiding them at all costs. Sadly, not everyone agrees. In 2012, Keith Levy, President of Mars Royal Canin USA told *Forbes* magazine 'the actual source of the protein is not important'.[21] While I, and surely every other nutritionist on the planet not working for a dry dog food company, would strongly disagree with this statement on many fronts, it was made in reference to Royal Canin announcing they were now using chicken feathers as the protein source in their allergy-control food. A result, apparently, of 'putting the dog at the heart of the innovation process'.

Just one of the reasons the source is vital, in the literal sense of the word, is that different foods offer different nutrient profiles. In particular, they differ in their amino acid profile. There are more than 30 amino acids and each species needs a different one. In fact, even within a species, an individual can need more of one than another, depending on their current physiological status. Of these, the following are EAAs for the dog:

> **Arginine** stimulates the immune system, induces growth hormone release and supports the liver by detoxifying ammonia.

Histidine releases histamines, is associated with pain control and widens small blood vessels to stimulate stomach acid secretion.

Isoleucine and **Leucine** - see Valine.

Lysine promotes bone growth in puppies and stimulates secretion of gastric juices.

Methionine assists gallbladder function, helps prevent fat deposits in the liver, balances the urinary tract pH and gives rise to taurine.

Phenylalanine related to appetite control, increases blood pressure in hypotension, works with minerals in skin and hair pigmentation and produces adrenalin and noradrenalin.

Threonine regulates energy draw, works in mood elevation or depression, manufactures adrenalin and pre-curses thyroid hormone.

Tryptophan produces serotonin that induces sleep.

Valine (and isoleucine and leucine) are EAAs that work together to regulate protein turnover and energy metabolism.

Taurine is involved in a large number of metabolic processes and can become essential under certain circumstances (although it remains up for debate if this is truly essential in dogs, as we will discuss).

Unsurprisingly, meat provides all the EAA's a dog needs to run his body correctly. Hence, they are termed *complete* proteins for dogs, unlike plant ingredients, which do not and are thus termed *incomplete* proteins for the dog (as they lack amino acids such as arginine, lysine, tryptophan and taurine). Nor is it as simple as just *animal* protein either. Like comparing skin to bone, beef muscle will obviously have an entirely different amino acid profile (and vitamin and mineral and chemical profile) to say beef liver. It might be duck and lamb that will offer far more tryptophan to your cat than chicken or turkey. Rabbit and lamb meat do not contain a whole lot of taurine. White meats like chicken and fish contain much more phosphorus than red meats, so up until recently, we tended to avoid them in a pet with kidney disease. And so it goes with each and every part of every animal out there.

Levy's point, we have to assume, is that whatever your ingredient mix lacks, you can add it in later in supplement form. However, as we will repeatedly show throughout this section, the notion of supplementing plant-based and thus nutrient-deficient dog food products with proteins, vitamins and minerals from jars appears to be something of a dark art. Studies show they are very consistently getting it wrong.

In 2001, hugely excessive methionine levels, considered one of the most limiting amino acids in animal feeds but also one of the most toxic of the EAA's if you don't get it right,[22] were included by the Iams Company resulting in the toxicosis of at least twenty-one dogs. According to the FDA report, which followed consumer complaints, the firm analysed their products and found the methionine concentration was in the range of 1.60-2.75%. AAFCO (2016)[23] recommends 0.33% methionine for adult dogs.

But of all the amino acids out there, taurine is surely the most famous.

Why Taurine is so Famous...

Taurine is a protein that is found in the muscle of every animal on the planet.[24] It is the second most abundant protein in muscle meat after glutamine. It supports neurological development and helps regulate the level of water and mineral salts in the blood. A taurine deficiency will cause a whole host of issues ranging from blindness, deafness and poor immune response, to abortions, lower number of foetuses, poor neonatal growth, reduced birth weights, reduced survival, as well as an increase in skeletal abnormalities such as curved spines, small stature and abnormal hind leg development. They don't call them *EAA's* for nothing. Something thousands of cats amply demonstrated for us, more than four decades ago.

In the 1970s, cats eating processed pet food began to go blind and die in great numbers from a new issue called Dilated Cardiomyopathy (DCM). First documented in the literature in 1970,[25] DCM is a condition where a thickening of the heart wall can result in decreased energy, cough, difficulty breathing and eventual death. At its peak, it is estimated that DCM was killing thousands of cats each year.[26] Typically, the blame was laid at the feet of the pet owners, that it was likely the feeding of dog food to cats that was causing the problem.[27] However once enough pets had suffered enough harm, public outcry grew loud enough not to be ignored. University of California, Davis began looking into it and found low plasma taurine in the affected animals to be the problem.[26]

Unlike dogs, taurine is an EAA in cats, which they must consume in their diet. Unfortunately for these cats, as meat is expensive, by the late 70s, cat food contained so little meat and it offered little by way of a dietary source of taurine to the cats. The manufacturers were soon convinced to up the taurine levels in their products, and the cats stopped dying,[28] which was nice. The same manufacturers now tend to say, 'after years of clinical research, we at Product X have discovered cats are carnivores and need taurine in their diet so this cat food has added taurine'. They have not necessarily added meat.

Taurine is deemed a nonessential amino acid for dogs, as they can manufacture some taurine from the more readily available dietary sulphur amino acids like cysteine and methionine.[24] Hence manufacturers are not required to include it in pet food. However, dogs are not particularly adept at the conversion. Sanderson *et al.* (2001)[29] fed protein-restricted diets to 17 beagles for 42 months. They noticed most suffered taurine depletion in some form, even when the diets were supplemented with cysteine and methionine to above adequate levels. It happens that DCM is also one of the most common heart conditions in dogs,[30] some of which are clearly genetic (Cavalier King Charles Spaniels, Dachshunds, Miniature and Toy Poodles, Doberman Pinschers, Boxers, Golden Retrievers and Miniature Schnauzers suffer DCM far in excess of others). However, despite lessons learned in the 70's, dry pet food continues to cause DCM in dogs fed *complete and balanced* dry foods.[31-33]

> ...[the] results suggest that consumption of certain commercial diets may be associated with low blood or plasma taurine concentrations and DCM in dogs. Taurine supplementation may result in prolonged survival times in these dogs...
>
> **Fascetti, 2003**[33]

Dry pet food can cause a taurine deficiency in your dog for a variety of reasons. First, there is the lack of meat ingredients (and thus taurine) in the mix. Next, as you will learn, manufacturers are consistently getting their methionine levels wrong, crucial to taurine production in the dog. High cooking temperatures can then destroy what little taurine is actually present in animal feed ingredients.[24] Furthermore, cooking degrades the protein in pet food into complexes that are resilient to digestion, feeding the wrong bacteria further down and these bacteria like to eat taurine.[34,35]

Another issue with kibble is that taurine is used in bile, which is excreted at the start of the intestinal tract to digest fats. Animals are generally excellent at recovering this taurine down the line by reabsorbing bile salts in the small intestines. However, common pet food filler ingredients, such as rice bran and beet pulp, leftovers of human food processing, are shown to bind bile salts, thus rendering them indigestible,[36] with beet pulp being the worst offender, further reducing available taurine for the animal.

Couple all these factors with breed dispositions and possibly larger body size (requiring a greater need of taurine) and you're asking for DCM. Studies show DCM often occurs in pets fed a *complete* cereal-based pet food, particularly those formulated using lamb,[32,37,38,] as lamb (and rabbit) meat offers the least amount of taurine.

The taurine issue is now so ingrained in the pet owner psyche that cat owners are still stressing about it even when feeding fresh meat-based diets, despite the fact most of these mixes contain a more than adequate taurine content in that department. Most, but not all.

Meat is high in taurine, but not all meat parts are equal. Organs like beef kidney, liver and lung contain significantly more taurine than beef muscle. As a whole though, that too depends on which muscle you're talking about.[24] That said, crucially for cat owners, some meats contain very little taurine and where they are fed the meat for too long, it can result in a taurine deficiency. Glasgow *et al.* (2002)[39] compared two groups of cats, one consuming nothing but rabbit meat (organs removed) and the other a Purina complete product. After 1 month, they showed significant benefits on the meat diet, including greater appetence, better stools and better-quality coats (although the latter was an observation and not measured). A cat on the rabbit diet was fatally struck down with DCM and 70% of the remainder on the rabbit-only diet was also affected. It is a sad cautionary lesson that: a) rabbit meat is low in taurine and b) the same, single-protein diet is not recommended for anything other than a short time. As we will highlight in our final section, variety is crucial to a well-balanced, species-appropriate diet.

If in doubt, it's always advisable for cat owners and owners of breeds at risk of DCM to limit the amount of low-taurine meats, just to be sure.

Why Protein Digestibility Is So Important

Source aside, another crucial consideration in protein quality is digestibility, as all the protein in the world is no good to you if you cannot digest and absorb it. Animal protein is more digestible than plant protein.[40,41] We can all testify to this. A less than enviable job I recall some people doing was when Dublin Bay was expanding in the 1980s and three divers were given the task of documenting the course of underwater currents prior to building. Their method was to track the path of undigested plant debris (mainly tomato seeds and corn kernels, apparently) coming from a sewage outlet that was discharging into Dublin Bay at the time.

While cooking increases the digestibility (and thus biological value) of vegetable items by breaking down tough plant fibre,[42] allowing an animal access to the goodies inside, it is the opposite with meat protein once temperatures exceed 110°C.[43] Processing can negatively affect amino acids in a variety of ways, through proteolysis (the breakdown of amino acids into smaller particles), protein cross-linking, oxidative reactions and Maillard reactions.[44] Of all processing factors, heat is the biggest enemy of protein as well as many heat-liable nutrients therein. High cooking temperatures increase the *mutagenicity* of meat and plant protein[45-47] by inducing a nonenzymatic reaction, often termed a Maillard reaction after its discoverer, between proteins and sugars, essentially making proteins, those proteins aggregate and cross-link. You can actually watch this mutation occurring slowly when your clear egg turns to white on the pan or those tasty, flame-grilled lines on your meat off the grill. In fact, that taste you are enjoying is a by-product of this Maillard reaction products or (MRPs). Taste aside, the problem is this reaction also makes meat more difficult to digest. Think about when you leave that bit of steak too long on the pan and you spend the next hour trying to chew your way through it. This process is eventuated by the loss of natural enzymes present in all animal cells. When you chew and eventually break down these cells in the stomach, enzymes leak out which help us to digest our meal,[48] giving us a digestive edge. However, heating meat much above 40°C (–40°F) destroys natural enzymes present in all raw meat cells.[48]

For these reasons, we know protein mutated by high heat is significantly more difficult to digest by humans,[49] cats,[50] dogs[51] and every other animal studied to date[3,52-59] which is something we have known since 1933.[60] This is why you must not feed cooked bones to dogs. X-rays show they are far more resilient to digestion in the gut.[61] Pointed, undigested fragments can pass into the intestine where they may build up, causing impaction in the dog or perforation of the intestinal wall.

The meat used in dry pet food is at least double or in the case of meat meal, triple-heat processed. Meat ingredients are first produced by rendering a mix of animal protein for at least 30 minutes under high temperature and pressure. This process is shown to drastically reduce the availability of amino acids present,[55, 62-64] rendering results in significant losses of lysine, methionine, threonine, leucine, taurine, valine, phenylalanine, cystine, serine and aspartic acid.[54] The protein soup that is harvested from this process is then dried to a powder under high temperature. Hence, rendered meat meal ingredients pale in comparison to fresh meat.[65] But we're not done yet. The meal is then transported to the pet food factory where it is cooked again at high temperature (121°C, 250°F) and intense pressure during the extrusion process, all of which further reduces the bioavailability of protein to the dog.[66] Unsurprisingly, cats are shown to digest significantly more dry matter, crude protein and energy on raw meat-based diets than kibble diets.[67,68] Similarly, the protein in raw dog food diets, which is found to be highly digestible,[69] is significantly better digested than the protein in dry kibbles.[70]

Reduced digestibility of protein is an important point. We know dogs need 18% crude protein (meaning total protein, CP) at an absolute *minimum* for normal function over 6 months (in a caged environment). Hence, nearly all 'complete' cereal-based dry food for adult dogs contains in or around this luxurious amount of protein. However, the CP on a pet food packet has been determined *in vitro* (in a laboratory) by combusting the entire sample by fire. In reality (*in vivo*), full digestion of all the protein present in these products rarely occurs, meaning not all of it is bioavailable to the dog. A number of factors contribute to this. Take, for example, the following premium puppy foods promoted by vets. We are told the average CP content of this food is around 23%. The first five ingredients are chicken meal, brown rice, rice, corn gluten meal and wheat gluten meal. In terms of bioavailability, the first issue here is the meal. We know dogs find chicken meal harder to digest.[52-54,66] In fact, not all meals are digested equally either. A study of three extruded pet food meals based on lamb meal, poultry meal or fish meal found that both dogs (and mink) digested as little as 71.5% of the crude protein available in lamb-based dry kibbles, compared to 80.2% and 87.0% of the poultry and fish meal-based foods, respectively.[71]

Second, not all the protein in this food comes from meat. The next two ingredients are rice, which is very largely carbohydrates although the brown rice will offer a very minor protein addition. The fourth and fifth ingredients, corn gluten and wheat gluten meal, are the by-products of human food manufacturing. We know they are almost entirely indigestible protein sources for dogs.[4,72] They are used here to boost the protein level on the side of the packet.

Again, proteins are the building blocks of life. Good quality protein is vital to the development of solid joints, organs and bones. Having enough of it is obviously crucial. According to the AAFCO (2016), 22.5% protein is the 'minimum required for normal development in a puppy'. With this in mind, how much of the CP stated on the pack is actually available to the puppy? Krogdahl *et al.* (2004)[73] examined this question of the crude (total) protein available to puppies. The authors tested a range of different dry food diets in mink, including Eukanuba Puppy, Proplan Puppy, Royal Canin Puppy and Hill's Puppy. They found that of the amount of protein stated, less than 75% of it was available to the animal. On average,

Eukanuba Puppy stated 27.9% protein, only 20.3% was actually available; Proplan Puppy stated 26.2% protein, only 20.1% was available to the test animals; Royal Canin Puppy stated 21.7% protein, only 16.7% was available; Hill's Puppy stated 26.8% protein, only 20.8% was available to the animal. In fact, Krogdahl *et al.*[73] further found no discernible difference in the nutrient content or protein quality or protein digestibility between lower-quality (cheaper) dry foods and these more premium products.

The Effect of Insufficient Protein on the Dog

In the very short term, there are a few perceivable adverse effects in your dog. In the long term, however, the effects of a protein deficiency are devastating for the animal. As protein functions in every single part and process of your body, victims of protein deficiency may expect a large array of issues. When protein intake is deficient, protein turnover in the dog slows and lean body mass is gradually depleted, leading to increased morbidity and mortality.[74] As early as 1968, studies showed that dogs maintained on the poor-quality protein are likely to suffer cartilage and bone issues, shortening of the villi and a reduction in the volume of the mucous membrane.[75] The study by Reynolds *et al.* (1996)[12] further elucidates this, when sled dogs fed 16%, 24%, 32% and 40% of ME from protein were seen to achieve a larger plasma volume and red blood cell mass during strenuous training, and less injury, the more protein they consumed. In fact, sled dogs have repeatedly demonstrated that working dogs need protein and fat. Kronfeld (1977)[76] demonstrated that his working sled dogs performed better on diets of protein/fat ratio of 1:1 compared to those on diets containing carbohydrates, a result of their ability to maintain higher serum concentrations of albumin, calcium, magnesium and free fatty acids during the racing season. They also exhibited the greatest increases in red cell count, haemoglobin concentration and packed cell volume. It should be pointed out that these are endurance dogs. Studies also show that a moderate protein and fat (24% ME from protein, 33% ME from fat and 43% ME from carbohydrate) might be more beneficial for sprint performance in dogs, as indicated by faster racing times (32.43 ± 0.48 versus 32.61 ± 0.50 s; $P < 0.05$) over a 500-m distance.[77] This is possibly a result of sprinting breeds having more fast-twitch muscles, as is normal for a sprinting animal, which the typical dog is not. Dogs are normally long-distance running machines and do better on more sustaining energy sources.[78]

A protein deficiency in the average dog is likely to be far more subtle than that. Burns *et al.* (1982)[40] studied the effects of dietary protein quantity and quality on the growth of dogs and rats. They concluded the rat is a useful model for examining the quality of proteins fed to dogs. With this in mind, Stewart *et al.* (1975)[79] tested a very marginal protein deficiency over the course of 12 generations of rats. They documented the proportion of small-for-gestational-age offspring 10 times higher in a malnourished colony than in a well-nourished colony. Furthermore, these rats suffered slower growth, delayed sexual maturation (especially in the females) and in adulthood, both sexes were significantly lighter and shorter than adults of the well-nourished colony. Platt and Stewart (1968)[75] found dogs maintained from weaning on diets of low protein value, grow slowly and develop changes in their bones, brains and behaviour.

Interestingly, Stewart *et al.* (1975),[79] note that in absolute terms organs weighed less, particularly brains, which were 53.5% lighter than those of the well-nourished animals. And this had an effect on their behaviour. Affected rats suffered increased sensitivity to noise, and as adults they showed marked differences in behaviour and learning patterns. 'It was difficult to attract and hold their attention.' As in humans and monkeys, a chronic lack of protein has been shown to cause behavioural disruption in dogs, resulting in behavioural and learning defects.[80,81] The researchers later found this to be due to a thinning of nerve walls called myelin sheaths,[75] most notably in the cerebellum where cell loss was greatest.

On top of growth, behavioural disruption and performance, dogs on poor-quality protein diets can expect disruption of the endocrine balance, producing marked aberrations in the control of carbohydrate metabolism,[82] which is of particular concern to dogs fed a high-carbohydrate diet – an issue that persisted even after rehabilitation on a proper diet.

A diet deficient in protein is expected to produce a poorer coat on a dog. Hence, coat condition is one of the top benefits cited by raw feeders. As you will find throughout this section, there are many potential reasons for this, including the lack of absorbable zinc and the lack of fresh fats. But by far, protein is the most important. Your dog's skin and coat are made up almost exclusively of protein. In fact, up to 30% of the protein your dog consumes goes into maintaining their skin and coat each day.[83] When you make a dog exist on the minimum amount of protein required for normal function, you starve less essential processes of the protein they need to look fabulous. Researchers at the University of California, Davis, ' observed that a raw meat and bone diet did produce a softer, fuller coat than complete, cereal-based dry food in cats,[39] although, sadly, they failed to measure it in any meaningful way.

Maillard Reaction Products

Then we come to the dangers of eating cooked meat as a long-term feeding strategy, bringing us back to Maillard reactions. Cooking meat under high temperature produces compounds termed MRPs, some of which you have been familiar with for a long time: the lovely smell a cooking steak gives off, the brown on the meat and the taste of a flame-cooked burger. All MRPs. You can be sure pet food manufacturers are more than aware of these little fellas. Sensory analysis of pet foods has been considered a highly important field of study for the pet food industry for, at least, the last three decades.[90] The industry has used certain MRPs for years to boost the flavour, palatability and thus consumption of their products.[84]

Their downside is when they try to kill you. In humans, a variety of MRPs are linked to cancer,[85] inflammatory and age-related degenerative processes,[86] as well as possibly playing a role in diabetes, and both renal and cardiovascular diseases.[87] With the recent rise of all meat-based dry foods for our pets, this is now an issue that needs immediate attention in pets.

Van Rooijen *et al.* (2014)[88] examined 67 extruded, canned and pelleted dog and cat foods used for growth and maintenance for the presence of a variety of harmful MRPs. They found that the average daily intake of certain MRPs were 122 times higher for dogs and 38 times higher for cats than the average intake for adult humans. The authors concluded the need for more research on the long-term health implications of MRP consumption by dogs and cats.

Gentzel (2013)[89] states that the bioaccumulation of advanced glycation end products, an MRP, is linked to chronic systematic inflammation and cancer in both humans and dogs. The MRP acrylamide has been studied intensively over the last decade, largely as it is so carcinogenic to humans,[85] and yet sadly so prevalent in many of the foods we enjoy each day. From chips and muffins to biscuits and breakfast cereal, where processed food is, you will often find acrylamides. Interestingly, they were first discovered when Dr. Eden Tareke was comparing acrylamide levels in wild animals and domesticated pets. She found unexpectedly high levels of acrylamides in pets attributable to consumption of highly processed food.[90]

Of particular interest, too, are Heterocyclic Amines (HCAs), the highly mutagenic and potentially carcinogenic by-products formed during meat browning.[49] HCA mutagens are also potent carcinogens in rodents and humans.[91-97] Researchers at the National Cancer Institute (www.cancer.gov) found that human subjects who ate beef rare or medium-rare, had less than one-third the risk of stomach cancer compared to those who ate beef medium-well or well-done. They recommend cooking meat below 100°C (212°F) to avoid HCAs. The vast majority of dry and canned pet food is cooked at 121°C (250°F) under great pressure for 30 minutes. Further, decreasing the water content of meat prior to heating increases mutagen formation.[98] This should all be very bad news for products using 4 times cooked meat meal as a protein source (once during rendering, again during drying, once during extrusion cooking, again during drying). Knize *et al.* (2003)[99] analysed 25 commercial pet foods for mutagenic activity (HCAs) and all but one gave a positive mutagenic response. The authors concluded that there is a connection between dietary HCAs and cancer in cats and dogs consuming these foods.

Worse still, these complexes can alter our immune-reactivity toward the food protein in question, increasing sensitivity, which can result in allergy to that protein in both humans[100] and cats.[50] Guildford *et al.* (1996)[51] found cooked, indigestible protein complexes are known to arouse the immune system around the dog's intestinal mucosa, resulting in gut complications.

Take note all you owners of dogs with a chicken or beef sensitivity. Processed ingredients are significantly more likely to illicit an immune response than the ingredients in their raw form. Vojdani (2009)[101] noted how IgE antibodies (central to the true allergy pathway) showed a three- to eight-fold increase in human patients challenged with a processed food antigen compared to the antigen in raw form. However, that is not to say dogs can't be sensitive to the raw form of a protein. Interestingly, Bethlehema *et al.* (2012),[102] using patch testing, found that some dogs can react to the raw version of a meat and not the cooked. Hence, when conducting elimination diets in suffering dogs, home-cooked diets should not be excluded entirely.

Interestingly, and unlike humans who are born with the condition, truly allergic, hypersensitive (IgE-mediated) reactions seem to suddenly materialise in dogs that did not exhibit issues previously, most often in dogs consuming the same diet for more than 2 years.[104] Termed spontaneously arising dietary hypersensitivity, it can arise to a variety of proteins but most commonly chicken and beef. There are two theories why this might be the case. The first is the vast amount of dry food is based on chicken or beef protein, it being the cheapest available. Should that animal develop a chronic gut issue following a life of ultra-processed food consumption, leaky gut is a potential end point of that disease. If chicken or beef is one of the major proteins of the mix, it will be one of the first through the gaps, alarming the body and resulting in a potential sensitivity to that dietary protein in the future.

The second theory concerns the gross over-vaccination of our dogs today. With little in the way of science for support, and contrary to the guidelines of the World Small Animal Veterinary Association guidelines, which state that every 3 years is fine, vets worldwide, guided by drug-manufacturer information, continue to *boost* animals annually, despite being adequately vaccinated for viruses as puppies. Yet we know vaccinations last in dogs, as they do in humans. A study funded by Pfizer found canine vaccinations elicit an immune response in dogs beyond 4 years, for all 5 antigens tested. Mouzin *et al.* (2004),[104] the authors, concluded by questioning the current one-year interval. The world's leading veterinary immunologist Dr. Ronald Schultz strongly agrees, documenting repeatedly using serology and challenge tests that the 3 core vaccines in dogs (parvovirus, adenovirus, distemper) last many years.[105] For this reason, veterinary immunologists think that a dog's immunity to many viruses is probably lifelong.[106] So there is little doubt vets are currently over-vaccinating them to no perceivable health benefit.

The problem is many boosters are made using chicken and beef blood serum[107] and this is injected straight into the bloodstream of the animal, instead of first being digested fully and passing through the gut wall in a form acceptable to the immune system. The desired, aggravated immune response may result in the body identifying that meat protein as a potential threat in the future. Supporting this, in October 2015, Arumugham published a study titled "Evidence that Food Proteins in Vaccines Cause the Development of Food Allergies and Its Implications for Vaccine Policy". With more than 20 studies in support (mostly of humans), it was stated:

> Numerous studies have demonstrated that food proteins contained in vaccines/injections induce food allergy. The IOM (Institute of Medicine)'s authoritative report has concluded the same. Allergen quantities in vaccines are unregulated. [...] The vaccine schedule has increased the number of vaccine shots to 30-40 and up to five vaccines are simultaneously administered to children. Vaccines also contain adjuvants such as aluminium compounds and pertussis toxin that bias towards IgE synthesis. Given these conditions, the predictable and observed outcome is a food allergy epidemic.

For all these reasons, the harsh heat treatment of protein in dry pet food production is considered a health risk to the pets consuming it. Many kibble brands are aware of this, or at least the public's desire to avoid such products and use higher pressure, known as *cold-pressing*, which lowers the required cooking temperature. These products often boast cooking temperatures of 40–70°C. However, and as with *dehydrated* or *air dried* treats, most use a high-temperature step at some stage as a necessary bacteria-kill step. How long they do that for is entirely up to them.

Reducing Protein in Senior Dog Diets Is Likely to Be Harmful

Senior diets, more often than not, contain even less protein than adult versions of the same food (please Google your favourite brand, for example, here). At this point, manufacturers hold up examples of when a low-protein diet can help in humans, such as those with some forms of kidney disease. It is most certainly true for patients suffering proteinuria, where protein has built in the blood to such an extent it risks poisoning them. However, it is not the case for all or even the majority of patients with kidney disease. After studying 1,524 severely ill patients with chronic kidney disease, Foque *et al.* (2006)[100] concluded that reduced protein diets helped in 31% of the cases. What effect the lower protein content had on the remaining 69% is unknown, but the results indeed suggest that, in some humans suffering chronic kidney disease, there may be some benefit. Also, some doctors recommend that patients about to undergo dialysis should reduce their protein intake prior to their first dialysis treatment but after that, actually increase the amount of high-quality protein in their diet. Outside of these instances, it is less often patients with kidney disease concern themselves with protein concentrations. And humans are omnivores.

While humans and dogs are used in comparative studies of disease progression such as cancer, as well as food sensitivities,[108] it must be remembered that digestively, dogs can differ markedly from humans. For one, dogs, as meat-eaters, have a more acidic stomach. They also have a shorter, more rapid digestive system and throughput time. Most importantly, as carnivores, they differ significantly in their ability to process and metabolise protein. Nowhere is this more apparent than in studies of the dog's kidney response to increases of protein in the diets. For 50 years we have known a meat-based diet benefits kidney function in previously dry-fed dogs by improving the glomerular filtration rate.[109] Studies of dogs with chronic kidney failure show the higher the protein content, the better off the dog is. Even when authors artificially removed 75–90% of their kidney function to replicate chronic kidney failure (CKF), those dogs that were fed a higher protein diet all fared better, without exception.[74, 110-112] Some did find lower phosphorus, 0.4% versus 1.4%, helped significantly, although we highlight in Section 4 that this cannot be construed as being equally relevant to dogs fed natural forms of phosphorus. Finco *et al.* (1994)[113] ran their trial for 2 years. Robertson *et al.* (1986)[110] ran their trial for 4 years. In dogs with chronic renal failure, clinical, haematological and biochemical responses to a combination of low protein (13-16% ME) and low phosphorus (0.4% DM) were negative in three out of four clinical trials.[114] Furthermore, there is no evidence of an age-related decline in digestive efficiency in dogs.[115] In perhaps the most damning of all studies to prove protein restriction is unnecessary in senior dogs, Finco *et al.* (1994)[113] nephrectomised thirty-one dogs of three breeds, all 7 to 8-year-olds, to increase the risk of renal damage associated with reduction of renal mass. The study, lasting four years, tested two diets differing in protein concentration, which were used to test the hypothesis that high dietary protein intake causes renal damage in ageing dogs. Sixteen dogs were fed a diet containing 18% protein; the other fifteen dogs were fed a diet containing 34% protein. After the forty-eight months, any dogs that survived the trial were euthanised and tissues were examined. Not only were no differences found in glomerular filtration rate, a good indicator of kidney function, but only 63% of Group A survived, compared to 87% of Group B. While this result was not statistically significant due to the number of dogs used, it suggests that even with massively decreased kidney function, older dogs still fare better on a higher protein diet than on a lower protein diet. This indicates that even in their later years, they are protein-digesting machines.

As numerous studies confirm that protein does not adversely affect their kidneys, even during many types of kidney failure and that dogs with CKF appear to do better on *higher* protein diets, the practice of reducing protein in older dogs for the 'benefit of their kidneys' or even in those dogs with CKF, appears highly questionable. In fact, rather than needing less, we have known for 50 years that healthy older dogs actually require 50% more protein in the form of higher-quality protein in their diets.[74,116]

> Protein restriction for healthy, older dogs is not only unnecessary it can be detrimental. Although their energy requirements tend to decrease, protein requirements actually increase by about 50% in older dogs. When insufficient protein is provided, it can aggravate the age-associated loss of lean body mass and may contribute to earlier mortality.
>
> **Laflamme, 2008**[74]

This information is unforgivably ignored by both the industry and those touting their nonsense. Reducing protein in older dogs' diets is nothing but an odious cash-saving technique at the detriment of senior dogs worldwide. And still it persists. If you feel as strongly as I do about this particular topic, I implore you to print out this section on protein and discuss it with your vet. You will be helping someone's old friend.

The Too Much Protein' Hypothesis

We know dogs are carnivores, meat protein-processing machines. They evolved upon lean meat diets, approximately four-parts animal protein to one-part fat. Given the choice, dogs choose to obtain their calories from protein and fat, not carbohydrates. Studies show dogs fed higher protein diets fare better in exercise and kidney function tests.

Despite this, the majority of Western dogs are fed low-protein, cereal-based dry food containing token *meat* addition. At best, these foods are formulated to provide the minimum amount of protein required for normal development. At worst, due to poor protein bioavailability (a result of the use of meat meal, heavy processing reducing digestibility and indigestible vegetable protein inclusions), dogs consuming these foods are consuming less than the minimum amount of protein required for normal development, certainly to the detriment of their health.

To suggest dogs can have a problem with higher meat-protein diets is today completely unsubstantiated and seems at this point highly unlikely. Despite this, the industry continues to push the myth that too much protein is potentially harmful to your dog, linking it to the rising incidence of kidney, skin or gut disease in the general (dry-fed) dog population, a myth that is sadly perpetuated by the veterinary industry.

Ironically, too much protein may well be a *possible* risk factor in these diseases, just not in the manner they suggest. It is not a matter of quantity, *per se*, but of protein *quality*. As we've already discussed, the cooking of meat in pet foods is shown to produce a variety of harmful MRPs. These are known to cause a variety of issues for the dog, from making the meat protein more difficult to digest to causing various maladies including gut issues, cancer and dietary sensitivity. When we know that the amount of antigen ingested at this point plays a significant role in the magnitude of the reaction in the patient,[124] and that poor meat protein ingredients, such as rendered meat meal, contain significantly more MRPs than fresh meat, then yes, it could be argued that 20% denatured and antigenic meat protein versus 30% might be a debate worth having.

TAKE-HOME POINTS

✓ Meat protein is the main portion of the dog's diet.

✓ Dogs evolved on a lean diet, comprising of approximately 60% protein and 10–15% fat. This gives us an ME ratio of roughly 7:3.

✓ The AAFCO states the *minimum* amount of protein a pet food producer can include in their adult pet foods and call them complete is 18% protein. This has become the benchmark for pet foods over time. The science supporting this figure is based on two feeding trials using a handful of caged Beagles fed a dry, ultra-processed diet.

✓ Sled dogs were maintained on a range of diets. It was found the more protein fed during training, the larger plasma volume and red blood cell mass they have during strenuous training. Moreover, dogs consuming the highest amount of protein were injury free.

✓ The source of the protein is vital.

✓ Meat by-products are everything except the meat from the carcass, including the organs such as the lungs, spleen, kidneys, liver, brain, ears, lips, tail, stomach and intestines freed of their contents (sort of), as well as the blood, bone and fatty tissue of the animal.

✓ Meat meal is a significantly poorer source of protein. It's an ultra-processed by-product of the rendering industry and arrives to the pet food factory as a grey powder.

✓ The rendering industry takes in waste meat that cannot be handled normally. In the United States, this includes hair, hoof, horn, hide, manure, spoiled animal carcasses (aka 4D meat – dead, diseased, dying, disabled meat), roadkill, supermarket and restaurant waste, and **euthanised pets**. The European Union do not render animals not fit for human consumption (eliminating spoiled meat, roadkill and pets) since the BSE crisis.

✓ A way to check for euthanised pets is to test for the presence of SPB. Dry food is constantly failing for the prescience of SPB. It remains the second most likely cause for dry and canned pet food recall in the United States.

✓ Fresh meat provides all the dogs EEAs, just not in every piece. Some pieces are higher (or absent) in certain proteins. You feed a variety of meat parts and meat types to achieve protein balance.

✓ In the 1970s, ultra-processed pet food was killing thousands of cats each year. The issue was later found to be DCM caused by a lack of taurine. Taurine is one of the most abundant amino acids in fresh meat. In keeping with the best canine nutrition principles of 'like feeds like', heart muscle is highest in taurine.

✓ Studies show dogs cannot utilise all the protein offered by these foods. First, many of the ingredients that add protein are practically indigestible (corn and wheat gluten). Second, the meat used in ultra-processed pet food is cooked under high temperature, often multiple times. High temperature cooking reduces the digestibility of meat for dogs by proteolysis (the breakdown of amino acids into smaller particles), protein cross-linking, oxidative reactions and Maillard reactions. This is a problem if you are feeding pet foods with the minimum amount of protein required to survive in a cage for 6 months, in line with the AAFCO standards.

✓ Chronic protein deficiency is likely to result in a decrease of fitness and lean body mass, a poorer coat, structural issues, organ failure and behavioural disruption.

✓ Cooked meat is tasty as high temperature produces compounds termed MRPs. MRPs are used in food processing to boost the smell, flavour and thus palatability of their products. Unfortunately, they are strongly linked to cancer, inflammatory and age-related degenerative processes, diabetes and both renal and cardiovascular diseases. Studies show pet food contains large amounts of MRPs. Cooking meat below 100°C is vital.

✓ Processed ingredients are significantly more likely to elicit an immune response in dogs.

✓ There is little evidence that high protein diets harm a dog's kidneys. Studies of dogs with replicated chronic kidney failure show a better prognosis the more protein you feed them.

> ✓ There is no age-related decline in digestive efficiency in dogs. In fact, healthy older dogs require 50% more protein in the form of higher quality protein in their diets.
>
> ✓ The industry practice of reducing protein in senior dog diets is likely harmful to the animal.

Chapter Eight References

1   Dierenfeld, E.S., Alcorn, H.L. and Jacobsen, K.L. (2002). *Nutrient Composition of Whole Vertebrate Prey (Excluding Fish) Fed in Zoos*. U.S. Department of Agriculture. Available online, www.researchgate.net

2   McWilliams, S. (2013). Non-destructive techniques to assess body composition of birds: A review and validation study. Journal of Ornithology, 154(3): 597–618

3   Mabee, D.M. and Morgan, A.F. (1951). Evaluation of dog growth of egg yolk protein and six other partially purified proteins, some after heat treatment. Journal of Nutrition, 43(2): 261–279

4   Neirinck, K., Istasse, L., Gabriel, A. *et al.* (1991). Amino acid composition and digestibility of four protein sources for dogs. Journal of Nutrition, 121: S64–S65

5   Hand, M.S., Thatcher, C.D., Remillard, R.L. *et al.* (2010). *Small Animal Clinical Nutrition*, 5th Edition. Published by the Mark Morris Institute, Topeka, KS

6   National Research Council (NRC, 1985). *Nutrient Requirements of Dogs*, Revised. National Academy Press,

7   Hand, M.S., Thatcher, C.D., Remillard, R.F. *et al.* (1998). *Small Animal Clinical Nutrition* (4th ed.). Topeka, KS: Mark Morris Associates

8   Romsos, D.R. and Ferguson, D. (1983). Regulation of protein intake in adult dogs. Journal of the American Veterinary Medical Association, 182: 41–43

9   Tôrres, C.L., Hickenbottom, S.J. and Rogers, Q.R. (2003). Palatability affects the percentage of metabolizable energy as protein selected by adult beagles. Journal of Nutrition, 133: 3516–3522

10   Serpell, J. (1995). The domestic dog: Its evolution, behaviour, and interactions with people. Cambridge, UK: Cambridge University Press

11   Cerundolo, R., Court, M.H., Hao, Q. *et al.* (2004). Identification and concentration of soy phytoestrogens in commercial dog foods. American Journal of Veterinary Research. 65(5): 592–596

12   Reynolds, A.J., Taylor, C.R., Hoppler, H. *et al.* (1996). *The effect of diet on sled dog performance, oxidative capacity, skeletal muscle microstucture, and muscle glycogen metabolism*. In: Carey, D.P., Norton, S.A., Bolser, S.M., eds. Recent Advances in Canine

and Feline Nutritional Research: Proceedings of the 1996 Iams International Nutrition Symposium. Wilmington OH: Orange Frazer Press, 181–198

13 Bryson, B. (2010). *At home: A short history of private life*. New York: Doubleday

14 AAFCO (Association of American Feed Control Officials) 2008. *Official feed terms*. Official Publication

15 Blakeslee, S. (1997). *Fear of disease prompts new look at rendering*. The New York Times. Published online, Mar 11th, available online, www.nytimes.com

16 O'Connor, J.J., Stowe, C.M. and Robinson, R.R. (1985). Fate of sodium pentobarbital in rendered products. American Journal of Veterinary Research, 46(8): 1721–1724

17 Martin, A.M. (2008). *Food pets die for: Shocking facts about pet food. 3rd Edition*. Newsage Press.

18 Eckhouse (1990). *How Dogs and Cats Get Recycled into Pet Food*. San Francisco Chronicle. Published online, Feb 19th, available online, www.sfchronicle.com

19 FDA (2001). *Dog Food Survey Results - Survey #1, Qualitative Analyses for Pentobarbital Residue*. Published online, Feb 28th, available online, www.fda.gov

20 Thixton, S. (2019). *When second place is very bad*. Published online, Mar 14th, 2019, www.truthaboutpetfood.com

21 Babej, M.E. (2013). *Dog Food Made From Feathers: A Win-Win for Royal Canin*. Published online, May 29th, available online, www.forbes.com

22 Ekperigin, H.E., Vora, P. (1980). Histological and biochemical effects of feeding excess dietary methionine to broiler chicks. Avian Diseases, 24(1): 82–95

23 AAFCO (Association of American Feed Control Officials) 2016. *Dog and Cat Food Nutrient Profiles*. Official Publication, See www.aafco.org

24 Spitze, A.R., Wong, D.L., Rogers, Q.R. *et al.* (2003). Taurine concentrations in animal feed ingredients; cooking influences taurine content. Journal of Animal Physiology and Animal Nutrition 87(7–8): 251–262

25 Ettinger, S., Bolton, G. and Lord, P. (1970). Idiopathic cardiomyopathy in the dog. Journal of the American Veterinary Association, 156: 1225

26 Pion, P.D., Kittleson, M.D., Rogers, Q.R. *et al.* (1987). Myocardial failure in cats associated with low plasma taurine: a reversible cardiomyopathy. Science, 237(4816): 764–768

27 Aguirre, G.D. (1978). Retinal degeneration associated with the feeding of dog foods to cats. Journal of American Veterinary Medical Association, 172(7): 791–796

28 Pion, P.D. And Kittleson, M.D. (1990). Taurine's role in clinical practice. Journal of Small Animal Practice, 31: 510–518

29 Sanderson, S.L., Gross, K.L., Ogburn, P.N. *et al.* (2001). Effects of dietary fat and L-carnitine on plasma and whole blood taurine concentrations and cardiac function in healthy dogs fed protein-restricted diets. American Journal of Veterinary Research, 62(10): 1616–1623

30 Tidholm, A. Haggstrom, J., Borgarelli, M. *et al.* (2001). Canine idiopathic dilated cardiomyopathy. Part I: Aetiology, clinical characteristics, epidemiology and pathology. The Veterinary Journal, 162(2): 92–107

31   Freeman, L.M., Michel, K.E., Brown, D.J. *et al.* (1996). Idiopathic dilated cardiomyopathy in Dalmatians: nine cases (1990-1995). Journal of the American Veterinary Medical Association, 209(9): 1592–1596

32   Tôrres, C.L., Backus, R.C., Fascetti, A.J. *et al.* (2003). Taurine status in normal dogs fed a commercial diet associated with taurine deficiency and dilated cardiomyopathy. Journal of Animal Physiology and Animal Nutrition (Berl), 87(9-10): 359–72

33   Fascetti, A. (2003). Taurine deficiency in dogs with dilated cardiomyopathy. Journal of the American Veterinary Medical Association, 223(8): 1137–1141

34   Hickman, M.A., Rogers, Q.R. and Morris, J.G. (1990). Effect of Processing on Fate of Dietary carbon-14 Taurine in Cats. The Journal of Nutrition, 120(9): 995–1000

35   Kim, S.W., Rogers, Q.R. and Morris, J.G. (1996). Maillard reaction products in purified diets induce taurine depletion in cats which is reversed by antibiotics. Journal of Nutrition, 126(1):195–201

36   Ko, K.S. and Fascetti, A.J. (2016). Dietary beet pulp decreases taurine status in dogs fed low protein diet. Journal of Animal Science and Technology, 58: 29

37   Delaney, S.J., Kass, P.H., Rogers, Q.R. *et al.* (2003). Plasma and whole blood taurine in normal dogs of varying size fed commercially prepared food. Journal of Animal Physiology and Animal Nutrition (Berl), 87(5-6): 236–44

38   Fascetti, A.J., Reed, J.R., Rogers, Q.R. *et al.* (2003). Taurine deficiency in dogs with dilated cardiomyopathy: 12 cases (1997-2001). Journal of the American Veterinary Medical Association, 223(8): 1137–1141

39   Glasgow, A.G., Cave, N.J., Marks, S.L. *et al.* (2002). *Role of Diet in the Health of the Feline Intestinal Tract and in Inflammatory Bowel Disease.* Center for Companion Animal Health, School of Veterinary Medicine, University of California, Davis, California

40   Burns, R.A., Le Faivre, M.H. and Milner, J.A. (1982). Effects of dietary protein quantity and quality on the growth of dogs and rats. Journal of Nutrition, 112(10): 1843–1853

41   Brown, R.G. (1989). Protein in dog food. Canadian Veterinarian Journal, 30(6): 528–531

42   Oste, R.E. (1991). Digestibility of processed food protein. Advanced Experimental Medical Biology, 289: 371–388

43   Teodorowicz, M., van Neerven, J. and Savelkoul, H. (2017). Food Processing: The Influence of the Maillard Reaction on Immunogenicity and Allergenicity of Food Proteins. Nutrients, 9(8): 835

44   Meade, S.J., Reid, E.A., Gerrard, J.A. (2005). The impact of processing on the nutritional quality of food proteins. Journal of AOAC International, 88: 904–922

45   Knize, M.G., Andressen, B.D., Healy, S.K. *et al.* (1985). Effect of temperature, patty thickness and fat content on the production of mutagens in fried ground beef. Food Chemistry Toxicology, 23: 1035–1040

46   Knize, M.G., Salmon, C.P., Pais, P. *et al.* (1999) Food heating and the formation of heterocyclic aromatic amine and polycylcic aromatic hydrocarbon mutagens/carcinogens. Advanced Experimental Medical Biology, 459: 179–193

47   Knize, M.G., Cunningham, P.L., Avila, J.R. *et al.* (1994). Formation of mutagenic activity from amino acids heated at cooking temperatures. Food and Chemical Toxicology, 32(1): 55–60

48   Townsend, W.E. and Blankinship, L.C. (1987). Enzyme profile of raw and heat-processed beef, pork and turkey using the "Apizym" system. Journal of Food Science, 52(2): 511–512

49   Oberli, M., Marsset-Baglieri, A., Airinei, G. *et al.* (2015). High true ileal digestibility but not postprandial utilization of nitrogen from bovine meat protein in humans is moderately decreased by high-temperature, long-duration cooking. The Journal of Nutrition, 145(10): 2221–2228

50   de Wit, M. (2013). *Immunological response to dietary proteins in cats*. Veterinary Medicine, Research Project at Massey University, Palmerston North, New Zealand. Veterinary Research Project. August 2013

51   Guildford, W. G., Center, S. A., Strombeck, D. R.*et al.* (1996). *Strombeck's Small Animal Gastroenterology (3rd ed.)* Philadelphia, PA: Saunders

52   Murray, S. M., Patil, A. R., Fahey, G. C. *et al.* (1997). Raw and rendered animal by-products as ingredients in dog diets. Journal of Animal Science, 75(9): 2497–2505

53   Johnson, M.L., Parsons, C.M., Fahey, G.C. *et al.* (1998). Effects of species raw material source, ash content, and processing temperature on amino acid digestibility of animal by-product meals by cecectomized roosters and ileal cannulated dogs. Journal of Animal Science, 76(4): 1112–1122

54   Pérez-Calvo, E., Castrillo, C., Baucells, M.D. *et al.* (2010). Effect of rendering on protein and fat quality of animal by-products. Journal of Animal Physiology and Animal Nutrition, 94(5): e154–e164

55   Hendriks, W.H., Emmens M.M., Trass, B. *et al.* (1999). Heat processing changes the protein quality of canned cat food as measured with a rat bioassay. Journal of Animal Science, 77: 669–676

56   Campbell, M.K. and Farrell, S.O. (2003). *Biochemistry* (4th ed.). Belmont, CA: Thomson Brooks/Cole

57   Kondos, A.C. and McClymont, G.L. (1972). Nutritional evaluation of meat meals for poultry. VII. Effect of processing temperature on total and biologically available amino acids. Australian Journal of Agricultural Research, 23(5): 913–922

58   Björck, I. and Asp, N.G. (1983). The effects of extrusion cooking on nutritional value – A literature review. Journal of Food Engineering, 2(4): 281–308

59   Johnson, M.L. and Parsons, C.M. (1997). Effects of raw material source, ash content, and assay length on protein efficiency ratio and net protein ratio values for animal protein meals. Poultry Science, 76(12): 1722–1727

60   Morgan, A F. and Kern, G.E. (1934). The effect of heat upon the biological value of meat protein. Journal of Nutrition, 7(4): 367–379

61   Lonsdale, T. (1992). *Raw meaty bones promote health*. Control and Therapy series no. 3323. Sydney, Australia: University of Sydney.

62   Wiseman, J., Jagger, S., Cole, D. J. A. *et al.* (1991). The digestion and utilization of amino acids of heat-treated fish meal by growing/finishing pigs. Animal Production, 53(2):215–225

63   Wang, X. and Parsons, C.M. (1998). Effect of raw material source, processing systems, and processing temperatures on amino acid digestibility of meat and bone meal. Poultry Science, 77(6): 834–841

64   Shirley, R.B. and Parsons, C.M. (2000). Effect of pressure processing on amino acids digestibility of meat and bone meal for poultry. Poultry Science, 79(12): 1775–1781

65   Cramer, K.R., Greenwood, M.W., Moritz, J.S. *et al.* (2007). Protein quality of various raw and rendered byproduct meals commonly incorporated into companion animal diets. Journal of Animal Science, 85(12): 3285–3293

66   Stroucken, W.P., van der Poel, A.F., Kappert, H.J. *et al.* (1996). Extruding vs Pelleting of a Feed Mixture Lowers Apparent Nitrogen Digestibility in Dogs. Journal of the Science of Food and Agriculture, 71(4): 520–522

67   Crissey, S.D., Swanson, J.A., Lintzenich, B.A. *et al.* (1997). Use of a raw meat-based diet or a dry kibble diet for sand cats (Felis margarita). Journal of Animal Science, 75(8): 2154–2160

68   Kerr, K.R., Vester Boler, B.M., Morris, C.L. *et al.* (2012). Apparent total tract energy and macronutrient digestibility and fecal fermentative end-product concentrations of domestic cats fed extruded, raw beef-based, and cooked beef-based diets. Journal of Animal Science, 90: 515–522

69   Beloshapka, A.N., Duclos, L.M., Vester Boler, B.M. *et al.* (2012). Effects of inulin or yeast cell-wall extract on nutrient digestibility, fecal fermentative end-product concentrations, and blood metabolite concentrations in adult dogs fed raw meat-based diets. American Journal of Veterinary Research, 73(7): 1016–1023

70   Algya, K.M. Cross, T.L., Leuck, K.N. *et al.* (2018). Apparent total tract macronutrient digestibility, serum chemistry, urinalysis, and fecal characteristics, metabolites and microbiota of adult dogs fed extruded, mildly cooked, and raw diets. Journal of Animal Science, 96(9): 3670–3683

71   Tjernsbekk, M.T., Tauson, A.H., Matthiesen, C.F. *et al.* (2016). Protein and amino acid bioavailability of extruded dog food with protein meals of different quality using growing mink as a model. Journal of Animal Science, 94(9): 3796-3804

72   Faber, T.A., Hernot, D.C., Parsons, C.M. *et al.* (2009). Protein digestibility evaluations of meat and fish substrates using laboratory, avian, and ileal cannulated dog assays. Journal of Animal Science, 88: 1421–1432

73   Krogdahl, A., Ahlstrøm, Ø. and Skrede, A. (2004). Nutrient digestibility of commercial dog foods using mink as a model. American Journal of Nutrition, 134: 2141S–2144S

74   Laflamme, D.P. (2008). Pet food safety: Dietary protein. Topics in Companion Animal Medicine, 23(3): 154–157

75   Platt, B.S. and Stewart, R.J.C. (1968). Effects of Protein-Calorie Deficiency on Dogs. Reproduction, Growth and Behaviour. Developmental Medicine & Child Neurology, 10(1): 3–24

76   Kronfeld, D.S., Hammel, E.P., Ramberg, C.F. *et al.* (1977). Hematological and metabolic responses to training in racing sled dogs fed diets containing medium, low or zero carbohydrate. American Journal of Clinical Nutrition, 30: 419-430

77   Hill, R.C., Lewis, D.D. and Scott, K.C. *et al.* (2001). Effect of increased dietary protein and decreased dietary carbohydrate on performance and body composition in racing Greyhounds. American Journal of Veterinary Research, 62: 440–447

78   Hill, D.E., Forbes, L., Zarlenga, D.S. *et al.* (2009). Survival of North American genotypes of *Trichinella* in frozen pork. Journal of Food Protection, 72(12): 2565–2570

79   Stewart, R.J.C., Preece, R.F. and Sheppar, H.A. (1975). Twelve generations of marginal protein deficiency. British Journal of Nutrition, 33: 233

80   Platt, B.S., Heard, C.R.C. and Stewart, R.J.C. (1964). *Experimental protein and calorie deficiency*. In N. H. Munro and J. B. Allison (Eds.), Mammalian protein metabolism. New York: Academic Press, Vol. 2, pp445–522

81   Chopra, J.S. and Sharma, A. (1992). Protein energy malnutrition and the nervous system. Journal of the Neurological Sciences. 110(1–2): 8–20

82   Heard, C.R.C. and Stewart, R.J.C. (1971). Protein-calorie deficiency and disorders of the endocrine glands. Hormones, 2: 40–64

83   Scott, D.W., Miller, W.H. and Griffin C.E. (2001). *Muller and Kirk's Small Animal Dermatology* 6th ed. Philadelphia, WB Saunders Company

84   Hagen-Plantinga, E.A., Orlanes, D.F., Bosch, G. *et al.* (2017). Retorting conditions affect palatability and physical characteristics of canned cat food. Journal of Nutritional Science, 6: e23

85   Olesen, P.T., Olsen, A., Frandsen, H. *et al.* (2008). Acrylamide exposure and incidence of breast cancer among postmenopausal women in the Danish Diet, Cancer and Health Study. International Journal of Cancer, 122(9): 2094–2100

86   Webster, J., Wilke, M., Stahl, P. *et al.* (2005). Maillard reaction products in food as pro-inflammatory and pro-arteriosclerotic factors of degenerative diseases. Zeitschrift für Gerontologie und Geriatrie, 38(5):347–353

87   Tessier, F.J. and Birlouez-Aragon, I. (2012). Health effects of dietary Maillard reaction products: the results of ICARE and other studies. Amino Acids, 42(4): 1119–1131

88   van Rooijen, C., Bosch, G., van der Poel, A.F.B. *et al.* (2014). Quantitation of Maillard reaction products in commercially available pet foods. Journal of Agricultural and Food Chemistry, 62(35): 8883–8891

89   Gentzel, J.B. (2013). Does contemporary canine diet cause cancer? A review. Veterinary World, EISSN: 2231-0916

90   Everts, S. (2012). The Maillard Reaction Turns 100. Chemical and Engineering News, 90(4): 58–60

91   Layton, D.W., Bogen, K.T., Knize. M.G. *et al.* (1995) Cancer risk of heterocyclic amines in cooked foods: an analysis and implications for research. Carcinogenesis, 16: 38–52

92   Skog, K., Johansson, M.A. and Jägerstadt, M.I. (1998). Carcinogenic heterocyclic amines in model systems and cooked food: a review on formation, occurrence and intake. Food Chemistry and Toxicology, 36: 879–896

93   Knize, M.G., Salmon, C.P., Pais, P. *et al.* (1999) Food heating and the formation of heterocyclic aromatic amine and polycylcic aromatic hydrocarbon mutagens/carcinogens. Advanced Experimental Medical Biology, 459: 179–193

94   Sinha, R., Chow, W.H., Kulldorff, M. *et al.* (1999). Well-done, grilled red meat increases the risk of colorectal adenomas. Cancer Research, 59: 4320–4324

95   Sinha, R., Kulldorff, M., Swanson, C.A. *et al.* (2000) Dietary heterocyclic amines and the risk of lung cancer among Missouri women.Cancer Research, 60: 3753–3756

96   Sinha, R., Kulldorff, M., Chow, W.H. *et al.*. (2001) Dietary intake of heterocyclic amines, meat-derived mutagenic activity and risk of colorectal adenomas. Cancer Epidemiology and Biomarkers Prevelance, 10: 559

97   Kikugawa, K. (2004). Prevention of mutagen formation in heated meats and model systems. Mutagenesis, 19(6): 431–439

98   Taylor, R.T., Fultz, E. and Knize, M.G. (1986) Mutagen formation in a model beef supernatant fraction. Elucidation of role of water in fried ground beef mutagenicity. Environmental Mutagen, 8(6): 65

99   Knize, M.G., Salmon, C.P. and Felton, J.S. (2003). Mutagenic activity and heterocyclic amine carcinogens in commercial pet foods. Environmental Mutagenesis, 539(1–2): 195–201

100   Foque, D., Laville, M. and Boissel, J.P. (2006). Low protein diets for chronic kidney disease in non-diabetic adults. Cochrane Database System Review, 19(2): CD001892

101   Vojdani, A. (2009). Detection of IgE, IgG, IgA and IgM antibodies against raw and processed food antigens. Nutrition and Metabolism, 6:22

102   Bethlehema, S., Bexley, J. and Muller, R.S. (2012). Patch testing and allergen-specific serum IgE and IgG antibodies in the diagnosis of canine adverse food reactions. Veterinary Immunology and Immunopathology, 145(3–4): 582–589

103   Day, M.J. (2005). The canine model of dietary hypersensitivity. Journal of the Nutrition Society, 64: 458–464.

104   Mouzin, D.E., Lorenzen, M.J., Haworth, J.D. *et al.* (2004). Duration of serologic response to five viral antigens in dogs. Journal of the American Veterinary Medical Association, 224(1): 55–60

105   Schultz, R.D. (2006). Duration of immunity for canine and feline vaccines: A review. Veterinary Microbiology, 117(1): 75–79

106   Bonagura, J.D. and Twedt, D.C. (2008). *Kirk's current veterinary therapy XIV*. Philadelphia, PA: Saunders

107 HogenEsch, H., Dunham, A.D., Scott-Moncrieff, C. *et al.* (2002). Effect of Vaccination on Serum Concentrations of Total and Antigen-Specific Immunoglobulin E in Dogs. American Journal of Veterinary Research, 63(4): 611–616

108 Wang, G.D., Zhai, W., Yang, H.C. *et al.* (2013). The genomics of selection in dogs and the parallel evolution between dogs and humans. Nature Communications, 4(1860)

109 O'Connor, J. and Summerhill, R.A. (1976). The effect of a meal of meat on glomular filtration rate in dogs at normal urine flows. Journal of Physiology, 256: 81–91

110 Robertson, J.L., Goldschmidt, M., Kronfeld, D.S. *et al.* (1986). Long-term renal responses to high dietary protein in dogs with 75% nephrectomy. Kidney International, 29: 511–519

111 Bovée, K.C. (1991) Influence of dietary protein on renal function in dogs. Journal of Nutrition, 121(11): Suppl. S128–S139

112 Hansen, B., DiBartola, S.P., Chew, D.J. *et al.* (1992). Clinical and metabolic findings in dogs with chronic renal failure fed two diets. American Journal of Veterinary Research, 53(3): 326–334

113 Finco, D.R., Brown, S.A., Crowell, W.A. *et al.* (1994). Effects of aging and dietary protein intake on uninephrectomized geriatric dogs. American Journal of Veterinary Research, 55: 1282–1290

114 Kronfeld, D.S. (1994). Dietary management of renal senescence and failure in dogs. Australian Veterinary Journal, 71(10): 328–331

115 Harper, E.J. (1998). Changing Perspectives on Aging and Energy Requirements: Aging and Digestive Function in Humans, Dogs and Cats. Journal of Nutrition, 128(12): 2632S-2635S

116 Wannemacher, R.W. and McCoy, J.R. (1966). Determination of optimal dietary protein requirements of young and old dogs. Journal of Nutrition, 88: 66–74

CHAPTER 9

Vitamins and Minerals

Introduction

The Association of American Feed Control Officials (AAFCO) set the bar for the nutrient content of your pet's food. All the good dry foods boast, on the front of their packets, they are in accordance with the AAFCO Nutrient Profiles. While we return to them later during our investigation of "Who are the pet food police?," for now it's important we understand the AAFCO Nutrient Profiles are, in fact, minimum requirements. To quote the AFFCO,

> "...finished product is compared to minimum nutritional values...
> **AAFCO 2016, "Dog and Cat Food Nutrient Profiles"**

That word 'minimum' rarely gets mentioned by the pet food reps, mind you.

At no point in the AAFCO Nutrient Profiles is optimum considered. In a way, this is understandable. Studies of optimum are highly complex. With so many variables at play, it would require thousands of dogs over years under varying conditions. So they are not done. Still today, we are yet to establish the optimum level of any nutrient in the dog or cat. Luckily for manufactures, the AAFCO only asks that their products reach the dizzying heights of the 'minimum level required for normal function' and they can use that 'complete' badge. So there's that.

More worryingly, as either their ingredients are lacking or their nutrient contents are processed out of existence, the ultra-processed pet food industry leans very heavily on synthetic nutrient inclusions. As you are soon to discover, such additions are not metabolised the same way as vitamins and minerals in their natural form. Poor absorption of such supplements often leads to deficiency while gross excesses regularly sicken and kill dogs and cats. It's thus worrying that only a handful of nutrient maximums get a mention in the AAFCO feed profile, and many of these seem to be disappearing. For instance, up until 2007, the maximum amount of crude zinc permitted was 1000 mg/kg of dry food (when minimum is 120 mg/kg of dry food). In 2007, the AAFCO decided to remove this maximum as it was based on 'the maximum tolerance concentration recommended for swine rations'[1] There is no maximum for zinc in place today. You can use as much as you like.

Up until 2007, the minimum and maximum iron content was 80 mg/kg and 3,000 mg/kg of dry food, respectively. This implies, 37 times your Recommended Daily Allowance (RDA) of crude iron per day is just about safe and anywhere between those two figures is assumedly fine for lifetime feeding. Then, in 2007, the AAFCO changed the minimum for dogs to 40mg/kg to bring it in line with National Research Council (NRC) (2006)[2] guidelines and once again eliminated the maximum amount of iron. They cited two reasons for doing this. First, they never actually had any data to indicate 3,000 mg/kg was safe for dogs; this figure again came from swine (and which, in 2005, was hastily reassessed as no long term safety studies were in place for pigs either).

The second reason stated was that they couldn't be sure of the digestibility of iron used in pet food. Normally, dogs source their iron in two forms – heme iron (from ingesting blood and meat products), and by far the most readily absorbed and non-heme iron (eating some plant material and where this iron is stored in the body of a herbivore). Both are chelated to a protein, meaning they are both readily absorbed by the body and at a predicable rate. Pet food manufacturers prefer iron oxide (aka rust) as it is not only cheap but can add a more reddish-brown colour to the normally grey kibble. The problem here is that iron oxides are not easily absorbed dogs. It is estimated that dogs on such mixes can absorb 10–20% of the iron in their mixes.When this is coupled with the fact that ingredients clash, further reducing the availability of iron and other minerals to the animal, the industry hasn't yet worked out how much exactly of this type of iron is actually safe for the dog. Considering what we know in humans, let's hope they get around to that one soon. The Institute of Medicine (2001) suggests a man's RDA of iron at 8 mg/day. However, likely due to our high meat consumption, we are averaging around double that, 16 mg/day of iron. The Institute stipulates that the tolerable upper intake level (UL) for iron is 45 mg/day of iron, not quite six times our RDA of iron, a level based on gastrointestinal distress as an adverse effect. Any more than that daily is predicted to have very negative consequences, indeed.

....as iron can form free radicals, its concentration in body tissues must be tightly regulated because in excessive amounts, it can lead to tissue damage...and possibly to neurodegenerative diseases

Abbaspour *et al.,* **2014**[3]

It's the same for copper. Commercial sources of copper are either copper oxide or copper sulphate. The latter is synthetically produced by treating either pure copper or more likely copper oxide with warm sulfuric acid to yield a blue salt called copper sulphate. The AAFCO (2014)[1] states 'because of very poor apparent digestibility, copper from oxide sources that are added to the diet should not be considered in determining the minimum nutrient concentration for copper'. Copper is a micro-mineral, meaning you need very little in your diet, but studies indicate dogs today are getting too much. Authors seeking to understand the higher incidence of liver disease in some breeds conclude 'we believe that the amount of copper in many commercial dog foods is excessive, and that Labrador Retrievers, because of their popularity as family pets, may be functioning as sentinels for trends in hepatic copper concentrations in the general pet dog population'.[4]

In fact, after more than 70 years of extruded dry pet food manufacturing, of the 12 minerals listed in the AAFCO Nutritional Profile, there are maximums in place for only four (calcium, phosphorus, iodine and selenium). Of the 11 vitamins listed they have maximums in place for just two. Incredibly, while excess salt stemming from ultra-processed foods attracts so much attention in human circles, somehow, the AAFCO haven't yet managed to set a single maximum for the taste-enhancers-but-kidney-rotting sodium, potassium or chloride in dogs or cats. Until they do, you can use as much as you like in your food and treats.

This is just a taste of where we are today with the specific vitamin and mineral requirements of dogs. Incredible, isn't it? And still, armed with pipettes and conical flasks, the pet food manufacturers assure us that thanks to 'science' your pet has never had his nutrient requirements so precisely met. I have to admit, I'm not so sure. To learn more, let's take a look at some of the issues facing pet food manufacturers as they attempt to navigate (and become the first to conquer, apparently) the George-Jetson-pill-approach to vitamin and mineral supplementation.

Erratic Vitamin Inclusions

From at least the time of Hippocrates (460–377 BC), the founder of modern medicine, we have suspected that items such as fruits and vegetables seem to contain *something* that bestows health on a person. We now know those little, bioactive compounds to be vitamins and minerals, but it wasn't until well into the 19th century that we realised this – it was thanks to sailors that we found them. Before then, sailors were dying in staggering numbers from lack of vitamin C, as much as 75% of 2,000 seamen on some voyages.[5] We simply had no idea that there were tiny vital molecules in some foods and not in others that bestowed life on us. Bryson highlights how slow the whole uptake of adequate nutrition was from that point. It wasn't until the end of the 19th century that a Dutch physician working in Java linked the two facts. People who ate wholegrain rice didn't get beriberi, while people who ate polished rice very often did. The aetiology of this disease, a chronic nerve wasting disorder resulting from a lack of thiamine (vitamin B_1), was discovered in 1912 by a Polish physician with the rather envious name of Cashmir Funk. Using dogs as his test subjects he was the first to identify the link between a vitamin deficiency and the onset of certain diseases, notably scurvy (vitamin C), pellagra (vitamin B_3) and rickets (vitamin D).

We now know that vitamins are positively vital to life. You need to eat your fill of them every day, but exactly how much and how often is still a matter of debate. For example, nobody paid much heed to the findings of Cashmir Funk (Why isn't that my name?) until 1939, when a Harvard Medical School surgeon, named John Crandon, apparently deprived himself entirely of vitamin C for as long as it took to make himself ill. This was a surprisingly long time. For the first 18 weeks, his only symptom was fatigue, but in the nineteenth week, he took a turn for the worse and would certainly have died, were it not for the intervention of his medical friends. They injected him with a high dose of vitamin C and Crandon was restored almost immediately.[1]

The above example highlights just how insidious a lack of a particular vitamin can be. Studies show vitamin C has a multiplicity of roles in dogs and humans. It is potent, immune-modulating and anti-inflammatory. It is essential for collagen: skin, tendon, bone, cartilage and connective tissue. It is an antioxidant, a flu fighter and a strengthener of tooth enamel.

Importantly, as it works on the nervous system, it calms the nerves and functions as a natural antidepressant. It helps fight the negative side effects of drugs and combats disease. Vitamin C is your front line in the fight against cancer. It is also the major anti-stress hormone. German researchers subjected 120 people to a sure-fire stressor – a public speaking task combined odiously with some complicated math problems. Half of the participants were given 1,000 mg of vitamin C beforehand. The others got a sugar pill. Stress was monitored and elevations in either blood pressure or the stress hormone cortisol were noted. Both were significantly higher in those who did not get the vitamin supplement.[6]

Yet despite Vitamin C being possibly the most important vitamin in our systems, certainly by quantity, you can apparently exist for 5 months without it with nothing but a little tiredness to show for it! If this is how long a total lack of our most important vitamin takes to materialise, it's easy to see how a simple deficiency of any one of them can sneak under the radar for so long. The effects are so mild, so chronic, that neither you nor your doctor will be able to pin an issue on the want of it. We all try to eat well (fresh food) and hope we're getting enough of the important bits. Copious amounts of studies and reports, though, are telling us that we Westerners are still getting it very wrong. Daily, we are both under-eating and over-eating in numerous vitamins and minerals.

Fully realising both their importance and our want of them, a vast industry has popped up to fill the gap. Instead of getting the diet right, a hassle at best, the market has isolated and purified vitamins and minerals for you and put them in a handy pill. Unfortunately, these manufactured nutritional supplements are not without their critics.

A colossal study by the US Preventive Task Force, published in the *Annals of Internal Medicine* (2016) combined every single study citing the benefits (or lack thereof) of vitamin and mineral supplements and included more than 450,000 participants. It found that with the sole exception of reported lower incidence of some cancers in men taking a multivitamin or mineral, supplements offered no consistent evidence of benefit for heart disease, cancer or longevity.

Worse still, their use has been linked to harm many times. A review published in 2012 examined the conclusions of 27 clinical trials assessing the efficacy of a variety of vitamin antioxidants and the results were far from favourable. Just seven studies reported that supplementation possibly led to some health benefit. Ten studies didn't see any benefit at all. The other 10 studies found many patients to be in a measurably worse state after supplementation, including an increased risk of lung and breast cancer.[7]

While vitamin supplements have had some successes, such as the taking of folic acid (vitamin B$_9$) to reduce birth defects in pregnant mothers,[8] as well as apparently reducing the chance of stroke[5] and some cancer in men,[9] many review studies looking at their long-term effects paint a different picture. For instance, in 2006, a study of postmenopausal women in the United States found that after 10 years of taking folic acid (vitamin B_9) every day, their risk of breast cancer increased by 20% relative to those women who didn't take the supplement.[10] This is a terrible dichotomy for many women hoping to conceive. To make things a little worse for them, a study of 35,000 mothers-to-be found that multivitamin use in the weeks before conceiving was associated with a modest increased risk of early foetal death.[11]

A study of 29,133 Finnish people in their 50s, all of whom smoked, found that those given a beta carotene vitamin supplement were 16% more likely to die of lung cancer.[12] Two years later, a study of more than 1,000 heavy smokers had to be terminated nearly 2years early when, after just 4 years of beta-carotene and vitamin A supplementation, there was a 28% increase in lung cancer rates and a 17% increase in deaths.[13]

Men who took multi-vitamins were twice as likely to die from prostate cancer compared to those who didn't,[14] a fact that was corroborated in 2011, when a study of 35,533 healthy men found that vitamin E and selenium supplementation increased prostate cancer by 17%.[15] A meta-analysis of sixty-seven randomised, controlled trials found that vitamin E, vitamin A and beta-carotene supplements may be associated with an increased incidence of mortality.[16]

While vitamin C is clearly a vital antioxidant, one particularly shocking finding was that taking too much vitamin C might actually *increase* your risk of cancer.[17] It is theorised that vitamin C protects *all* cells from the often pesky and damaging effect of free radicles, both good and bad alike. Researchers are calling this the 'the antioxidant paradox'.

Thus, while Western nutrition may now recognise that fruits and vegetables confer beneficial disease-preventing properties, scientists attempting to isolate single components from these foods and incorporate them into a 'magic pill' for disease prevention struggle to confer the same benefits as when they are consumed from whole food sources. Sadly, this doesn't stop our drug-addicted culture believing the George Jetson magic pill for health. Around 50% of Americans are taking dietary supplements for health benefits, and the number of users is rapidly increasing.[13] After all, popping a pill is a lot easier than avoiding pizza, eating vegetables and going for a nice, long walk. Couple this need to believe with copious amounts of in-house 'scientific' trials and polish it all off with fancy jargon, and you have marketing gold.

According to the US Food and Drug Administration (FDA) and *Nutritional Business Journal*, in 2012, sales of nutritional supplements alone generated close to $32 billion in revenue. By 2020 sales were projected to double to above $60 billion, supporting more than 450,000 jobs nationwide.

Quite clearly, the synthetic vitamin supplementation of humans is still very much a work in progress. Their use is still something of a dark art with unpredictable consequences. Something that, at best, has had some benefits, and, at worst, is misleading and clearly dangerous. The dry pet food industry is almost wholly reliant on synthetic vitamin and mineral supplementation, a dual effect of their choice of ingredients and the detrimental effects of processing.

If this is the current state of knowledge in our own vitamin requirements, what we know of canine vitamin requirements is in the dark ages. We have not a single *optimum* vitamin content for the dog. Thus far, we have been operating on the minimum level required for normal function. Those sorts of studies are highly complex, so they're not done in dogs. All we have an idea of are the minimums and some maximums. Currently pet food manufacturers are only required to include vitamins at the *minimum level required for normal growth*.

Before we consider what the negative effects of heat and storage might be on these minimum values, take a look at the list below. Try to identify one nutrient that you would be happy your child was consuming at the required minimum for normal development over 6 months.

Fat-soluble Vitamins

Vitamins A, D, E and K, commonly found in meat and meat products, are transported around the body in fat. Any excesses are stored by your body in the liver and fatty tissues. This means you don't need to get them from food sources every day.

Vitamin A: Essential for the eyes and other organs, such as the skin. Also important for the bones, teeth, hair and immune system.

Vitamin D: Known to humans as the sunshine vitamin (and actually a hormone), dogs and cats can't synthesise their own vitamin D from the sun as humans can. Even so, all animals need it for bone growth as it regulates the absorption of calcium and phosphorus by the body. This is why a deficiency of vitamin D materialises as bone and joint issues, including rickets. But, like the others, vitamin D is vital to most areas of the body including the eyes, heart, kidneys, glandular and nervous systems, skin and teeth!

Vitamin E: Known as the age fighter, vitamin E is the body's main antioxidant. It combats free radicals in the body (formed when fat goes rancid), which are responsible for ageing. Dry food manufacturers spray their fats on the outside of their pellets before storing to encourage dogs to eat the product. With subsequent long storage periods, there is a high potential for fat rancidity. Heat and storage destroy vitamin E (hence dry-fed dogs require vitamin E supplementation in abundance, approximately 10–20 mg per kilo of body weight, per day).

The AAFCO (2016) requires 50 IU of vitamin E per kilo of dry matter. While most prey animals seem to have just enough vitamin E in this respect, some important prey species, including whole domestic rabbits, are seen to fall very short, averaging less than 20 IU/kg of Vitamin E DM.[18] That said, while many synthetic vitamins seem to be handled by the body just as efficiently, even more so with some versions, this is not the case with vitamin E. Studies of humans and various farm animals all show that natural forms of vitamin E are absorbed and utilised twice as efficiently as it's synthetic form in dietary supplements.[19] Sadly, as studies of dogs fed nutrients in their normal form are not conducted by the industry, we can't be sure how much natural vitamin E is actually required by dogs day to day. There are also some differences in the utilisation of natural and synthetic beta carotene (the vitamin A precursor), vitamin D and vitamin K, in this regard.[19]

Vitamin K: The anti-haemorrhagic vitamin, vitamin K functions in blood clotting as well as in healthy skin and bones. It is made by bacteria, which live in your intestines. Thus, faeces can be a great source of vitamin K (one of the causes of coprophagy in dry-fed dogs.) The vitamin is not included in dry dog food as dogs can synthesise their own (when healthy).

Water-Soluble Vitamins

Vitamins B and C, found in a range of foodstuffs including meat, fish, fruit, vegetables and whole grains, are transported around the body in water. This means that your body can't store them because you pass the excess through urine. You need to eat foods containing these vitamins every day. Water-soluble vitamins are the first to be destroyed by cooking; so steam/grill rather than broil.

B Complex Vitamins: So, called because there is a variety of them, B complex vitamins are essential to energy production as well as mental and emotional wellbeing. In humans, B vitamins are used in the treatment of depression,[20] ADHD[21] and hyperactivity[22] to name but a few. In fact, Harding *et al.*[22] found doses of B complex to be as effective as Ritalin in curbing hyperactivity in children. The study of this one vitamin alone gave rise to a new avenue of science – psycho-dietetics, which essentially studies the relationship between food and emotional health.[23] As they cannot be stored, you need a constant fresh supply for good emotional health.

Vitamin B_1 (thiamine): The brain requires thiamine to help convert glucose (blood sugar) into fuel. It is thus essential for the brain and nervous system's operation. Without it, the brain rapidly runs out of energy. This can lead to fatigue, depression, irritability and general anxiety. Deficiencies can also cause memory problems, loss of appetite, insomnia and gastrointestinal disorders. The consumption of refined (processed) carbohydrates drains the body's thiamine supply and may be a significant cause of behavioural upset.

Vitamin B_2 (riboflavin): Riboflavin is used to make the enzymes that release energy to the cells. It is particularly important for healthy skin and vision. It also helps to boost the body's immune system.

Vitamin B_3 (niacin): Niacin supports energy production and many chemical reactions. It aids in sleep and memory function as well as sex hormone production. Pellagra disease, which produces psychosis and dementia, is caused by niacin deficiency. A niacin deficiency may materialise as agitation and anxiety, as well as mental and physical slowness.

Vitamin B_5 (pantothenic acid): Like the other B vitamins, pantothenic acid supports energy production and strengthens the immune system. It is vital to the breakdown of fats and uptake of amino acids. Pantothenic acid is needed for hormone formation and the brain chemical acetylcholine, which combine to prevent certain types of depression. Symptoms of deficiency will thus include fatigue, chronic stress and depression.

Vitamin B$_6$ (pyridoxine): Again, with a supportive role in energy production, this vitamin aids in the processing of amino acids so the body can use them. It boosts immune system function and is vital in the manufacture of hormones such as serotonin, melatonin and dopamine, the three head honchos in emotional health and well-being. Thus, a Vitamin B$_6$ deficiency causes impaired immunity, skin lesions and mental confusion.

Vitamin B$_9$ (folic acid): Folic acid has a direct role in cell growth and maintenance. It is needed for DNA synthesis and immune system function. It rose to stardom with the discovery of its importance to pregnant females, to prevent neural tube defects in the developing foetus.

Vitamin B$_{12}$ (cobalamin): Only found in animal products, Vitamin B$_{12}$ is vital to red blood cell formation and maintaining both immune and nervous system function. It is also essential to support the brain tissue. Deficiency is linked to a variety of neurological issues including irritability, confusion, dementia or mania. These deficiencies take a long time to develop as the liver can store a 3-to 5-year supply.

Vitamin C (ascorbic acid): Vitamin C has multifunctionality. It is THE vitamin for the immune system, acting as an antioxidant and anti-inflammatory agent. It is also the building block of collagen (skin, tendon, bone, cartilage, connective tissue). It is the major anti-stress hormone helping to fight the negative side effects of drugs. It combats disease.

Despite its importance, vitamin C is usually not included in dry food pellets, given that healthy dogs can manufacture very small amounts for themselves,[2] even if they don't seem to be that good at it. For instance, dogs have much lower rates of ascorbic acid production than other animals, such as goats, cows, rats and rabbits.[24] For this reason, some authors believe there to be little benefit in giving additional vitamin C to a normal, healthy dog.[25] Indeed, vitamin C supplementation might even hamper the performance of racing greyhounds.[26] However, it's neither normal nor racing dogs that we're concerned about in this instance. It is sick ones. The rate of Vitamin C synthesis in the dog's liver tissue is lower than other animal species.[24] Authors note that during stress or intense exercise, the requirement of vitamin C may exceed the synthetic capacity of their liver.[2] Should a problem arise down the road for your dry-fed dog, a period of sickness, stress or injury, when a little vitamin C boost would very much benefit them, this vitamin boost will never arrive. This is likely why sick dogs, such as those with canine distemper virus, can benefit significantly from vitamin C supplementation. Belfield (1967)[27] described how 10 dogs struck down with distemper appeared to benefit from 1-2 g/day of intravenous Vitamin C over three days. Stimulated by these findings and using 16 dogs, Leveque (1969)[28] increased their chances of survival from 5-10% to 44%. These types of vitamin boosts are eternally unavailable to sickly, dry-fed dogs.

For this reason, many natural vets recommend that dogs on a dry diet should be supplemented with 50-100 mg/kg body weight (BW) per day (under slight stress: 100 mg/kg BW; under moderate stress: 200 mg/kg BW; under heavy stress: 300 mg/kg BW; under very heavy stress: 350 mg/kg BW.[29] You cannot overdose on vitamin C, although some diarrhoea can occur at high doses. When supplementing with vitamin C, use the ascorbic acid form – this way you are not adding all the additional calcium, sodium or magnesium that you will find in the ascorbate form.

Biotin: Other vitamins exist, such as biotin (part of the B complex), which our bodies are full of. But we still don't know exactly what they do, or how a deficiency materialises. We could be going around with less memory, 5 fewer IQ points, shorter fingers – who knows? We suspect it functions in the bone marrow, glandular and metabolic systems, muscles, hair and skin. For dogs,the the AAFCO[30] only recently allowed for some in 'complete' pet food (0.07 mg/kg of BW) while FEDIAF (The European Pet Food Industry Federation, a French acronym) claims it is not necessary for dogs at all.

The problem processed pet foods have is that heat is the enemy of water-soluble vitamins. It is why we should not 'overcook the goodness' out of our green vegetables. Lešková et al. (2006)[31] found significant losses (>33%) of the heat-liable vitamins retinol, vitamin C, folate and thiamine during the cooking of food at just 100°C (212°F). Dry food is subjected to heat of at least 120°C (250°F) for 30 minutes during the extrusion process, and studies repeatedly show this process positively obliterates vitamin content.[32-35] In their review of the extrusion process, Björck and Asp (1983),[32] noted significant loss of the heat-labile vitamins B_1, B_5, B_{12} and C in dry food. Mooney (2010)[35] found that in all cases, the concentration of vitamins in extruded pet food exiting the extruder and dryer were lower than target levels. Hoffmann LaRoche and Nutley (1995)[34] noted a 34% decrease in carotene after processing, a 15% decrease in vitamin E after processing dry food at 110°C for thirty minutes (20°C cooler than normal temperatures).

Worse still, Mooney (2010)[35] noted the quantity of vitamins in extruded pet food declined by approximately 50% over six months storage in ambient conditions. Hofmann La Roche[36] found that after just 6 months storage, Vitamin B_1 fell by more than 57%, vitamin B_2 fell by more than 32%, vitamin B_{12} fell by 34%, vitamin C fell by 14% and vitamin E fell by 29%. Unbelievably, these authors documented 100% vitamin C destruction, a vitamin B_6 loss of 89% and vitamin A, vitamin B_1 and biotin losses of 50% in canned dog foods. In fact, Mooney (2010)[35] found that most nutrients were negatively affected after just 6 weeks of stressed shelf life testing.

This is worrying. We are now forced to ask how much of what is written on the side of the bag will actually be absorbed by my dog from this food product? A product manufactured many months ago, taken from a paper bag that has travelled thousands of miles, has sat in hot cargo holds, pet shop floors and is open in the cupboard for a few weeks? This is something we cannot know. And what is their solution to all this nutrient destruction? Add in lots and lots of the most sensitive vitamins from a conical flask to make sure at least some make it to your dog.

As covered extensively by Anne Martin in her book *Food Pets Die For* (2007), this practice of artificial supplementation by manufacturers is far from an exact science. In her case, it caused the hypervitaminosis (with vitamin D) and unfortunate death of her little dog. Martin then pursued the particular company in a court battle for the $120 veterinary fee. The company agreed to pay, but Martin was required to sign a disclaimer, essentially banning her from shouting from the rooftops, which might prevent them selling the product elsewhere.

Thankfully, Martin did not accept this offer. The company then employed three solicitor firms and spent over $50,000 to keep her quiet. This is the power of the industry, but thankfully this belligerence by the industry created an ardent voice for dog owners in the form of Martin.

Nor is she alone. In their review titled "Class I and Class II Pet Food Recalls Involving Chemical Contaminants from 1996 to 2008" Rumbeiha and Morrison (2011)[37] note that there were a total of 22 Class I and II pet food recalls (the most serious form of recall, where illness has been documented, production must cease, product must be recalled immediately and, in so far as possible, customers be informed of what's going on). Of these, 27% were due to excessive chemical adulterants, the majority being for excessive or insufficient chemical vitamin supplementation resulting in the injury and death of numerous pets. These included excess cholecalciferol (Vitamin D) in dry pet food in 1999, which injured or killed at least 25 dogs and again in 2006, this time in four different products made by Royal Canin, causing toxicosis in at least six dogs and five cats.

This Vitamin D saga continues to this day. Recently, following dangerously high levels of Vitamin D, Hill's Pet Food was involved in a colossal recall of much of their range. It involved the following products:

Hill's Prescription Diet c/d Multicare Canine Chicken & Vegetable Stew

Hill's Prescription Diet i/d Canine Chicken & Vegetable Stew

Hill's Prescription Diet i/d Canine

Hill's Prescription Diet i/d Low Fat Canine Rice, Vegetable & Chicken Stew

Hill's Prescription Diet z/d Canine

Hill's Prescription Diet g/d Canine

Hill's Prescription Diet j/d Canine

Hill's Prescription Diet k/d Canine

Hill's Prescription Diet w/d Canine Vegetable & Chicken Stew

Hill's Prescription Diet w/d Canine

Hill's Prescription Diet z/d Canine

Hill's Prescription Diet Metabolic + Mobility Canine Vegetable & Tuna Stew

Hill's Prescription Diet Derm Defence Canine Chicken & Vegetable Stew

Hill's Science Diet Adult 7+ Small & Toy Breed Chicken & Vegetable Stew

Hill's Science Diet Puppy Chicken & Barley Entrée

Hill's Science Diet Adult Chicken & Barley Entrée Dog Food

Hill's Science Diet Adult Turkey & Barley Dog Food

Hill's Science Diet Adult Chicken & Beef Entrée Dog Food

Hill's Science Diet Adult Light with Liver Dog Food

Hill's Science Diet Adult 7+ Chicken & Barley Entrée Dog Food

Hill's Science Diet Adult 7+ Beef & Barley Entrée Dog Food

Hill's Science Diet Adult 7+ Turkey & Barley Entrée

Hill's Science Diet Adult 7+ Healthy Cuisine Braised Beef, Carrots & Peas Stew Dog Food

Hill's Science Diet Adult 7+ Youthful Vitality Chicken & Vegetable Stew Dog Food

Hill's Prescription Diet k/d Kidney Care with Lamb Canned Dog Food

Hill's Prescription Diet c/d Multicare Urinary Care Chicken & Vegetable Stew Canned Dog Food

Hill's Prescription Diet c/d Multicare Urinary Care Chicken & Vegetable Stew Canned Dog Food

Hill's Prescription Diet i/d Digestive Care Chicken & Vegetable Stew Canned Dog Food

Hill's Prescription Diet i/d Low Fat Canine Rice, Vegetable & Chicken Stew

Hill's Prescription Diet i/d Low Fat Digestive Care Rice, Vegetable & Chicken Stew Canned Dog Food

Hill's Prescription Diet g/d Aging Care Turkey Flavour Canned Dog Food

Hill's Prescription Diet w/d Digestive/Weight/Glucose Management Vegetable & Chicken Stew Canned Dog Food

Hill's Prescription Diet w/d Digestive/Weight/Glucose Management with Chicken Canned Dog Food

Hill's Prescription Diet r/d Canine

Hill's Prescription Diet Digestive Care with Turkey Canned Dog Food

Hill's Science Diet Adult Chicken & Barley Entrée Canned Dog Food

Hill's Science Diet Adult Beef & Barley Entrée Canned Dog Food

Hill's Science Diet Adult Chicken & Beef Entrée Canned Dog Food

Hill's Science Diet Adult 7+ Beef & Barley Entrée Canned Dog Food

Hill's Science Diet Adult 7+ Healthy Cuisine Roasted Chicken, Carrots & Spinach Stew Dog Food

Hill's Science Diet Healthy Cuisine Adult Braised Beef, Carrots & Peas Stew Canned Dog Food

Hill's Science Diet Healthy Cuisine Adult 7+ Braised Beef, Carrots & Peas Stew Canned Dog Food

Hill's Science Diet Adult Perfect Weight Chicken & Vegetable Entrée Dog Food

In terms of a single brand, with one million cases of pet food recalled, it's now one the biggest pet food recall in history. While Hill's tried to blame their vitamin premix supplier, the FDA said Hill's failed to follow company procedures for consistently verifying the quality of ingredients in its pet foods (FDA warning letter to Hill's MARCS-CMS 576564, find online). At the end of the day, Hill's produced 22 million cans of pet food and didn't check a *single can* before it left the factory.

While the FDA has yet to reveal how many pets died as a result of this most recent slip, *The Washington Post* notes that Hill's Pet Nutrition Facebook and Twitter pages were overwhelmed with replies from distressed pet owners, many of whom claimed their dogs had gotten extremely sick or died after consuming the food. Some said they'd paid thousands in medical bills as a result of the accompanying illness.[38] In 2019, a judicial panel consolidated 35 lawsuits against Hill's Pet Nutrition into a single federal legal action.[39] Thiamine (Vitamin B_1) appears to be one of the trickiest nutrients for manufacturers. The AAFCO (2016)[30] states:

> ...because processing may destroy up to 90% of the thiamine in the diet, allowance should be made to ensure the minimum nutrient level is met after processing...

Manufacturers thus include lots of thiamine mononitrate to replace all the Vitamin B_1 that they know will be destroyed during processing. Sadly, analysis of major pet food recalls over the 8 years to 2017, for just vitamin deficiency/ excess, all of which occurred in dry and canned pet food, reveals that thiamine is at the centre of five of them. (For more details, see www.fda.gov "Animal and Veterinary Recalls Archive.")

- 2017 JM Smucker Company (twice). Possible low levels of thiamine (vitamin B$_1$).

- 2016 Addiction Pet foods, elevated levels of vitamin A.

- 2016 Fromm Family Foods, elevated levels of vitamin D 2016 Nestlé Purina, 'may not contain the recommended level of vitamins and minerals'.

- 2015 Ainsworth Pet Nutrition voluntarily recalled their cat food for 'potentially elevated vitamin D levels'.

- 2014 Natura Pet recalled cat food due to vitamin insufficiency.

- 2013 Premium Edge, Diamond Naturals and 4health dry cat food formulas voluntarily recalled due to possibility of low levels of thiamine (vitamin B$_1$).

- 2012 Nestlé Purina voluntarily recalls their therapeutic canned cat food due to a low level of thiamine (vitamin B$_1$).

- 2011 Wellpet LLC voluntarily recalls canned cat food due to less than adequate levels of thiamine (vitamin B$_1$). WellPet decided to recall 'out of an abundance of caution'.

- 2010 Blue Buffalo Company recalls their dry dog food because of possible excess of vitamin D. Blue Buffalo learned of this potential condition in its products when it received reports of thirty-six dogs diagnosed with high vitamin D levels after feeding on these products.

- 2010 P&G recalls canned cat foods due to low levels of thiamine (vitamin B$_1$).

- 2009 Diamond Pet foods announces recall of Premium Edge Adult Cat and Premium Edge Hairball Cat Food for the potential to produce thiamine deficiency. Twenty-one cases were confirmed in cats eating this product.

Of course, this is only IF an issue is detected. For example, it was astute researchers at Michigan State University's Diagnostic Center for Population and Animal Health (DCPAH) that led to the recall of Blue Buffalo dry food in 2010 for dangerously high levels of vitamin D. They began receiving samples from all over the country from hypercalcaemic dogs. DCPAH endocrinologist

Kent Refsal thankfully noticed a pattern and the team investigated further by telephoning the individual vets in charge of each case. Once the common factor was identified, they shook the FDA awake and alerted them to the issue. Four years on the situation in dry food is no better. Markovich *et al.* (2014)[40] observed a wide range of thiamine concentrations in pet foods evaluated. Twelve of 90 pet foods were below the minimum protocol set out by the AAFCO. They concluded that clinicians should consider thiamine deficiency as a differential diagnosis in cats with acute neurologic dysfunction.

It stands that not one dry food manufacturer can tell you reliably the vitamin content of your dog's food. Perhaps this wouldn't be so bad if the food wasn't labelled as 'complete' and therefore suitable to feed to your dog as his sole nutritional input for the rest of his life. You just need one nutrient level to be off (later we will demonstrate just how often that occurs), and over time your dog will suffer. When that problem does pop up, you and your vet will almost certainly be oblivious to the actual cause.

It is telling that when vitamins are added to 'complete' dry foods, dogs are seen to benefit. Mentioned earlier addition of vitamin C significantly increased the survival times of dry-fed dogs with distemper. Chew *et al.* (2000)[41] found that dogs, on a commercial Iams dry food but that were supplemented with beta-carotene (vitamin A), enjoyed heightened cell-mediated and humoral immune response to challenge. When dogs on 'nutritionally complete and balanced' Mars Pet Foods were supplemented on a daily basis with a vitamin mix of vitamin C, vitamin E, beta-carotene and lutein (as well as the protein lycopene and amino acid taurine), they achieved sustained increases in circulating levels of antioxidants that exerted a protective effect by decreasing DNA damage, leading to improved immunological performance.[42] These authors also reported that over an 8-week rabies vaccination course, the supplemented dogs demonstrated significantly higher vaccine-specific virus-neutralising antibody levels, with a tendency toward establishing a vaccine-specific antibody response quicker than did the control group of dogs. Khoo *et al.* (2005)[43] fed groups of puppies on 'complete and balanced' pet food. To one group they added an antioxidant vitamin mix containing vitamin E, vitamin C, beta-carotene and selenium. To both groups, they then administered a standard vaccination protocol consisting of canine parvovirus (CPV) and distemper (CDV) vaccine, at 2 and 4 weeks. The results showed that animals supplemented with these simple vitamin antioxidants had significantly increased memory cells and serum E concentrations compared to the control group, which the authors note "may help to provide longer-lived protection against infections." Crucially, Khoo *et al.* (2005)[43] conclude:

> The minimum AAFCO recommendation for dietary Vitamin E (50 IU/kg) may not be sufficient to protect cells during periods of immune stress.

In other words, while the AAFCO has defined the minimum amount of dietary vitamin E (50 IU/kg) for pups, should these pups need a little extra antioxidant oomph in times of sickness, stress or vaccination, it won't be there for them. This is a crucial issue with complete diets. Complete for whom? And when?

Despite the fact we know processing and storage times destroy the vitamin content of pet food over time; despite the fact their products are constantly being recalled for insufficient and excessive vitamin doses at the cost of pet's lives; despite the fact we know when 'complete' foods are supplemented with some vitamins dogs benefit; and despite the fact the whole human supplement industry is fraught with alarming issues, it's interesting (but not surprising) that pet food manufacturers still boldly claim to have created 'complete' food products for all dogs that are not only as good as, but *better* than, fresh ingredients. This is an amazing feat, as even NASA can't come up with a complete diet for their astronauts, with fluctuating vitamin availabilities being their biggest concern. In an article titled "How to Feed an Astronaut: A Talk with NASA",[44] Michelle Perchonok was asked how NASA maintains the nutritional value of foods when they require a shelf life of a year. She replied:

> …That is a huge, huge challenge and we're still not there…some of the vitamins are significantly lost…we do know the methods we're using to preserve the foods are part of the culprit for losing the nutrition…and, of course, nutrition gets lost over time…

The idiots at NASA could save themselves a lot of time and money if they asked the science arms of the pet food industry for some of their trade secrets.

The Problems with Mineral Supplementation

Mineral is just another word for those chemical elements that the body needs to function. They include calcium, iron, sodium, iodine, zinc and magnesium. Vitamins and minerals are really peas in a pod. The only real difference is that vitamins come from living things such as plants and bacteria while minerals do not.

Like most vitamins, minerals are not made in the body; we must consume them. They are divided into two groups – macro- and micro-minerals. The macro-minerals, so called because we need relatively more of them, are big-ticket items such as calcium, phosphorus, sodium, potassium and magnesium. Their weight is normally measured in milligrams. Micro-minerals, aka trace elements, include iron, copper, zinc, manganese and iodine. We need much smaller amounts of these in our daily diet.

Again, as with vitamins, we cannot do without minerals for a long period of time and expect to be ok. Mineral deficiency results in growth retardation, osteoporosis and anaemia (caused by a lack of zinc, calcium and iron, respectively). While this is happening to all of us, all of the time, Western society is also plagued with a dangerous excess of minerals – salt, NaCl, sodium chloride, being the headline issue for the last few decades.

Excess salt comes from the processed food we eat, where manufacturers use sodium and potassium chloride to artificially boost the flavour of their tasteless products. I mean, who would have thought a kilo of corn flakes contains more salt than a kilo of salted peanuts? Twice as much in fact, just one serving contains half your RDA.

Minerals are really interesting. For instance, the human body contains enough iron to make a 3-inch nail, enough sulphur to kill all the fleas on an average dog, enough carbon to make 900 pencils, enough potassium to fire a toy cannon and enough phosphorus to make 2,200 match heads.[5] After that, it gets a bit hazy. You have enough bromine in your body to fill a thimble, but what it's for – nobody is really sure. Most nutritionists agree that arsenic, sourced in celery and asparagus, plays some role in digestion. Yet it is so poisonous that a match-head amount of it will cause sudden death.

And for all our fussing over them, we still suffer gross mineral insufficiencies and excesses. We are all grossly under-eating in magnesium, magnesium and manganese (as we're not eating enough fresh food) and grossly over-eating in other minerals such as calcium and sodium, reflecting our move toward animal protein sources (milk, cheese) and processed foods in general.

In fact, in terms of zinc, calcium and sodium, it appears the same is happening in our dogs.

Again, while we have all the minimums, some of the maximums are missing and except in the case of calcium and phosphorus, we are entirely without optimums in the dog. However, considerably less is known of the more obscure micro-minerals such as copper, manganese, zinc, iodine and selenium. This is evident in the fact the AAFCO[30] recommends that adults and pups need the same amounts of these in their diet. Now obviously this can't be right. For optimal development, growing pups and older dogs undoubtedly need different levels of each one of these. It's just that the science isn't there, yet. While we can easily study the effects of diets wholly void of these nutrients, the effects of a mere deficiency are much harder to pin down. If we leave aside the basic humanity of it, which you must do should you sell your soul and test on animals, you would need a much greater number of dogs, caged for years in various stages of mineral deficiency. This rapidly becomes financially unviable.

A Note on Dry Food Calcium and Phosphorus Contents

Just as we say crude protein to denote all the types of protein used in ultra-processed food, digestible or otherwise, the same applies to calcium and phosphorus. Crude calcium (Ca) and crude phosphorus (P) denote all the Ca and P naturally occurring from the ingredients used but also the Ca and P that are added in supplement form by the manufacturer.

The amount of crude Ca and P used in ultra-processed pet food today is of major concern. Although the figure is constantly being reviewed downward, the general consensus is that these nutrients in dog food should not exceed the required 0.8% crude Ca and 0.69% crude P per kilogram of dry matter (DM) for the normal growth of puppies in both small and large breeds (although this figure likely exceeds metabolic requirements in giant breeds).[45-48] These authors all stipulate that a crude Ca:P ratio of 1.2:1 in ultra-processed pet food is important.

Despite these findings, AAFCO's (2016)[30] current guidelines of 1.2% crude Ca and 1% crude P DM for growth are approximately 50% higher than the aforementioned authors. Worse, the highly influential NRC (2006)[2] permits up to 2% crude Ca in pet food. Worse still, until the AAFCO recently revised their figures downwards, they permitted 2.5% Ca in pet food, more than three times the crude Ca recommended by the authors above each and every day of your dog's life, presumably before it becomes a danger. Specifically, the NRC (2006)[2] state:

> ...For most breeds of dogs, the maximum tolerable dietary calcium concentration is 2%. Most breeds of dogs will suffer a reduction in food intake and growth if diet calcium exceeds 2.3%.

Sadly, while the maximum crude Ca concentration is now set at 1.8 or 2%, the AAFCO (2016)[30] and NRC (2006)[2], respectively, note that even the top brand, premium pet foods very regularly exceed this figure. Thixton (2015)[49] conducted an in-depth analysis of the top brands of pet food, including Royal Canin, Hill's, Science Diet, Caesar and many other brands. The author ordered 12 different brands of pet food online and had them sent directly to a lab, a smart way of avoiding any accusations of handler bias. They found a Nestlé Purina cat food to contain 3.14% crude Ca, and Mars dog food (Caesar) with 3.17% crude Ca. Incredibly, they noted 7.7% crude Ca and 4.1% crude P in a Hill's Prescription Diet for urinary tract health in dogs. With levels of crude Ca and P 10 times that recommended, all of which must be removed by the kidneys, this is staggeringly dangerous for what is already a kidney-ill animal.

We know it's a common problem. You might note on your bag of dry food that Ca is often phrased as 'containing *no less* than 1% Ca and 0.8% P'. Even the most popular, most expensive and veterinary-prescribed large-breed puppy food here in Ireland boasts (at the time of writing) a crude Ca concentration of 1.4% and a crude P content of 1.1% which, it is claimed, fosters the 'healthy development' of your pup.

Before we discuss the effect of consuming such a consistently high doses of crude Ca and P each day, we need to ask why manufacturers would include more crude Ca and P than is absolutely necessary, especially when studies repeatedly demonstrate it's best to keep crude Ca at the lower level in pet food, or risk growth deformities.[46,48,50-56]

The answer likely lies in the amount of meat and bone meal used by the manufacturer. As well as adding a cheap 'meat' portion to the product, desirable on the label, meat and bone meal powder contains a lot of the minerals that must be listed on the side of the pack, most notably Ca and Pas well as the micro-minerals such as selenium, iron, copper and magnesium that manufacturers need their mixes to contain. Unfortunately, the more meal you add, the more Ca gets into your mix as meat meal would be more accurately called bone meal. Precious little 'meat' makes its way to the rendering vat. A balancing act thus ensues between the need for cheap animal protein ingredients and excess Ca in the mix.

But focusing on the vet-prescribed large-breed puppy food containing 1.4% crude Ca and 1.1% crude P, what is the effect on the developing pup that consumes 75% more than their RDA of supplemented Ca, and 38% more than their RDA of supplemented P, every day of its developing life? Every available independent study to date attests that the implications are absolutely dire for the dog.

Unlike adult dogs, puppies appear to have inefficient mechanisms for regulating how much dietary Ca they absorb from their food. During times of high dietary Ca, pups will both absorb and retain more Ca.[52,57] Lauten *et al.* (2002)[48] show that increasing Ca and P concentrations in pet food are rapidly reflected in the bone mineral content, lean mass and body fat of young pups (less than 6 months). Excess Ca and P in the blood combine to form hard deposits, known as calcifications, in the soft tissues of the body. These can gather in joints, making them stiff and painful, or more worryingly, they can move to block blood vessels resulting in heart and lung disease in the animal. Constantly higher intakes of Ca (sometimes only by small fractions) and P are very detrimental to the development of an immature skeleton, particularly in large breeds. Studies show bones become thicker and denser, where excessive growth creates troublesome spurs of bone growth and joint development problems, particularly fragmented coronoid process (FCP), osteochondritis dessicans (OCD) and canine hip dysplasia (CHD).[46,50,52-55,58]

While maintaining a lower crude Ca and P content and indeed a crude Ca/P ratio of 1.2:1 that appears to be crucial in ultra-processed pet food, it is less likely to apply to real food. The problem is the type of minerals used, in particular the presence of calcium carbonate (an inexpensive source of Ca, but here it also acts as a preservative and a colour retention agent) and dicalcium phosphate (a Ca and P supplement but also a tartar control agent that improves the texture of the product).

As metals, albeit often soft ones, minerals are part of the inorganic group of natural elements. In other words, it doesn't come from the land of the living. As you might suspect, inorganic elements are relatively difficult to absorb. The gut does not readily grant them free passage through for absorption by themselves. They must be in an organic form, that is, bound to a protein (a carbon molecule). The body recognises this more natural protein complex and allows the whole compound to pass through. It's sort of like bringing your friend to a private party.

Without you, your friend mightn't have gotten in – even though he's the one with the tunes!

Organic minerals are thus far better absorbed and utilised by the body than inorganic minerals.[1,57] It is for this reason that some of the best man-made supplements are based on chelated minerals. This is where an inorganic mineral is artificially bound to a carbon molecule in the laboratory. Unfortunately, the process is very expensive, so these types of minerals are rarely if ever included in this form in human supplements let alone pet food.

Napoli *et al.* (2007)[59] divided 183 women into three groups – one group (the 'diet' group) consumed at least 70% of their daily Ca from real food, another (the 'supplement' group) consumed at least 70% of their Ca from tablets or pills (exact source of Ca unspecified) and a third whose Ca-source percentages fell somewhere in between these ranges. They found that the 'diet' group took in the least Ca, an average of 830 milligrams per day and yet this group had higher bone density in their spines and hip bones than women in the 'supplement' group, who consumed about 1,030 milligrams per day.

It is the same for P. Historically, we were told ultra-processed pet food high in P is a risk factor for kidney disease. But what kind of P? Contrary to inorganic P more commonly used in dry foods (monosodium and dicalcium phosphate), P occurring naturally in food items such as meat or vegetables seems to have little to no effect whatsoever on postprandial plasma P in cats.[60,61]

It stands to reason that the body can better deal with greater fluctuations of naturally occurring minerals in the diet. Minerals never present to an animal uniformly in nature. A meal of carcass will be high in bone. A meal of rabbit will differ greatly to a meal of squirrel. And even within species, animals will differ throughout the year. In fact, no prey animals that I can find has a Ca/P ratio of 1.2:1. The lowest I can find is 1.4:1 in young cows and deer,[65] which would be largely unavailable to a feral dog except in carcass form. Most potential prey animals exhibit significantly higher ratios, with C/P ratios of 1.7 and 1.8:1 Ca to P for rabbits and rats while mice, squirrels and frogs appear to average approximately 2:1 Ca:P.[18]

Are we to worry that the puppy eating one or two meaty bones a week (and thus blowing their weekly Ca allowances out the window) might turn into a bone statue? The body regulates, if presented with the right nutrients. It has to. Let that pup munch *ad lib* on Ca supplements twice a week and the result would surely be graver down the line.

Unfortunately, we do not have figures for how much organic Ca and P a dog requires in his diet. All the studies pertain to dry-fed dogs. What we do know is that Ca supplements should never, ever be used in developing dogs of any type but particularly dry-fed dogs unless under the supervision of a vet who has had some formal training in nutrition.

Zinc

While it may seem ridiculous now, as recently as 1977, zinc was thought to have no role in diet at all.[62] Now we know that zinc is vital to your dog's skin, coat and bone growth. It plays a vital role in almost every form of growth in your body and that of your dog's. And like the rest of us, they can't store it. So, you need a plentiful supply in the diet.

As we saw with the amount of protein stated on the side of the packet, not all the zinc in dry dog food is bioavailable to your dog. The problem is zinc absorption will vary in accordance with the source of zinc used in the diet.[63-65] Chelated zinc, that is, zinc acetate or zinc citrate, is far easier absorbed by the body and deemed more bioavailable as a whole, compared to the cheaper, inorganic versions of zinc, including zinc sulphate and zinc oxide. Unfortunately, but perhaps unsurprisingly, it is the latter you will find in ultra-processed pet food as it is significantly cheaper to produce. Despite authors noting that zinc oxide is poorly utilised by the dog[66] and that natural zinc is utilised 60–80% better,[67,68] zinc oxide remains the zinc of choice for dry pet food manufacturers. Authors repeatedly demonstrate that dogs fed diets containing zinc oxide have poorer hair growth and coat condition.[69]

To make matters worse, zinc availability in dogs is subject to the presence or absence of dietary antagonists, such as calcium.[67] Excess calcium, particularly in the presence of phytates (found in cereals), binds zinc, impairing growth and mineral utilisation in rats and dogs,[70-76] which is bad news considering the amount of Ca and cereal used in pet food.

Also, as we have discussed previously, phytic acid found in cereal is known to bind significant amounts of zinc, magnesium and iron from the diet, drastically reducing availability for humans, retarding skeletal growth and inducing both rickets and osteomalacia in virtually every animal studied, including dogs.[77-83]

Simply including more zinc oxide is not the answer either, as excess zinc can result in interaction with other minerals, reducing availability of intrinsic copper for example, among other elements.[72]

Thus, adding zinc, in a form that is very poorly utilised by the dog, to a product that is attempting to be 'complete', is expected to cause serious problems. A zinc deficiency in pups will impair mineral utilisation and lead to poor, abnormal growth and dry flaky skin with possible lesions (particularly in foot pads) with secondary skin infections, thick crusts on the elbows and dull coat.[77,84,85] A quick, temporary solution for this condition is to rub the affected area with any seed or nut oil (very high in zinc and Vitamin E), such as coconut or almond oil, although nothing replaces a diet containing adequate amounts of the most readily absorbed form of nutrition.

It's interesting to note that another symptom of a zinc deficiency in humans is known as hypogeusia, where your taste buds stop working and render food tasteless.[86] Mind you, this is a potential advantage for pets living on a dry pet food diet.

The poor absorption of zinc in ultra-processed pet food has dry dog food manufacturers in a bind.

Up until 2016, the AAFCO wanted to see 120 mg of zinc per kilo minimum in 'complete' dry food for puppies. In their revised version, this figure drops to 100 mg/kg. But even at this you will struggle to find a single prey animal that offers anything close to this zinc content.[18] This means, should you be formulating a 'complete' raw dog food using whole prey, your dog or cat might be viewed as deficient in zinc as per the AAFCO standards, and you have to run around finding other ingredients to boost the zinc content of your whole foods to keep your more species-appropriate fresh product compliant with the nutritional principles of the synthetic pet food industry. How does this make sense?

Excess Salt

Excess salt is a taste enhancer, a time-old practice of processed food companies to make their tasteless products more appealing. It's just one of the reasons we are told to reduce our processed food intake. As carnivores, dogs and cats have an innate preference for salty food.[87,89] Palatability tests reveal that dogs prefer the taste of a moist food as the salt content increases. However, it appears this effect is not as evident with dry food. One reason put forward by the Small Animal Clinical Nutrition (SACN) (2010)[87] is that palatability enhancers are added topically to this product which 'probably masks any taste effects of sodium chloride or any other salts'. And still, it is used liberally in dry pet food. Unfortunately, finding out the salt content of dry pet food is not easy, not helped by the fact it, like carbohydrates, is not required to be disclosed on the label.

The guide dogs in Australia are fed Mars Advance Pet Food, as of 2016

> To ensure their health from puppy to adulthood, ADVANCE is used exclusively to rear, feed and nourish Guide Dogs around Australia.
> **Advance Website, 2016, www.advancepet.com.au/breed-profiles/**
> **dog-breeds/guide-dogs.asp.**

Here are the first 13 ingredients of their chicken-flavoured puppy growth food, as of 2016:

Chicken, Maize Gluten, Chicken Fat, Rice, Maize, Sorghum, Natural Flavour (Chicken), Tuna, Beet Pulp, Sunflower Oil, **Iodised Salt**, **Potassium Chloride**, Inulin.

In bold type are the salt additions. They are obliged to state the sodium content. This product has 0.6 g sodium per 100 g. That is the equivalent of 1.5 g of salt per 100 g, as salt (NaCl) is 40% sodium and 60% chloride. Potassium chloride is a popular sodium-free taste enhancer of processed foods. They are not obliged to state the amount of potassium chloride, which is the next ingredient in the mix by order of weight.

Potassium chloride's toxicity, in a healthy person, is approximately equal to that of table salt and it has the same effect on your kidneys.[89] I contacted Mars to find out how much potassium chloride was in the mix but this was, sadly, sensitive information that I was not permitted to know. What we are told by the label is that there is 0.5 g of inulin in the mix. Therefore, there must be between 0.5 g and 1.5 g potassium chloride in there (those figures being the stated inulin and iodised salt concentrations, respectively). Let's give them the great benefit of the doubt and go with the lowest possible value of 0.5 g potassium chloride.

This now equates to a salt content of 2% (1.5% sodium chloride + 0.5% potassium chloride). To put this figure in some context, this would make this dry food twice as salty as salted peanuts (approximately 1% salt) and 20 times saltier than fresh meat (roughly 0.1% salt).

The sodium (Na) requirements of the adult dog lies between 4.6 mg/kg and 11.5 mg/kg of body weight.[51] If we take the upper level for this example then, a 30 kg Lab requires 0.35 g of sodium per day, or, **0.86 g** of salt per day, for normal function.

Excluding the 0.5% potassium chloride content of this product for a moment, at 1.5% sodium chloride a 30kg Labrador, eating the recommended 440 g of this food, would be consuming **6.6 g** of salt per day (2.64 g of sodium).

Thus, at 6.6g of salt per day, a 30-kg lab is consuming nearly eight times what he needs for normal function, each and every meal of its life, and this is before we include their other salt ingredients, such as potassium chloride.

This is permitted by the industry. Here is the AAFCO's statement on why they haven't set a maximum for sodium in pet food:

> As noted by the 1990 CNES [The AAFCO Canine Nutrition Expert Subcommittee], because palatability and food consumption would decline due to excess sodium before adverse health effects were observed, setting a maximum concentration for sodium was not of practical concern.
>
> **AAFCO, 2014**[90]

Ok then! So, what might be the effect of eating eight times your RDA of salt per day? Well, the average human (75 kg) is recommended to consume no more than 6 g of salt a day, but UK adults are now averaging at least 9 g a day[91] or 1.5 times their RDA of salt. In their review of all the science available on the subject, the WHO cites this level of salt intake in humans is linked to a significant increase in hypertension, cardiovascular disease, osteoporosis, stomach ulcers, cancer, kidney and bone disease.[91] The bottom line is; we are very strongly advised to get our salt content below 6 g per day.

Unless dogs have evolved a mechanism of exuding salt through their skin or spitting it from their nose like a marine iguana, you would be forgiven for thinking that nearly eight times their RDA of salt is going to do significantly more damage in dogs than 1.5 times the RDA in humans, especially when we know that an excess ingestion of salt induces hypertension in dogs[92] just as it does in humans. And that hypertension is associated with obesity, chronic renal disease and many endocrinopathic diseases such as hypo and hyperthyroidism in dogs.[93-97] Also, as 43% of the sodium that a dog consumes is stored in their bones,[2] we can expect it to have the same detrimental effect on their bones and joints, as it does on ours.

You would hope the industry has some seriously supportive science at the ready to put our minds at ease over these high salt contents.

Are you getting used to being disappointed yet?

Professor Scott Brown, a highly qualified US vet with 24 years' experience in internal medicine and renal pathophysiology, currently Professor of Physiology at the University of Georgia and winner of the Royal Canin Award in 2010 for his contribution to small animal medicine, wrote a piece for Royal Canin/Mars titled "Salt, Hypertension and Chronic Kidney Disease".[101] Published in the journal *Veterinary Focus* (owned by Mars Inc.), Professor Brown lays out the argument for dogs being able to cope with very high salt concentrations, concluding:

> ...while it is likely there will be individual animal variation due to genetic, environmental, and disease factors, normal dogs and dogs with stages I–III CKD appear unlikely to be particularly salt-sensitive...
>
> **Brown (2007)**[98]

This is heartening. But if you were a curious soul and wanted to know the actual studies used to back up this statement, you might feel a little less easy.

The two references used to support this opinion are Krieger *et al.* (1990)[99] and Greco *et al.* (1994).[100] Krieger *et al.* (1990)[99] used six caged dogs and ran the test for 7 days. Not mentioned in the article was the fact that these authors did find a significant increase in cardiac output (CO or heart rate) by Day 2. To offset this effect, the dog's system decreased total peripheral resistance (TPR), ultimately allowing the blood to flow more easily. CO and TPR returned to control values only when low salt was resumed.

This test lasted only a week. Increased heart rate is linked to heart disease and susceptibility to other diseases *over time*. Okin *et al.* (2010)[101] studied 9,000 cardiac patients and concluded that physicians need to track the pattern of increasing heart rate over years, and not just consider single readings. Salt is a long, slow killer. It's not the first salty chip that gets you, but just try eating salty chips for breakfast and dinner for a few years. So, if anything, that study would serve to worry me, not pacify. Let's hope the second study is a little more enlightening.

Greco *et al.* (1994)[100] used 8 dogs but this time ran the trial for a slightly better 4 weeks. They first partially nephrectomized the dogs (removed 75% of their kidney function), then fed one group low, then high, then low (LHL) sodium feeds and the other high, then low, then high (HLH) sodium feeds, to test if dogs with kidney failure are sensitive to fluctuations in sodium in their diet. Mean arterial blood pressure was considerably higher in the LHL group, although it was not statistically significant.

Can you imagine a food company, today, bringing out a 'complete' food for humans that would result in you consuming 48 g of salt per day instead of the advised 6 g? And then, to defend their high-salt product, they produce two studies, the first using 6 people and lasting only a week (where a significant increase in cardiac output was noted) and the second 8 people for a month (where mean arterial blood pressure was higher, just not significantly)?

The authorities would have a heart attack.

A final note about salt: while the grossly excessive use of salt is sure to end your life quicker, I must point out that salt plays a crucial role in our health. I mean, have you seen what those Ibex do to get their salt fix on the wall of the Cingino dam in Italy?! Utterly terrifying.

While high-salt diets have been incriminated in the past, it's important to note that low-salt diets have their issues, too. A large pooled analysis of some 133,118 individuals (63,559 with hypertension, 69,559 without hypertension) found that, compared with moderate sodium intake, high sodium intake is indeed associated with an increased risk of cardiovascular events and death in earlier populations with hypertension. However, no effect was seen in people without hypertension. On the other hand, low sodium intake is associated with increased risk of cardio-vascular events and death in both those with or without hypertension.[102]

It's all to do with electrolytes. There are seven major electrolytes in the body including sodium ($Na+$), chloride ($Cl-$), potassium ($K+$), magnesium ($Mg++$), calcium ($Ca++$), phosphate ($HPO4-$) and bicarbonate ($HCO3-$). These guys play a whole lot of crucial roles in the body and we are under-eating in many of them. Electrolytes are like spark plugs, chemical substances that help the electric nervous systems to function. They make it possible for the cells to generate energy, pumping hearts and brains and muscles. They also control the acid/base balance, something our body is constantly trying to maintain. They control cell wall structure and the movement of water in and out of the cell. In this way, a good quality salt in moderation can be a nutritious addition to your cooking and to your dog. The Himalayan type is pretty good. Best is unrefined, nonoxidised (not air-dried) sea salt.

In fact, you may try a little home experiment, but not in a dry-fed dog already consuming dangerously high amounts of salt. Facebook groups are popping up in support of the fact that salt therapy can help ill or itchy dogs. It's a simple approach. You offer your dogs two types of water, one is plain, filtered water. The other is plain filtered water with a teaspoon of high quality salt dissolved into it.

Now, let your dog approach the bowls and watch what he does. Dogs have amazing noses, hundreds to thousands of times better than yours, depending on who you talk to. Think about that figure for a second. Imagine a nose twice as good as it is now. Or even three times better? It's hard to imagine. But hundreds of times better is impossible to comprehend, just as it would be to imagine having the vision of an eagle (8 times better than ours) who can not only spot a camouflaged rabbit on the wing from 2 miles but can actually zoom in on their prey once targeted! Dogs perceive the world in a way that we cannot comprehend. It is universally accepted that dogs can smell the vitamins and minerals in water much like a shark can detect a drop of blood in an Olympic swimming pool, which is just one of the reasons why they practice selective coprophagy (poo-eating to top up some elements of their diet that may be lacking) or pick only certain stems of grass. In this way, it is thought that if the dog requires electrolytes, they will select that water over the plain stuff.

I have seen this simple step significantly reduce itch and skin redness overnight, among a range of other interesting observations such as: more energy and increasing appetite. I always recommend clients try this little experiment on their raw-fed dog when a stubborn inflammatory issue arises (as long as they're not already on hugely excessive salt diets). People always feel better when they have little experiments to do and remedies they have to make themselves. It also might be useful to raw-fed dogs' after post-work activties, for example: sprinting, sledding, agility and shepherding.

TAKE-HOME POINTS

✓ We still know relatively little about our own mineral requirements. It stands that knowledge of the dog's requirements, particularly of the micro minerals (copper, manganese, zinc, iodine, selenium, etc.) are all but in the dark ages.

✓ While vitamins are from the land of the living, such as plants and bacteria, minerals are not.

✓ The Ca and P content of pet food arises from both the ingredients used but also the man-made additives included at the mixing stage, including calcium carbonate and dicalcium phosphate. The body does not treat both forms of nutrients the same. For now, we will include both under the term crude Ca or P.

✓ For now, the general consensus is that the ideal crude Ca and crude P content of ultra-processed dry food is 0.8% crude Ca and 0.69% crude P for growing puppies (though this possibly exceeds requirements in giant breeds). The Ca/P ratio 1.2:1 is important in ultra-processed pet food.

✓ Until very recently, the AAFCO permitted 2.5% crude Ca in pet food, three times the ideal amount of crude Ca in pet food. They have recently dropped that to 1.8% crude Ca. And still, dry pet food companies very regularly exceed that level, likely due to the level of bone meal used.

✓ Studies show too much crude Ca in ultra-processed foods leads to joint issues in dogs, particularly large breeds; hence, maintaining lower levels of Ca and P are advised.

✓ However, this is unlikely to apply to natural forms of Ca. Minerals in their 'natural' form, that is, chelated or bound to a carbon molecule, are significantly better absorbed and utilised by the body than synthetic minerals produced in a laboratory.

✓ The same applies to P where naturally occurring P in food items such as meat or vegetables seems to have little to no effect on postprandial plasma phosphorus in cats.

✓ Minerals rarely present to an animal uniformly in nature. For instance, no prey animal has a Ca/P ratio of anything close to 1.2:1. The average appears closer to 1.8:1.

✓ Zinc oxide remains the zinc of choice by dry pet food manufacturers despite it being poorly utilised by the dog. Dogs fed diets containing zinc oxide have poorer hair growth and coat condition.

✓ Phytic acid from cereal and excess Ca further bind available zinc from the diet. Adding extra zinc to overcome this won't work as it reduces the availability of copper.

✓ A zinc deficiency will materialise as a poor skin and coat, poor growth, skin infections, thick crusts on elbows. Rubbing with any seed or nut oil can greatly help the latter.

✓ Large amounts of salt are used as a taste enhancer and preservative in dry pet food.

✓ Some of the leading dry foods contain 2% salt (sodium chloride, potassium chloride), making them twice as salty as salted peanuts, 20 times saltier than fresh meat.

✓ Taking the 1.5% sodium chloride (NaCl) portion used by most pet foods, this results in a Labrador consuming 6.6g of NaCl per day, or eight times their RDA for salt every day.

✓ If we humans eat 1.5 times our RDA for salt we die quicker from hypertension, cardiovascular disease, osteoporosis, stomach ulcers, cancer, kidney and bone disease.

✓ There are no studies of any value supporting the safety of such high salt inclusions.

✓ The AAFCO continues not to put in place a maximum for salt inclusion in pet food.

✓ While salt gets a bad rap, good salt is beneficial in moderation as it is full of electrolytes. Consider doing the saltwater experiment on a raw fed dog using good quality salt.

- ✓ Vitamins are essential for life. You need them constantly. However, you can go long periods without them before anything too dramatic happens; so, a deficiency can be very hard to spot.

- ✓ Scientists attempting to isolate single components from foods, such as vitamins, and incorporate them into a synthetic 'magic pill' for disease prevention, struggle to confer the same benefits as when they are consumed from whole food sources.

- ✓ Most vitamins are affected negatively by heat processing but the water-soluble vitamins (B complex, C) are particularly sensitive to heat and storage time.

- ✓ B vitamins are added synthetically to the food during mixing. Thiamine (Vitamin B_1) appears to be a particularly tricky one for ultra-processed food as it explains multiple large-scale recalls annually.

- ✓ Vitamin C is not required in pet food as dogs can make it themselves, albeit they are quite poor at it. The vitamin C requirement of stressed and sick dogs is likely their ability to synthesise it. Studies show some sick dogs benefit from added vitamin C in their daily fare. On a diet of the same ultra-processed pet food, this vitamin boost will never come.

- ✓ The recommended vitamin C doses are:

  - 100 mg/kg BW under slight stress

  - 200 mg/kg under moderate stress

  - 300 mg/kg BW under heavy stress

- ✓ The incorrect vitamin D supplementation of ultra-processed pet food remains a lethal threat to pets, evident most recently with the colossal Hill's recall.

- ✓ As it stands, not one dry food manufacturer can tell you reliably the vitamin content of your dog's food by the time they eat it.

- ✓ Multiple studies show dogs living on ultra-processed pet food benefit from added vitamins in their diet.

Chapter Nine References

1   AAFCO (Association of American Feed Control Officials) 2014. Proposed Revisions Edited per Comments for 2014 Official Publication. Available online, www.aafco.orf

2   National Research Council (NRC, 2006). *Your dog's nutritional needs. A Science-Based Guide For Pet Owners*. National Academy of Sciences.

3   Abbaspour, N., Hurrell, R. and Kelishadi, R. (2014). Review on iron and its importance for human health.Journal of Research in Medical Sciences, 19(2): 164–174

4   Johnston, A.N., Center, S.A., McDonough, S.P. *et al*. (2013). Hepatic copper concentrations in Labrador Retrievers with and without chronic hepatitis: 72 cases (1980–2010). Journal of the American Veterinary Medical Association, 242(3): 372–380

5   Bryson, B. (2010). *At home: A short history of private life*. New York: Doubleday

6   Brody, S. Preut, R., Schommer, K. *et al*. (2002). A randomized controlled trial of high dose ascorbic acid for reduction of blood pressure, cortisol, and subjective responses to psychological stress. Psychopharmacology, 159(3): 319–324

7   Villanueva, C. and Kross, R.D. (2012). Review: Antioxidant-Induced Stress. International Journal of Molecular Science, 13: 2091–2109

8   Milunsky, A., Jick, H., Jick, S.S. *et al*. (1989). Multivitamin/Folic Acid Supplementation in Early Pregnancy Reduces the Prevalence of Neural Tube Defects. Journal of the American Medical Association, 262(20): 2847–2852

9   Wang, X., Qin, X., Demirtas, H. *et al*. (2007). Efficacy of folic acid supplementation in stroke prevention: A meta-analysis. The Lancet, 369(9576): 1876–1882

10   Kim, Y.I. (2006). Does a High Folate Intake Increase the Risk of Breast Cancer? Nutrition Review, 64(10): 468–475

11   Nohr, E.A. Olsen, J., Bech. B.H., Bodnar, L.M., Olsen, S.F., Catov, J.M. (2014). Periconceptional intake of vitamins and fetal death: A cohort study on multivitamins and folate. International Journal of Epidemiology, 43(1): 174–184

12   The Alpha-Tocopherol Beta Carotene Cancer Prevention Study Group (1994). The Effect of Vitamin E and Beta Carotene on the Incidence of Lung Cancer and Other Cancers in Male Smokers (1994). New England Journal of Medicine, 330:1029–1035

13   Omenn, G.S., Goodman, G.E., Thornquist, M.D. *et al*. (1996). Risk Factors for Lung Cancer and for Intervention Effects in CARET, the Beta-Carotene and Retinol Efficacy Trial. Journal of the National Cancer Institute, 88(21): 1550–1559

14   Bjelakovic, B. and Gluud, C. (2007). Surviving Antioxidant Supplements. Journal of the National Cancer Institute, 99(10): 742–743

15   Klein, E.A., Thompson, I.M., Tangen, C.M. (2011). Vitamin E and the Risk of Prostate Cancer. The Journal of the American Medical Association, 306(14): 1549–1556

16   Bjelakovic, G., Nikolova, D. and Gluud C. (2013). Meta-regression analyses, meta-analyses, and trial sequential analyses of the effects of supplementation with beta-carotene, vitamin A, and vitamin E singly or in different combinations on all-cause mortality: Do we have evidence for lack of harm? PLoS One, 8(9):e74558

17   Soni, M.G., Thurmond, T.S., Miller, E.R. *et al*. (2010). Safety of Vitamins and Minerals: Controversies and Perspective. Toxicological Sciences, 118(2): 348–355

18   Dierenfeld, E.S., Alcorn, H.L. and Jacobsen, K.L. (2002). Nutrient Composition of Whole Vertebrate Prey (Excluding Fish) Fed in Zoos. U.S. Department of Agriculture. Published online, www.researchgate.net

19   Levin, E. (2005). Vitamin E isn't helpful and may be harmful. British Medical Journal, 330: 0–f

20   Mikkelsen, K., Stojanovska, L. and Apostolopoulos, V. (2016). The Effects of Vitamin B in Depression. Current Medicinal Chemistry, 23(38): 4317–4337

21   Harding, K.L, Judah, R.D. and Gant, C.E. (2003a). Outcome-Based Comparison of Ritalin versus Food-Supplement Treated Children with AD/HD. Alternative Medicine Review, 8(3): 319–330

22   Harding, K. L., Judah, R. D. and Gant, C. E. (2003b). Nutrient supplementation is as effective as ritalin for curing ADHD and hyperactivity. Alternative Medicine Review, 8(3): 319–331

23   Cheraskin, E., Ringsdorf, W. M., Brecher, A. (1981). *Psychodietetics. Food as the key to emotional health.* Stein & Day Publishers

24   Chatterjee, A. Majumder, B. Nandi, N. Subramanian (1975). Synthesis and some major functions of vitamin C in animals. Annals of the New York Academy of Science, 258: 24–47

25   Hesta, M., Ottermans, C., Krammer-Lukas, S. *et al.* (2009). The effect of vitamin C supplementation in healthy dogs on antioxidative capacity and immune parameters. Animal Physiology and Animal Nutrition, 93(1): 26–34

26   Marshall, R.J., Scott, K.C., Hill, R.C. *et al.* (2002). Supplemental vitamin C appears to slow racing greyhounds. Journal of Nutrition, 132(6, Suppl 2): 1616S–1621S

27   Belfield, W.O. (1967). Vitamin C in treatment of canine and feline distemper complex. Veterinary Medicine in Small Animal Clinics, 62(4): 345–348

28   Leveque, J.I. (1969). Ascorbic acid in treatment of the canine distemper complex. Veterinary Medicine in Small Animal Clinics, 64: 997–1001

29   Billinghurst, I. (1993). *Give your dog a bone.* Self-published.

30   AAFCO (Association of American Feed Control Officials, 2016). Dog and Cat Food Nutrient Profiles. Official Publication, See AAFCO.org

31   Lešková, E., Kubíková, J., Kováčiková, E. *et al.* (2006). Vitamin losses: Retention during heat treatment and continual changes expressed by mathematical models. Journal of Food Composition and Analysis, 19(4): 252–276

32   Björck, I. and Asp, N. G. (1983). The effects of extrusion cooking on nutritional value – A literature review. Journal of Food Engineering, 2(4): 281–308

33   Killeit, U. (1994). Vitamin retention in extrusion cooking. Food Chemistry, 49(2): 149–155

34   Hoffmann LaRoche, F.T. and Nutley, N.J. (1995). Paper presented at the Science and Technology Center, Hill's Pet Nutrition, Inc, Topeka, KS, on vitamin stability in canned and extruded pet food, 1995

35   Mooney, A. (2010). *Stability of Essential Nutrients in Petfood Manufacturing and Storage.* Masters Thesis. Kansas State University

36   Hoffmann LaRoche, F.T. (1995). Paper presented at the Science and Technology Center, Hill's Pet Nutrition, Inc, Topeka, KS, *Vitamin stability in canned and extruded pet food*. Cited in Hand *et al.* 2010, Chapter 8

37   Rumbeiha, W. and Morrison, J. (2011). A Review of Class I and Class II Pet Food Recalls Involving Chemical Contaminants from 1996 to 2008. Journal of Medical Toxicology, 7(1): 60–66

38   Brice-Saddler, M. (2019). *A dog food company recalled its products, but these grieving pet owners say it's too late*. Washington Post. Published online, Feb 9th, www.washingtonpost. com

39   Wall, T. (2019). *35 lawsuits combine over Hill's vitamin D dog food recall*. Pet Food Industry Magazine. Published online, Oct 10th, www.petfoodindustry.com

40   Markovich, J.E., Freeman, L.M. and Heinze, C.R. (2014). Analysis of thiamine concentrations in commercial canned foods formulated for cats. Journal of the American Veterinary Medical Association, 244(2): 175-179

41   Chew, B.S., Park, J.S., Wong, T.S. *et al.* (2000). Dietary carotene stimulates cell-mediated and humoral immune response in dogs. Journal of Nutrition, 130: 1910–1913

42   Heaton, P., Reed, C.F., Mann, S.J. *et al.* (2002). Role of dietary antioxidants to protect against DNA damage in adult dogs. Journal of Nutrition, 132: 1720S–1724S

43   Khoo C., Cunnick J., Friesen K. *et al.* (2005). The role of supplementary dietary antioxidants on immune response in puppies. Vet Therapeutics, 6:43–56

44   Hernandez-Sherwood, C. (2010). *How to feed an astronaut: A talk with NASA's space food manager*. Published online Nov 18 2010 www.zdnet.com

45   Hazewinkel, H.A.W. (1985). Influences of Chronic Calcium Excess on the Skeletal Development of Growing Great Danes, Journal of the American Animal Hospital Association, 21: 377–391, 1985

46   Nap, R.C., Hazewinkel, H.A.W. and Voorhout, G. (1993). The influence of the dietary protein content on growth in giant breed dogs. Journal of Veterinary and Comparative Orthopaedics and Traumatology, 6: 1–8

47   Goodman S.A., Montgomery R.D., Lauten S.D. *et al.* (1997). Orthopedic observations in Great Dane puppies fed diets varying in calcium and phosphorus content—A preliminary report. Veterinary and Comparative Orthopaedics and Trauma, 10: 75

48   Lauten, S.D., Cox, N.R., Brawner, W.R. *et al.* (2002). Influence of dietary calcium and phosphorus content in a fixed ratio on growth and development in Great Danes. American Journal of Veterinary Research, 63(7): 1036–1047

49   Thixton, S. (2015). *The Pet Food Test Results*. Published online, Jan 4th, www. truthaboutpetfood.com

50   Hedhammar, A., Krook, F. W. Whalen, J. P. *et al.* (1974). Over nutrition and skeletal disease: An experimental study in growing Great Dane dogs. Cornell Veterinarian, 64(2, suppl. 5): 1–159

51   Goedegebuure, S.A. and Hazewinkel, H.A.W. (1986). Morphological findings in young dogs chronically fed a diet containing excess calcium. Veterinary Pathology, 23(5): 594–605

52   Hazewinkel, A.W. (1991). Growth and Skeletal Development in Great Dane Pups Fed Different Levels of Protein Intake. The Journal of Nutrition, 121: S107–S113

53   Hsu, C. H. (1997). Are we mismanaging calcium and phosphate metabolism in renal failure? American Journal of Kidney Disease, 29(4): 641–649

54   Richardson, D. C. and Toll, P.W. (1997). Relationship of nutrition to developmental skeletal disease in young dogs. Veterinary Clinical Nutrition, 4: 6–13

55   LaFond, E., Breur, G.J. and Austin, C.C. (2002). Breed susceptibility for developmental orthopedic diseases in dogs. Journal of the American Animal Hospital Association, 38(5): 467–477

56   Hazewinkel, H.A.W. (2004). *Nutritional Influences on Hip Dysplasia*. 29th Annual Congress of World Small Animal Veterinary Association

57   Hazewinkel, H. and Mott, J. (2006). *Main nutritional imbalances in osteoarticular diseases.* In P. Pibot, V. Biourge and D. Elliott (Eds.), Encyclopaedia of canine clinical nutrition (p348–383). Castle Cary, UK: Royal Canin

58   Tryfonidou, M.A., van den Broek, J., van den Brom, W. E. *et al.* (2002). Intestinal calcium absorption in growing dogs is influenced by calcium intake and age but not by growth rate. Journal of Nutrition,132: 3363–3368

59   Napoli, N., Thompson, J., Civitelli, R. *et al.* (2007). Effects of dietary calcium compared with calcium supplements on estrogen metabolism and bone mineral density. American Journal of Clinical Nutrition, 85: 1428-1433

60   Alexander, J., Stockman, J., Atwal, J. *et al.* (2018). Effects of the long-term feeding of diets enriched with inorganic phosphorus on the adult feline kidney and phosphorus metabolism. British Journal of Nutrition, 21: 1–21

61   Coltherd, J.C., Staunton, R., Colyer, A. *et al.* (2019). Not all forms of dietary phosphorus are equal: an evaluation of postprandial phosphorus concentrations in the plasma of the cat. British Journal of Nutrition, 121(3): 270–284

62   Ho, S.K. and Hdiroglou, M. (1977). Effects of dietary chelated, sequestered zinc and zinc sulphate on growing lambs fed a purified diet. Canadian Journal of Animal Science, 57: 93–99

63   Ashmead, H.D., Graff, D.J. and Ashmead, H.H. (1985). Intestinal absorption of metal ions and chelates. Springfield, IL: CC Thomas

64   Wedekind, K.J. and Baker, D.H. (1990). Zinc bioavailability in feed grade sources of zinc. Journal of Animal Science, 68: 684–689

65   Mertz, W. and Roginski, E.E. (1971). *Newer trace elements in nutrition.* New York: Marcel Dekker

66   Hallberg, L. and Rossander-Hulthen, L. (1993). Factors influencing the bioavailability of iron in man. In U. Schlemmer (Ed.), Bioavailability '93: Nutritional, chemical and food processing implications of nutrient availability (pp. 23–32). Ettlingen, Germany: Federation of European Chemical Societies

67   Lowe, J.A., Wiseman, J. and Cole, D.J.A. (1994a). Absorption and retention of zinc when administered as an amino-acid chelate in the dog. Journal of Nutrition, 124: 2572–2574.

68 Lowe, J.A., Wiseman, J. and Cole, D.J.A. (1994b). Zinc source influences zinc retention in hair and hair growth in the dog. Journal of Nutrition, 124: 2575S–2576S

69 Wedekind, K.J. and Lowry, S.R. (1998). Are organic zinc sources efficacious in puppies? Journal of Nutrition, 128(12), 25935–25955

70 Robertson, B.T. and Burns, M.J. (1963). Zinc metabolism and zinc deficiency syndrome in dogs. American Journal of Veterinary Research, 24: 777–1002

71 Hoff, J.E. (1945). The influence of phytic acid on the absorption of Ca and Ph. Biochemical Journal, 40: 189–192

72 Forbes, R.M., Parker, H.M. and Erdman, J.W., Jr (1984). Effects of dietary phytate, calcium and magnesium levels on zinc bioavailability to rats. Journal of Nutrition, 114: 1421–1425

73 Van den Broek, A. and Thoday, K. (1986). Skin diseases in dogs associated with zinc deficiency: A report of 5 cases. Journal of Small Animal Practice, 27: 313–323

74 Sousa, C.A., Stannard, A.A., Ihrke, P. J. et al. (1988). Dermatosis associated with feeding generic dog food: 13 cases (1981–1982). Journal of the American Veterinary Medicine Association, 192(5): 676–680

75 Huber, T.L., Laflamme, D.P., et al. (1991). Comparison of procedures for assessing adequacy of dog foods. Journal of American Veterinary Medical Association, 199: 731–734

76 Larsen, T. and Sandström, B. (1992). Effect of calcium, copper, and zinc levels in a rapeseed meal diet on mineral and trace element utilization in the rat. Biological Trace Element Research, 35(2): 167–184

77 Watson, T.D.G. (1998). Diet and skin disease in dogs and cats. Journal of Nutrition, 128(12): 2783S–2789S

78 Ewer, R.F. (1973). The carnivores. London: Weidenfield and Nicolson

79 Nap, R.C. and Hazewinkel, H.A.W. (1994). Growth and skeletal development in the dog in relation to nutrition; a review. Veterinary Quarterly, 16(1): 50–59

80 Weaver, C.M., Peacock, M. and Johnston Jr., C.C. (1999). Adolescent Nutrition in the Prevention of Postmenopausal Osteoporosis. The Journal of Clinical Endocrinology & Metabolism, 84(6): 1839–1843

81 Mann, J. and Truswell, S.A. (2002). Essentials of Human Nutrition, 2nd Ed. Editors Oxford University Press

82 Hurrell, R.F., Reddy, M.B., Juillerat, M.A. et al. (2003). Degradation of phytic acid in cereal porridges improves iron absorption by human subjects. American Journal of Clinical Nutrition, 77: 1213–1219

83 Hellanda, S., Denstadlib, V., Wittena, P.E. et al. (2006). Hyper dense vertebrae and mineral content in Atlantic salmon (Salmo salar L.) fed diets with graded levels of phytic acid. Aquaculture, 261(2): 603–614

84 Mahajan, S.K., Prasad, A.S., Lambujon, J. et al. (1980). Improvement of uremic hypogeusia by zinc: a double-blind study. The American Society for Clinical Nutrition, 33(7): 1517–1521

85 Denton, D.A. (1967). Salt appetite. In Handbook of Physiology, Vol. 1. cited in Serpell, J. (1995). The domestic dog: Its evolution, behaviour, and interactions with people. Cambridge, UK: Cambridge University Press

86 Rozin, P. and Kalat, J.W. (1971). Specific hungers and poison avoidance as adaptive specialisations of learning. Psychological Reviews, 78: 459–486

87 Hand, M.S., Thatcher, C.D., Remillard, R.L. *et al.* (2010). *Small Animal Clinical Nutrition*, 5th Edition. Published by The Mark Morris Institute, Kansas, U.S

88 Scientific Advisory Committee on Nutrition (2003). Salt and Health. The Stationery Office. London. https://www.gov.uk/government/publications/sacn-salt-and-health-report

89 Gupta, B.N., Linden, R.J., Mary, S.G. *et al.* (1981). The influence of high and low sodium intake on blood volume in the dog. Quarterly Journal of Experimental Physiology, 6: 117–128

90 AAFCO (Association of American Feed Control Officials, 2014). Proposed Revisions Edited per Comments for 2014. Official Publication. Available online, www.aafco.org

91 World Health Organisation (WHO, 2013). *A global brief on hypertension: silent killer, global health crisis*. Official Publication. Available online www.ish-world.com

92 Anderson, L.J. and Fisher, E.W. (1968). The blood pressure in canine interstitial nephritis. Research in Veterinary Science, 9: 304–313

93 Cowgill, L.D. and Kallet, A.J. (1986). *Systemic hypertension*. In: Kirk RW, ed. Current Veterinary Therapy IX. Philadelphia, PA: WB Saunders Co, 360–364

94 Rocchini, A.P., Moorehead, C.P., Wentz, E. *et al.* (1987). Obesity-induced hypertension in the dog. Hypertension, 9(3): 64–-68

95 Littman, M.P. (1990). Chronic spontaneous systemic hypertension in dogs and cats. In: Proceedings. Eighth Veterinary Medical Forum, American College of Veterinary Internal Medicine, Washington, DC, May: 209–212

96 Ross, L.A. (1992). *Endocrine hypertension*. In: Kirk RW, Bonagura JD, eds. Current Veterinary Therapy XI. Philadelphia, PA: WB Saunders Co., 309–313

97 Simpson, F.O. (1979). Salt and hypertension: a skeptical review of the evidence. Clinical Science (London), Supplement 5: 463s–480s

98 Brown, S.A. (2007). Salt, hypertension and chronic kidney disease. Veterinary Focus, 17(1): 45

99 Krieger, J.E., Liard, J.F. and Cowley, A.W. (1990). Hemodynamics, fluid volume, and hormonal responses to chronic high-salt intake in dogs. American Journal of Physiology, 259: H1629–H1636

100 Greco, D.S., Lees, G.E., Dzendzel, G. *et al.* (1994). Effects of dietary sodium intake on blood pressure measurements in partially nephrectomized dogs. American Journal of Veterinary Research, 55: 160–165

101 Okin, P.M., Kjeldsen, S.E., Julius, S. *et al.* (2010). All-cause and cardiovascular mortality in relation to changing heart rate during treatment of hypertensive patients with electrocardiographic left ventricular hypertrophy. European Heart Journal, 31(18): 2271–2279

102 Stolarz-Skrzypek, K., Kuznetsova, T., Thijs, L. *et al.* (2011). Fatal and Nonfatal Outcomes, Incidence of Hypertension, and Blood Pressure Changes in Relation to Urinary Sodium Excretion. The Journal of the American Medical Association, 305(17): 1777–1785

CHAPTER 10

Fats

Good Fats and Bad Fats

If I were to ask you which fat might be better for you – some fat scooped off the top of a rendering vat containing a variety of meat waste from a land far away, cooked up in a kibble a year ago, chemically preserved, left sitting in a bag for months in a warehouse and pet shop floor at varying temperatures only to sit in an open bag in a cupboard for a couple of weeks OR the fat from the flesh of a sardine recently pulled from the sea, which would you say?

Let's not dignify that with a response but as with the question, 'Fancy some of my cheap dry food made from old boots and soiled saw dust?' We need to get people thinking about the quality of the fats they are feeding their pets. And a little perspective helps this process.

For the last two decades, fat has been the enemy of the masses and low-fat products have been all the rage. Unfortunately, this ultimately led to more carbohydrates and sugar in our factory food diets, giving us our obesity, diabetes and heart disease epidemics. Then we started to discover that fresh fat is actually vital to our health and metabolic process. For starters, and somewhat ironically, we now know that fat plays a crucial role in weight control.[1,2] Fat forms the outside of your cells and, as such, communicates with insulin, regulating the cells blood sugar and consequently your hunger. Some fats turn on genes that are responsible for burning fats, while at the same time turning off genes that store fat. Omega-3s are also involved in regulating thyroid hormone function, which regulates body fat. Finally, when teamed up with a good dose of protein, fat is filling, with medium chain fats like coconut oil being the most satiating of all.

But it doesn't stop there. Your skin is made up of lots of fat, as are your eyes. The right fats promote their good health. Good fats play a pivotal role in your metabolism and the whole inflammation process, which makes it central to disease. The right fats fight cancer while the wrong fats fuel it.[3] Fat is critical to the reproductive process whereby the wrong fats can result in complications with PMS and menopause. In men, a lack of good fat reduces testosterone and androgen hormones, all critical for reproductive health and body growth. Fat plays a crucial role in bone mineral density and osteoporosis.[1] Your brain runs on cholesterol and fat; in particular, docosahexaenoic acid (DHA). Good fats here result in better moods with less risk of depression. In fact, lower cholesterol levels in the brain are associated with an increase in suicidal tendencies, an almost direct result of decreased levels of the neurotransmitter serotonin (the feel-good hormone) in the blood.[4]

Of all the fats out there, some of the most discussed are omega-3 and omega-6. These two polyunsaturated fatty acids have sprung to prominence as copious amounts of studies amply demonstrate their importance for good health. Omega-3 is the anti-inflammatory fatty acid, which reduces inflammation in joints and eases the symptoms of arthritis, as well as plays a crucial role in the nervous system, vision and learning, fat burning and fat storage. Omega-6 is not only essential to brain function but also to growth and development. It is vital to bone health, hair and nail growth and repair and skin. Plus, it maintains the reproductive system, as well as has crucial roles in energy metabolism.

So, if it's a nice lean body you're after, with good skin, good vision, strong bones, less cancer, better moods and a robust reproductive process, then good fat needs to be consumed regularly.

This brings forth the question: what is *bad* fat? Awhile back, in the late 20th century, saturated fats (meat, dairy, coconut oil) received a lot of bad press based on some confused science. We started lowering saturated fat intake and, unfortunately, replacing it with carbohydrates, thereby exasperating the very issues we were trying to avoid, such as diabetes and obesity.

However, as with most things fat, we have now backtracked on this one. A meta-analysis, which pooled data from 21 studies, including nearly 348,000 adults, found no difference in the risks of heart disease and stroke between people with the lowest and highest intakes of saturated fat.[5]

We now know that saturated fats are the building blocks of cell membranes and hormones. They are carriers for the fat-soluble vitamins A, D, E and K. They help lower cholesterol levels. They help prevent cancer. They even act as antiviral agents.

Trans fats, mentioned earlier, are positively nasty. They are the ones that stop margarine going hard. They are commonly found in cookies, cereals, pastries, salad dressing, fried foods and other such tasty items. While trans fats do occur naturally in tiny amounts in meat and dairy, it was when we began creating them ourselves, in a lab using a process called hydrogenation (the adding of hydrogen to liquid oil to create solid fats thereby increasing a product's shelf life and stability) and consuming them in great quantity that the lard hit the fan.

In 1911, Proctor & Gamble recognised the potential of this hydrogenation process, established the patent and began their marketing campaign to sell their new miracle trans fat product called Crisco Shortening. World War II and the butter shortage gave this campaign the boost it needed and solid margarine products became a norm in our fridge. Experts then weighed in with 'evidence' that not only told us saturated fats were bad for us but that trans fats were the answer, which was great news for Proctor & Gamble. By the late 1980s, the massive anti-saturated fat PR campaign proved effective, with trans fats replacing saturated fats in virtually all processed foods. Everyone jumped on board, even the (industry-funded) American Heart Foundation began awarding their official 'Heart Healthy' badge to calorie-and-trans-fats-laden foodstuffs, including Frosted Flakes and Pop-Tarts.

It turns out the evidence produced in support was somewhat misguided. We now know trans fats fuel chronic inflammation in the body.[6] Over time, they increase the likelihood of heart disease, stroke, diabetes, and other chronic conditions.[7] And it doesn't take much of them. In their review of the subject, Mozaffarian *et al.* (2006)[7] show that for every 2% of calories from trans fats consumed daily, the risk of heart disease rises by 23%. These authors note that eliminating industrially produced trans fats from the US food supply could prevent between 6% and 19% of heart attacks and related deaths, or as many as 200,000 souls each year. It doesn't end there either. Trans fats also increase the amount of 'harmful' low-density lipoprotein (LDL) cholesterol in the bloodstream[7] and this leads to one of the biggest misunderstandings in human nutrition.

For years, we thought the cause of heart disease was all the cholesterol we saw clogging the arteries of heart attack victims. Like the notion eating fat makes you fat, this makes sense, right? But for more than 20 years we have known that in most individuals, diet has very little to do with it.[8,9] What we were actually witnessing was a body desperately trying to heal itself. Most of your 'harmful' LDL cholesterol, approximately 80% of it, in fact, is produced by your own liver and intestines. LDL cholesterol produces a range of vital functions to the body, including cell membrane integrity, but it also works to reduce inflammation in the body. In essence the cholesterol is like the foam from a fire extinguisher. It was trying to put out the fire resulting from your bad diet and lifestyle (trans fats aren't alone in spiking your blood cholesterol – anything that causes chronic inflammation will do that, including obesity, diabetes, smoking and lack of exercise). Typical of modern medicine, we saw the symptoms and worked on reducing cholesterol via a change in diet but also cholesterol-lowering drugs that quickly grew into a $20 billion market by 2016. Despite knowing for more than twenty years cholesterol is not the enemy *per se*, it seems the world's seniors are now on cholesterol-lowering drugs. How quick they were to come in, how slow they are to go.

For all these reasons, trans fats are quite clearly something to be avoided. In 2015, the Food and Drug administration (FDA) decreed that trans fats were so dangerous that they must be entirely removed from our foods by January 1, 2020. To date, they are still being used in some margarines and vegetable oils and thus, fried fast food, but also vegetable shortening and thus many baked products that use shortening in the mix.

So, good fats promote good health. The bad ones do not. But it is not just good and bad fats either. We must also pay close attention to fat quality, as good fats can be made very bad indeed. You've heard of rancidity? This is the oxygenation of fats. When good fats are exposed to the air, they oxidise and turn rancid, creating free radicals. These are bad little particles that go whirring around reaping destruction on healthy cells. To contain and neutralise these free radicals, the body must employ its antioxidants such as vitamins A, C, D and E. This leaves fewer of these resources available to your body for cellular repair and disease prevention. And if the levels get too low or free radicals overwhelm the body's ability to regulate them, a condition known as 'oxidative stress' ensues and disease sets in, resulting in a weakening of the immune system, cancer, cardiovascular issues, skin and liver damage.[10]

Then you have to consider the effects of heating on fat. The oxygen in deep frying fat reacts with oil[11] in a process known as thermal oxidation. The problem is not only the formation of free radicals but also the creation of aldehydes. Scientists have linked these aldehydes in vegetable oils used in frying to numerous illnesses including cancer, heart disease and dementia, with corn and sunflower the worst offenders.[12-14] Even the fumes from cooking vegetable oils are linked to lung cancer in Chinese women.[15]

To summarise, here's the story with fat in ten words:

Fresh fats in whole, natural form good. Factory fats bad.

Dogs Benefit from Good Fat Additions

While the concept of good and bad fats is appropriate for human health, dogs seem to work a little differently. They are better able to handle a greater quantity of fat than us. Our 'bad' fats don't seem to affect them in the same way. Studies so far suggest that dogs (and cats) can remain in a near perpetual state of having more high density lipoprotein (HDL) cholesterol than low density lipoprotein (LDL) cholesterol, no matter what types of fats they consume.[16] Furthermore, they appear entirely resistant to the development of hypercholesterolemia (high cholesterol) and atherosclerosis (where plaque builds up in the arteries and veins, ultimately leading to a heart attack or stroke). This is the opposite of what you would expect in humans in this state.

But that does not mean that fat quantity and quality do not matter to the dog. It absolutely does. Just like humans, dogs suffer vitamin, protein and fat deficiencies when exposed to rancid fat. That's how we discovered these things for ourselves in the first place.[17] And that is why they prefer their fat to be as fresh as possible. When presented with dry diets varying in fat rancidity, they always choose the dry food with the least rancid fat.[17]

Moreover, dogs are seen to immediately benefit from the addition of good fat in the form of omega-3. Supplementing dry-fed dogs with omega-3 is proven to aid skin repair, to enhance the development of the nervous system and overall cognition, to significantly reduce steroid need and fight cancer in dogs.[18-25] Supplementing 'complete' commercial dry dog foods with good quality fatty acids such as linoleic acid (a type of omega-6) is proven to improve coat condition and quality in dogs.[26] Heinemann *et al.* (2005)[27] found that supplementing a lactating bitch that was consuming a dry, 'complete' and balanced product made by Nestlé Purina Pet Care with omega-3, significantly improved visual performance in pups after twelve weeks. In a study on the use of dry, 'hypoallergenic' pet foods over regular dry foods in dogs suffering pruritus, Ricci *et al.* (2009)[28] hypothesised the reason behind the partial amelioration of clinical symptoms on hypoallergenic diets because they contain fats from fish oil.

So, good quality omega-3 is a vital addition to your dog's diet. But a bit more detail than that is necessary. Omega-3 and omega-6 are actually group names for a collection of fatty acids, including linoleic acid (LA), an omega-6 fatty acid), alpha-linolenic acid (ALA), an omega-3 fatty acid), eicosapentaenoic acid (EPA), an omega-3 fatty acid) and docosahexaenoic acid (DHA), an omega-3 fatty acid).

In humans, LA and ALA are termed essential fatty acids as our body cannot make them by itself, they must be consumed in the diet. As we are physiologically able to make the others (EPA and DHA) from ALA,[29,30] they are not considered truly essential fatty acids in humans.

EPA and DHA are deemed essential fatty acids for dogs (and cats). While they both seem to be able to fulfil their omega-6 requirements from both plant oils or animal fat additions,[31] dogs and cats are practically unable to carry out the ALA conversion. To be specific, while dogs are poor at it, requiring several enzymatic steps to convert it into EPA,[16,31] cats entirely lack one of the metabolic enzymes to carry it out at all. Therefore, both dogs and cats must get their omega-3 from animal sources, best sourced from fat, including oily fish, but also from cartilage and fatty organs such as brains and eyes.

In this way, EPA and DHA are vital to dogs. Studies show supplementing pups with fish oils rich in DHA following weaning improved cognitive, memory, psychomotor and immunologic and retinal functions in growing dogs.[32] Hadley *et al.* (2017)[33] found that DHA supplementation supports healthy brain function in dogs by improving shape discrimination learning associated with visual processing.

Despite this, authors note that 25% of the best-selling, 'complete' dry foods tested contain zero or practically zero EPA and DHA.[34]

Fats Used in Pet Food

If you are wondering why pets on 'complete' food benefited from the addition of good fat, then look no further than the fat used in pet food.

The majority of fat used in most cereal-based pet food comes from a rendering plant. Ideally, the pet food label would be able to state the name of the animal used, such 'beef fat' or 'chicken fat'. This is more desirable than the more ominously vague term 'animal fat' where they can't even tell you where the fat comes from. The AAFCO (2008)[35] permits some worrying fats to be included in the rendered fat used to supply pet food companies. Unlike the EU, the US permits diseased meat to be rendered. This is a concern when we know this fat tissue stores most man-made lipophilic chemicals.[36] This will include many of the drugs used to try keep that animal alive and/or to kill it.[37] Rotting animal flesh aside, that cooking oil and grease from restaurants is permitted in both the EU and US is astounding. With the rapid expansion of fast food restaurants across the earth and huge grease bins a regular feature in every recycling facility that I have been to, there is great potential for a worrying quantity of nasty fat being used in pet food.

We know that oil repeatedly heated to high temperature is highly dangerous stuff.[12-14] An earlier study reported that over 54 weeks, there was no adverse effect on dogs given oil previously used in the food industry for deep fat frying.[38] But more recently, a diet consisting of 'red meat' and used grease from restaurants was fed to hunting dogs resulted in retinal degenerations and lipofuscin (fatty residues found in the liver, kidney, heart muscle, retina, adrenals, nerve cells and ganglion cells that result from ageing and wear and tear accumulation) in intestinal smooth muscle and neurons in dogs.[39] From this authors perspective, it's hard to see how the red meat could be implicated here.

The rendered mix is stewed under high heat and pressure, something fat hates. Hence rendering lowers the quality of fat.[40] This fat is then sprayed on the outside of the dry dog food pellet as it comes out of the extruder. Dogs find it tastier this way[16] but it creates another problem, as fat hates oxygen. Thus, the fat on the pellet needs to be chemically preserved to prevent oxidation.

Pet food manufacturers use a rich tapestry of synthetic chemicals to prevent fat breakdown. Some of the more unnatural kind, butylated hydroxyanisole (BHA), butylated hydroxytoluene (BHT) and ethoxyquin, have received more than their fair share of bad press. Carcinogenicity tests showed that addition of the antioxidant BHA to the diet of rodents for twenty-four weeks induced high incidences of papilloma and squamous cell carcinoma of the fore-stomach of both sexes.[41] The authors referenced note their results indicate that BHA should be classified in the category of 'sufficient evidence of carcinogenicity'. In their review of the subject, Kahl and Kappus (1993)[42] found 'all published findings to date agree with the fact that BHA and BHT are tumour promoters.' Long-term studies reveal these chemicals promote tumour growth, typically in the stomach and liver. Despite this Kahl and Kappus (1993)[42] conclude that the 1990s level of BHA and BHT in human food was 'probably harmless' and both the FDA in the United States and European food governing bodies state something similar, with the latter approving BHA as a food additive while at the same time considering it a 'possibly carcinogenic to humans (category 2B),' as well as a category one potential endocrine disruptor (European Food Safety Authority, 2011). The US Department of Health and Human Services, National Toxicology Program's 2011 Report on Carcinogens, states BHA "is reasonably anticipated to be a human carcinogen".

For these reasons, BHA and BHT are falling out of favour in human food manufacturing, but they are still found in tiny quantities in butter, cereal, chewing gum and snack foods. I think, considering the ever-rising cancer rates in humans and dogs, the fewer possible carcinogens in the diet, the better.

Still, the fat in dry dog food must be preserved. Studies show the likes of BHA greatly out-perform some of the more natural preservatives such as mixed tocopherols like vitamins C and E.[17] Unfortunately, fats preserved with more natural methods tend to go rancid within months at ambient temperature.[17] When the referenced authors stored a variety of dry foods for 12 months in warm temperatures, they noted that dogs would opt for the dry foods preserved with BHA as the products preserved with mixed tocopherols (vitamin E) had gone significantly more rancid. Hence, powerful synthetic preservatives such as BHA and BHT remain very popular chemicals in the dry pet food sector today.[43]

Ethoxyquin is another dangerous one. A very versatile chemical, ethoxyquin can be used as a pesticide, a preservative or a rubber stabiliser. It is banned for use in the United States, European Union and Australia as a direct additive in foods meant for human consumption. In 1988, the FDA's Centre for Veterinary Medicine (CVM) began receiving reports from pet owners and veterinarians of suspected health issues possibly linked to ethoxyquin. The CVM wasted no time and *only 9 years later* asked the pet food industry if they would mind lowering their ethoxyquin usage from 150 ppm to 75 ppm, considering the EPA had now determined that dogs showed raised liver enzymes on 160 ppm, not to mention they're eating it every day, and puppies and nursing bitches eat even more per body weight. Thankfully, the industry eventually obliged.

What is the chronic effect of eating 75 ppm of ethoxyquin every single meal? Not sure, but it's surely not *as bad* as 150 ppm.

In his piece for the *Journal of Nutrition* titled "Safety of Ethoxyquin in Dog Foods"*, Dzanis, (1991)[44] states the reported signs of ethoxyquin toxicity in dogs include liver, kidney, thyroid and reproductive dysfunction, teratogenic and carcinogenic effects, allergic reactions and a host of skin and hair abnormalities. It is interesting to note that of the types of dog food affected, the 'premium' brands were most incriminated. Dzanis notes many anecdotal reports, which stated a dog's condition was resolved after replacement of ethoxyquin-containing diets with diets free of ethoxyquin. However, while pet food companies may not be adding ethoxyquin themselves, due to 'inconsistencies in labelling of pet food products,' they cannot rule out its inclusion in the product's ingredients.

Safety aside, the chemical preservation of fat in pet food seems reasonably effective. Studies show that when dry pet food is stored for 3 months under ambient conditions, you can expect a total loss of EPA, DHA and total fatty acids of 17%, 9% and 11%, respectively.[45] However, somewhat incredibly, I cannot source any information on the rate of fat oxidisation in a bag of kibble that has been opened by the pet owner and exposed to the air.

Getting the Fat Balance Right

With omega-6 and 3, it is important to note that it's not so much a matter of quantity, but of ratio. Humans evolved on a diet with ratios of omega-6 to omega-3 of close to 1:1.[46] But Westerners today are far out of sync in this regard. The problem is that not all foods are balanced in their omega-6 and omega-3 concentrations. Most vegetable oils, but not all, are much higher in omega-6, while the likes of fish oil and animal fat is much higher in omega-3.

We all know how good the Mediterraneans have it, with their oily fish diet. In comparison, Westerners are consuming far too many grains and vegetable oils, resulting in ratios more like 15:1 or 16:1.[46] This is an out of whack ratio. Hugely excessive amounts of omega-6 in our modern diets, is thought to play a role in the pathogenesis of many diseases, including cardiovascular disease, cancer and inflammatory and auto-immune diseases.[46] This has been suspected since the 1970s when researchers studied the Greenland Inuit Tribe. The Greenland Inuit consumed large amounts of fat from fish and yet displayed virtually no cardiovascular disease. The high level of omega-3 fatty acids consumed by the Inuit reduced triglycerides, heart rate, blood pressure and atherosclerosis,[47] albeit a great number of other factors could be at play here. That said, DiNicolantonio (2016),[48] notes how a recent shift in Inuit diet toward a more Western diet, one higher in refined carbohydrates and sugar, is sadly bringing them more in line with Western cardiovascular disease rates.

Simopoulos (2002)[46] highlights how recent studies noted a ratio of 5:1 had a beneficial effect on human patients with asthma, a ratio of 4:1 decreased mortality by 70% in the secondary prevention of cardiovascular disease, while a ratio of 2.5:1 reduced cell proliferation in colorectal cancer patients and significantly eased the suffering in patients with rheumatoid arthritis. In fact, the literature suggests that beginning at 5:1, the closer this ratio gets to par in patients suffering pretty much any type of inflammation, including issues ranging from dermatitis, eczema and psoriasis to arthritis, asthma, coeliac disease, cardiovascular disease, irritable bowel syndrome, cystitis, cancer and diabetes, the better off the patient will be. This means less processed plant oils (chips, let's face it!) and as much fresh omega-3 laden foods such as oily fish, olives, nuts and seeds as possible.

Despite its importance in humans, unfortunately, a reliable omega-6 /omega-3 ratio is yet to be established for dogs. The AAFCO (2016)[49] unhelpfully recommends that the omega-6 to omega-3 fatty acid ratio should be less than 30:1. Now, this may seem *extremely* high based on what we've learned in omnivorous, almost herbivorous humans, allowing too much room for cereal-based dry products to be obscenely high in omega-6. The result will surely be increased inflammation in the dog. Supporting this, in their review of the fatty acid composition in 11 commercial dog foods, Ahlstrøm *et al.* (2004)[34] concluded that dry dog foods vary substantially in their omega-6/omega-3 ratios and that it was these differences that may explain some of the differences in biological responses reported by dog owners.

To ascertain what the *ideal* omega-6/omega-3 ratio might be in a dog fed normally, we should look to the nutrient content of typical wild prey animals. Paulsen *et al.* (2014)[50] investigated the fatty acid composition of a range of prey animals. Their omega-6/omega-3 ratios ranged from 2:1 (for the European hare), approximately 3:1 for many deer, 4:1 for wild pheasant (as is wild rabbit), 5:1 for wild duck and pheasant, 6:1 for grouse, 8:1 for wild boar (compared to 13:1 for domestic pigs) and 11:1 for domestic chicken. Thus, the more natural, 'wild' and organic the animal you are using, the better the omega-6/omega-3 fatty acid ratio will be. A ratio range of somewhere around 4:1–5:1 would thus be pretty good for the average raw-fed dog, temporarily lower if they are inflamed.

Some Fat Recommendations

Analysis of prey commonly consumed by dogs indicates that the dog, a lean, long-distance running animal, evolved on a very lean diet. Using the rabbit as an average meal, this would be a meal of approximately four-parts protein to one-part fat[51] or a metabolisable energy (ME) ratio of approximately 2:1 protein to fat, with wild prey expected to be far leaner again. While higher fat diets might be used in pups and reproducing bitches and certainly in working dogs, until we know more we must assume a low-fat diet is optimum for the average, adult dog, breed differences aside (huskies surely evolved upon fattier diets).

The question becomes what *type* of fat is best to feed them. We know that for humans the fresher the fat, the better. When we are fed fresh, whole, unadulterated fats we are healthier, and we live longer than those societies consuming processed fats. Unfortunately, dogs today are largely receiving old, heavily processed fats. It is a practical impossibility for a dry pet food, manufactured many months ago, using rendered animal fat, to supply much by way of good fats to your dog. Despite heavy chemical use, fats will denature during rendering, during storage and when you open the bag. We know this to be the case as when good fats are added to a dog's 'complete' dry diet, they are consistently seen to benefit.

As we know, one in four top-selling dry foods contain practically zero EPA and DHA; the rest can have omega-6/omega-3 ratios as high as 30:1. Anyone buying cereal-based dry pet food should consider some form of omega-3 supplementation for their pet. Up until recently, the easiest way to do this was to add fish oil tablets. I do not recommend salmon oil from farmed salmon. It is one of the dirtiest, drug heavy industries out there and destroying the environment.

That said, regular fish oil tablets too have come in for some bad press recently. The oils therein are extremely sensitive and very prone to oxidative damage if not handled correctly. Fish oil may be a source of heavy metals such as dioxins and polychlorinated biphenyls (PCB's) but it's also unsustainability of it all. It's estimated 20–25 million tonnes of fish are extracted from our seas each year for agricultural meal and oil alone; that is the combined weight of every single American citizen every year. In my opinion, they are still more friend than foe, certainly the better types. Instead of generic 'fish oil' tablets maybe go for a named species such as wild Atlantic salmon oil (avoid generic salmon oil, it comes from salmon farms, huge chemical usage and environmentally disastrous) or better still or better still anchovy, sardine or pollock oil (the smaller the fish, the less heavy metals they accumulate). There are other sources of animal omega-3 too. Of late, attentions have shifted toward other omega-3 sources, such as Antarctic krill. A keystone prey species of whales and the entire Antarctic ecosystem, krill is clearly not ideal long-term either. Phytoplankton is now the product of choice for many pet owners. While it is pricey, you get a lot of EPA/DHA for your buck, so it almost balances out.

In my opinion, the best of the bunch for a general day-to-day might be a 'refined fish oil'. This means there's more of the good stuff in there (EPA&DHA) and less filler oil used. Avoid the fish oil supplements with added vitamins A & D. This is common for human supplementation but these vitamins are stored by the liver and require more careful dosing in dogs. If I was supplementing to help ease stiff joints, I would jump to a CO_2-extracted green lipped mussel extract as it has a very high potency of omega's and studies show it's particularly effective at relieving arthritic pain in dogs.[52]"

Still, nothing replaces fresh, whole oily fish such as sardines, a fantastic and relatively sustainable source of excellent quality protein and fats. Another great idea is a bag of frozen mussels. A little handful of these fired out into the grass make a great treat and they are packed full of quality omega-3's and other goodies, even if you have to buy the canned versions. Important here though – if you're going to eat oily fish from a can, don't use the ones in sunflower oil as it is high in (cooked) omega-6, which will totally negate the benefits of whatever omega-3 is in there. Like putting sugar (inflammatory) in probiotic drinks meant to benefit a troubled gut, the food industry repeatedly demonstrates that whether the product is of any actual benefit to the consumer matters little, 'contains Omega-3' looks good on the label and moves units. Brine (pour the excess off) or fresh water is much better.

For basic function, dogs require around 20 to 30 mg of EPA and DHA per kilo of body weight daily. A tin of sardines/mackerel contains up to 300 mg of, albeit cooked, EPA and DHA.

TAKE-HOME POINTS

✓ Good fat is crucial to a range of your body's systems. It is central to both the inflammatory and reproductive process, in the fight against cancer and to control weight. Fat plays a crucial role in bone mineral density and osteoporosis. It even boosts your mood.

✓ Examples of good fat is omega-3. This is the anti-inflammatory fatty acid, easing symptoms of arthritis, playing a crucial role in the nervous system, vision and learning, fat burning and fat storage.

✓ Another good fat is omega-6. It is essential to brain function, growth and development. It is vital to bone health, hair and nail growth and repair and skin.

✓ Bad fats are the ones that have been produced by humans. One type is produced by a process called hydrogenation. These are the trans fats and they are positively nasty, linked to increasing inflammation, heart disease, stroke, diabetes and other chronic conditions.

✓ Bad fats also arise when you expose good fats to light, air or heat. High temperature cooking, such as deep fat frying, results in thermal oxidation and this in turn produces free radicals that are linked to cancer, skin and liver issues but also aldehydes; they are among the most cancerous food substances out there. The more you repeatedly heat it, the worse it gets.

✓ The majority of animal fat used in pet food comes from a rendering plant. In the United States, that means meat from dead, diseased, dying and disabled meat and the lipophilic toxins therein. Both the United

---

States and the European Union permit waste oil from restaurants to be used – fat that we know can result in retinal degenerations and lipofuscin in dogs.

✓ Dogs fed a 'complete' ultra-processed diet are seen to benefit greatly from good fat additions, showing improvements in coat quality, amelioration of skin conditions and increased visual performance in pups when fed to a pregnant mother.

✓ The animal sourced omega-3 fatty acids EPA and DHA are essential to dogs and cats. 25% of the best-selling, 'complete' dry foods tested, contain zero or practically zero EPA and DHA.

✓ As fat is so unstable, a variety of synthetic chemicals are used to prevent fat breakdown, including BHA, BHT and ethoxyquin, all of which have very bad reputations, if just for cancer.

✓ Fats preserved 'naturally' with vitamin E do not last.

✓ A dietary omega-3/omega-6 fatty-acid ratio of 4–5:1 is about right for the average dog. Lowering this ratio during periods of inflammation is right.

✓ When dosing with fish oil best use the oil of a smaller fish, such as sardine or anchovy, or a refined fish oil which contains more EPA&DHA and less filler.

✓ While fresh sardines are infinitely superior, any oily fish from the can is Ok. Avoid the ones in oil.

Chapter Ten References

1   Rosen, C.J. and Klibanski, A. (2009). Bone, Fat, and Body Composition: Evolving Concepts in the Pathogenesis of Osteoporosis. The American Journal of Medicine, 122(5): 409–414

2   Hooper, L., Abdelhamid, A., Moore, H.J. *et al.* (2012). Effect of reducing total fat intake on body weight: systematic review and meta-analysis of randomised controlled trials and cohort studies. British Medical Journal, 345: e7666

3   WHO, World Health Organisation (2013). *A global brief on Hyper tension. Silent killer, global public health crisis*. Official Publication. Available online, www.who.int

4   Engelberg, H. (1992). Low serum cholesterol and suicide. The Lancet, 339(8795): 727–729

5   Siri-Tarino, P.W., Sun, Q., Hu, F.B. *et al*. (2010). Meta-analysis of prospective cohort studies evaluating the association of saturated fat with cardiovascular disease. American Journal of Clinical Nutrition. 91(3): 535–546

6   Lopez-Garcia, E., Schulze, M.B., Meigs, J.B. *et al*. (2005). Consumption of trans fatty acids is related to plasma biomarkers of inflammation and endothelial dysfunction. Journal of Nutrition, 135(3): 562–566

7   Mozaffarian, D., Katan, M.B., Ascherio, A. *et al*. (2006). Trans fatty acids and cardiovascular disease. New England Journal of Medicine, 354(15): 1601–1613

8   McNamara, D.J. (1995). Dietary cholesterol and the optimal diet for reducing risk of atherosclerosis. Canadian Journal of Cardiology, Suppl G: 123G–126G.

9   Ravnskov, U., Lorgeril, M.D, Diamond, D.M. *et al*. (2018). LDL-C does not cause cardiovascular disease: a comprehensive review of the current literature. Expert Review of Clinical Pharmacology, 11:10

10   Lobo, V., Patil, A, Phatak, A. *et al*. (2010). Free radicals, antioxidants and functional foods: Impact on human health. Pharmacognosy Reviews, 4(8): 118–126

11   Peers, K.E. and Swoboda, A.T. (1982). Deterioration of sunflower seed oil under simulated frying conditions and during small-scale frying of potato chips. Journal of the Science of Food and Agriculture, 33: 389–395

12   Esterbauer, H. (1993). Cytotoxicity and genotoxicity of lipid-oxidation products. American Journal of Clinical Nutrition, 57(5): 779S–785S

13   Tang, M.S., Wang, H.T., Hu, Y. *et al*. (2011). Acrolein induced DNA damage, mutagenicity and effect on DNA repair. Molecular Nutrition Food Research, 55(9): 1291–1300

14   Grootveld, M., Ruiz-Rodado, V. and Silwood, C.J.L. (2014) Detection, monitoring and deleterious health effects of lipid oxidation products generated in culinary oils during thermal stressing episodes. Inform, American Oil Chemists' Society, 25(10): 614–624

15   Metayer, C., Wang, Z., Kleinerman, R.A. *et al*. (2002). Cooking oil fumes and risk of lung cancer in women in rural Gansu, China. Lung Cancer, 35(2): 111–117

16   Hand, M.S., Thatcher, C.D., Remillard, R.L. *et al*. (2010). *Small Animal Clinical Nutrition*, 5th Edition. Torpeka, KS: Mark Morris Institute,

17   Gross, K.L., Bollinger, R., Thawnghmung, P. *et al*. (1994). Effect of three different preservative systems on the stability of extruded dog food subjected to ambient and high temperature storage. Journal of Nutrition, 124(12): 2638S–2642S

18   Scott, D.W., Miller, W.H., Jr, Decker, G.A. *et al*. (1992). Comparison of the clinical efficacy of two commercial fatty acid supplements (EfaVet and DVM Derm Caps), evening primrose oil, and cold water marine fish oil in the management of allergic pruritus in dogs: A double-blinded study. Cornell Veterinarian, 82(3): 319–329

19   Scott, D.W. and Miller, W.H. (1993). Nonsteroidal anti-inflammatory agents in the management of canine allergic pruritus. Journal of South African Veterinary Association, 64(1): 52–56

20   Scott, D.W., Miller, W.H., Jr, Griffin, C.E. (1995). *Structure and function of the skin*. Muller and Kirk's Small Animal Dermatology (5th ed.). Philadelphia, PA: Saunders (pp. 1–54)

21   Scott, D.W., Miller, W. H., Reinhart, G. A. *et al.* (1997). Effect of an omega-3/omega-6 fatty acid-containing commercial lamb and rice diet on pruritus in atopic dogs: Results of a single-blinded study. Canadian Journal of Veterinary Research, 61(2): 145–153

22   Logas, D. (1995) Systemic nonsteroidal therapy for pruritus: the North American experience. Proceedings of 19th WALTHAM/OSU Symposium Dermatology, p32–36

23   Sture G.H., Lloyd D.H. (1995). Canine atopic disease: therapeutic use of an evening primrose oil and fish oil combination. The Veterinary Record, 137: 169–170

24   Watson, T.D.G. (1998). Diet and skin disease in dogs and cats. Journal of Nutrition, 128(12): 2783S–2789S

25   Lenox, C.E. (2015). Timely topics in Nutrition: An overview of fatty acids in companion animal medicine. Journal of the American Veterinary Medical Association, 246(11): 1198–1202

26   Marsh, K.A., Ruedisueli, F.L., Coe, S.L. *et al.* (2000). Effects of zinc and linoleic acid supplementation on the skin and coat quality of dogs receiving a complete and balanced diet. Veterinary Dermatology, 11(4): 277–284

27   Heinemann, K.M., Waldron, M.K., Bigley, K.E. *et al.* (2005). Long-chain (n-3) polyunsaturated fatty acids are more efficient than alpha-linolenic acid in improving electroretinogram responses of puppies exposed during gestation, lactation, and weaning. Journal of Nutrition, 135(8):1960–1966

28   Ricci, R., Berlanda, M., Tenti, S., *et al.* (2009). Study of the chemical and nutritional characteristics of commercial dog foods used as elimination diet for the diagnosis of canine food allergy. Italian Journal of Animal Science, 8: 328–330

29   Brenna, J.T. (2002). Efficiency of conversion of alpha-linolenic acid to long chain n-3 fatty acids in man. Current Opinion in Clinical Nutrition and Metabolic Care, 5(2): 127–132

30   Harris, W.S. (2010). *Omega-3 fatty acids*. In: Coates PM, Betz JM, Blackman MR, *et al.*, eds. Encyclopedia of Dietary Supplements. 2nd ed. London and New York: Informa Healthcare: 577–586

31   National Research Council (NRC) (2006). *Nutrient requirement of dogs and cats*. Washington, DC: National Academies Press

32   Zicker, S.C., Jewell, D.E., Yamka, R.M. *et al.* (2012). Evaluation of cognitive learning, memory, psychomotor, immunologic, and retinal functions in healthy puppies fed foods fortified with docosahexaenoic acid–rich fish oil from 8 to 52 weeks of age. Journal of the American Veterinary Medical Association, 241(5): 583-594

33   Hadley, K.B., Bauer, J. and Milgram, N.W. (2017). The oil-rich alga *Schizochytrium* sp. as a dietary source of docosahexaenoic acid improves shape discrimination learning associated with visual processing in a canine model of senescence. Prostaglandins, Leukotrienes and Essential Fatty Acids, 118: 10–18

34   Ahlstrøm, Ø., Krogdahl, Å., Gregersen Vhile, *et al.* (2004). Fatty acid composition in commercial dog foods. Journal of Nutrition, 134: 2145S–2147S

35   Association of American Feed Control Officials (AAFCO, 2008). Official feed terms. Official Publication. Available online, www.aafco.org

36   Lee, Y.M., Kim, K.S., Jacobs, D.R. *et al.* (2016). Persistent organic pollutants in adipose tissue should be considered in obesity research. Etiology and Pathophysiology/Toxicology, 18(2): 129–139

37   O'Connor, J.J., Stowe, C.M. and Robinson, R.R. (1985). Fate of sodium pentobarbital in rendered products. American Journal of Vet Research, 46(8): 1721–1724

38   Nolen, G.A. (1973). A feeding study of a used, partially hydrogenated soybean oil, frying fat in dogs. Journal of Nutrition, 103: 1248–1255

39   Davidson, M.G., Geoly, F.J., Gilger, B.C. *et al.* (1998). Retinal degeneration associated with vitamin E deficiency in hunting dogs. Journal of American Veterinary Medical Association, 213: 645–651

40   Pérez-Calvo, E., Castrillo, C., Baucells, M.D. *et al.* (2010). Effect of rendering on protein and fat quality of animal by-products. Journal of Animal Physiology and Animal Nutrition, 94(5): e154–e164

41   Ito, N., Fukushima, S. and Tsuda, H. (1985). Carcinogenicity and Modification of the Carcinogenic Response by BHA, BHT, and Other Antioxidants. Critical Reviews in Toxicology, 15(2)

42   Kahl, R. and Kappus, H. (1993). Toxicology of the synthetic antioxidants BHA and BHT in comparison with the natural antioxidant vitamin E. Zeitschrift für Lebensmitteluntersuchung und Forschung, 196(4): 329–338 [Paper in German, summary in English]

43   Chanadang, S., Koppel, K. and Aldrich, G. (2016). The Impact of Rendered Protein Meal Oxidation Level on Shelf-Life, Sensory Characteristics, and Acceptability in Extruded Petfood. Animals, 6(8): 44

44   Dzanis, D.A. (1991) Journal of Nutrition Nov;121(11 Suppl):S163-4. *Safety of ethoxyquin in dog foods*

45   Mooney, A. (2010). *Stability of Essential Nutrients in Petfood Manufacturing and Storage.* Masters Thesis. Kansas State University

46   Simopoulos, A.P. (2002). The importance of the ratio of omega-6/omega-3 essential fatty acids. Biomedecine & Pharmacotherapy, 56(8): 365–379

47   Dyerberg, J., Bang, H.O. and Hjorne, N. (1975). Fatty acid composition of the plasma lipids in Greenland Eskimos. American Journal of Clinical Nutrition, 28(9): 958–966

48   DiNicolantonio, J.J. (2016). Increase in the intake of refined carbohydrates and sugar may have led to the health decline of the Greenland Eskimos. Open Heart, 3(2)

49   Association of American Feed Control Officials (AAFCO, 2016). Dog and Cat Food Nutrient Profiles. Official Publication, see www.aafco.org

50   Paulsen, P., Bauer, A. and Smulders, F.J.M. (2014). *Trends in game meat hygiene.* Wageningen Academic Publishers. Chapter 28: Lipids in tissues of wild game

51   Dierenfeld, E.S., Alcorn, H.L. and Jacobsen, K.L. (2002). *Nutrient Composition of Whole Vertebrate Prey (Excluding Fish) Fed in Zoos.* U.S. Department of Agriculture. Available online www.researchgate.net

52   Bierer, T.L. and Bui, L.M. (2002). Improvement of Arthritic Signs in Dogs Fed Green-Lipped Mussel (Perna canaliculus). The Journal of Nutrition, 132(6): 1634S–1636S

CHAPTER 11

Teeth

Bacteria love warm, damp, dark environments. Give them food here and they thrive. So, your mouth is an ideal place for them. You always have bacteria in your mouth. On your teeth they form a sticky, invisible layer called plaque. Unfortunately, as you'd expect, they cause a bit of trouble when they're not kept under control.

The first indication that all is not well, in the buccal cavity of a person or dog, is a bad smell. What you can smell is the sulphurous by-product of the bacteria flourishing in the mouth, essentially bacteria farts. But smelly breath (*halitosis*) is just the tip of the iceberg for the sufferer, as the other by-product is acid. Plaque's stickiness helps keep the acid against the teeth where it begins to strip down the enamel, and over time damages the teeth and gums. Allowed to persist, bacterial toxins will attack the gums, bone and ligaments surrounding the teeth, causing shrinkage of the gums and loosening of the teeth. This is *periodontitis*.

If left to fester for an extended period, plaque can solidify into a hard, yellow layer called tartar. From underneath this hard and hard-to-remove shell, bacteria can safely attack the gums, every minute of every hour of every day. The gums are full of blood and the bacteria want in. The body absolutely does not want this to happen, so it sends the troops out to the site to defend the body from invasion, resulting in inflammation along the gum line (that little red line you see above a sore tooth). This inflammation (*gingivitis*, meaning infection at the gums) is not only painful for the afflicted animal but it is a constant drain on resources, leaving it less able to deal with other threats. Thus, afflicted dogs will be immuno-compromised[1] and more susceptible to disease as a result.

Nor does it end there. All this immuno-debris must be cleared away by the kidneys, which puts them under significant, daily pressure. In this way animals presenting with poor teeth almost always exhibit decreased kidney function. De Bowes *et al.* (1996)[2] studied 45 dogs with periodontal disease. They found histopathologic changes (refers to the microscopic examination of tissue in order to study the manifestations of disease) in kidney, myocardium (papillary muscle of the heart) and the liver.

A foul mouth is never OK in a dog, young or old. At the very least, there are bad breath, mild discomfort, damaged gums and teeth, a depletion of resources and an increased susceptibility to disease, as well as unsightly tartar, which will require a dental scrape, normally under anaesthesia. At worst, it's agony – heart, kidney and liver disease, with major surgery needed.

It thus comes with some concern that the American Veterinary Dental College states that, 'by three years of age, most dogs and cats have some evidence of periodontal disease'.[3] And Dr René Carlson, president of the American Veterinary Medical Association states, 'It's estimated that by the age of two, 80% of dogs have some form of periodontal disease.'[4] The same figure, cited in the study by Lonsdale,[5] is given by Dr. Susanne Penman, President of British Veterinary Dental Association, who states that nine in 10 dogs have some form of gum disease by 3 years of age.

If the issue is so serious and so very common, you'd be forgiven for wondering why this is happening in our dogs and what might the solution be.

Let's begin with wild carnivores. How do they keep their gnashers so brilliantly white? The answer is abrasion.

The biting, tearing and crunching of whole meat pieces is long since known to keep dental disease at bay.[6-8] Pavlović *et al.* (2007)[8] studied the incidence of dental disease in wild wolves. Of 34 skulls examined, 9% had dental issues. Only two wolves had any form of periodontitis and that was a result of broken teeth, which would result in the wolf avoiding the tooth when chewing thus allowing tartar buildup.

Fagan (1980),[7] a veterinary dental consultant, presented a paper called "Diet Consistency And Periodontal Disease In Exotic Carnivores," to the Meeting of the American Association of Zoo Veterinarians in Washington DC. He highlighted a massive body of work by British scientist Sir Frank Colyer who, vexed by the observation that the relocation of wild animals from their natural habitats into a captive environment brought about radical changes in the environment of its oral cavity, began researching the dental disease of captive animals. This work resulted in an exhaustive, 700-hundred-page text on the subject called "Variations and Diseases of the Teeth of Animals."[6] After examining thousands of individual cases of oral pathology in exotic animals, Colyer came to the following conclusions:

- The disease is caused by an alteration in the animal's diet characteristics as being either a physical or a chemical nature – in other words, by a departure from natural diet and conditions.

- Foods of firm consistency will increase the number, distribution and tone of the capillaries in the gingival tissue, which in turn improves the metabolism and vitality of all of the supporting and surrounding structures.

- The degree of keratinisation of the stratified squamous epithelium, which affords protection against trauma and other injurious agents, is affected by the frictional qualities of the diet.

Colyer was emphatic that diet consistency and texture play a regulatory role in the aetiology of oral disease. Fagan (1980)[7] concludes that zoo veterinary medical staff must heed this advice, that anyone caring for captive exotic animals should take careful note of both the food preferences of the animal in the wild, as well as the occupational therapy value of food items that are not necessarily related to nutritional value.

> ...animals need more *hassle factor* per mouthful of nutrients. The best kept secret of the last fifty years is that we must eliminate the pre-processed, the over-cooked, the smashed, the blended and the pureed foods, and feed our animals a more appropriate diet duplicating the feeding habits of feral conditions... not predigested TV dinners...
>
> **Fagan, 1980[7]**

In 1984, Haberstroh *et al.*[9] fed captive Amur tigers, normally on an all frozen-meat-based diet, beef bones twice a week and reduced dental plaque and calculus accumulation and improved gingival health. Clarke and Cameron (1998)[10] compared the dental calculus scores in domestic cats eating commercially available canned and dry foods with those in feral cats consuming a diet consisting of small mammals, birds, reptiles and insects. Unsurprisingly, the dental calculus scores were significantly better in feral cats than domestic cats.

And it's the very same in dogs. We have known for years that the solution to periodontal disease in dogs, aside from having to actually physically brush their teeth every day (in which case Tromp *et al.* (1986)[11] found brushing 3 times a week is sufficient), is a diet with more 'hassle factor'. Firmer diets reduce dental calculus,[12] and promote healthier gums[13] in dogs. Gray (1923)[14] highlighted how the problem, greater in smaller dogs, was a result of dogs fed soft diets with insufficient dental activity, when compared to a normal diet that required 'the cutting and tearing of raw flesh, breaking or crunching bones, and using their teeth in ratting and rabbiting, etc.' Brown and Park (1968)[15] periodically replaced the moist kibble ration fed to thirty dogs displaying dental calculus and tooth loss, with oxtail. Two-thirds of their calculus was removed by 24 hours after the first oxtail feeding; calculus dropped to 5% by end of Week 2. Interestingly, the same authors note that oxtails, consisting of hard spinal vertebrae, were fed to over 200 dogs for more than 6 years and 'no harmful effects were observed'. Marx *et al.* (2016)[16] investigated the use of two types of beef bone (cortical or solid bone and epiphyseal or 'spongy' marrow bone) to control dental calculus in beagles. Chewing cortical bone reduced dental calculus by 36% after just 3 days and by 71% after 12 days. Chewing marrowbone reduced dental calculus by 57% after 3 days and by 82% after 12 days. Again, no complications such as tooth fractures, pieces of bone stuck between teeth or intestinal obstructions were observed during the studies.

Thus, active chewing plays a central role in the gum disease process. Authors found less accumulation of calculus, less gingival inflammation and less periodontal bone loss in dry-fed dogs that were given access to a variety of chewing materials.[17] In this respect, it's hard to get away from the failings of kibble, in terms of dental hygiene – 8/10 dogs have gum disease by the time they are three years of age. It just so happens that approximately 8/10 dogs are fed kibbled dog food! Many breeds largely swallow the small pieces whole, barely glancing off the teeth. When kibble diameter is increased by just 50%, there is a 42% calculus reduction in dogs.[18]

Pet food manufacturers are not stupid. They are aware of this lack of abrasion, so they respond with a special 'pro-dental' shape, designed to better clean teeth. While some authors note dental-type dry foods can out-perform normal dry dog food in terms of teeth cleaning,[19] Capik (2007) reviewed these special dental diets and found they didn't *significantly* reduce dental plaque in dogs.

Thankfully, pet food manufacturers have again come up with an answer they can sell us in the form of dental sticks and 'jumbo bones', (items that are as large as bones, are flavoured like bones and are often as hard as fresh bones; indeed they are bone shaped but *crucially* they are not actually real bones which are not only genuinely nutritious but cost nothing!). Here are the ingredients of a popular jumbo bone:

Rice flour, glycerine, sugar, cellulose powder, wheat flour, propylene glycol, sodium caseinate, natural poultry flavour, dried meat by-product, potassium sorbate, vitamins and minerals.

The second and third ingredients, which are in order of weight, are both sugar, without which the dog wouldn't eat it. Sugar. In a product for teeth?! When they're often made by candy manufacturers, perhaps we shouldn't be so surprised.

To analyse these ingredients further, the sixth ingredient, propylene glycol, essentially keeps it rubbery. Sodium caseinate is essentially casein, the protein from milk. It is a natural, glue-like substance. Casein protein breaks down to casomorphins, as the name implies, morphine type compounds, which act as a histamine releaser and contribute to negative reactions in 75% of humans on the planet who consume it. Your chances of being in that 75% depends on how long your gene pool has been drinking from cows' udders, with Europeans faring the best. Dogs, entirely ill adapted to the breakdown of dairy from 12-weeks-old, are expected to be as good with casein as they are with gluten, and that is not very good at all. Certainly, not better than humans, who have been trying to digest the stuff for thousands of years.

Dental stick products have similar ingredients but lean a lot heavier on the salt to make them palatable to dogs:

Rice Flour, Wheat Starch, Glycerin, Gelatin, Gum Arabic, Calcium Carbonate, Natural Poultry Flavor, Cellulose Powder, Sodium Tripolyphosphate (**Salt**), **Salt** (Iodised), Potassium Chloride (**Salt**)…

As of July 25, 2015, Pedigree pet food state on their website:

…74% of vets recommend Pedigree Dentastix as being good for oral health…
        ***based on a March 2011 survey of 3,214 UK and Republic of
                                                                Ireland vets**

Like most things when it comes to nutrition, I'm going to go against the majority of vets on this one and say I strongly recommend *not* relying on these types of products for canine dental hygiene.

Meat on the bone or raw, meaty bones themselves are clearly the answer. This subject has been covered extensively by Tom Lonsdale,[1,5] who cites Dr. Coles, President of the Australian Veterinary Dentist Society in 1997, as saying, 'chewing bones twice a week helps to prevent dental disease'. In his review of periodontal disease in dogs and cats, Watson (2006)[21] recommends supplementing the diet with raw bones with meat and connective tissue attached.

It's important to note, however, that not all studies appear in agreement. One study stands alone in direct conflict with the above findings. Buckley *et al.* (2011)[22] surveyed a colossal 17,184 dogs and 6,371 cats over a decade and found there was a significant effect of diet on the oral health of our pets. Most notably, the feeding of home-prepared diets actually increased the probability of an oral health problem in both cats and dogs. They conclude, 'feeding only a dry diet was beneficial for oral health in cats and dogs."

What this home-prepared diet consisted of was not mentioned (and home-prepared diets done incorrectly can certainly have their own problems) but I was surprised enough to do a little digging. This study was organised by the Polish Small Animal Veterinary Association and published in the prestigious *British Journal of Nutrition*. This was encouraging. A little more digging revealed the study was part of the "Pet Smile" campaign and was funded by the commercial pet food industry. The Pet Smile website provides the following information:

- In 2003 and 2004 the campaign was funded by Nestlé Purina.

- In 2006 and 2007, the campaign was supported by Mars (Royal Canin and Pedigree Dentastix) together with Petplan Insurance.

- In 2008, the major sponsors were Mars, Colgate-Palmolive (Hill's) and Petosan.

- In 2009, it was funded by Mars (Whiskas Dentabits joined Pedigree Dentastix).

Two years later the study's findings were published. This is not to say the findings are wrong, it's just that they jar so badly with what would seem to be the expected outcome based on all the other evidence above.

Another study, at first glance, appears to weaken the whole natural-diet-for-cleaner-teeth argument. Steenkamp and Gorrel (1999)[23] found 41% of African Wild Dogs had periodontal disease, mostly through cracked and fractured teeth. The authors note that they found "mild calculus" on only two of the skulls. This study is often used to argue that a natural diet would not be protective against periodontal disease in domestic dogs.[24] Of course, as Section 1 discussed, the

African Wild Dog (*Lycaon pictus*), while most certainly a canid, has been separate from wolves (*Canis lupus*) and thus dogs, for more than 5 million years, around the time our ape ancestors were climbing down from the trees.[25] Furthermore, African Wild Dogs, very omnivorous compared to feral domestic dogs, are known to regularly consume sugary fruits.[26] Thus comparing them to meat and bone-eating domestic dogs is akin to comparing leaf-eating chimps to hotdog eating humans. This doesn't perturb www.DentalVets.co.uk which praised the study as an 'elegant work,' concluding it was 'a useful counterweight to the entrenched opinions of the Raw Meaty Bone lobby'.

That aside, it's a fact that wild animals break and fracture teeth. A study of feral cats found 62% of skulls (186 of 301 skulls) had some degree of periodontal disease, although only 9% of them had any calculus.[27] We can absolutely expect wilder animals to have a harder time catching their dinner than the majority of our pets who, at most, have to perform, sit and wait. Wild animals do not sit around and wait to be eaten. They shake and kick, quite vigorously, as you can imagine. Prey struggle free and teeth clash. Legs are ripped from clenched jaws. Hooves and heads and knees make regular contact with jaws. It's a hazardous job catching dinner with your face, especially when it's fighting back. Domestic dogs under our care are not threatened in this way. And this is all before we consider the bone mineral densities of wild animals to those of the significantly less exercised baby animals reared in our confined meat sector. In fact, bone density is another factor in tooth fracture in carnivores, in particular, the age of the bone. Studies show carnivores incur greater tooth damage when attempting to consume older carcasses.[28-30] As we will come back to in Section 4, a lot of the issues vets are seeing with bone consumption by dogs today are as a result of cooked bones. You must never feed cooked bones.

It follows that if you want to reduce tartar build up in dogs, you need to introduce some hassle factor to their diet and this is best done with meat on the bone or raw meaty bones, once or twice a week. Take a few minor precautions (please see our raw feeding section) and you can reduce the risk of tooth fracture to very close to zero.

TAKE HOME POINTS

✓ Plaque is the invisible, sticky layer of biofilm on your teeth. Allowed to persist, it can degrade the teeth and gums. This is periodontitis.

✓ If left to fester, the plaque can solidify into hard yellow tartar. From here the bacteria attempt to invade the blood capillaries in the gums daily. This is gingivitis and is visible as a red line on your dog's gums just above the teeth. It can result in kidney, heart and liver disease.

✓ By just 3 years of age, 80% of dogs have some form of periodontal disease.

✓ Studies show it is the biting, tearing and crunching of whole meat pieces (hassle factor) that keeps dental disease at bay in most carnivores and certainly in dogs.

✓ Feeding raw meaty bones not only cleans the dog's teeth but few, if any ,harmful effects are observed.

✓ Studies of the dental fractures in omnivorous canids such as African Wild Dogs, bear little relevance to the domestic dog. In fact, as most domestic dogs no longer catch large, struggling quarry with their faces, comparing their dentition to wolves isn't accurate either.

✓ 'Dental' products made by the manufacturers of ultra-processed pet food generally contain large amounts of salt and sugar and are absolutely not advised.

✓ Cooked bones are never ever to be fed to dogs.

Chapter Eleven References

1   Lonsdale, T. (1992). *Raw meaty bones promote health*. Control and Therapy series no. 3323. Sydney, Australia: University of Sydney

2   De Bowes, L.J., Mosier, D., Logan, E. *et al.* (1996). Association of periodontal disease and histologic lesions in multiple organs from 45 dogs. Journal of Veterinary Dentistry, 13(2): 56–60

3   Diogo Pereira dos Santos, J., Cunha, E., Nunes, T. *et al.* (2019). Relation between periodontal disease and systemic diseases in dogs Research in Veterinary Science, 125: 136–140

4   San Fillippo, M. (2012). *Your pet's bad breath is no laughing matter.* AVMA Press Release. Published online, www.avma.org

5   Lonsdale, T. (2001). *Raw meaty bones promote health.* Wenatchee, WA: Dogwise Publishing

6   Colyer, F. (1936). *Variations and Diseases of the Teeth of Animals*, p. 677. John Bale, London,

7   Fagan, D.A. (1980). *Diet consistency and periodontal disease in exotic carnivores.* Prepared for the Meeting of the American Association of Zoo Veterinarians, Washington D.C., Oct 18, 1980. Published online www.citeseerx.ist.psu.edu

8   Pavlović, D., Gomerčić, T., Gužvica, G. *et al.* (2007). Prevalence of dental pathology in wolves (*Canis lupus L.)* in Croatia—a case report. Veterinarski Arhiv, 77:291–297

9   Haberstroh, LI., Ullrey, D.E., Sikarski, J.G. *et al.* (1984). Diet and oral health in captive Amur tigers (*Panthera tigris altaica*). Journal of Zoo Animal Medicine, 15: 142–164

10   Clarke, D.E. and Cameron, A. (1998). Relationship between diet, dental calculus and periodontal disease in domestic and feral cats in Australia. Australian Veterinary Journal, 76(10): 690–693

11   Tromp, J.A.H., Jansen, J. and Pilot, T. (1986). Gingival health and frequency of tooth brushing in the beagle dog model. Clinical Periodontology, 13(2): 164–168

12   Egelberg, J. (1965). Local effect of diet on plaque formation and development of gingivitis in dogs. I. Effect of Hard and Soft Diets. Odontology Review, 16: 31–41

13   Burwasser, P. and Hill, T. J. (1939). The effect of hard and soft diets on the gingival tissues of dogs. Journal of Dental Research, 18: 398

14   Gray, H. (1923). Pyorrhoea in the dog. Veterinary Record, 3: 167–169

15   Brown, E.N. and Park, J.F. (1968). Control of dental calculus in experimental beagles. Laboratory Animal Care, 18: 527–535

16   Marx, F.R., Machado, G.S., Pezzali, J.G. *et al.* (2016). Raw beef bones as chewing items to reduce dental calculus in Beagle dogs. Australian Veterinary Journal,. 94(1-2): 18–23

17   Harvey, C.E., Shofer, F.S., Laster, L. (1996). Correlation of diet, other chewing activities and periodontal disease in North American client-owned dogs. Journal of Veterinary Dentistry, 13(3): 101–105

18   Hennet, P., Servet, E., Soulard, Y. *et al.* (2007). Effect of pellet food size and polyphosphates in preventing calculus accumulation in dogs. Journal of Veterinary Dentistry, 24(4): 236–239

19   Logan, E.I., Finney, O. and Hefferren, J.J. (2002). Effects of a Dental Food on Plaque Accumulation and Gingival Health in Dogs. Journal of Veterinary Dentistry, 19(1): 15–18

20   Capik, I. (2007). Periodontal health vs. different preventative means in toy breeds – clinical study. Acta Veterinaria Brno, 79(4) : 637–645

21   Watson, A.D.J. (2006). Diet and periodontal disease in dogs and cats. Australian Veterinary Journal, 71(10): 313–318

22   Buckley, C., Colyer, A., Skrzywanek, M. *et al.* (2011). The impact of home-prepared diets and home oral hygiene on oral health in cats and dogs. British Journal of Nutrition, 106(S1): 124–127

23   Steenkamp, G. and Gorrel, C. (1999). Oral and dental conditions in adult African wild dog skulls: A preliminary result. Journal of Veterinary Dentistry, 16(2): 913–918

24   Larsen, J.A. (2010). Oral products and dental disease. Compendium, 32(9): E1–3

25   Vilà, C., Savolainen, P., Maldonado, J.E. *et al.* (1997). Multiple and ancient origins of the domestic dog. Science, 276(5319): 1687–1689

26   Sillero-Zubiri, C., Hoffmann, M. and MacDonald, D.W. (2004). *Canids: Foxes, wolves, jackals and dogs. Status survey and conservation action plan.* Gland, Switzerland: IUCN. Available online, www.researchgate.net

27   Verstraete, F.J., van Aarde, R.J., Nieuwoudt, B.A.*et al.* (1996). The dental pathology of feral cats on Marion Island, part II: periodontitis, external odontoclastic resorption lesions and mandibular thickening. Journal of Comparative Pathology, 115(3): 283–297

28   Mech, L.D. and Frenzel, L.D. Jr (1971). *Ecological studies of the timber wolf in Northeastern Minnesota.* Minnesota: US Department of Agriculture. Available online www.fs.usda.gov

29   Carbone, C., Frame, L., Frame, G. *et al.* (2005). Feeding success of African wild dogs (*Lycaon pictus*) in the Serengeti: The effects of group size and kleptoparasitism. Journal of Zoology 266(2): 153–161

30   Vucetich, J.A, Vucetich, L.M. and Peterson, R.O (2012). The causes and consequences of partial prey consumption by wolves preying on moose. Behavioral Ecology and Sociobiology, 66(2): 295–303

CHAPTER 12

Chemicals

If you can't pronounce it, don't eat it. That is the throwaway nutritional rule you hear in many circles. There's a lot of truth to it, certainly when you consider some of the chemical additives that are making their way into pet food, some on purpose, others accidentally during processing or storage thereafter. We have discussed many already. To recap, we know that sodium pentobarbital (SPB), a chemical that is used to put dogs and cats asleep, is the second most common reasons for pet food recall in the United States. This chemical is still being found in great abundance in these products today. We have learned that the incorrect chemical supplementation of pet foods with vitamin and mineral supplements is repeatedly causing serious illness and deaths in pets. Furthermore, to achieve long storage times, fats are preserved with questionable chemical preservatives such as butylated hydroxyanisole (BHA), butylated hydroxytoluene (BHT) and ethoxyquin. Sadly, there are many, many more chemicals to come.

With more agents than the FBI, pet food manufacturers are permitted by the Food and Drug Authority (FDA) to include anti-caking agents, antimicrobial agents, curing, drying and firming agents, oxidising and reducing agents, pH control agents and surface-active agents. Other chemicals such as synergists and texturisers, emulsifiers, humectants and stabilisers control the exact texture of the pellet. One of these texturisers, a thickener called sodium carboxyl-methylcellulose, is a plastic filler once used to thicken milk shakes but now banned by the FDA for human consumption. But it seems it's *fine* for pet food. None of these substances are required to make the ingredients panel.

For the non-GRAS (Generally Recognised as Safe) ones, they are not permitted to use them *ad lib*. Here's the process, as laid out and referenced by Patrick (2006),[1] where CVM (Centre for Veterinary Medicine) is the FDA branch responsible for animal feed (italics added by Patrick for effect).

For non-GRAS additives the pre-market approval process requires the submission of a food additive petition to the FDA [47]. The petition generally contains, among other information, a description of the chemical identity of the additive, the manufacturing process and controls, human food safety data, target animal safety data, and product labelling [48]. Interestingly, CVM "has used regulatory discretion and *not* required food additive petitions for substances that do not raise any safety concerns" [49]. CVM explains that since food additive approval is time-consuming, regulatory action will only be taken if the label is inconsistent with the accepted intended use of the additive or if new data 'received' raises concerns regarding safety or suitability of the additive [50]. One has to wonder how closely the CVM monitors the 'intended use' of the additive considering they have already chosen not to use their resources for pre-market approval *as mandated by Congress* in the FFDCA. Moreover, it is unclear from where the CVM expects to 'receive' data that calls into question the 'safety' of the additive. Certainly, it will not be provided by the pet food manufacturer.

Then there are the chemicals they don't mean to put in themselves. A lot of undesirable meat and carcasses used in rendering plants, such as 4D meat (dead, diseased, dying, disabled), are denatured by chemicals to ensure that they exit the human food chain. Meat inspectors are advised that the meat to be denatured must be in 'pieces no larger than 4 inches' to allow for maximum contact of the denaturing chemical.[2] This denaturing involves covering the meat with any number of toxic substances, creosote being a particularly nasty one. A tar-oil derivative, creosote was until recently used as a disinfectant or to preserve wood but has since been removed from the market due to it being a known carcinogen as well as causing kidney and liver disease, seizures, skin irritation similar to chemical burns, rashes, mental disarray and death. Listed as a known poison and carcinogen by the United States Health and Safety Administration, by the International Agency for Research on Cancer and the Environmental Protection Agency, it is concerning to hear the following words from Dr Wendell Belfield, former United States Drugs Association Vet:

> As a veterinary meat inspector, we denatured with carbolic acid (a potentially corrosive disinfectant) and/or creosote (used for wood-preservation or as a disinfectant). Both substances are highly toxic. According to federal meat inspection regulations, fuel oil, kerosene,

crude carbolic acid and citronella (an insect repellent made from lemon grass) are all approved denaturing materials. Condemned livestock carcasses treated with these chemicals can become meat and bone meal for the pet food industry.

***Food Not Fit for a Pet*, Wendell O. Belfield, DVM. *Let's Live Magazine*, May 1992**

Interestingly, when Dr. Belfield was asked which commercial pet food he would recommend, his reply was 'my standard answer is *none*'.[2]

There was an interesting case settled on the steps of the courts on January 2, 2017. It made plain just how nasty the chemical adulterants used in pet food can be. However, this time we are not talking about the effects these chemicals had on dogs but on the employees making the stuff. The petition for damages, filed by eight plaintiffs (Boyd versus Mars Pet Care), in Jasper County, Missouri, on August 23, 2012, was taken against a Mars Petcare kibble manufacturing facility. The claim was that Mars Petcare was 'negligent and careless' in preventing employee exposure to pesticides and other toxins used during the pet food manufacturing process.

Reported in *The Joplin Globe* newspaper,[3] the crux of the claim was over phosphine gas, a rodenticide and pesticide. It was also used in chemical bombs during World War I to kill humans. The problem many pet food manufacturers have is that they use poor-quality grain in their mixes. Dina Butcher, Agriculture Policy Advisor for the North Dakota Governor Ed Schafer, investigated the wheat quality used in dry dog food and concluded 'the grain that would go into pet food is not a high-quality grain'.[4]

Poor-quality grain is prone to containing some very toxic moulds, most notably aflatoxin, something you'll be learning more about later. Phosphine is used on these stockpiles of wheat to stop it from going bad. Toxic to humans in tiny doses, it was reported that phosphine monitors in the Mars factory normally sounded a warning alarm at 0.2 parts per million (ppm) in the air. Company records allegedly indicated that on two days there was a personal monitoring reading of 5.85 ppm, almost 30 times higher than safe levels.

The following to and fro is taken from sworn testimony provided in deposition by Mr Joey Tyree from the Boyd v. Mars Petcare lawsuit, a man that was working with these rail cars from 2006 to 2011. The original court documents were provided by a whistle-blower to Susan Thixton and published on her platform www.TruthAboutPetFood.com on May 15, 2007.

Q. Now, aeration, I've talked about, that is – uses the term clearing of rail cars; is that right?

A. Yes.

Q. What is clearing of a rail car mean?

A. Basically it's – it's getting – the product is good to go.

Q. So you've cleared it to enter the plant; is that right?

A. Yes.

Q. And you're aerating the poisonous gas phosphine gas out of these rail cars; is that right?

A. Yes.

Q. And can you help me with some other terms? We've talked about clearing. What's the term under gas mean?

A. Under gas means it's – it's fumigating at that time.

Q. And tell us what fumigation means.

A. Means you're putting the poisonous gas inside something and you have to measure it by cubic feet and square feet. If you put that much gas in there, it's supposed to kill everything inside that for a period of time. And then you pull it out and air it out.

Q. Did you ever use a mask or respirator when you did your aerating?

A. One time, whenever Occupational Safety and Health Administration (OSHA) was there, is the only time I ever used it.

Q. So Presto-X was — knew you were aerating rail cars but did not provide you with a respirator?

A. Correct.

Q. Did you get a respirator then when it was — when OSHA came in 2012 to do the plant inspection?

A. Yes.

Q. That was the first time you got a respirator?

A. Yes.

Later Tyree testifies he saw a grey residue on the corn after the fumigation process was finished. This is OK for pet food.

And these are the chemicals they mean to put in there. In 2011, Vollmer *et al.* tested 119 dry foods from the German pet food market, for the migration of mineral oil hydrocarbons from the packets into the foods. The limit for mineral oil saturated hydrocarbons in human food is 0.6 mg/kg.[4] Vollmer *et al.* found that levels in dry food were frequently exceeded by a factor of 10–100. Most dry foods sampled were merely 2 to 3 months old and far from the end of their shelf life, which is usually 1 to 3 years. Unsurprisingly, products in paper or polyethylene bags fared the worst with foil providing the best protection. About a quarter of the migrating mineral oil was from printing ink used for decorating the bag.

Bisphenol A (BPA) is commonly used to coat metal surfaces that will be holding food and is suspected to be an endocrine disruptor with oestrogenic activity and the proliferation of cancer cells, although at what concentration is yet to be determined. As humans move to avoid all products containing the plastic, the same duty of care is not afforded pets. The pet food industry uses a variety of plastic lacquers on their cans. Studies show these compounds can migrate into the food, with smaller cans possibly posing a bigger risk due to the amount of surface area the food is exposed to per gram. Researchers in Japan tested 15 tinned cat foods and eleven tinned dog foods for the presence of BPA. Leeching was found to occur at varying levels in all the samples.[5] BPA is known to inhibit thyroid function,[6] particularly in cats, as they are slower to eliminate BPA than dogs. Edinboro *et al.* (2004)[6] seemed to confirm this link between tinned pet food (particularly ring-pull cans) and hyperthyroidism in cats (especially females). They concluded that owners should avoid such products, although the benefits of such a move might not be seen for years as cats may have already developed irreversible thyroid damage.

Of all chemical adulterations, the 2007 melamine scandal was by far the worst. This time the problem arose from contaminated Chinese wheat gluten and rice protein. It was suspected they were using melamine, a hard, highly poisonous chemical substance produced from coal and used in the manufacturing of plastic but also in this case to artificially boost the protein content of animal feed ingredients.

In their piece titled "Filler in Animal Feed Is Open Secret in China", Barboza and Barrioneuvo (2007)[7], note how Chinese companies regularly buy melamine scrap to add to animal feed, such as fish, pigs, poultry and pets as 'there's no regulation that says not to do it'. Animal feed manufacturers there actually advertise online that they are looking to source melamine, which is exactly what one of the companies implicated in this scandal was doing the month before the link was made. With price differences of $1.20 for melamine compared to $6 for protein, and no legislation to stop it, it's easy to see how this occurred.

This particular scandal ended up affecting over 100 companies including Menu Foods, Nestlé Purina, Hill's Science Diet and Royal Canin.[8] In the United States, Australia, Europe and South Africa, 5,300 products and more than sixty million packages of pet food were recalled,[7, 8] highlighting for us the fact that most of these products use the same ingredients and are about as different from each other as fur and hair.

The effect on companion animals was colossal. Cathy Langston, a vet from New York's Animal Medical Centre (the veterinary equivalent of the Mayo Clinic) noted two hundred cases of kidney failure in animals over just one weekend.[9] That's one vet, from one hospital, in one country. In April, The *New York Times* reported that the US FDA alone had received more than 14,000 reports of pets sickened by products containing poisoned Chinese ingredients.[7] By May, 3 months after the recall began, 4,000 complaints of pet deaths had been reported to the United States FDA.[10] Reuters could confirm only 16 of these deaths. In fact, a survey by the American Association of Veterinary Laboratory Diagnosticians found only 347 cases from April to June 2001 that met the diagnostic criteria for 'pet food-induced nephrotoxicity'. As with most other recalls, linking pet death and subsequent financial claims to a particular company proved virtually impossible. Thus, the exact numbers of cats and dogs injured and killed by this particular scandal remains unknown as there is no adverse reporting system for pet foods.[11] However, the number must have been very high, at least for cats. One of the many companies responsible (and there were more than 100 large companies caught) tested their products on 40 to 50 pet dogs and cats – seven of them died.[12] Banfield Hospital, a group with access to the health reports of millions of cats and dogs in the United States, estimated as many as 39,000 cats were injured or killed upon eating melamine-tainted pet food.

Unbelievably, even though some companies knew their products were contaminated, no action was taken. A press release by the FDA (April 12, 2007) highlighted how they, in an effort to test how well the pet food companies were complying to the recall, conducted approximately 400 checks of retail stores across the country. The FDA noted that some companies still had not recalled their product from the shelves. In other words, they knew what was going on, yet these highly toxic products continued to be sold.

Senator Maria Cantwell was so appalled at the situation, she had to petition the US FDA to name the two companies that were known to have received the contaminated rice protein but were not coming forward to alert pet owners as to the danger from their products. The press release[13] simply wanted the FDA to publish the names of all pet food manufacturers it had on file who received shipments of contaminated ingredients, so pet owners could avoid them. Cantwell also petitioned the FDA to push manufactures to trace and recall all pet food made using potentially contaminated ingredients and inspect all suspect pet food ingredients imported from China and other countries. In other words, this sort of compliance is not done voluntarily, nor quickly. Money and reputations are at stake!

If it wasn't patently clear before, this should be ample demonstration that pet food companies can do what they want, as they are rich and powerful, while regulators are weak and cash strapped. With so much pressure from so many dead pets in so many congressional districts, the federal government eventually passed the Food Safety Modernization Act in 2010, three years after the event. The bill expanded the FDA's power, granting the agency the ability to implement mandatory recalls. Until then, all were technically 'voluntary' actions taken by the companies themselves. It also instructed the FDA to up the basic standards for pet food sanitation and force manufacturers to ensure their supply chain was at least safe. But as the next section demonstrates, so underfunded are they, that only a tiny percentage of suppliers, never mind their products, are currently checked. So, it's hard to see this one making much of a difference.

> ...As a result of the 2007 scandal, according to information provided by the accounting firm Heffler, Radetich & Saitta LLP in Philadelphia, $12,357,277 was estimated to have been paid to 20,229 US and Canadian aggrieved pet owners, a mere $611 per claim....

As for China's part, ConsumerAffairs.com (September 14, 2007) highlighted how China repeatedly blocked requests from the FDA to inspect the facilities suspected of producing the contaminated products. Ignoring melamine for a moment, this is worrying as China has an appalling safety record when it comes to food. In the past they have been implicated in a variety of scandals including fake baby food (can it get *more* fake?), soy sauce made from human hair, cuttlefish being soaked in ink to improve their colour and eels that were fed contraceptive pills to make them grow long and slender.[7] Not that an appalling safety record for food (certainly meat) quality has put off pet food manufacturers. As we highlighted previously, determined to keep costs down, the very next year after this scandal, imports of Chinese ingredients by American pet food companies *continued to grow*. In fact, in 2007, when the scandal was in full flow, these American pet food companies were importing 55,000,000 lbs of Chinese chicken for use in their products. By 2011, this figure had increased by 56% to 85,800,000 lbs.[14]

The problem for the consumer is trying to identify the origin of the ingredients used. Each multinational producer has factories around the world – always including one in Asia. The citing of manufacture aside, where each individual ingredient comes from, is none of your business. As dry food manufacturers are not rewarded for the quality of the ingredients they use in their mixes, they will opt for the cheapest, which invariably involves the cheapest labour and the most deplorable conditions for the animals in question. Today, that still means Asia, although the new US system of Concentrate Animal Feed Operations (CAFOs), which now produce the majority of their meat, is not far behind in terms of minimal space, dire welfare and indeed high chemical usage. The European Union do not permit the import of meat meals that were formulated using anything but human-grade meat waste, which excludes dead, diseased, dying, disabled animals and dogs – although how they actually verify and patrol this is unknown.

It clearly matters to your dog that they do, however. Chemical additives used in dry food are now shown to be second only to dietary protein in causing adverse food reactions in your dog.[15,16] Scientists have discovered chemicals in commercially available pet foods that have detrimental effect on sperm quality in dogs and also negatively affected male/female ratios and litter size over the last 30 years.[17] They also found an increased incidence of cryptorchidism in male offspring, a condition in which the testes fail to correctly descend into the scrotum. The environmental contaminants that are responsible for these effects, most notably diethylhexyl phthalate (DEHP) and polychlorinated biphenyl 153 (PCB153), were found in dry dog food and the dogs' testes, 'at concentrations reported to perturb reproductive function in other species. Testicular concentrations of DEHP and PCB153 perturbed sperm viability, motility and DNA integrity *in vitro*'.[17] And before genetics are blamed, the researchers concluded that due to the rate of deterioration and because their research was carried out over a relatively short period of time, genetics were not at play.

TAKE-HOME POINTS

✓ Dry food contains a dizzying amount of chemicals, the majority of which, such as anti-microbial agents, anti-caking agents, all the curing, drying and firming agents, any oxidising and reducing agents, pH control agents and surface-active agents. Not to mention synergists, texturisers, emulsifiers, humectants and stabilisers are not required to be listed on the pet food label.

✓ Sodium pentobarbital, the chemical used to euthanise pets, is the second most common cause of pet food recall in the United States.

✓ Waste meat destined for the meat and bone industry can be chemically denatured before rendering. The chemicals permitted include fuel oil, kerosene and carbolic acid.

✓ Employees have sued pet food producers following exposure to highly toxic phosphine gas, a rodenticide and pesticide that were sprayed on the grain as it arrives in the factory, presumably in an effort to reduce mycotoxins on poorly handled grain.

✓ The melamine scandal was the worst atrocity to affect dogs in living memory. Chinese wheat was being purposely contaminated with melamine, an oil derivative used in the plastics industry, in an effort to boost its protein content. Thousands of pets were killed. One hospital group alone estimated 39,000 cats were injured or killed. Despite some companies knowing the threat, they still didn't recall their products from shelves. The FDA would not inform owners who those companies were. It's still going on.

✓ Chemical additives used in dry food are now shown to be second only to dietary protein in causing adverse food reactions in your dog.

✓ Studies show chemicals in commercially available pet foods have detrimental effect on sperm quality in dogs and have also negatively affected male/ female ratios and litter size over the last 30 years.

Chapter Twelve References

1   Patrick, J.S. (2006). *Incestuous Pet Food Regulation Allows Consumers to Feed Ring Dings and Krispy Kremes.* Dissertation thesis. Available online, www.harvard.edu

2   Martin, A.M. (2007). *Food pets die for: Shocking facts about pet food.* Troutdale, OR. Newsage Press

3   Kennedy, W. (2014). *Recent report cites findings at former Mars Petcare plant; workers' lawsuit remains pending.* Joplin Globe Online, published Jan 20, www.joplinglobe.com

4   WHO (World Health Organisation, 2002). *Evaluation of certain food additives. Fifty-Ninth Report of the Joint FAO / WHO Expert Committee on Food Additives.* Official Publication. Available online, www.who.int

5   Kang, J.H. and Kondo, F. (2002). Determination of bisphenol A in canned pet foods. Research in Veterinary Science, 73, 177–182

6   Edinboro, C.H., Scott-Moncrieff, C., Janovitz, E. *et al.* (2004). Epidemiologic study of relationships between consumption of commercial canned food and risk of hyperthyroidism in cats. Journal of the American Veterinary Medical Association, 224(6): 879–886

7   Barboza, D. and Barrioneuvo, A. (2007). Filler in Animal Feed Is Open Secret in China. April 30, 2007. New York Times. Published online, Apr 30th, www.nytimes.com

8   Weise, E. and Schmit, J. (2007). *FDA limits Chinese food additive imports.* USA Today. Published online, Apr 30th, www.usatoday.com

9   ABC News (2007). *Doctors caution thousands more pet deaths expected.* ABC News. Published online, Mar 23, www.abcnews.go.com

10   Heavey, S. (2007). *U.S. Pet food Recall Widens amid Cross-contamination.* Reuters. Published online, May 4th, available online, www.reuters.com

11   Rumbeiha, W. and Morrison, J. (2011). A Review of Class I and Class II Pet Food Recalls Involving Chemical Contaminants from 1996 to 2008. Journal of Medical Toxicology, 7(1): 60–66

12   Wade McCormick, L. (2007). Tainted Dog Food Still Killing Dogs. Published online, Jan 10th, www.consumeraffairs.com

13   Cantwell, M. (2007). *Cantwell Presses FDA to Reveal All Companies That Received Contaminated Pet food Ingredients.* Published online, Apr 23rd, www.cantwell.senate.gov

14   USDA Global Agriculture Trade System. Sourced online, www.fas.usda.gov

15   Roudebush, P. (1999). *Hypoallergenic Diets for Dogs and Cats.* In Kirk's Current Veterinary Therapy XIII, Bonagura, J.D. (ed.), W.B. Saunders Co., Philadelphia, 1999. p530-536

16   Kennis, R. (2006). Food allergies: Update of pathogenesis, diagnoses, and management. Veterinary Clinics of North America: Small Animal Practice, 36(1): 175–184

17   Lea, R.G., Byers, A.S., Sumner, R.N.*et al.* (2016). Environmental chemicals impact dog semen quality *in vitro* and may be associated with a temporal decline in sperm motility and increased cryptorchidism. Scientific Reports, 6: 31281

CHAPTER 13

Hazardous Microbiologic Contamination

One of the standout reasons, we are told, to choose heavily processed, chemically preserved pet food over fresh meat-based products for our dogs is microbiological safety. This message resonates, in part, as history has taught us that fresh ingredients necessitate some care. Millions of food poisoning incidents (of humans) each and every day amply demonstrate that fresh ingredients handled poorly can put you on your ass or, at the very least, pooing a lot out of it.

Species-appropriate raw diets are compiled using meat and bone from the human food sector. The problem is the meat sector is positively rife with potentially harmful bacteria, with the United States leading the charge, thanks in no small part to the fact that the majority of their cases arise from concentrated animal feeding operations (CAFOs). These desperate, unhygienic, overcrowded hell holes are nasty bacteria heaven. They are, in fact, the breeding ground for the vast majority of our antibiotic resistant bacteria today. Here's how the Animal Legal section of the Michigan State University College of Law put it:

> CAFOs raise animal welfare, environmental degradation, and human health concerns. In terms of animal welfare, one of the greatest concerns is the close confinement and crowdedness of the animals. These conditions create boredom and stress in the animals, as well as physical and mental illnesses. In terms of environmental degradation and human health concerns, the number one problem is animal manure, which is produced in such massive quantities that the soil cannot absorb the waste, thus leaving it to run off fields and pollute the surrounding soil and water, including human drinking water. Additionally, methane emissions from CAFOs both contribute to greenhouse gases and create adverse

physical and mental health impacts in humans. CAFOs also increase the prevalence of antibiotic resistant diseases, due to the antibiotics regularly given to the animals.

Overcash 2011[1]

To keep the CAFOs going, the US is now seen to have some very worrying food hygiene policies. For instance, unlike *Escherichia coli* 0157, *Salmonella* isn't classified as an 'adulterant' under US law, meaning producers have no obligation to withhold contaminated batches. In 2015, the United States Department of Agriculture's (USDA's) Food Safety and Inspection Service introduced a new testing regime for US chicken slaughterhouses.[2] Among a number of rulings, they declared that up to 9.8% of chicken carcasses are permitted to fail for *Salmonella* by the end of the kill line (a line that includes a lovely bath in chlorine wash to kill bacteria, another step not permitted in the European Union) while no more than 15.6% are permitted to test positive for *Campylobacter.* They're a bit more flexible with 'chicken parts' where up to 15.4% may test positive for *Salmonella*. In fact, even when the USDA was petitioned by Laura MacCleary of US Regulatory Affairs (a food safety watchdog) to at least include antibiotic-resistant forms of *Salmonella* on the adulterant list, the USDA refused (published on the USDA website, FSIS-response-CSPI-020718.pdf).

Not that Europe is entirely off the hook here either. What began in Asia and was perfected by the Americans is now percolating across the pond, as it tends to do. There are more than 800 'mega farms' in Britain alone.[3] Pigs in the Netherlands are reared in such deplorable conditions that workers in the sheds are 760 times more likely to test positive for MRSA that the general public.[4] But at least the European Union has a zero tolerance policy for pathogenic bacteria such as *Salmonella* and *E. coli*, which reduces the threat somewhat.

Back in 2000, 22% of US raw retail chicken meat harboured some form of *Salmonella*[5] compared to just 6% of retail chicken in the United Kingdom.[6] 39% of United States chicken samples yielded *E. coli* (as well as 19% of the beef samples, 16% of the pork samples, 12% of turkey samples)[7] while the United Kingdom again is but a fraction of these figures. Even today the *Salmonella* content of United States poultry remains stubbornly high at 25%.[8]

The inevitable result is that a lot of Americans are going to get sick. One-in-seven of the United States population suffers from food-borne illnesses annually (though the CDC have it at roughly one of eight,[9] ten times the rate seen in the United Kingdom.[10] *Salmonella* infections alone result in 23,000 hospitalisations,

450 deaths and an estimated \$365 million in direct medical costs in the United States.[11]

It stands to reason, if you have to work with these contaminated ingredients, you're going to have problems. There are going to be a number of ways to cleanse your meat product of microbiological contamination, most importantly here cooking and chemicals. The raw dog food sector, by definition, is not supposed to employ either. This is good news for guts, nutrient content and digestibility, but it exposes products to bacterial contamination, certainly if you're manufacturing a product made on US meat. This is made all the worse by the pieces of meat raw dog food producers actually use.

Those furthest away from the gut cavity are least likely to suffer *Salmonella*. These include breast meat, steak, leg and shoulder meats, etc. The reason being, *Salmonella* (and *E. coli*) live inside the gut of the animal. When they are eviscerated, which in poultry is usually done by sucking the innards out with a vacuum-like machinery, snapping the gut tube and the neck and anus. The inevitable result is some digesta may spill into the surrounds. Giant cattle-slaughtering facilities suffer the same hygiene issues, all a result of the desire to process as much as possible as quickly as possible. Thus, while breast meat, leg and shoulder cuts are not always immune they are less likely to have issues.

Unfortunately, these are the parts consumed by humans and thus fetch a higher price on the market. All raw dog foods are made from cheaper cuts including wings, drumsticks and thighs (often less likely to have *Salmonella*) but also necks, carcass and, crucially, organ meats, all of which are more likely to pose problems. Exact pieces aside, manufacturers are free to source old, spent hens which are more likely to harbour *Salmonella* due to their physiological state.[12] And, as we discovered, loopholes exist, at least in the United States, that permit pet food manufacturers to use meat that hasn't passed veterinary inspection.

It should thus come as no surprise that numerous studies have detected *Salmonella* and *E. coli* in raw dog food products.[13-16] A Food and Drug Authority (FDA) investigation spanning two years (2010-2012) found that 8% (15/196) of raw dog food samples tested positive for *Salmonella*, 16% (32/196) for *E.coli*.[17] The FDA declined to mention which of the more than 2,500 serotypes of *Salmonella* they detected (as only 100 are pathogenic to humans). What they did highlight was "raw pet foods may harbour food safety pathogens, such as...*Salmonella*". Unfortunately, while the FDA and the USDA permit more than 15% of human food samples to fail for this pathogen, since 2013 they decided to impose a zero-tolerance restriction for the bug in pet food (see the FDA's "Compliance Policy

Guide for *Salmonella* in Food for Animals") – A tough deal for manufacturers there, considering the ingredients they have to work with.

However, it's not just the United States we see problems. In the Netherlands, van Bree *et al.* (2018)[18] analysed 35 commercially frozen raw dog foods from eight different suppliers. *Salmonella* was present in 20% of samples. *E. coli* O157 was isolated from 23% of samples. *Listeria monocytogenes* was present in 54% of samples. Worse still, and documented in the literature for the first time, 6% contained *Toxoplasma gondii* (a parasite that has now infected approximately 40 million Americans). Also, again for the first time, 11% contained the single celled parasite *Sarcocystis cruzi* and *Sarcocystis tenella*. *S. cruzi* is hosted by the dog and *S.tenella* by the cat, although it is nonpathogenic to both. The parasite is simply using them as a 'definitive host', a place where they reproduce and cast-off eggs in the faeces in order to get to their ultimate target animal, which is the cow and sheep, respectively. Neither of these parasites can infect humans. Another first occurred in 2019 when 13 cats were infected with five later dying from TB, allegedly after consuming a wild venison-based raw pet food product made by Natural Instinct in the United Kingdom.[19] On their website (naturalinstinct.com/venison, as of 2019), the company notes 'our suppliers of the wild venison offal had not had the offal inspected in line with European Union requirements'.

Focusing on just *Salmonella*, while it is clearly undesirable in any product that might share a fridge with human food, you need not be overly concerned for your dog. Dogs do not normally suffer salmonellosis, even when they are fed meat contaminated with it.[15,20] That said, it would be incorrect to say it never occurs. While it is suspected that more dogs might experience a subclinical form,[21] salmonellosis has been reported, albeit very rarely, in both cats and dogs fed both dry and raw dog food as well as gone off table ingredients.[21-25] An underlying sickness or stress is always suspected in these cases as we know dogs house *Salmonella* normally in their intestines to no ill harm,[26] albeit most species are of a nonvirulent strain. This is a normal trait of meat eaters. Big and small cats,[27] multiple free-ranging sea mammals[28] and even omnivores such as badgers and foxes[29] are all known to house *Salmonella* in their intestines *subclinically* (with no outward sign of disease). While obviously our intensively reared domestic animals are a major reservoir for the pathogen, wild prey including various game,[30] wild boar,[31] rodents[32] and numerous wild birds[33] are all potential carriers. In fact, some of what we consider the nastier species meat-eaters. Writing for *Nature*, Callaway (2014)[34] highlighted how various pathogenic microbes 'some of which are flesh-eating', help vultures and other carrion eaters to process their hazardous meals, akin to probiotics in humans.

I think it's fair to say that if your diet consists of fresh, *whole* animals and sometimes not-so-fresh meat, it simply wouldn't do to get sick from consuming it. Those individuals died out a long time ago. It's thought the dog has a number of protective measures in place including antibacterial saliva, extremely low stomach acids and undoubtedly a gut flora more than capable of keeping pathogenic bacteria such as *Salmonella* in place. This is why dogs can take their bone out to the back yard, put it down on the less than sterile ground, chew it for a bit, leave it for a while to warm in the sun and come back to it later. After a few hours they might bury it. After a few days, should they remember where they put it, they may dig it up again for a rechew. I know mine does. At this stage, the bone would be highly dangerous from a human point of view, yet your dog is happily chewing away with no ill effects.

The prevalence of *Salmonella* in clinically healthy dogs is estimated to range from 0–44 %[35,36] The higher figures are generally reserved for populations of greyhounds as these guys tend to be fed notoriously poor-quality meat. In one study, 112 samples of commercial raw meat for greyhounds were cultured for *Salmonella*.[37] and 45% were positive with *S. typhimurium*, a common pathogen of humans. Carter and Quinn (2000)[35] reviewed multiple studies from Iran, United Kingdom and the United States. They found that more than thirty serovars of *Salmonella* were found in healthy dogs, some of them pathogenic to humans. They note that 0–15% of household pets were shedding *Salmonella* compared to 16–24% of strays (in Iran and Sudan). This difference in prevalence between the two is understandable, considering their lifestyles.

The problem is when dogs consume foods contaminated with *Salmonella* there is a small (2–6%) to very good (44%) chance they will shed that *Salmonella* in their faeces for up to 7 days afterward.[13,20,38] It is for this reason, a dog shedding the wrong sort of *Salmonella* (dogs and cats naturally house numerous *Salmonella* species in their intestines, few of which are pathogenic) is considered to be a human health risk by some authors.[13,15,36,39]

While it's indisputably true your raw-fed dog *may* thus be a possible vector of harmful bacteria, it's interesting to note that so far it seems to be proving quite unlikely. In regard to salmonellosis, at the time of writing, with millions now fresh feeding their pets worldwide, there has only ever been four documented instances of a virulent species of *Salmonella* identified in both patient and product, the first occurring in 2018.[40,41] However, whether it was from the food itself in the fridge, poor food handling by their parents, the dog's bowl or their stool is unknown. An enormous survey of raw feeders by DogRisk, a research group from the

University of Helsinki, Finland, set out to examine the rate of food-transmitted pathogens in raw-feeding households. They had 16,475 households respond from 81 countries.[41] While 24 of those households had suspected contamination from pet food, only three analysed the meat fed to their pets and identified the same pathogen that infected the individual. All were *E. coli*. This means that, even allowing for the unverified suspicions, more than 99.6% of households feeding their pets raw food did not report any pathogens being transmitted from the food to humans. Crucially, this was over the entire time they had been feeding raw food to their pets, which ranged from several weeks to 65 years. If we pluck an average figure of just 5 years, with 1.5 meals per day (some adults get one, some get two, pups get many), across 16,475 households, that is more than 45 million raw meals!

This suggests the feeding of raw dog food is quite safe, at least when compared to the rate of *Salmonella* in the general population. Perhaps this is because most of us are equipped with a healthy respect of raw meat from a young age. As a raw meat-based product, this care in handling is naturally shifted to raw dog food products that can now share our fridge. Unfortunately, that care and indeed history of owner safety does not extend to dry pet food.

Wait…what? Didn't your vet warn you?! Yes, commercial dry dog food is not only a potential source, but also it seems people are far more likely be infected with *Salmonella* as a result of handling it.

When Carter and Quinn (2000)[35] were reviewing the incidence of *Salmonella* in healthy dry and raw-fed dogs around the world, they list the potential food sources of *Salmonella* to be uncooked offal and bones, raw eggs, raw chicken and *commercial dry dog foods*. The reason being dry dog food can contain *Salmonella*. In fact, it is the top cause of dry dog food recall today, by a considerable degree. In just the first 5 years of this decade (2010–2015) there were 19 colossal dry and canned pet food recalls due to *Salmonella* contamination, involving many thousands of tonnes of pet food. Taken from *www.fda.org* animal and veterinary recalls archive, these were as follows:

- 2015 Bravo recalls select chicken and turkey pet foods because of possible *Salmonella* after issues were detected separately by the New York and Colorado State Departments of Agriculture.

- 2014 Hill's Pet Nutrition voluntarily recalls Science Diet Adult Small & Toy Breed due to possible *Salmonella* contamination. "All 17 affected customers have been contacted by Hill's, and there have been no reported illnesses related to this product to date."

- 2014 Pro-Pet LLC recalls dry dog and cat foods because of possible *Salmonella*.

- 2014 PMI Nutrition recalls cat food due to possible *Salmonella*. The issue was detected after routine testing by the FDA Detroit District Office identified possible *Salmonella* contamination, upon which the company recalled their product 'out of an abundance of caution'.

- 2014 Bravo issues nationwide recall of 8 different pet foods for dogs and cats due to possible Listeria. The issue was detected when 'an independent lab detected the bacteria in a sample during a recent review'.

- 2013 Nestlé Purina voluntarily recalls Purina White Meat Chicken and Whole Barley Recipe adult dry dog food bags due to possible *Salmonella* health risk.

- 2013 P&G voluntarily recalls 11 types of Eukanuba and 18 types of cat and dog food due to possible *Salmonella* health risk.

- 2013 Natura Pet issues voluntary recall of Specialised Inova and Evo dry pet foods after the FDA identified possible *Salmonella* health risk.

- 2012 Breeder's Choice Pet food recalls AvoDerm Natural Lamb Meal & Brown Rice adult formula because of possible *Salmonella* health risk.

- 2012 Solid Gold Health Products for pets recalls for possible *Salmonella* health risk.

- 2012 Apex Pet Foods initiates voluntary recall of dry pet food due to the potential for *Salmonella*.

- 2012 Natural Balance Pet foods initiates voluntary recall of dry pet foods due to the potential for *Salmonella* contamination.

- 2012 Diamond Pet Foods recall dry dog food, chicken soup for pets and Diamond Puppy Formula due to possible *Salmonella* contamination.

- 2011 Nestlé Purina recalls One Vibrant Maturity 7+ Dry cat food recall due to potential *Salmonella*.

- 2010 P&G voluntarily recalls dry cat food due to potential *Salmonella* exposure.

- 2010 P&G voluntarily recalls Iams and Eukanuba specialised dry pet foods due to potential *Salmonella* health risk.

- 2010 P&G voluntarily recalls Prescription Renal Diet cat food due to a possible *Salmonella* health risk, detected by the FDA.

- 2010 Natural Balance Pet Foods Inc. voluntarily recalls Natural Balance Sweet Potato & Chicken dry dog food due to a possible *Salmonella* health risk, detected by the FDA.

- 2010 Feline's Pride issues nationwide recall of its Natural Chicken Formula cat food due to *Salmonella* contamination.

With nobody discussing this elephant in the room, it follows that people are going to get sick and the figures sadly reflect that. In 2007, Schotte *et al.* (2007)[42] linked an outbreak of illness in staff who were looking after military kennels in Montevideo, Uruguay to contaminated dry commercial feed. In another incident, following a major outbreak of *Salmonella schwarzengrund* in the United States a colossal study was undertaken by Behravesh *et al.* (2010),[43] who found dry dog *and* cat food to be the cause for the outbreak. However, it took the two teams 3 years to establish this. In that time seventy-nine people in twenty-one states were poisoned with *Salmonella schwarzengrund* – half of them were children under 2 years of age. The issue was traced back to Mars Pet Care who ended up recalling over 23,000 tonnes of pet food sold under 105 different brand names.[44] In 2012, the CDC in the United States reported that 53 people from around the United States and Canada had contracted *Salmonella infantis* from dry dog food (or their dry-fed dogs), 20 of whom were again children under 2 years of age. One in three ended up in hospital.[45]

This means, since 2007, at least 132 people are known to have contracted *Salmonella* from dry food, despicably half them were children under two years of age, compared to possibly four adults from a raw dog food product (as of Sep 2020). And yet, despite the colossal recalls and the very real possibility of toddlers getting infected, has a single vet group anywhere *ever* warned these families of the potential risk sitting on the floor of their cupboard?

Nor is it just *Salmonella* you should watch out for with dry food. Susan Thixton's group, the Association for Truth in Pet Food (ATPF), advocates for pet owner rights. In 2016, two of their members sat on the board of The Association of American

Feed Control Officials (AAFCO) who set the guidelines for pet food production, an unbelievably privileged position for a fresh food advocate, considering who might populate the rest of the board (more on AAFCO later). In 2016, the ATPF decided to assess just how bad the microbial situation was in ultra-processed pet food. They published the first publicly funded analysis of 12 top brand pet foods (six cat and six dog foods). These included Hill's, Royal Canin, Science Diet, Prescription Diets and Cesar.[46] Cleverly, to avoid accusations of handler bias and threat of court action, the products were ordered online and shipped directly to the laboratory for testing. They were tested for nutrient excesses, dangerous bacteria and toxic fungi. All failed in some respect, many on all three counts. In relation to pathogenic bacteria, 9 of the 12 products contained bacteria the FDA terms as 'qualifying pathogens'. Included were *Streptococcus* (of strep throat fame, seven of the 12 ultra-processed pet foods tested), *Staphylococcus* (common cause of food poisoning in humans, 10 of the twelve of the ultra-processed pet foods tested), *Bacillus* spp. (common cause of food poisoning, 10 of the 12 ultra-processed pet foods tested).

Another level of concern, considering the quality of meats permitted for use in this sector, is drug-resistant bacteria. Chaban *et al.* (2010)[47] investigated the shedding of *Campylobacter* by apparently healthy (n=70) and diarrhoeic (n=65) dogs. The diets of all the healthy dogs were recorded and fifteen of them ate some or all raw meat and bone. They found that 58% (41 of 70) of the healthy dogs were shedding *Campylobacter* (97% of the diarrheic dogs were shedding the bug, though sadly the authors neglected to record a single piece of information regarding their diet at the time). So, even if all the raw-fed dogs were shedding *Campylobacter* (unlikely), at least half of the dry-fed dogs were, too. And, unlike raw dog food, authors have isolated the same species of drug-resistant *Campylobacter jejuni* from a dog fed a commercial dry diet as detected in a girl infected with the same species.[48] Similarly, Leonard *et al.*[49] assessed the antimicrobial resistance patterns of *Salmonella* and *E. coli* recovered from pet dogs (n=132) in Ontario between 2005–2006. They found 96% were shedding antimicrobial resistant *E. coli* in their faeces. Unless every owner in Ontario was raw feeding back in 2005, then it's more than clear that commercial diets are not sorting that problem out either. Worse, 41 of those *E. coli* samples were resistant to two or more drug classes. This is not to say drug-resistant bacteria will not be found in raw dog food but as they must use ingredients that were fit for human consumption, it is hoped the threat will be less, at least in the European Union.

The truth is, it seems, when it comes to harmful bacteria there are no safe choices. However, unlike raw dog food, it's not just bacteria you need to watch out for in dry pet food. These products contain a whole host of pathogens that you probably have never heard of and some of them, particularly a toxic group of moulds, are among the most pathogenic natural substances on the planet.

Mycotoxins are poisonous chemical compounds produced by certain moulds that live on various foods, including nuts, fruits, soy, cereals and grain, when they are handled, transported and stored incorrectly. We know the grain used in pet food is subpar.[50] In fact, it is firmly established that cereal by-products are diverted to animal feed even though, due to processing methods, they are known to contain mycotoxins at concentrations greater than raw cereals.[51,52] Moreover, cooking offers no protection.[53] Even after production, bags of dry food must then be transported great distances in varying conditions to sit on warm shelves for months. Then the client opens the bag and exposes the contents to air, warmth and humidity, and leaves it sitting in his cupboard for weeks. It should come as no surprise then, that despite manufacturers employing various chemical antifungal measures, such as spraying incoming ingredients with the deadly phosphine gas, the majority of dry, cereal-based pet foods contain some amount of mycotoxins.[51] When Thixton's group tested eight foods for the presence of these toxic moulds, *all* tested positive (four were low-risk, two were medium risk, two were high risk). Some of the nastier mycotoxins found in high numbers by the authors included *Aspergillus* (can cause tremors and convulsion, bloody diarrhoea and lower immune response), *Fumonisins* (can cause lower food intake, digestive disorder, impact liver function, lowering immune response) and *Zearalenone* (impacting reproduction and sexual maturity, can cause irregular heats, pseudo-pregnancy and abortions).

Authors repeatedly show that long-time exposure to low levels of the mycotoxins found in pet foods will pose a health risk to dogs.[52,54-56] We have known this for some time. In their study titled "Mycotoxins: Hidden Killers In Pet Foods", Devegowda and Castaldo (2000)[57] highlight that as early as 1952, a case of hepatitis in dogs was directly linked to the consumption of mouldy pet food. Boermansa and Leungb (2007)[58] use numerous studies to show the consumption of mycotoxins, including aflatoxins, ochratoxins, trichothecenes, zearalenone, fumonisins and fusaric acid by our pets, can result in "chronic diseases such as liver and kidney fibrosis, infections resulting from immunosuppression, and cancer".

Of all the mycotoxins you should worry about, aflatoxin is by far the most dangerous to you and your dog. It is among the most carcinogenic substances known to man.[59] It only rose to prominence in the 1960s when 100,000 turkeys and ducks died after consuming contaminated peanut meal. Unfortunately, we find dry pet food is rife with aflatoxin.[53,57,60,61,62] In fact, in just four years, there have been six major dry pet food recalls for aflatoxin:

- 2013 Hy-Vee issues voluntary recall of certain dry dog food products due to elevated levels of aflatoxin, detected by the Iowa State Department of Agriculture.

- 2011 Advanced Animal Nutrition recalls Dog Power dry dog food due to above acceptable levels of aflatoxin.

- 2011 O'Neal's Feeders Supply recalls Arrow Brand dry dog food for above acceptable levels of aflatoxin.

- 2011 Cargill Animal Nutrition recalls River Run and Marksman dry dog foods for above acceptable levels of aflatoxin.

- 2011 P&G voluntarily recalls dry dog food for above acceptable levels of aflatoxin.

- 2010 Kroger recalls pet foods as products may contain aflatoxin.

Sadly, dogs are especially susceptible to its toxic effects.[61] In 1998, 55 dogs died in Texas after eating dog food containing levels of aflatoxin that varied only between 150 and 300 parts per billion.[60] In 1998, aflatoxin killed at least twenty-five dogs.[63] The Pet food Recalls of www.FDA.org tells us that over one million pounds of dog and cat food manufactured in the United States were recalled following the discovery of this toxin. In 2006, corn aflatoxin killed perhaps 100 dogs.[64] These pets died with symptoms ranging from enlarged, pale yellow livers, cirrhosis, chronic hepatopathy, hepatic lipidosis, portal fibroplasias and biliary hyperplasia. Untold more suffered but survived following bouts of anorexia, lethargy, vomiting, jaundice and diarrhoea.

> The actual number of pets affected by adulterated pet food is not known because hitherto there was no adverse reporting system for pet foods
> **Rumbeiha and Morrison, 2011**[63]

This is why authors repeatedly note that mycotoxin contamination in pet food poses one of the most serious health threats to pets today.[53,55,57,58,62] Even the mouthpiece for the pet food sector, www.PetfoodIndustry.com, seems to be in agreement. In 2013, when addressing the rise of vegan dry foods, they published a piece on mycotoxins, which concluded as follows:

> Pet foods with plant-derived proteins may also contain more harmful toxins than pet foods with traditional fish and meat proteins, according to new research from the University of Guelph.
>
> **www.pet foodindustry.com, 23 August, 2013**

In a piece titled "Cancer-Causing Toxin Found In Hong Kong Pet Food Sparks Alarm", the *South China Morning Post* (July 20, 2017) reported how a Hong Kong consumer association tested numerous brands of dry kibble pet foods and found that multiple US-made pet foods contained aflatoxins, including Nestlé Purina, Mars Pedigree, Hill's Science Diet and KiteKat, albeit under the acceptable threshold. The paper reported the Purina manufacturer as stating the carcinogen aflatoxin was an 'unavoidable natural contaminant'.

It gets worse. The same group found two US-made pet foods contained melamine (Gold Adult Dog Food and Iams Chicken Cat Food) and cyanuric acid (found in Purina Pro Plan), which you should remember caused the deadly 2007 Chinese melamine scandal.

It's still going on, 10 years after this terrible scandal broke.

Nor is it just aflatoxin. There have been recalls for vomitoxin which, as its name implies, will leave you very, very sick. Like aflatoxin, vomitoxin loves grain – wheat, barley, oats, rye and corn. But, unlike aflatoxin, it is not carcinogenic. While it will irritate the gastrointestinal tract immensely and possibly give you stomach ulcers, it's unlikely to kill you. The FDA has established a level of 1 ppm restriction of vomitoxin in the human food chain, a 5 ppm restriction in dogs and cats, even though we are many times bigger than they are. Go figure!

In 1995, Nature's Recipe were forced to pull thousands of tonnes of dog food, costing the company approximately $20 million, when pet owners complained that their dogs began to vomit and lose their appetite. The incident prompted the FDA's Agriculture Policy Advisor, Dina Butcher, to step in to investigate. She concluded humans need not fear as, needless to say, 'the grain that would go into pet food is not a high-quality grain' (Knight Ridder 1995 – yes, that's his real name!)

Then there are storage mites. Brazis *et al.* (2008)[65] note how storage mites such as *Tyrophagus*, *Acarus* and *Lepidoglyphus* are important potential allergens in dogs with atopic dermatitis.

They opened 10 different premium commercial dry dog foods, (one actually formulated for dogs with skin disorders) and stored them for 6 weeks under two different environmental conditions. After 5 weeks, mites were detected in 9 out of ten of the diets. Mites are a human health risk too. In a piece titled, "When Mites Attack: Domestic Mites Are Not Just Allergens", Ciu (2014)[66] highlighted how storage mites, (separate from dust mites, as they occur widely in and contribute to the deterioration in quality of stored products like grains and foodstuffs) can cause diseases in the mouth but also in the pulmonary, intestinal and urinary systems of humans.

For all these reasons, to suggest that dry food is a *safer* alternative to fresh food from an infection point of view, for them or us, is ignorant (at best) to blatantly misleading. This stance pushes consumers blindly towards a product that repeatedly demonstrates it will gravely sicken children and maim and kill your dogs, often with bugs that do not exist on meat-based products.

It thus comes with some dismay that, in 2012, the American Veterinary Medical Association (AVMA), one of the most influential veterinary groups on the planet (proudly cash-sponsored by Hill's Pet Food), came out with their "Resolution #5 Policy on Raw or Undercooked Animal-Source Protein in Cat and Dog Diets" for vets. It states:

> …several studies reported in peer-reviewed scientific journals have demonstrated that raw or undercooked animal-source protein may be contaminated with a variety of pathogenic organisms…

This we know is true. Raw food products have had their share of recalls for *Salmonella* and *E. coli* over the last decade. However, we also know the reverse is true, yet zero space was given by the AVMA to this crucial point. In fact, one of the references the AVMA cites in support of their statement, Strohmeyer *et al.* (2006)[16] analysed twenty raw dog foods as well as two dry and concluded *both* product types contained *E. coli*. Sadly, this was deemed irrelevant by the AVMA scientists.

The AVMA goes on to say:

> …secondary transmission of these pathogens to humans (e.g., pet owners) has also been reported…

Now this was interesting, that in 2012, I was aware of no such study or report of any kind. The very first *suspected* case materialised in the literature in 2018. To support this crucial statement the AVMA uses four studies. The first study[13] didn't note any transfer of pathogens to humans. It found *Salmonella* in raw-fed dog stool and stated, "dogs fed raw chicken *may* therefore be a source of environmental contamination".

The second study, titled "Human Health Implications Of Salmonella-Contaminated Natural Pet Treats And Raw Pet Food",[15] states the fourth line of their summary 'no confirmed cases of human salmonellosis have been associated with these diets'. Hmmm, so no joy there either.

The third supportive study[15] was of two cats with unknown health histories, that contracted salmonellosis. The authors concluded, 'this report provides evidence that the practice of feeding raw meat-based diets to domestic cats may result in clinical salmonellosis'. No mention of sick humans there either.

The fourth and last study[39] shows there is a risk that humans can become infected with *Salmonella* after handling contaminated meat products intended for dogs, such as pet shop bones and pigs' ears dog treats. So, not raw dog food then.

Thus, of the four studies the AVMA used to support their widely referenced statement that 'secondary transmission of these pathogens to humans (e.g., pet owners) has also been reported', none make any such conclusion whatsoever. Largely as, at their time of publication, there was no such evidence in existence, only multiple cases of dry dog food causing Salmonellosis in humans, which again, was somehow missed by the AVMA.

On this sort of evidence, the AVMA rules out fresh ingredients as a whole for all dogs and cats, recommending that vets worldwide 'never feed inadequately treated animal-source protein to cats and dogs'.

This is clearly science of the poorest kind. I wonder what would happen if I showed the AVMA the 2015 CDC report on food poisoning in people,[9] which highlights that 48,000,000 Americans suffer from a food-borne illness each year and 3,000 are killed by it. And the top food culprits? You guessed it – fresh fruit and vegetables.

Seedy vegetables, such as tomatoes or zucchini, and fruit accounted for 18% and 12% of *Salmonella* cases, respectively. (Eggs and chicken account for 12% and 10%, respectively, with beef accounting for 9% and pork 8%). Leafy vegetables accounted equally for more than a third of all *E. coli* cases. Fruit accounted for half of all *Listeria* illnesses. And yet, with the obvious dangers of fruit and vegetables so clearly established, nobody is calling for a blanket ban on fresh vegetables, leafy greens and antioxidant rich fruit, in favour of something processed, pulverised, preserved and packaged by a candy company.

The dry pet food industry knows its ingredients are contaminated; it's why they try ever more inventive ways of killing the bugs. A recent idea was irradiating the food. Unfortunately, this didn't work out too well for the animals eating it. Between June 2008 and March 2009, 87 cats in Australia developed hind limb paralysis on eating an imported, irradiated dry pet food.[67] Following their investigation of dry pet food products causing *Salmonella* poisoning in the United States, Behravesh *et al.* (2010)[43] concluded their study with the following crucial advice that you won't hear repeated by the average vet:

> …this outbreak highlights the importance of proper handling and storage of pet foods in the home to prevent human illness, especially among young children…

It's a small wonder people are getting sick from the stuff. Who here has handled dry dog food without washing their hands? Back in my training days, I've had it in my pockets to use as treats. I've eaten it! We store big open sacks of it on the floor where smaller humans crawl and get dangerously sick as a consequence. We treat dry food complacently because nobody is warning us, despite the literature showing it is often crawling with potential pathogens, many of which you will not find in a raw meat-based dog food product.

I honestly believe, to help reeducate the masses, both raw *and* dry pet food (and pet shop treats such as pigs' ears) should come with a health warning. At the very least, as with raw dog food, you should keep dry pet food out of the reach of children, wash your hands and surfaces after each use and make sure to pick up your pet's stools daily.

> You will always make more money exploiting people's irrationalities than you can by fixing them.
> **Richard Thaler, Winner of the Noble Prize for Economics, 2017**

TAKE-HOME POINTS

✓ The meat industry is rife with pathogenic bacteria. The issue is significantly worse in the United States than in the European Union.

✓ Raw dog food manufacturers making raw products based on the carcass, neck and organs from this industry are very exposed to microbiological contamination. Tests show pre-made raw dog foods often fail micro testing, with *Salmonella* present in 8–20% of samples taken in the United States and the European Union.

✓ Your dog is a meat eater, a carcass scavenger, a poo eater. *Salmonella* in their food (and in their intestines) is a very normal phenomenon for them. While healthy dogs are safe, the more they consume, the more they will pass out in their faeces.

✓ Of domestic pet dogs, 0–15% are thought to shed *Salmonella* normally. Authors note potential sources for this contamination is raw meat and bones, eggs and commercial dry food.

✓ With all the focus on raw, we must keep in mind *Salmonella* is the number one cause of dry pet food recall today. From just 2010 to 2015, there were 19 colossal dry and canned pet food recalls for the issue.

✓ In just the last 8 years (2012–2019), 68,000 tonnes of dry food have been recalled for pathogenic bacteria. During the same time, only 900 tonnes of raw were recalled for the same issue, and that is with the FDA looking *only at raw* from 2015.

✓ Since 2007, 132 people are known to have contracted *Salmonella* from ultra-processed pet food, half of them toddlers under 2 years of age.

✓ Dry pet food is also known to contain a variety of other human pathogens, including *Streptococcus*, *Staphylococcus* and *Bacillus*.

✓ Nearly 50% of dry-fed dogs also shed *Campylobacter.* Authors have isolated the same species of drug-resistant *Campylobacter jejuni* from a dog fed a commercial dry diet as detected in a girl infected with the same species.

- ✓ Apparently healthy dry fed dogs appear to shed *E. coli*, with many samples resistant to two or more drug classes.

- ✓ The quality of grain used in pet food is of very poor quality. Manufacturers know this and treat it with chemicals to prevent fungal growth. Despite this, studies show dry food is positively rife with mycotoxins such as aflatoxin and vomitoxin, among the most pathogenic natural substances on the planet. Authors show their consumption by pets can result in chronic diseases of the liver and kidney, immunosuppression and cancer.

- ✓ Open bags of dry food are very prone to storage mites, which are a human health risk.

- ✓ Misleading statements focusing on the microbiological threat of raw dog food by influential groups such as the AVMA inadvertently push people toward the ultra-processed dry foods, whose threat level is never discussed by these groups, let alone checked. As our vets remain oblivious to the threat, both pets and people are going to continue to get sick.

- ✓ Dry pet food has contributed to the deaths of thousands and thousands of pets in the last decades. This is compared to a tiny handful on fresh/raw dog food, with most stemming from people feeding poorly balanced meals to their pets. No pre-made raw food to date is documented to have killed a single pet.

- ✓ Fresh fruit and vegetables are the top causes of *Salmonella*, *E. coli* and *Listeria* in humans, not meat. This is not a reason to exclude such food items from your diet. It is a warning that you need to clean up the food chain and take some simple precautions.

Chapter Thirteen References

1   Overcash, E.A. (2011). *Overview of CAFOs and Animal Welfare Measures*. Michigan State University College of Law, Animal Legal & Historical Center. Available online, www.animallaw.info

2   USDA (2015). *Changes to the Salmonella and Campylobacter verification testing program: Proposed performance standards for Salmonella and Campylobacter in not-ready-to-eat comminuted chicken and turkey products and raw chicken parts and related agency procedures*. Published online, www.federalregister.gov

3   Wasley, A. and Davies, M. (2017). *The rise of the "megafarm": How British meat is made.* The Bureau of Investigative Journalism. Published online, Jul 7th, www.thebureauinvestigates. com

4   Voss, A., Loeffen, F., Bakker, J. *et al.* (2005). Methicillin-resistant *Staphylococcus* aureus in pig farming. Emerging Infectious Diseases, 11(12): 1965–1966

5   Schlosser, W., Hogue, A., Ebel, E. *et al.* (2000). Analysis of *Salmonella* serotypes from selected carcasses and raw ground products sampled prior to implementation of the Pathogen Reduction; Hazard Analysis and Critical Control Point Final Rule in the US. International Journal of Food Microbiology, 58: 107–111

6   FSA (Food Standards Agency) Report (2001). *UK-wide Survey of Salmonella and Campylobacter Contamination of Fresh and Frozen Chicken on Retail Sale.* Published online, www.food.gov.uk

7   Zhao, C., Ge1, B., De Villena, J. *et al.* (2001). Prevalence of *Campylobacter* spp., *Escherichia coli*, and *Salmonella* serovars in retail chicken, turkey, pork and beef from the greater Washington, D.C., Area. Applied Environmental Microbiology, 67(12): 5431–5436

8   Kindy, K. (2014). *Foster farms outbreak sparks legal petition to outlaw dangerous pathogens.* Washington Post. Published online, Oct 1st, www.washingtonpost.com

9   Interagency Food Safety Analytics Collaboration (2018). *Foodborne illness source attribution estimates for 2015 for Salmonella, Escherichia coli O157, Listeria monocytogenes, and Campylobacter using multi-year outbreak surveillance data, United States.* GA and D.C.: U.S. Department of Health and Human Services, CDC, FDA, USDA-FSIS. 2018. Published online www.cdc.gov

10   Wasley, A. (2018). *Dirty meat: Shocking hygiene failings discovered in US pig and chicken plants.* The Guardian Newspaper. Published online, Feb 21st, www.theguardian.com

11   Sjolund-Karlsson, M., Howie, R.L., Blickenstaff, K. *et al.* (2013). Occurrence of beta-lactamase genes among non-Typhi *Salmonella enterica* isolated from humans, food animals, and retail meats in the United States and Canada. Microbial Drug Resistance, 19(3): 191–197

12   USDA (2005). *ANNEX B - Distribution of Salmonella Prevalence in Hens and Eggs.* Sourced online https://www.fsis.usda.gov

13   Joffe, D. J. and Schlesinger, D. P. (2002). Preliminary assessment of the risk of *Salmonella* infection in dogs fed raw chicken diets. Canadian Veterinary Journal, 43: 441–442

14   Weese, J.S., Rousseau, J. and Arroyo, L. (2005). Bacteriological evaluation of commercial canine and feline raw diets. Canadian Veterinary Journal, 46: 513–516

15   Finley, R., Reid-Smith, R. and Weese, J.S. (2006). Human health implications of *Salmonella*-contaminated natural pet treats and raw pet food. Clinical Infectious Diseases, 42: 686–691

16   Strohmeyer, R.A., Morley, P.S., Hyatt, D.R. *et al.* (2006). Evaluation of bacterial and protozoal contamination of commercially available raw meat diets for dogs. Journal of American Veterinary Medical Association, 228: 532–542

17   Nemser, S., Doran, T., *et al.* (2014). Investigation of *Listeria*, *Salmonella*, and toxigenic *Escherichia coli* in Various Pet Foods. Foodborne Pathogens and Disease, 11: 706–709

18 van Bree, F.P.J., Bokken, G., Mineur, R. *et al.* (2018). Zoonotic bacteria and parasites found in raw meat-based diets for cats and dogs. Veterinary Record, 182(50)

19 Kelly, R. (2019). *Feline tuberculosis cases in the UK traced to raw cat food.* VIN News Services. Published online, May 15th, www.news.vin.com

20 Finley, R., Ribble, C., Aramini, J. *et al.* (2007). The risk of *Salmonellae* shedding by dogs fed *Salmonella*-contaminated commercial raw food diets. Canadian Veterinary Journal, 48: 69–75

21 Morse, E.V., Duncan, M.A., Estep, D.A. *et al.* (1976). Canine salmonellosis: A review and report of dog to child transmission of *Salmonella enteritidis*. American Journal of Public Health, 66(1): 82–83

22 Stacker, C.L., Galton, M.M., Cowdery, J. *et al.* (1952), *Salmonellosis in dogs. II. Prevalence and distribution in greyhounds in Florida.* Journal of Infectious Diseases, 91: 6–11

23 Stiver, S.L., Frazier, K.S., Mauel, M.J. *et al.* (2003). Septicemic salmonellosis in two cats fed a raw-meat diet. Journal of American Animal Hospital Association, 9: 538–542

24 Wright, J.G., Tengelsen, L A., Smith, K.E. *et al.* (2005). Multidrug-resistant *Salmonella typhimurium* in four animal facilities. Emerging Infectious Diseases, 11(8): 1235–1241

25 Selmi, M., Stefanelli, S., Bilei, S. *et al.* (2011). Contaminated commercial dehydrated food as source of multiple *Salmonella* serotypes outbreak in a municipal kennel in Tuscany. Vet Italiana, 47: 183–190

26 Burnie, A.G., Simpson, J.W., Linsay, D. *et al.* (1983). The excretion of *Campylobacter*, *Salmonellae* and *Giardia lamblia* in the faeces of stray dogs. Veterinary Research Comment, 6:133

27 Pretorius, A.M., Kuyl, J.M., Isherwood, D.R. *et al.* (2004). *Bartonella henselae* in African Lion, South Africa. Emerging Infectious Diseases, 10(12): 2257–2258

28 Gilmartin, W.G., Vainik, P.M. and Neill, V.M. (1979). *Salmonellae* in feral pinnipeds off the Southern California coast. Journal of Wildlife Disease, 15:511–514

29 Chiari, M., Ferrari, N., Giardiello, D. *et al.* (2014). Isolation and identification of *Salmonella* spp. from red foxes (*Vulpes vulpes*) and badgers (*Meles meles*) in northern Italy. Acta Vet Scandinavia, 56(1): 86

30 Magnino, S., Frasnelli, M., Fabbi, M. *et al.* (2011). *Game Meat Hygiene in Focus.* Wageningen: Wageningen Academic Publishers. *The monitoring of selected zoonotic diseases of wildlife in Lombardy and Emilia-Romagna, northern Italy*; p223–244

31 Wacheck, S., Fredriksson-Ahomaa, M., König, M., Stolle, A. *et al.* (2010). Wild boars as an important reservoir for foodborne pathogens. Foodborne Pathogens and Disease, 7:307–312

32 Lapuz, R., Tani, H., Sasai, K. *et al.* (2008). The role of roof rats (*Rattus rattus*) in the spread of *Salmonella Enteritidis* and *S. Infantis* contamination in layer farms in eastern Japan. Epidemiology and Infection, 136(9): 1235–1243

33 Pennycott, T.W., Park, A., and Mather, H.A. (2006). Isolation of different serovars of *Salmonella enterica* from wild birds in Great Britain between 1995 and 2003. Vet Record, 158: 817–20

34   Calloway, E. (2014). Microbes help vultures eat rotting meat. Nature. Published online, Nov 26th, www.nature.com

35   Carter, M.E. and Quinn, J.P. (2000). *Salmonella infections in dogs and cats*. In: Wray C, Wray A, editors. *Salmonella in domestic animals*. Wallingford, UK: CAB International; 2000. p231–244

36   Sanchez, S., Hofacre, C.L., Lee, M.D. *et al.* (2002). Animal sources of salmonellosis in humans. Journal of the American Veterinary Medical Association, 221: 492–497

37   Chengappa, M.M., Staats, J., Oberst, R.D. *et al.* (1993). Prevalence of *Salmonella* in raw meat used in diets of racing greyhounds. Veterinary Diagnostics and Investigation, 5(3): 372–7

38   Lenz, J., Joffe, D., Kauffman, M. *et al.* (2009). Perceptions, practices, and consequences associated with foodborne pathogens and the feeding of raw meat to dogs. Canadian Veterinary Journal, 50(6): 637–643

39   LeJeune, J.T. and Hancock, D.D. (2001) Public health concerns associated with feeding raw meats to dogs. Journal of the American Veterinary Medical Association, 219: 1222–1225

40   FDA (2018). *FDA investigates outbreak of Salmonella infections linked to raws for paws ground turkey food for pets*. Published online, Feb 9th, www.fda.gov

41   Anturaniemi, J. (2018). *The relationships between environment, diet, transcriptome and atopic dermatitis in dogs*. Doctoral dissertation. Faculty of Agriculture and Foresty, University of Helsini. Available online, www.helda.helsinki.fi

42   Schotte, U., Borchers, D., Wulff, C. *et al.* (2007). *Salmonella montevideo* outbreak in military kennel dogs caused by contaminated commercial feed, which was only recognized through monitoring. Veterinary Microbiology, 119(2–4): 316–323

43   Behravesh, B., Ferraro, A., Deasy, M. *et al.* (2010). Human *Salmonella* infections linked to contaminated dry dog and cat food, 2006–2008. Pediatrics, 126(3): 477–483

44   Reinberg (2008). *Salmonella* outbreak tied to dry dog food continues. ABC News. Published online, Nov 7th, www.abcnews.go.com

45   US Centre for Disease Control and Prevention (CDC, 2012). Multistate outbreak of human *Salmonella infantis* infections linked to dry dog food (Final Update). Published online, July 18th, www.cdc.gov

46   Thixton, S. (2015). The Pet Food Test Results. Published online, https://truthaboutpetfood.com/the-pet-food-test-results

47   Chaban, B., Ngeleka, M. and Hill, J.E. (2010). Detection and quantification of 14 *Campylobacter* species in pet dogs reveals an increase in species richness in feces of diarrheic animals. BMC Microbiology, 10:73

48   Damborg, P., Olsen, K.E.P, Nielsen, E.M. *et al.* (2004). Occurrence of *Campylobacter jejuni* in pets living with human patients infected with *C. jejuni*. Journal of Clinical Microbiology, 42(3): 1363–1364

49   Leonard, E.K., Pearl, D.L., Finley, R.L. *et al.* (2012). Comparison of antimicrobial resistance patterns of *Salmonella sp.* and *Escherichia coli* recovered from pet dogs from volunteer households in Ontario (2005–06). Journal of Antimicrobial Chemotherapy, 67(1)

50   Corbin, J. (1996). Pet foods and feeding. Feedstuffs, 17 July: 80–85

51   Sharmaa, M. and Márquez, C. (2001). Determination of aflatoxins in domestic pet foods (dog and cat) using immunoaffinity column and HPLC. Animal Feed Science and Technology, 93(1–2): 109–114

52   Scudamore K.A., Hetmanski M.T., Nawaz S. *et al.* (1997). "Determination of mycotoxins in pet foods sold for domestic pets and wild birds using linked-column immunoassay clean-up and HPLC". Food Additives and Contaminants. 14 (2): 175–186

53   Aquino, S. and Corrêa, B. (2011). Aflatoxins in pet foods: A Risk to Special Consumers. Universidade Nove de Julho, Intech, pdf 22032

54   Leung, M.C., Díaz-Llano, G. and Smith, T.K. (December 2006). Mycotoxins in pet food: a review on worldwide prevalence and preventative strategies. Journal of Agricultural and Food Chemistry. 54 (26): 9623–9635

55   Böhm, J., Koinig, L., Razzazi-Fazeli, E. *et al.* (2010). Survey and risk assessment of the mycotoxins deoxynivalenol, zearalenone, fumonisins, ochratoxin A, and aflatoxins in commercial dry dog food. Mycotoxin Research, 26(3): 147–153

56   Streit, E., Schatzmayr, G., Tassis, P. *et al.* (2012). Current situation of mycotoxin contamination and co-occurrence in animal feed-focus on Europe. Toxins, 4(10): 788–809

57   Devegowda, G. and Castaldo, D. (2000). *Mycotoxins: hidden killers in petfoods. Is there a solution?* In: Technical Symposium on Mycotoxins. Alltech Inc, Nicholasville, Kentucky, USA.

58   Boermansa, H.J. and Leung, M.C. (2007). Mycotoxins and the petfood industry: Toxicological evidence and risk assessment. International Journal of Food Microbiology, 119(1–2): 95–102

59   Hudler, G. (1998). *Magical mushrooms, mischievous moulds*. Princeton, NJ: Princeton University Press.

60   Bingham, A.K., Huebner, H.J., Phillips, T.D. *et al.* (2004). Identification and reduction of urinary aflatoxin metabolites in dogs. Food and Chemical Toxicology, 42(11): 1851–1858

61   Stenske, K.A., Smith, J.R., Newman, S.J. *et al.* (2006). Aflatoxicosis in dogs and dealing with suspected contaminated commercial foods. Journal of the American Veterinary Medical Association, 228(11): 1686–1691

62   Maxwell, C. K., Díaz-Llano, G. and Smith, T.K. (2006). Mycotoxins in Petfood: A Review on Worldwide Prevalence and Preventative Strategies. Journal of Agricultural Food Chemistry, 54 (26): 9623–9635

63   Rumbeiha, W. and Morrison, J. (2011). A Review of Class I and Class II Pet Food Recalls Involving Chemical Contaminants from 1996 to 2008. Journal of Medical Toxicology, 7(1): 60–66

64   Muirhead, S. (2006). Pet food varieties recalled (Food and Drug Administration and state feed regulatory agenices investigation of dog deaths). Feedstuffs, 78(3): 3

65   Brazis, P., Serra, M., Sellés, A. *et al.* (2008). Evaluation of storage mite contamination of commercial dry dog food. Veterinary Dermatology, 19(4): 209–214

66   Cui, Y. (2014). When mites attack: domestic mites are not just allergens. Parasitic Vectors, 7: 411

67   Child, G., Foster, D.J., Fougere, B.J. *et al.* (2009). Ataxia and paralysis in cats in Australia associated with exposure to an imported gamma-irradiated commercial dry pet food. Australian Veterinary Journal, 87(9): 349–351

CHAPTER 14

The Argument for Raw Feeding

You may remember from my introduction that I was a little put out when the local vets in Perth, Western Australia, had no interest in my small raw dog food test which resulted in some of their most 'allergy-prone' dogs getting fully better in a matter of weeks. Perhaps even harder to take was when I couldn't convince my boss at the time via a lengthy and characteristically detailed presentation (which soon became my first canine nutrition seminar later that year) that dry food was likely not in the interest of our dogs. This was particularly unforgiveable as I was showing them the results of another Australian Guide Dog organisation that was not only feeding raw to their entire colony but was now reporting some incredible things about their vet bills.

Encouraged by a small test of their own, and while all other Guide Dog schools were and still to this day are sponsored by Mars Pet Food in Australia, Guide Dogs Queensland (GDQ) decided to go their own way. In 2009, under the guiding hand of their formidable CEO, Chris Laine, they moved their entire working colony (approximately 216 dogs at the time, circa 2009) to all-raw-fed. The results after *just 1 year* were staggering. In recent correspondence with Chris, I was reassured their vet bills fell by some 80,000 Australian dollars. By all accounts, the incidence of skin, ear and gut conditions in the Brisbane dogs plummeted, the very same as my dogs in Perth. The dogs were weeing less, and urinary tract infections were resolved (all Australian working dogs are fed Mars Advance pet food, then and now in 2020. We analysed this product's salt content in Chapter 10). They also had some interesting things to say about joint issues and panosteitis, two things Guide Dogs really fear as it can take a dog out of training.

A piece in the Brisbane newspaper, *The Courier Mail* documents the switch as follows:

A plague of health issues persuaded chief executive Chris Laine that change was needed, and since then she says there have been some remarkable results. Healthcare costs have dropped 82 per cent, despite the colony expanding. Serious skin and digestive issues have all but vanished and healthier teeth and gums have been observed, along with reduced body odour and fresher breath. The switch is all the more notable because the group, a registered charity stretched for funds, was offered free dry food if it endorsed a brand.

Murray, 2011[1]

The last line in relation to offers of free food in return for endorsement is something most large dog organisations can testify to. I remember a previous boss of mine saying a top pet food company offered them free food if we would go on record saying it helped our dogs focus better. I would love to name the brand but, like so many of these anecdotal stories, it wouldn't be in this book's interests.

It got even better for GDQ. Very quickly, Laine made another leap by having their own brand of raw dog food manufactured. They called it Leading Raw and it took off. Who wouldn't buy pet food recommended by a guide dog organisation? Very soon GDQ was not only feeding a top quality raw for next to nothing but they were making serious money. It was a brilliant move, ensuring the financial future of their organisation for years to come, to the great benefit of the thousands in need of their services. A real success story.

The last social media post I can find on the GDQ Facebook page pertaining to Leading Raw pet food was December 14, 2014. It said they were expanding their range to include natural treats. And then, nothing. There is no farewell. No announcement regarding the sale of the product range back to the manufacturer. Not a single scandal on the product or the organisation. Nothing. In 2015, Chris Laine was replaced with a new CEO and GDQ was immediately back to feeding Mars Advance pet food, in line with the rest of the guide dog schools in Australia. Leading Raw lasted 5 years.

What happened? I asked Chris Laine the same thing recently. She replied:

…I believe my contract wasn't renewed because I would not conform and sign the Mars contract with the other states… I was already getting free RAW food for the colony so I saw no benefit to the contract with Mars... only an unhealthy down side.

Chris Laine in email to me, 2020

When Chris left GDQ, many other key employees, particularly those working with the dogs, left soon after. It is hard to overstate how committed you get to the health and welfare of these phenomenal dogs, especially when you spend 24/7 with them.

One of those staff members was Lauren Elgie. Lauren is the only geneticist and animal breeding specialist working in canine colony management and service dog reproduction in the southern hemisphere. Equipped with a deep knowledge of canine breeding, she now owns and is managing director of Career Dogs Australia, a seed breeding program for various Service Dog organisations both in Australia and around the world. When Lauren talks about breeding a solid pup, we should listen. On the GDQ controversy, Lauren says:

> Even though raw-feeding the dog colony at GDQ was a massive success it was always controversial at the board level and with our general practice vets. The organisation enjoyed extremely significant savings with respect to colony vet expenses, but lacking vet support it was always going to be hard for the program to confidently stand over the practice long term.
> **Lauren Elgie to me, *personal correspondence***

Lauren feeds exclusively raw food to their breeding stock. They wean all their pups on to raw and support their pregnant and lactating broods with a highly nutritious raw food blend developed from Lauren's years of experience feeding raw to the GDQ colony. In Lauren's opinion, it gives them the best chance at optimal growth, digestive health, orthopaedic health and fertility prospects.

> Unfortunately, when we place our stock into various service dog organisations, they are inevitably fed kibble, which is a little disappointing as I feel they may not reach their potential with respect to optimal growth and health. I also believe that raw feeding positively and significantly impacts a dog's general state and behaviour.

One important point to remember is that there are many guide dog schools in Australia. There are five schools under the Royal Guide Dogs Associations of Australia umbrella dotted around the country. Mars sponsors them all, as it does Australian Seeing Eye Dogs (two major schools in Australia). In fact, it seems Mars is one of the biggest sponsors of Guide Dog schools the worldwide.

Still, at some point someone somewhere surely would have needed more than simply Mars's' bruised ego to make such a move on such an adored organisation.

In that respect, I'm confident the positional statement on raw made by the American Animal Hospital Association (AAHA) just months previously did not help matters. A quick Google search reveals how it scuppered fresh feeding for so many service dogs in the United States at the time, much to the dismay of countless owners who value their dog's health far beyond such organisations or the companies investing in them. For clarification, I have shortened the following statement for berevity and added italics for effect.

> Past proponents of raw food diets *believed* that this was the healthiest food choice for pets. It was… also *assumed* that feeding such a diet would cause no harm to other animals or to humans. There… have subsequently been *multiple studies* showing both these premises to be false. Based on… *overwhelming scientific evidence*, AAHA does not advocate or endorse feeding pets any raw or… dehydrated non-sterilised foods, including treats that are of animal origin… It is especially important… that therapy pets involved in AAI fed raw protein diets.
>
> **AAHA 2014 Positional Statement on Raw Feeding**[2]

The AAHA is the second major veterinary governing body in the United States, the other being the American Veterinary Medical Association (AVMA). It happens that, much like the AVMA's positional statement on raw that erroneously claimed raw was harming humans, the AAHA's short piece on raw feeding is replete with unsubstantiated claims and unforgivable errors. But it is the last line, where the AAHA eliminates the use of fresh food for the service dogs of America based on "overwhelming scientific evidence" that angers me the most. This highly influential and yet completely unreferenced statement (granted, they did put a handful of studies below for us to wade through and attempt to attribute to each point) is an excellent example of the selective application of science to make a point. Because of the damage it has done and as it will set up so well for what is to follow in the third section, I'm going to pull apart this statement, line by line.

Their use of the word *believed* in the very first line is terribly ironic. It is an attempt to imply that the matter, presumably that cereal-based pet food made by candy manufacturers is the healthier choice for dogs and cats, has been put to bed. However, the *fact* remains, among all their noise and cries of 'science' and 'the need for evidence' there is not *a single* head-to-head study of any value available to us which suggests this unnatural, ultra-processed, high carbohydrate diet outperforms a fresh, species appropriate diet for these meat eaters.

I'll give you a second to take in the implications of that statement.

The very basics of evidence-based science is proving in a set manner that something is better than a control. A control group is where you expect the *normal* results. It gives you a vital standard to compare your test group against. In pharmaceuticals, the control group will not be receiving a treatment (or, more likely, they would be given a sugar pill, called a placebo). In this case, the control group would be the usual, established method – a fresh, species-appropriate diet. And yet, despite having more than adequate resources to get the job done and seven decades to do it, the dry pet food sector has never, EVER found it necessary to produce a *single peer-reviewed work* comparing a 'complete' dry food to a suitably 'complete' premade raw dog food. This is real *evidence* and it is conspicuous by its total absence in the literature. Worse still, it seems, the entire *evidenced-based* veterinary community has never required it. That the dogs in their clinic seem OK is enough for them. Unfortunately, science isn't interested in speculation.

Take my best friend for example, the picture of health and irritatingly good at football, far better than I was (I'm confident he won't be reading this). Our manager said he was our most valuable player. It happens that he smoked, and I didn't. What does that tell us about smoking? The answer is nothing at all. Any more than my holding up (almost literally) my 94-year-old Granny, a chronic alcoholic, as a testament to the effects of drinking (Granny wasn't an alcoholic, though by all accounts she was addicted to tea and French fancies). If you want to see firsthand the effects of smoking, you pitch eleven smokers against eleven nonsmokers of equal ability, allow no substitutions and watch the eleven non-smokers finish them in the second half.

This is clearly a crucial point and we will spend more time looking at 'pet food science' in the next section. For now, we can be thankful that they are not the only ones looking at the problem.

Numerous circumstantial works indicate a high cereal diet may not be to the dog's advantage. We have already shown obesity is better controlled, that sled dogs incur less injury and that dogs with chronic kidney failure all appear to do better on diets containing more (animal) protein. But many works are now emerging that point to the benefit of feeding dogs a species-appropriate, fresh, raw diet (SAFR diets?!). Leading the way in such studies is the veterinary department of the University of Finland, otherwise known as DogRisk*. Their first foray into the benefits of raw began with an exploratory work that analysed the voluntary information submitted by 632 clients of a raw dog food company. [3] The participants were given a blank box in which to write their comments. A total of 206 reported that their dogs had had skin related issues. Of these, 152 (74%) voluntarily reported total recovery from symptoms while a further 36 (17%) voluntarily reported 'significant recovery' from symptoms after their change to a raw dog food diet. That's 91% of dog owners reporting a significant to total recovery following their move to raw dog food (for reasons we will elaborate on shortly). One hundred and forty five dogs had gastrointestinal problems prior to their dietary change,while 127 of those (88%) enjoyed a complete recovery following a change to raw (with a further 6% experiencing 'significant recovery'). That's 94% reporting significant to total recovery of gut issues. Of these, 38 dogs had eye-related issues. Seventy nine percent of these experienced total recovery (with a further 8% enjoying 'significant recovery' from their symptoms) following their move to raw. Fifteen had urinary tract problems and 53% had complete recovery from symptoms (with a further 13% seeing 'significant recovery') following their move to raw. Twelve pet owners avoided the euthanising of their pet. These are not insignificant results.

Inspired by these findings, the team of vets began investigating further. Next, they focused on the incidence of canine hip dysplasia (CHD) in German Shepherd dogs (GSD) using data from their files. Genetics aside, several environmental factors contribute to the development of CHD, nutrition (and overfeeding) being two.

Grundström (2013)[4] examined the hypothesis that feeding a species-appropriate raw diet might protect large-breed dogs from CHD. Their poster was presented at the Waltham Nutritional Symposium in 2013. They analysed information from 287 GSD owners ranging in age from 2–6 months (54 with CHD, 103 without) and 6–18 months (49 with CHD, 81 without) and found that feeding a species-appropriate diet consisting of raw meat, raw offal, raw bone and raw cartilage, raw fish, raw egg and raw tripe could protect GSD from CHD. The data further showed that even if only a part of a kibble-fed dog's diet is supplemented with raw food, it could help protect puppies from CHD. Interestingly, the study found that feeding cooked meat, bone and cartilage might increase the risk.

In 2015, DogRisk was back with their most convincing work to date[5] as it involved a head-to-head of raw and dry-fed dogs with atopy (exhibiting a heightened immune response to common allergens). This time they measured the metabolite levels in dogs suffering atopy. In particular, they were looking at homocysteine, a by-product of the metabolism, which is related to a number of diseases, but dogs suffering allergy/immune responses have higher levels of it in the blood. It's fair to say it's something you'd like to see less of in the body.

What they found was indicative of everything we have discussed previously. First, dogs eating raw food had 0.17 nM homocysteine in their blood. Dry-fed dogs had 1.57 nM, nearly a ten-fold increase. But even more remarkably, when raw dry-fed dogs were moved to raw they suffered a near five-fold increase in homocysteine (from 0.17 nM to 0.77 nM) while dry-fed dogs changed to raw enjoyed a five-fold decrease in homocysteine (from 1.57 nM to 0.30 nM).

They followed up this work with a paper presented at 42nd WSAVA Congress in 2017. They found that compared to raw, dogs eating a dry diet showed a highly changed regulation of genes in the skin, proving dry food seems to have a dramatic impact on skin gene expression. These findings were verified by Anderson *et al.* (2018),[6] using peripheral blood mononuclear cell (PBMC) gene expression, microarray profiling. This catchy named technique is a minimally invasive tool commonly used in human diet intervention studies. They concluded that a meat diet was associated with a decrease in cytokine gene and receptor expression compared to a kibble diet. The kibble-fed dogs had increased expression of immune-related genes/pathways and elevated plasma IgA concentrations.

This work paints a very clear picture – in comparison to raw dog food, dry food is likely causing a lot of inflammation in dogs. Whether this is due to its high cereal content, high chemical content, the types of protein used, the lack of fresh fats or maybe even processing technique, remains unknown.

The DogRisk* group followed up this work with a colossal cross-sectional questionnaire of more than 8,000 dogs. They investigated if diet, in this case if an ultra-processed carbohydrate-based diet (UPCD) or a non-processed meat-based diet (NPMD), might be associated with the development of canine atopic dermatitis.[7] They found feeding UPCDs resulted in a significantly higher risk of canine atopic dermatitis. Feeding NPMDs during the prenatal and early postnatal periods had a significant negative association with the incidence of canine atopic dermatitis in adult dogs (aged above 1 year).

Author's note:

DogRisk is a phenomenal canine research group hailing from the University of Helsinki, Finland. They exist on donations. The more of these they get, the more studies they will produce. It is vital for dogs the world over that they continue their excellent work. Please consider donating just $1 a month or even a year. Every little bit helps. Please visit their website: www.dogrisk.com.

In the same year, Iowa State University evaluated four commercially manufactured raw meat and bone diets (RMBDs) formulated for canids in zoos by using domestic dogs as a model owing to the functional and digestive anatomical similarities between the domestic dogs and their wild counterparts. They set out to assess, 1) the digestibility of the diets, 2) the microbial risk to humans and 3) that there be no adverse health implications on canine health as a result of feeding the RMBDs. They found:

> …overall, nutrients in RMBDs were highly digested by domestic dogs and diets did not result in clinical signs of gastrointestinal upset/distress. Further, RMBDs did not negatively influence general health status in dogs as measured by serum chemistry, electrolytes, complete blood count (CBC), and histology of gastrointestinal tract and associated tissues… using chamber evaluation of intestinal integrity and barrier function indicated possible benefit of feeding RMBDs to dogs.
>
> **Iennarella-Servantez, 2017**[8]

In fact, in response to comments by one Dr. Buffington in 2008, who stated that there was no evidence to suggest there was anything wrong with feeding dry, cereal-based pet food to meat eaters, Dr. MacMillan (2008)[11] promptly sourced seventy veterinary research papers that directly blamed pet food for causing cancer, kidney failure, cystitis, dilated cardiomyopathy, struvite crystals and calcium oxalate stones, among many other illnesses. MacMillan concludes:

> …Veterinarians who make money out of the sale of pet foods and from the illnesses they create are betraying pets and pet owners by failing to tell them that feeding such poor-quality nutrition will eventually cause illness in the pet…
>
> **MacMillan, (2008)**[9]

As we slowly come to learn the devastating effects of a life spent on such a poor food substrate, one area that is now harnessing a lot of attention is the impact on gut flora. Algya *et al.* (2018)[10] took four types of pet food diets including dry kibble, two types of cooked tray products and raw dog food, and compared them for macronutrient digestibility, serum chemistry, urinalysis and faecal characteristics, including metabolites and microbiota. They found that raw diets were highly palatable and highly digestible. Crude protein was better digested when presented raw than dry; raw-fed dogs exhibited reduced blood triglycerides (fat in the blood), maintained faecal quality and serum chemistry, and adapted their faecal microbial community to their new diet.

A stable, healthy gut flora is central to your health. It's incredible to think you are more bacteria cells than human cells; in fact, on a DNA basis, they outnumber you 10 to 1. You have around 1.5 kg of them happily living in your gut. They do the house cleaning, consuming not only all the undigested food and symbiotically providing for us some vitamins and useful by-products, but also sloughed epithelial cells and mucus that lines our guts. But we now know their role goes far beyond simply providing us with vital nutrition. They are a defensive barrier from pathogens, educating and working alongside our immune system from the time we are born to keep us and ultimately themselves in business. They can interfere with the adherence of pathogens to the intestinal mucosa by signalling for more mucous production. Their by-products reduce the growth of potential pathogens. They fix up any gaps in the gut membrane, prevent leaky gut and reduce our susceptibility to food allergies. The gut flora is now known to play roles in a myriad of diseases from weight gain and diabetes to heart disease and cancer. But it's their role in behaviour that personally interests me the most.

> You have two wolves constantly battling inside you, one is bad and one is good. Which one wins? The one you feed.
> **Adapted from a Cherokee Native American Proverb**

When we think of the gut flora, we assume it is simply bacteria. However, in there you have a myriad of bacterial communities, fungi, all sorts of single-celled protozoans and numerous viruses all whizzing around, living in something close to harmony, a harmony brought about by competition. When all is well, the good guys (commensal microbes) keep the bad guys (pathogenic microbes) in check. The payoff for feeding them has positive repercussions for your health – a perfect symbiotic relationship carefully developed since you first crawled from the primordial ooze. However, should something upset that balance (dysbiosis), and the bad guys have a chance to flourish, their presence and by-products tend to come at the expense of host fitness. The disruption of normal digestion alone can result in a myriad of health issues for the animal. There will be less house cleaning, less gut repair, more inflammation. You will suffer less protection from pathogenic bacteria. Above all, you will absorb less of the beneficial by-products normally produced by the commensals. As your gut flora is responsible for more than 90% of the feel-good hormone serotonin in the body, the inevitable consequence is a negative impact on behaviour. Studies show disrupting the gut flora has negative psychological consequences in practically every animal studied, including dogs.[11,12]

The good news is we can eat our way out of a funk, too. We know the consumption of probiotic yoghurts, fermented vegetables and kefir, foods that contain life, has enormous physical and mental health benefits, that's why we call them probiotics,which is Latin meaning "for-life". Behaviour in rats and humans can be significantly improved in the low individual by feeding probiotics.[13,14] While kibble manufacturers boast their products are chemically barren of any life whatsoever, whole food proudly contains life. Animals on dry food will never enjoy the obvious health benefits of consuming probiotics from their food.

Nor is it simply the chemical anti-life in kibble negatively impacting the dry-fed dog's biome. Harsh processing measures denatures protein, making it more resilient to digestion. Different bacterial communities now thrive on this new food source, fueling dysbiosis in cats.[15,16] Section 2 reveals how fibre, both soluble and insoluble, slows the passage of digesta and feeds certain bacterial groups, radically shifting the gut flora of dogs.

Kichoff *et al.* (2019)[17] compared the faecal biome of 31 dogs rescued from a dog fighting ring, 21 of whom were displaying problem behaviours. Analysis revealed an association between gut biome and aggression. Feeding raw dog food results in a more balanced growth of bacterial communities and a positive change in the readouts of healthy gut functions in comparison to extruded diet in eight boxers[18]. These changes are expected to be good but measuring that is complex. Sandri *et al.* (2016)[18] noted a high correlation for short-chain fatty acids (SCFA's) in the stools of meat-fed dogs, in particular butyrate. Largely produced by the microbiota, butyrate has been shown to have profound central nervous system effects on mood and behaviour in mice, acting like an antidepressant.[19] Similarly, BARF diets have been found to increase faecal levels of gamma-aminobutyric acid (GABA) in dogs.[20] GABA is a major inhibitory neurotransmitter of the mammalian central nervous system. It decreases certain activity in your brain, turning certain processes off, calming you down. It follows that decreased levels of GABA are implicated in the pathophysiology of several neuropsychiatric disorders, including hyperactivity and attention deficit disorder, anxiety and depression.

Nor are these the only behavioral concerns with feeding kibble. Vitamin B$_6$ (pyridoxine) is required for the conversion of tryptophan to serotonin (a now-famous relaxing neurotransmitter) and melatonin (a nice, relaxing hormone). Other

B vitamins are required for the efficient absorption of B_6. So, vitamin B complex is very important for a calm mind. Processing, certainly extrusion, destroys heat liable vitamins such as B complex. Hoffmann LaRoche (1995)[21] examined the effect of dry food storage times of just six months, vitamin B_1 fell by more than 57%, Vitamin B_2 fell by more than 32%, Vitamin B_{12} fell by 34%. But unbelievably, they noted a Vitamin B_6 loss of 89% in canned dog foods. Mooney (2010)[22] noted serious vitamin B losses after just 6 weeks of stressed shelf-life testing.

Then there is the power of fat. Omega-3, in particular EPA and DHA, are essential for normal brain development, playing a pivotal role in the regulation of synaptic plasticity and neurogenesis as well as dopamine neurotransmission. Rat diets deficient in omega 3's result in aggression and stress behaviours, while decreasing learning ability[23]. It's the same in dogs. A study of 18 aggressive German Shepherds showed lower omega-3 concentrations and higher omega-6 concentrations (from the copious plant ingredients), resulting in a higher omega-6/omega-3 ratio.[24] Despite this, Hadley et al. (2017)[25] found one in four best-selling, 'complete' dry foods tested contain zero or practically zero EPA and DHA. DHA deficiency in pregnant and lactating bitches affects the brain development of puppies[23]. Simply supplementing dry diets with fish oil containing high levels of DHA improves the learning capability of puppies compared to those fed low-level DHA fish oil.[25,26]

And what of carbohydrates? Kids after a birthday party – is it the sugar or the chemicals? It's hard to say. Cereal-based pet food, with its high carbohydrate load and rapid digestion, is a very high glycaemic food, not unlike a children's breakfast cereal. A study measured the impact of breakfast cereals of different glycaemic loads on the mental performance of children (where high glycaemic foods contain a lot of carbohydrates that are easily digested, delivering their sugar payload rapidly into the blood). Memory was assessed by asking the candidates to recall a series of objects. The ability to sustain attention was measured by asking for a response after various delays. The incidence of negative behaviour was recorded when playing a video game that was too difficult to allow success. It was found that a low glycaemicload breakfast resulted in better memory and attention spans, with fewer signs of frustration, and more time was spent on task.[13] There is a reason behaviour is one of the first improvements noted by owners when changing from kibble to fresh, species-appropriate dog food (author comment) but sadly, it remains the least studied. It remains a facet of health of zero concern to the pet food industry. It does not factor in pet food formulation, regulation or manufacturing. Thus, in terms of revealing literature, we have little to go by. Published in the Journal of Small Animal Practice, Mugford (1987)[27] noted how eight agitated Golden Retrievers that changed from commercial dry or canned diets to home-prepared meals made of beef and rice showed improvements in behaviour. The authors concluded that in most cases, people who have dogs with behavioural problems should move their pets from a normal commercial diet toward a home-prepared one.

Anderson and Mariner (1971)[28], of the University of Durban-Westville, South Africa, studies 100 dogs exhibiting negative behaviours, of which 86% were dry-fed. The dogs were permitted to feed *ad lib* on fresh meat (minced offal, beef, chicken, tripe) and cooked vegetables. Raw meaty bones were provided two to three times per week. of these clients, 98% reported 'dramatic' improvement. The authors concluded that an appropriate diet (coupled with restricted exercise, in the case of hyperactivity) is 'unequivocally therapeutic in treating a wide cross-section of behaviour problems'.

Now, to the second line of the AAHA statement above–it was assumed such a diet would cause no harm to animals (who assumes that?) or to humans (or that?!) which they follow up with 'there has been multiple studies showing both these premises to be false'. As we highlighted with the AVMA statement which stated the very same thing, at the time the AAHA went to press with their positional statement on raw (2014), there was not a single incident on record of a human being harmed by raw dog food. The references they include underneath do not support that statement. Instead, it seems the AAHA is happy to direct pet owners toward a product that has poisoned at least 130 people with *Salmonella* in the last decade alone, half of them toddlers under 2 years of age.

To support their point regarding raw causing harm to animals, the AAHA referenced some instances of nutrient imbalances resulting from members of the public feeding some pretty bad home-prepared mixes to their pets (such as just chicken breast to cats for a long period of time or 80% white rice to German Shepherd pups) resulting in harm and a very small number of pet deaths to which we will return later. With all its focus on the potential hazards of fresh pet food to both pet and human health alike, the AAHA appeared to have little time to address the very real threat posed by dry pet food. This means no mention of any one of the innumerable instances we have highlighted above where dry pet food has maimed and killed sometimes hundreds, sometimes thousands and sometimes tens of thousands of pets in the past, unlike premade raw dog food.

One of the reasons for the high death toll in pets fed 'complete' dry foods is that users, often under advice from their vet, rarely move from their product of choice, day in day out. Unfortunately, we know a staggering number of these 'complete' ultra-processed foods fail to meet the minimum nutritional standards as set out by The Association of American Feed Control Officials (AAFCO). This ensures sickness in the animal over time.

Hodgkinson *et al.* (2004)[29] analysed 33 brands of dry food for growing dogs available in Chile. Among a range of issues, the authors found two products contained inadequate levels of calcium, seven had an incorrect calcium to phosphorus ratio, seven had insufficient zinc, twelve had too little iodine and thirteen had too little potassium. Overall, only 4 of the 33 dog foods contained adequate levels of protein, EAA's, fat (including linoleic acid) and minerals. In total, the authors concluded, only nine (27%) of the 33 dog foods might provide adequate nutrition for dogs at specified maintenance level.

A study of cat foods revealed drastically unpredictable adherence to labelling requirements and nutrient requirements. Nine of 20 cat foods did not adhere to their 'guaranteed analysis' and eight did not adhere to the standards for nutrient composition.[30] On top of this, the authors noted various deficiencies and excesses of crude protein, crude fat, fatty acid and amino acids in the majority of the products.

A New Zealand study compared the nutrient composition of 29 wet cat foods to the AAFCO cat maintenance nutrient profile. They found nine of the foods did not meet the AAFCO nutrient profiles, four contained excessive levels of methionine, 5 contained inadequate taurine. In all, 60% of the budget, 18% of the premium and 43% of the super-premium foods failed to meet the AAFCO standards.[31]

In the most shocking of all, Davies *et al.* (2017)[32] tested more than 170 dry and canned pet foods sold in the UK. They found that a staggering 94% of the 'complete' canned food and 62% of the 'complete' dry foods were not compliant with FEDIAF/AAFCO's minimum guidelines.

When Semp (2014)[33] conducted blood trials of dogs fed complete, cereal-based pet food (n=20), they observed 7/20 (35%) of the dogs were outside their reference range (RR) for vitamin B_{12}, 5/20 (25%) were outside the RR for folic acid, 5/20 (25%) were outside the RR for iron, 12/20 (60%) were outside their RR for L-carnitine and 2/20 (10%) were outside their reference range for protein (5.4–7.6 g/dl).

In my opinion, the steadfast belief of the veterinary sector in the 'completeness' of dry food belies how unequipped they are to have a serious nutritional conversation. It's nonsense to assume that a single food, day in day out, will best suit every animal at every point in time. Ignoring the complete and unnecessary tedium of it, we know that exposure to different challenges and maladies throughout life create varying energy and nutrient requirements through time.

Euthenics is the study of an individual's metabolic requirements instead of the population. It shows us that individual animals will vary greatly in their need for vitamin, nutrient and energy requirements depending on their metabolic state and genetic makeup. Even though humans are approximately 99.9% identical at the genetic level, the 0.1% difference in the genetic sequence is sufficient to produce phenotypical differences, such as varying eye colours, height, susceptibility to diseases and responses to bioactive components of food. This implies, for optimal health, diets would be personalised to each individual's needs. In the wild, vertebrate predators demonstrate they will regulate their intake of certain prey items at certain times to balance the gain of macro-nutrients, and that failure to do so can result in fitness penalties.[34-36]

Moreover, study after study shows that adding pretty much anything to these 'complete' products results in some form of benefit to the animal. We have already shown how adding something such as blueberries to 'complete' pet food can increase the performance of sled dogs. Fish oil can vastly improve the health of dogs suffering arthritis and inflammatory skin conditions. Milgram *et al.* (2005)[37] preserved the cognitive abilities of senior dogs over 2 years simply by adding some antioxidants and a mix of spinach flakes, tomato pomace, carrot granules, citrus pulp and grape pomace to their 'complete' dry food. A remarkable study in Scottish Terriers revealed that by simply replacing a significant proportion of their kibble diet with vegetables including leafy greens and yellow/orange vegetables three times a week reduced the risk of these dogs developing transitional cell carcinoma (bladder cancer) by a staggering 90% and 70%, respectively.[38] Khoo *et al.* (2005)[39] found that supplementing a pup's 'complete' dry food with more antioxidant, in this case more vitamin E, improved their immune response to vaccinations, concluding 'the minimum AAFCO recommendation for dietary vitamin E (50 IU/kg) may not be sufficient to protect cells during periods of immune stress'.

How can these simple additions benefit a dog if his original meal was already 'complete' at the time? For dogs fed the same 'complete' meal each day, this vital health boost in a time of need, via some simple dietary additions, will never come. It seems the only thing extra we are permitted to feed is drugs to treat the disease that will inevitably kick in following the absence of the aforementioned nutrients.

> Virtually all pet foods contain unsubstantiated claims for safety, completeness and balance that no human food in the world would ever be able to.
>
> **Dr Elizabeth Hodgkins, Once Director of Technical Affairs at Hill's Pet Nutrition, Hodgkins, 2007**[40]

I always put this question to the crowd during a seminar: can you name a single processed food for humans that is better than the ingredients it was made from? It's amusing to watch the gears turning. I still haven't come up with anything. The reason I ask is because the answer is so telling. Every single one of the millions of species on earth thrive on fresh, biologically appropriate food. Only humans, dogs and cats consume ultra-processed food and we humans are advised to avoid it at all costs.[41-44]

And still, on the back of such unsupported nonsense and in the face of some working dog organisations reporting both health and thus financial improvements with its use, one of the most influential veterinary governing bodies in the world removes fresh, species appropriate food from what are some of most precious dogs on the planet. How can such a vacuous, misleading statement be accepted by our entire veterinary sector? Why aren't more vets speaking up for fresh food here? Something rotten is going on... and I'm about to show you what.

TAKE-HOME POINTS

- ✓ Queensland Guide Dogs once used raw dog food to feed their colony. During that time the CEO reported major health and financial benefits. The CEO was removed in 2015 and dry feeding was reinstated, in line with all other Australian guide dog schools.

- ✓ Ironically the *evidence-based* veterinary industry favours the use of dry, ultra-processed, cereal-based pet food over fresh, species appropriate meals for meat eaters without a single head-to-head comparison of any merit suggesting it's a particularly smart thing to do. Not one.

- ✓ A survey of 632 raw fed dogs shows that 67% of owners jumped to raw in the hope it might help fix their pets maladies. The results showed that 74% of skin issues, 88% of gut issues, 79% of eye issues and 53% of urinary tract issues were resolved.

- ✓ Inspired by the findings, Dog Risk of University Helsinki, Finland dug deeper. They showed that a species-appropriate raw diet was protective to canine hip dysplasia. In fact, if just a little kibble was replaced with raw dog food, it had a protective effect for puppies.

- ✓ The same group measured the stress metabolites of dry and raw fed dogs. Dry-fed dogs had nearly a 10-fold increase in stress metabolites at rest than raw fed dogs. When raw-fed dogs were moved to dry food, they suffered a five-fold increase in stress metabolites. When dry fed dogs were moved to raw food, they enjoyed a five-fold decrease in stress metabolites. It was later found that a raw meat diet is associated with a decrease in cytokine gene and receptor expression.

- ✓ The same group followed this up with a large survey of more than 8,000 dogs. They noted a decrease in the incidence of atopy and allergies in dogs fed a raw food diet.

- ✓ Iowa State University found the nutrients of raw meat and bone diets were highly digestible and did not result in gastrointestinal upset.

- ✓ Studies find raw dog food both highly palatable and digestible. Crude protein is better digested in raw compared to dry pet food. The dogs safely adapt their gut flora to their new diet. Faecal quality is maintained.

- ✓ Disrupting the gut flora leads to a myriad of health issues for the individual, including negative psychological consequences. Consuming foods that contain probiotics helps to right the unbalance.

- ✓ Dry food contains chemical anti-life, difficult to digest protein and large amounts of fibre. All have been shown to disrupt the gut flora.

- ✓ Raw dog food increases faecal butyrates and GABA, which are expected to have anti-depressive and calming health benefits, respectively, for the dog.

- ✓ Raw is also replete with vitamins such as B-complex as well as the animal fats (EPA and DHA) and low in sugar, all of which are expected to fuel positive behavioural outcomes in the dogs

- ✓ Studies suggest dogs fed home-prepared meals of fresh meat (minced offal, beef, chicken, tripe) and cooked vegetables are calmer.

- ✓ Like the AVMA, in 2012 the American Animal Hospital Association (AAHA) released a deeply erroneous but well shared denouncement of raw feeding. In it they claim some people have harmed their pet by feeding them poorly formulated homemade diets, which is true, but then implied that this food has harmed humans, which was absolutely false at their time of writing.

- ✓ Studies show 'complete' dry pet food repeatedly fail to meet the minimum requirements of AAFCO. Davies *et al.* (2017) tested more than 170 dry and canned pet foods sold in the United Kingdom and found that 94% of the 'complete' canned food and 62% of the 'complete' dry foods were not compliant with the AAFCO's guidelines.

- ✓ If pet food was truly 'complete' then we shouldn't be able to add various real ingredients and see such immediate payoffs. Blueberries increase the performance of sled dogs. Fish oil reduces inflammatory skin and joint issues in dogs. Sprinklings of various vegetable ingredients improve the cognitive performance in senior dogs. Replacing some kibble with leafy greens and orange/yellow vegetables three times a week reduced cancer risk in Scottish Terriers by upward of 70%.

- ✓ The AAHA used their erroneous positional statement to rule out fresh food for thousands of service dogs across the United States and likely the world.

Chapter Fourteen References

1   Murray, D. (2011). *Pet food laced with dangerously high levels of sulphur dioxode, tests reveal*. Courier Mail. Published online, Jul 17th, www.couriermail.com.au

2   American Animal Hospital Association (AAHA, 2014). American Animal Hospital Association's positional statement on raw feeding. AAHA Official Publication, published online www.aaha.org/about-aaha/aaha-position-statements/raw-protein-diet/

3   Hielm-Björkman, A., 2013. Exploratory study: 632 shared experiences from dog owners changing their dogs' food to raw food (BARF) diet. Published online, University of Helsinki, Finland, website https://www2.helsinki.fi/sites/default/files/atoms/files/kokemuksia_raakaruokinnasta.pdf

4   Grundström, S. (2013). *Influence of nutrition at young age on canine hip dysplasia in German Shepherd dogs*. The WALTHAM International Nutritional Sciences Symposium (WINSS) 2013, Oregon, USA.

5   Roine, J., Roine, M. Velagapudi, V. *et al.* (2015). *Metabolomics from a Diet Intervention in Atopic Dogs, a Model for Human Research?* 12th European Nutrition Conference (FENS) 2015, Berlin, Germany

6   Anderson, R.C., Armstrong, K.M., Young, W. *et al.* (2018). Effect of kibble and raw meat diets on peripheral blood mononuclear cell gene expression profile in dogs. The Veterinary Journal, 234: 7–10

7   Hemida, M., Vuori, K.A., Salin, S. *et al.* (2020). Identification of modifiable pre- and postnatal dietary and environmental exposures associated with owner-reported canine atopic dermatitis in Finland using a web-based questionnaire. PLoS One, 15(5): e0225675

8   Iennarella-Servantez, C.A. (2017). *Evaluation of raw meat diets on macronutrient digestibility, fecal output, microbial presence, and general health status in domestic dogs*. Graduate Theses and Dissertations, 15537

9   MacMillan, F. (2008). Who is responsible for the efficacy and safety of pet foods? Canadian Veterinary Journal, 49(10): 945–946

10   Algya, K.M., Cross, T.L., Leuck, K.N. *et al.* (2018). Apparent total-tract macronutrient digestibility, serum chemistry, urinalysis, and faecal characteristics,metabolites and microbiota of adult dogs fed extruded, mildly cooked, and raw diets. Journal of Animal Science, 96(9): 3670–3683

11   Cryan, J.F. and Dinan, T.G. (2012). Mind-altering microorganisms: the impact of the gut microbiota on brain and behaviour. Nature Reviews Neuroscience, 13(10): 701–712

12   Foster, J.A. and McVey Neufeld, K.A. (2013). Gut-brain axis: how the microbiome influences anxiety and depression. Trends in Neuroscience, 36(5):305–312

13   Benton, D., Williams, C. and Brown, A. (2007). Impact of consuming a milk drink containing a probiotic on mood and cognition. European Journal of Clinical Nutrition, 61: 355–361

14   Messaoudi, M., Lalonde, R., Violle, N. *et al.* (2011). Assessment of psychotropic-like properties of a probiotic formulation (Lactobacillus helveticus R0052 and Bifidobacterium longum R0175) in rats and human subjects. British Journal of Nutrition, 105: 755–764

15   Hickman, M.A., Rogers, Q.R. and Morris, J.G. (1990). Effect of Processing on Fate of Dietary carbon-14 Taurine in Cats. The Journal of Nutrition, 120(9): 995–1000

16   Kim, S.W., Rogers, Q.R. and Morris, J.G. (1996). Maillard reaction products in purified diets induce taurine depletion in cats which is reversed by antibiotics. Journal of Nutrition, 126(1):195–201

17   Kirchoff, N.S., Udell, M.A.R. and Sharpton, T.J. (2019). The gut microbiome correlates with conspecific aggression in a small population of rescued dogs (Canis familiaris). Peer J. 2019; 7: e6103

18   Sandri, M., Dal Monego, S., Conte, G., et al (2016). Raw meat based diet influences faecal microbiome and end products of fermentation in healthy dogs. BMC Veterinary Research, 13(1).

19   Schroeder F.A., Lin CL, Crusio W.E. et al. Antidepressant-like effects of the histone deacetylase inhibitor, sodium butyrate, in the mouse. Biol Psychiatry. 2007;62:55–64

20   Pilla R., Guard B.C., Steiner J.M. et al. Administration of a synbiotic containing Enterococcus faecium does not significantly alter fecal microbiota richness or diversity in dogs with and without food-responsive chronic enteropathy. Front Vet Sci. (2019) 6:277

21   Hoffmann LaRoche, F.T. (1995). Paper presented at the Science and Technology Center, Hill's Pet Nu-trition, Inc, Topeka, KS, on "Vitamin stability in canned and extruded pet food". Cited in Hand et al. 2010, Chapter 8.

22   Mooney, A. (2010). Stability of Essential Nutrients in Petfood Manufacturing and Storage. Masters Thesis. Kansas State University

23   Bosch, G., Hagen-Plantinga, E.A. and Hendriks, W.H. (2015). Dietary nutrient profiles of wild wolves: insights for optimal dog nutrition? British Journal of Nutrition, 113: S40–S54

24   Re, S., Zanoletti, M. and Emanuele, E., 2008. Aggressive dogs are characterized by low omega-3 polyunsaturated fatty acid status. Veterinary research communications, 32(3), pp.225–230

25   Hadley, K.B., Bauer, J. and Milgram, N.W. (2017). The oil-rich alga Schizochytrium sp. as a dietary source of docosahexaenoic acid improves shape discrimination learning associated with visual processing in a canine model of senescence. Prostaglandins, Leukotrienes and Essential Fatty Acids, 118: 10–18

26   Zicker, S.C., Jewell, D.E., Yamka, R.M. et al. (2012). Evaluation of cognitive learning, memory, psychomotor, immunologic, and retinal functions in healthy puppies fed foods fortified with docosahexaenoic acid–rich fish oil from 8 to 52 weeks of age. Journal of the American Veterinary Medical Association, 241(5), pp.583–594.

27   Mugford, R.A. (1987). The influence of nutrition on canine behaviour. Journal of Small Animal Practice, 28: 1046–1055

28   Anderson, G. and Mariner, S. (1971). The Effect of Food and Restricted Exercise on Behaviour Problems in Dogs. Canine Academy, KwaZulu Natal, South Africa; Zoology Department of the University of Durban-Westville, South Africa

29 Hodgkinson, S., Rosales, C.E., Alomar, D. *et al* (2004). Chemical nutritional evaluation of dry foods commercially available in Chile for adult dogs at maintenance. Archivos de Medicina Veterinaria, 36(2): 173–181

30 Gosper, E.C., Raubenheimer, D., Machovsky-Capuska, G.E. *et al* (2016). Discrepancy between the composition of some commercial cat foods and their package labelling and suitability for meeting nutritional requirements. Australian Veterinary Journal, 94(1-2): 12–17

31 Hendriks, W.H. and Tarttelin, M.F. (1997). Nutrient composition of moist cat foods sold in New Zealand. Proceedings of the Nutrit ion Society of New Zealand, 22: 202–207

32 Davies, M., Alborough, R., Jones, L. *et al* (2017). Mineral analysis of complete dog and cat foods in the UK and compliance with European guidelines. Science Reports, 7: 17107

33 Semp, P.G. (2014). Vegan Nutrition of Dogs and Cats. Master's Thesis, Veterinary University of Vienna, Vienna, Austria

34 Mayntz, D., Nielsen, V.H., Sørensen, A.,*et al* (2009). Balancing of protein and lipid by a mammalian carnivore, the mink (*Mustela vison*). Animal Behaviour, 77: 349–355

35 Hewson-Hughes, A.K., Hewson-Hughes, V.L., Miller, A.T., Hall, S.R., Simpson, S.J. and Raubenheimer, D. (2011b). Geometric analysis of macronutrient selection in the adult domestic cat, *Felis catus*. Journal of Experimental Biology, 214: 1039–1051

36 Kohl, K.D., Coogan, S.C.P. and Raubenheimer, D. (2015). Do wild carnivores forage for prey or for nutrients? Evidence for nutrient-specific foraging in vertebrate predators. Bioessays, 37(6): 701–709

37 Milgram, N.W., Head, E., Zicker, S.C. *et al* (2005). Learning ability in aged beagle dogs is preserved by behavioral enrichment and dietary fortification: a two-year longitudinal study. Neurobiological Aging, 26: 77–90

8 Raghavan, M., Knapp, D.W., Bonney, P.L. *et al* (2005). Evaluation of the Effect of Dietary Vegetable Consumption on Reducing Risk of Transitional Cell Carcinoma of the Urinary Bladder in Scottish Terriers. Journal of American Veterinary Medical Association, 227(1): 94–100

30 Khoo C., Cunnick J., Friesen K. *et al* (2005). The role of supplementary dietary antioxidants on immune response in puppies. Veterinary Therapeutics, 6: 43–56

40 Hodgkins, E.M. (2007). Your cat: Simple New secrets to a longer, stronger life. New York:Thomas Dunne Books.

41 Moodie, R., Stuckler, D., Monteiro, C. *et al* (2013). Profits and pandemics: prevention of harmful effects of tobacco, alcohol, and ultra-processed food and drink industries. The Lancet, 381(9867): 670–679

42 Monteiro, C., Moubarac, J., Levy, R. *et al*. (2017). Household availability of ultra-processed foods and obesity in nineteen European countries. Public Health Nutrition, 1–9

43 Fiolet, T., Srour, B., Sellem, L. *et al* (2018). Consumption of ultra-processed foods and cancer risk: results from NutriNet-Santé prospective cohort. British Medical Journal, 360

44 Kelly, B. and Jacoby, E. (2018). Special issue on ultra-processed foods. Public Health Nutrition, 21(1): 1–4

SECTION THREE

Why all the confusion?

CHAPTER 15

Veterinary Nutritional Training

Before we discuss the problems in our veterinary sector, I would like to repeat the caveat that this is not a criticism of individual vets. The guys at the coalface, the men or women you meet face-to-face, helping you with your sick pet, allowing for the few bad eggs, are invariably there with the very best of intentions. We have to assume vets pursue this field as they love animals and they worked extremely hard to make that dream a reality. Contrary to popular belief, they're not all charging what they like and whizzing around in Porsches. In fact, in my opinion, the majority of independent vets are not paid enough for the hours and stress they put into their practice. Instead, my personal ire is directed wholly at the machine that is now producing these vets. As we are about to show, the last few decades have seen veterinary science being replaced by the veterinary *industry*.

> We should never attribute to malice that which is adequately explained
> by neglect.
>
> **Hanlon's Razor**

I studied science for 8 years in college, the first 4 years as part of an honour's degree, the second 4 conducting my doctorate. The degree generally involves some core subjects at the start (for example, in first year, I studied biology, chemistry, math, geology and botany) and over time you drop some in favour of the ones you prefer. For me it was all about animals. I wanted to study them alone as quickly as humanly possible. By my third and fourth years, biology itself became specialised into various subjects. In my case I homed in on zoology which involved a lot of time spent on evolution, entomology, parasitology, marine ecology, behaviour, genetics, immunology, anatomy, physiology, environmental impact assessment and, no doubt, many other subjects that I have now all but forgotten. You would usually spend a full academic year studying each subject, involving perhaps 20–30 lectures. These would be split between two semesters, with perhaps half the lectures before Christmas and half after. Each semester also included up to 10 accompanying practicals. It was a massive workload. When my friends in other subjects were facing somewhere between 10–15 hours of curricular activity each week on their courses of choice, we science folk were largely facing a timetable that was at least 35 hours a week in the first two years. And that is before you were expected to finish the often-terrible amount of extracurricular homework. All in all, a general honour's degree in science, while utterly enthralling in parts, is quite a foreboding task, often with some of the highest dropout rates, at least in Ireland when I was doing it back in 1998. The common line was :'look left, look right, one of you three will not be here next year'. It is certainly no small undertaking. And then you begin your doctorate.

The point to all this is that I would have spent a reasonable amount of time studying, for example, geology in my first year but today I can tell you very little about it. I certainly shouldn't be tasked with explaining it to anyone, let alone making big decisions based on my understanding of it. In fact, I think I actually failed the course by a narrow margin but as my other subjects were OK, I managed to scrape through based on some form of allowance permitted me. I was an 18-year-old, so you can understand that sketching rocks did not quite top my list of priorities at the time. And I can say this for quite a number of the subjects I took back then but have spent little time since trying to stay abreast of in any real way.

It is the dizzying expanse of science and every subject in it that explains why people usually specialise further and further into tiny corners of it. In human medicine we call our local doctor a GP, a general practitioner, a jack-of-all-trades. Their knowledge is crucially broad but rarely specialised. We hope, should the issue be serious, their expansive knowledge quickly pinpoints the potential problem and refers us to the correct specialist consultant, be they experts of the brain, eyes, ears, throat, arms, legs, joints, reproductive organs, kidneys, pancreas, liver, blood, lymphoid, hormonal and neural systems, or joint and muscle rehabilitation in the young or the old.

We have specialised nutritionists such as public health and clinical dietitians and food allergy specialists. We have gastroenterologists and experts in dietetics (the effect of nutrition on behaviour), most of whom may have spent more than 4,000 hours (30 hours a week, 35 weeks a year for 4 years) studying their discipline of choice before even leaving college.

While vets are excellent generalists, no doubt, it is clearly a mental impossibility for an 18-year-old to master all subjects – anatomy, chemistry, physiology, physiotherapy, dentistry, nutrition, pathology, oncology, immunology, cardiology, entomology, parasitology, bacteriology, epizoology, anaesthesiology not to mention a lot of pharmacology and any other *ology* you can think of, in *all* parts of *all* animals – dogs, cats, cows, sheep, horses, fish, birds, reptiles, rodents and amphibians, in just 5 short academic years.

After college our young vets are catapulted into veterinary practice where they are taught the numerous surgical tasks they may be expected to perform and how to run a business. This they learn in 2 years and off they go, sink or swim. From this point, vets are obliged to keep up their education via Continuing Veterinary Education courses; however, this is less than forty hours a year (and the vast majority of which are corporate food and drug presentations).

How can we expect a kid, with this sort of workload, to fully grasp the enormity of any one of these subjects? To suggest they can, in *every* respect, does an enormous disservice to people who do take the time to study, in-depth, just one of these disciplines. But to suggest they should be the *only* persons *ever* dispensing information in *all* of these fields is irresponsible in the extreme.

Respect where respect is due, it is a savage workload, but it surely contributes to the sad fact many young vets today have unacceptably high depression and suicide rates. Data collated over the last three decades involving the death records of more than 11,600 US veterinarians reveal female vets are 3.5 times more likely to die by suicide than members of the public,[1] while males are 2.1 times more likely. From 2000 to 2015, roughly 10% of deaths among female veterinarians could be attributed to suicide (in the United States, 1.7% of their more than 2.8 million deaths per year are linked to suicide). Depression, anxiety and burnout are the chief factors at play, with the authors specifically noting 'long work hours, work overload, practice management responsibilities, client expectations and complaints, euthanasia procedures, and poor work-life balance' as the contributing issues. Nett *et al.* (2015)[2] note that anxiety and depression are common among veterinarians, as are related personality traits such as perfectionism, which must be torment in the face of such a daunting workload and a tide of knowledge they have been swimming against since setting their targets on veterinary medicine in school as a child.

Author's note:

I don't like to put out problems without voicing some solutions. In this case, would it not make more sense that, very much like the science degree, the general veterinary student enters something of a funnel system, where the degree starts off broad but the student is permitted to specialise according to their field of choice? Why should a farm vet have to waste so much time on the smaller animals? They do not intend to be a small animal vet. Doesn't it make sense that a town full of veterinary surgeons would not be all offering the same broad service? What about one for dogs, one for cats, one for skin and guts, one for broken limbs, one for surgery, one for dentistry, each top of their game.

The world's leading veterinary nutritionists state a knowledge of nutrition is *vital* for veterinarians in order to inform owners about the care of *healthy* animals as well as both the prevention and treatment of disease.[3] This is why all veterinary governing bodies, including the The European Association of Establishments for Veterinary Education (EAEVE), the Royal College of Veterinary Surgery (RCVS) and American Veterinary Medical Association (AVMA), have set standards for veterinary nutritional competency in their new graduates, a skill that, according to the AVMA, falls under 'treatment planning, health promotion, disease prevention, food safety, and case management skills'. In 2011, the World Small Animal Veterinary Association (WSAVA) dictated that nutritional assessment was a 'fifth vital sign', meaning it must be conducted *every time* a pet is presented to a veterinarian. And yet, many veterinarians do not perform this vital nutritional assessment.[4] A 2003 survey revealed that while 90% of dog and cat owners wanted dietary recommendations from their vet, only 15% perceived that they had actually received them.[5] It seems very few pet owners are having nutritional conversations with their vet. If it is so important, why is this not happening? The evidence suggests they are unable to hold such conversations.

Those on the outside looking in, most of them vets themselves, note that the level of nutritional knowledge in vets today is utterly dismal, bordering on entirely absent[6-8] Nestle and Nesheim (2010)[9] called all the accredited veterinary schools in the United States and found that 22 out of the 27 offer only elective or minimal nutrition courses (e.g. one credit hour per year) and five do not offer any nutritional training at all. A 1996 survey of veterinarians in the United States found that 70% thought their nutritional education was inadequate.[8] In 2013, only

16% of 134 small animal veterinarians felt they had received enough nutritional training in college.[10]

> Vets today are less than adequately versed in canine and feline nutrition and dietary options.
>
> **Remillard, 2008**[11]

My own personal experience over the years writing this book verifies this sad fact. I have spoken with many newly qualified vets the world over in both a formal and informal capacity. They often tell me they can't remember a single canine nutrition lecture in their 5 years studying outside of the pharmacological use of some vitamins and minerals with certain diseases. When we talk it is clear that outside of the physiology of how the gut works, for example, these young vets are hopelessly adrift when discussing the most basic of nutritive concepts. They appear unable to formulate a suitable meal plan for a healthy dog or cat, let alone a therapeutic diet for a sick one.

This is alarming. When the deans of 63 separate veterinary schools in the European Union, Middle East and Russia were asked about this apparent knowledge gap, 97% of respondents agreed that as nutrition was a modifiable risk factor for major chronic diseases and therefore an integral component of disease management, nutritional assessment should be a core competency of new veterinary graduates.[3] And yet, 41% of vet school deans were either not very satisfied or not at all satisfied with the nutritional skills of their graduates. In terms of hours spent teaching clinical nutrition, at 19 hours in total, it appears the EU schools are spending significantly longer on the subject than the US schools.[3] When the deans were pressed for how much more time should be spent on small animal nutrition, they said a further 28 hours. One of their main problems is not having someone to teach it to the students. According to 71% of deans, a requirement for including an additional teaching faculty member who is focused and trained in small-animal nutrition presents a common problem: small-animal nutrition was being taught by non-vets or by faculty members with training only in production-animal nutrition. The colleges worried that the instructors' knowledge and interest in nutrition was likely to be weak if they are not trained in nutrition.

Some more interesting details were harvested by the author. As 48 of the 63 of the veterinary schools participate in a pet feeding program sponsored by a pet food company, Becvarova *et al.*[3] reveal that the majority of veterinary schools in the European Union, Middle East and Russia have some form of relationship with a pet food company. When the deans mentioned that some *non-branded* textbooks might help, the authors suggested the Mark Morris Institute as a resource, a group they describe as 'a non-profit veterinary education foundation' who provide "feline, canine, and equine nutrition lectures and laboratories to 45 veterinary schools in seven countries". Not mentioned was the fact that the Mark Morris Institute is owned by Hill's pet food, an oversight made all the more strange by the fact the study's lead author is an employee of Hill's Pet Nutrition, Inc. in Topeka, Kansas.

A chronically heavy workload, in part, explains the dearth of nutritional knowledge in the average vet today. But the knowledge gap appears to extend to the very top levels of veterinary nutrition.

> Some animals won't eat a therapeutic diet get stuck doing a home-cooked diet,"…"It can be really tedious for pet owners to make their own food, especially when you're dealing with a large-breed dog. Owners need to be aware of the amount of work that it may entail. It should be *under the guidance of a veterinary nutritionist*, and if they're going to be on a home-prepared diet long term it needs to be complete and balanced.
> **Martha Cline, DVM, DACVN to Veterinary Practice News 2018**
> **President of the American Academy of Veterinary Nutrition**
> **2017-2019**
> **https://www.veterinarypracticenews.com/**
> **the-trials-of-therapeutic-diets/**

We are constantly told that pet owners seeking a therapeutic diet should only do so under the guidance of a board-certified veterinary nutritionist (VN), as that vet has undertaken further studies in small-animal nutrition. As opposed to a generic brand dry food that claims to suit great swathes of the dog population, a therapeutic diet is designed to meet a specific need in your pet. It is expected to have a functional outcome for the animal. This includes anything from weight loss to the relief of recurring digestive upset.

To obtain this most rudimentary nutritional information, the advice is not to go to the local vet but to seek out your local VN. Herein lies the problem. There are just over 100 VNs registered with the American College of Veterinary Nutrition (ACVN), but not all of these are actually available to us. Many are employed directly by dry pet food companies. Many others are employed directly by university vet departments and are tied up in research duties there. According to the ACVN, 24 of them are available for the average pet owner to contact. Correspondence with a random selection of VNs indicated the basic price for this *casual* (non-specific) chat on nutrition ranges from $100 to $400 per hour. However, should you need advice tailored to your pet's health needs, termed therapeutic advice, it requires the VN to study the pet's health records. Of the 33 VNs in the ACVN database that offer a 'remote consultation with a veterinarian' service, only 28 reside in the United States. As this process requires a referral from your vet you must pay for their time too. Unsurprisingly, the fee for a specific, therapeutic diet for your pet rises very sharply at this point.

This, according to the ACVN, is the very best way to disseminate what is some very rudimentary dietary information to owners of overweight pets, a disease that now affects approximately 60% of America's 160 million dogs and cats. If each patient requires just an hour's assessment, it would mean 28 VN's splitting the 96 million cases between them. This means each has 3.43 million hours of obesity work ahead of them. If they each ignore all their other cases and dedicate six hours a day to obesity, five days a week, and as long as no more pets get fat in the meantime, they would clear this backlog in just shy of 2,199 years.

As of 2020, of the 69 VNs that specialise in small animal nutrition, 58 live and work in the United States and yet less than half of the 30 US vet schools have a VN on the books (the results of an unpublished survey by VNs Chandler and Dobbins 2003). The figures are even worse in the European Union where only 30% of schools employ a VN.[12] Of the eight veterinary schools in the United Kingdom, only the Royal Veterinary College actually employs a VN. They actually have two of the three available. Unfortunately, as of March 2020, neither provide remote consultations to owners or to referring veterinary surgeons. This means the majority of UK veterinary students risk being taught animal nutrition by teachers equipped with little more than a veterinary degree level of understanding of the complexities of the mammoth subject that is nutrition (in case you were wondering – Ireland and Australia each have a single VN, England and New Zealand both have two and France, the home of Mars Royal Canin, has three, all of whom are employed by Royal Canin and none of whom provides consults for vets or pet owners). The only other VN available to British vets and pet owners is in Scotland. Her name is Marge Chandler, DVM, MS, MANZCVSc, DACVN, DACVIM, DECVIM-CA, MRCVS. The intimidatingly qualified Chandler does offer remote vet referrals for Irish and UK vets but sadly not for pet owners.

Dr. Chandler, is chair of the American College of Veterinary Nutrition Education Committee, co-chair of the WSAVA Global Nutrition Committee, founder of the European Veterinary Nutrition Educators Group and a member of the European Pet Food Industry Federation (FEDIAF) Scientific Advisory Board. It's fair to say, when Chandler speaks on nutrition, the veterinary community listens. Sadly, she is a very outspoken critic of feeding pets fresh, species-appropriate food. As such, she is often the voice and indeed face of many free educational/marketing seminars hosted by major dry pet food producers. It was during one such seminar for Webinarvet in 2015 (now owned by Nestlé), titled "Feeding Raw Food Diets to Dogs and Cats: What is the Evidence?", that Dr. Chandler bemoaned the sad state of the scientific evidence in support of the notion of feeding dogs and cats fresh, species-appropriate food to the 300 vets in attendance. Webinarvet is a well-run, profitable and influential platform so we must assume Dr. Chandler prepared well for this live-but-recorded and still readily available seminar. You're always going to bring your good stuff to these things, aren't you? This veterinary heavyweight starts off by highlighting that no amount of *anecdotal* examples of success and good health make up a single fact. While this itself is highly debatable, it does set the tone for the rest of the seminar. Dr. Chandler then went on to speak for an hour on the many hazards of raw feeding, herself using an astounding amount of anecdotes. During the hour, Dr. Chandler spent 7 minutes talking about a study of a *single* Shetland Sheepdog fed an unspecified 'raw diet' that suffered cranial cervical myelopathy, hypocalcaemia, hypophosphataemia, rickets and suspected nutritional secondary hyperparathyroidism. She then spent 6 minutes on a tragic story about 'one poor kitty' that suffered a great range of illnesses after consuming 'raw', most importantly toxoplasmosis. Now while this cat was not raw fed *per se* her owner informed Dr Chandler that as she was such an avid hunter she sometimes gave her a piece of fresh meat. From this Dr Chandler managed to isolate the chance that the source of toxoplasmosis was not any one of the hunted rodents and birds but the piece of meat the owner might have given her beforehand, implying toxoplasmosis is a big concern in the UK meat sector, which it is not, certainly not when compared to wild rodents. Dr. Chandler then spent 5 minutes on the dangers of feeding bones as both "she and her friend have removed a bone from a dogs mouth". *One time*, apparently, Dr. Chandler claims this bone was raw.

That's nearly a third of a single terrifying lecture with the word *evidence* in the title supported by anecdotal testimony. But it has to be the way as evidence of actual risk from premade raw dog food, manifesting as pet injury or death, is incredibly rare. As far as I can tell, when Dr. Chandlers' webinar went live in 2015, there was exactly zero instances of dogs harmed by premade, 'complete' raw dog food. The first record of that was in 2019 when five cats were killed following the consumption of raw venison contaminated with TB. Compare this to the tens of thousands of pets killed and untold numbers harmed following the consumption of ultra-processed pet food for reasons ranging from insufficient to excessive nutrient inclusions, mycotoxins, melamine and irradiation in just the last few decades alone. An incredible oversight, and one that further ignores the fact that, in the decade previous to that statement, 132 humans contracted *Salmonella* from dry pet food, half them toddlers under 2 years of age. Numbers of humans ever harmed by premade raw dog food prior to Dr. Chandler's statement? Zero.

D. Chandler wasn't finished. She then spent another five minutes talking about the potential dangers of raw-hide chews – a product we all agree is probably one of the worst things you can feed to your pet-but as it uses the word 'raw' in its title, it went with the raw conversation regardless. Much of the rest of the lecture was spent convincing the attendees that bones do not clean a dog's mouth, that the only way to do this was by brushing. Incredibly, of the 300 people in attendance at this webinar, the majority being vets, nurses and students, 98% of them agreed that brushing a dog's teeth when they got dirty was the ONLY way to keep teeth clean, bar perhaps some magic 'dental formula' dry food, implying that other non-dental forms are a potential risk factor for gum disease. I asked 'if 8/10 dogs are dry fed and 8/10 have gum disease by the time they are three years of age, might the diet possibly be a factor here, as it is in humans?' but the question was ignored.

In terms of the evidence for feeding pets fresh, species-appropriate food, this is what Dr. Chandler chose to present to the 300 vets in attendance. Nor is Dr .Chandler alone among VNs. While I'm sure it has happened somewhere, as of May 2020, I have yet to read of any VN anywhere offering some balance to the terror campaign by warning pet owners about the inherent dangers posed by the feeding of dry pet food to animal or human. In fact, just under the paragraph stating neither of the VNs employed by The Royal Veterinary College are available for remote consults, the RVC provides some links to assist any vets or pet owners with their queries. There are links to seven frequently asked questions provided. The first is 'What is a board certified veterinary nutritionist?' The second question is 'Are raw pet foods better than canned or kibble (dried) foods?' For that to be the second question the RVC is asked is quite telling in itself. When we click the link we are redirected to the ACVN' (acvn.org) frequently asked questions section, implying veterinary nutrition experts on both sides of the pond agree. On the potential benefits of fresh, species-appropriate ingredients in pets, the ACVN gives us two paragraphs. Here's the first (italics added by me for effect):

Raw diets, both home-prepared and commercial, have become more popular. Advocates of raw diets claim benefits ranging from improved longevity to superior oral or general health and even disease resolution (especially gastrointestinal disease). Often the benefits of providing natural enzymes and other substances that may be altered or destroyed by cooking are also cited. However, proof for these purported benefits is currently restricted to testimonials, and no published peer-reviewed studies exist to support claims made by raw diet advocates. *No studies have examined differences in animals fed raw animal products to those fed any other type of diet (kibble, canned, or home cooked) with the exception of looking at the effects on digestibility.* Typically raw meats (but not other uncooked foods like grains or starches) are slightly more digestible than cooked meat.

www.acvn.org/frequently-asked-questions/#canned

Ignoring the fact studies of raw versus dry do now exist, the no-studies-exist line clearly works both ways. Incredibly, the ACVN and all of their members appeared stubbornly fixated on a product that lacks a single study demonstrating it can outperform a fresh, species-appropriate diet.

And on the potential benefits of fresh food, that's all we are given. The very next paragraph gets into the potential 'risks and concerns' of fresh feeding, including nutritional imbalances and microbiological concerns, two things that are not only very common in ultra-processed food but evidently far more lethal. The ACVN urges consumers that 'safe and proper handling of raw foods is crucial for reducing the risk, but safety cannot be guaranteed'. That's a fair statement, but let's compare all this to the information provided by the ACVN to the very next question on the list: 'Are commercially available pet foods safe and healthful?'(Italics are added by me for effect).

Safety problems (with regard to both nutritional adequacy and toxin/ microbiological contamination) are occasionally documented…most manufacturers utilize *sophisticated mechanisms* for *quality control and food safety*, including screening and reporting systems. As such, commercial foods remain a consistent, safe, and healthful option for feeding pets.

In relation to sophisticated mechanisms, raw dog food companies are regulated by the very same authorities as the ultra-processed pet food sector, the same rules and requirements, and the same pathogenic microbiology load (e.g. zero *Salmonella* and *E. coli*). Furthermore, as you're about to find out, if you're a raw processor in the United States you are far more likely to be checked up on compared to your dry counterparts. And as for quality control, the recent Hill's recall for incorrect vitamin D tells us all we need to know about how the very best in the business are operating in that regard – 22 million cans of pet food left the world's vets' favourite dry food company without anyone checking the ingredients coming in or the product going out.

Despite the melamine scandal of 2007, the Hill's recall highlights that major holes still exist in the reporting of such events to the public. In a piece titled "Hill's Aims To Repair Reputation Amid Vitamin D-Related Recall", Hill's tells Vets In the News, one of the largest vet information websites in the world, that its *first priority* was to reach pet owners in an effort to stop dogs from eating the recalled products.[13] That was February 15, 2019. Hill's contaminated products had been on the shelves since October 2018. The first recall was January 31, 2019. Their second was February 8, 2019. And yet, on March 15, 2019 – 6 weeks after the problem was first identified – VIN News releases a piece titled "Veterinarians Want Transparency From Hill's About Vitamin D Recall".[14] In it they highlight how one frustrated vet, after hearing about the Hill's scandal from another pet food rep, became 'fed up with a lack of information from the company' and started testing products off the shelf herself. Two weeks later that test came back – four to five times the maximum safety level of vitamin D was found. The same piece highlights how message boards on the Veterinary Information Network, an online community for the profession, revealed this vet was not alone. Numerous vets were reporting they were 'blindsided with clients' concerns long before hearing from Hill's directly'. It seems there's room for improvement here.

But it is the ACVN's use of the word *safety* that irks most of all. Comparison of pet harm and death figures aside, I find it incredible that we are now at a point nutritionally in dogs that pet food manufacturers' use of synthetic nutrients to replace nutrients missing in their premixes, coupled with various chemicals and ultra-harsh processing techniques to reduce pathogenic load of the mix, is supposed to put our minds at ease! The raw sector employs no such measures. They instead are forced to ensure the ingredients they use from the outset have everything the animal will need, higher-quality ingredients that are necessarily free of such bacteria (which they must test rigorously, lacking the chemical and processing 'safety net'). Thereafter, normally absorbed nutrients at normal levels ensure imbalances are far less likely to kill, and even that is further avoided by the tendency of raw feeders to feed a highly varied diet.

As it stands today, the vast majority of VNs are very clearly primarily concerned with feeding dogs dry, cereal-based pet food. I contacted a number of VNs asking for their opinion on feeding pets fresh, species-appropriate food. For what was largely concerns over safety, the majority were still very much against the notion in 2020. A small handful were very much for 'fresh food' but not *raw* dog food, where they mean fresh-upon-inclusion but then cooked, the very opposite to what most would assume to mean as fresh. Still, this is expected to be a major step forward for these animals, in my opinion, particularly when managed by someone as capable as a VN when it comes to supplementation.

In terms of raw, there was also a glimmer of light. In personal correspondence with now ex-president of the ACVN, Martha Cline as previously quoted above, when asked 'fresh or raw food for dogs, yes or no', the answer was yes to both. Nor was she alone in offering her valuable time to at least converse on the matter. I had friendly and frank conversations about fresh feeding pets with a small number of VNs. But the fact remains that approximately 20% of UK dog owners who now feed fresh, species appropriate food to their pets, are on their own. They must educate themselves and studies show they are doing exactly that, at the cost of the client-vet relationship. A 2016 study from an oncology referral service showed that 90% of owners made diet changes after a diagnosis of cancer in their pet.[15] Of these changes, 63% involved exclusion of a conventional diet and 54% involved inclusion of a homemade component. This study out of Ontario, Canada highlighted that while 85% of owners highly valued the opinion of their veterinarian, 51% expressed some distrust of conventional diets and only 28% agreed that conventional pet food companies place high priority on pet health and well being.

A recent survey of raw-feeding pet owners found 20% got the information they needed online.[16] Another 14% used published references. Just 8% sought the advice of their vet before making a decision. In fact, when asked if they trusted their vet's opinion on nutrition, just 13% of raw feeders had complete faith, compared to 55% of dry feeders. This damaged their overall faith in their vet with 36% of raw feeders fully trusting their vet compared to 64% who do not raw feed. Morgan *et al.* (2017)[16] incorrectly trot out the often repeated line that the high level of distrust of veterinarians as a resource for pet nutrition 'may be an indication of poor communication between veterinarian and clients'. We have already discussed that 85% of pet owners report never having had a nutritional assessment by their vet, something that is required by most vet governing bodies (EAEVE, RCVS, AVMA and WSAVA). Crucially, if this was done and the pet was found to be in good health, it would verify to the vet that what the pet owner is doing is scientifically sound. Morgan *et al.* (2017)[16] wrap up their work far more accurately (italics added by me) as follows:

> These results may indicate deficiencies in veterinarian's comfort with discussing nutrition with their clients, which *may be a consequence of insufficient/inadequate training in nutrition* during veterinary school and from continuing education following graduation.
>
> **Morgan *et al.*, 2017**[16]

As more species-appropriate ways of feeding dogs continue their takeover of the market, trust in conventional vets is going in the opposite direction. This is not only a sad state of affairs for the average vet, who almost certainly wants the best for your dog, but it is going to prove dangerous for pets. Among some more reliable sites and forums, there are now a vast number of groups on both sides demonstrating a poor understanding of the processes involved. Many don't even use their real names, which can mask hidden agendas.

We have always lived in a world where he who shouts loudest gets heard. Initially it was television. In the 2000s, we had exciting, if poorly informed, roller-blading dog trainers teaming up with National Geographic to set force-free dog training back a couple of decades. Now, we have the internet and attention spans are dropping further still. Your info needs to be quick, catchy and, most importantly, visually pleasing. Just the mention of a study conducted by someone, someplace, is enough for most, busy vets and public alike. Well-meaning websites now employ a fleet of copy writers and graphic designers to put out beautiful, easy to understand and thus infinitely shareable content. While the theory behind much of it can often be sound, how it is picked up and employed by the receiver is anyone's guess. Unfortunately, there are instances when their information can be grossly off target.

In 2014, a natural dog forum with more than a million followers online put up a post citing that it didn't matter what your dog was fed, from dry food to fresh food to some form of George Jetson supplement pill diet, as there have been instances of dogs living long lives on all diet types. I commented with my 94-year-old, chain-smoking, alcoholic granny analogy. They didn't hear from me again until I was alerted to another article the same group published in 2017 that was teaching people how to make species-appropriate raw dog food at home. In their recipe they failed to include any organ meat, cartilage or bone (but did include half a teaspoon of dried ginger powder!), a diet that is now undoubtedly still being employed by many dog owners today. When I again highlighted the flaws in their approach, I was banned from further participation in the group. It's never good to look bad on social media. This well-organised group now offers one of the most popular online courses to train people in canine nutrition. For just a few hundred dollars, they can make you a canine nutrition 'expert' in a matter of hours! You get a cert and everything!

Without veterinary input, poorly prepared pet owners are sleepwalking into a field they know little about and some pets are going to get sick. The literature is already peppered with instances of people feeding grossly inappropriate, home-prepared diets. A cat suffered hypervitaminosis A after being fed a diet containing little more than pork liver.[17] A litter of German Shepherd puppies suffered phosphorus-induced secondary hyperparathyroidism from a diet containing 80% rice.[18] Some dogs were fed large amounts of beef gullet (and thus beef thyroid) and suffered hyperthyroidism.[19] Ten cats suffered pansteatitis (inflammation of body fat) following a very high-fat diet of pigs' brains or oily fish for too long.[20] There are also a handful of individual case reports of single and sometimes two animals fed mineral deficient, home-prepared diets.[21-23] In all these cases, the most rudimentary knowledge of canine or feline nutrition would have very certainly avoided these unfortunate occurrences, information that could easily be passed on when the owner presents the puppy for her initial vaccinations. In fact, such a service is an added revenue stream for the clinic.

At this point you can't help but wonder, with the importance of real, fresh, whole ingredients in our diet now firmly ingrained in our psyche, when we know processed food should factor as little as possible in our own diets, when farm and zoo animals are healthiest when fed fresh, species-appropriate nutrition, with the sheer volume of issues established in Section 2 with their product of choice, how is that vets, our brightest minds, remain steadfast in their pious devotion to a product that lacks a single head-to-head of any value in support?

To understand what is going on, we need to take a brief step back and look at what is happening with our own health care system, to the doctors within it and the scientific foundation that underpins the whole kit and caboodle.

TAKE-HOME POINTS

✓ While vets are excellent generalists, no doubt, it is a mental impossibility for an 18-year-old to master all health disciplines in all animals in just five years. Such a daunting workload surely contributes to the immense pressure young vets are under today.

✓ The world's leading vet governing bodies have legislated that a knowledge of nutrition is *vital* for veterinarians in order to inform owners about the care of *healthy* animals as well as both the prevention and treatment of disease. Unfortunately, pet owners are not receiving this information.

✓ There is strong consensus that the level of nutritional knowledge in conventional vets today is far from adequate.

✓ Pet owners are told to consult VN's for advice concerning therapeutic diets but this is a practical if not financial impossibility for most pet owners today.

✓ VNs are chiefly concerned with feeding dry, ultra-processed diets. With nowhere else to turn, pet owners are going elsewhere for their information, with a mixed bag of results. In this way, there is potential for pets to be harmed.

Chapter Fifteen References

1   Tomasi, S.E., Fechter-Leggett, E.D., Edwards, N.T. *et al.* (2019). Suicide among veterinarians in the United States from 1979 through 2015. Journal of the American Veterinary Medical Association, 254(1): 104–112

2   Nett, R.J., Witte, T.K., Holzbauer, S.M. *et al.* (2015). Risk factors for suicide, attitudes toward mental illness, and practice-related stressors among US veterinarians. Journal of the American Veterinary Medical Association, 247(8): 945–955

3   Becvarova, I., Prochazka, P., Chandler, M.L. *et al.* (2016). Nutrition Education in European Veterinary Schools: Are European Veterinary Graduates Competent in Nutrition? The Journal of Veterinary Medical Education, 43(4): 349–358

4   Baldwin, K., Bartges, J., Buffington, T. *et al.* (2010). AAHA nutritional assessment guidelines for dogs and cats. Journal of the American Animal Hospital Association, 46(4): 285–96

5   AAHA (2003). *The path to high-quality care: practical tips for improving compliance.* Lakewood, CO: American Animal Hospital Association

6   Martin, A.M. (2007). *Food pets die for: Shocking facts about pet food.* Troutdale, OR: Newsage Press

7   Schultz, K.R. (1998). *Natural nutrition for dogs and cats.* Carlsbad, CA: Hay House

8   Lonsdale, T. (2001). *Raw meaty bones promote health.* Wenatchee, WA: Dogwise Publishing

9   Nestle, M. and Nesheim, M.C. (2010). *Feed Your Pet Right: The Authoritative Guide to Feeding Your Dog and Cat.* Free Pr: S. & S.

10   Buffington, C.A. and LaFlamme, D.P. (1996). A survey of veterinarians' knowledge and attitudes about nutrition. Journal of the American Veterinary Medical Association, 208(5): 674–675

11   Remillard, R.L. (2008). Homemade diets: Attributes, pitfalls, and a call for action. Topical Companion Animal Medicine, 23(3): 137–142

12   Abood, S.K. (2008). Teaching and assessing nutrition competence in a changing curricular environment. Journal of Veterinary Medical Education, 35(2): 281–287

13   Fiala, J. (2019a). *Hill's aims to repair reputation amid vitamin D-related recall.* VIN News Service, published online, Feb 15th, www.news.vin.com

14   Fiala, J. (2019b). *Veterinarians want transparency from Hill's about vitamin D recall.* VIN News Service. Published online, Mar 15th, www.news.vin.com

15   Rajagopaul, S., Parr, J.M., Woods, J.P. *et al.* (2016). Owners' attitudes and practices regarding nutrition of dogs diagnosed with cancer presenting at a referral oncology service in Ontario, Canada. Journal of Small Animal Practice, 57(9): 484–490

16   Morgan, S.K., Willis, S. and Shepherd, M.L. (2017). Survey of owner motivations and veterinary input of owners feeding diets containing raw animal products. PeerJ, 5:e3031

17   Polizopoulou, Z.S., Kazakos, G., Patsikas, M.N. *et al.* (2005). Hypervitaminosis A in the cat: a case report and review of the literature. Journal of Feline Medical Surgery, 7(6): 363–368

18   Kawaguchi, K., Braga, I.S., Takahashi, A. *et al.* (1993). Nutritional secondary hyperparathyroidism occurring in a strain of German shepherd puppies. Japanese Journal of Veterinary Research, 41: 89–96

19   Köhler, B., Stengel, C. and Neiger, R. (2012). Dietary hyperthyroidism in dogs. Journal of Small Animal Practice, 53: 182–184

20   Niza, M.M.R.E., Vilela, C.L. and Ferreira, L.M.A. (2003). Feline pansteatitis revisited: Hazards of unbalanced homemade diets. Journal of Feline Medicine and Surgery, 5: 271–277

21   Becker, N., Kienzle, E. and Dobenecker, B. (2012). Calcium deficiency: a problem in growing and adult dogs: two case reports. Tierarztl Prax Ausg K Kleintiere Heimtiere, 40(2): 135–139 [Article in German. Abstract in English]

22   Hutchinson, D., Freeman, L.M., McCarthy, R. *et al.* (2012). Seizures and severe nutrient deficiencies in a puppy fed a homemade diet. Journal of the American Veterinary Medical Association, 241(4):477–483

23   Moon, S.J., Kang, M.H. and Park, H.M. (2013). Clinical signs, MRI features, and outcomes of two cats with thiamine deficiency secondary to diet change. Journal of Veterinary Science, 14(4): 499–502

The Science of the Human Food and Drug Industries

Despite Jenner first discovering vaccines in 1796, it's fair to say modern medicine didn't really kick off until nearly a century ago with the discovery of antibiotics. Alexander Fleming, it seems, did not maintain the most orderly of labs but it was this very fact that helped him to discover penicillin, saving many millions of lives in the process. Apparently, Fleming returned from holidays one day in 1928 and noticed he had left a window open. Through it blew in some *Penicillium notatum* spores which contaminated a culture plate of *Staphylococcus* bacteria he had also accidentally left uncovered. Thankfully, he was skilled enough to notice the ring around the fungus where the bacteria could not grow. This was the start of antibiotics, and it was this discovery, together with our new fascination with chemistry as a whole, that really jump-started our current slavish addiction to all things chemical.

We are told today that when you get sick, modern medicine has never been better equipped to save you. There's a lot of truth to that and we are all suitably appreciative when it happens. The advances in medicine over the last century have been incredible. We moved from vaccines and sanitation in the 19th century to anaesthesia, germ theory and antibiotics by the start of the 20th century. By the 1950s, we had organ transplants, stem cell therapy and a plethora of incredible drugs, from various vaccines and antivirals to steroids and antiinflammatories. We are now in an era of artificial intelligence and nanobots. Modern medicine now ensures that you are not only quite likely to survive most maladies but live longer than ever before after the event. There has literally never been a better time to be sick. This is lucky because so many of us are doing exactly that.

Today, while it is casually accepted that one in two Americans will be diagnosed with cancer in their lifetime, thankfully only 185 per 100,000 will actually die of it. This is a disease where more than 90% of cases are attributed to environmental factors, most of them ingested. Cancer, heart disease, obesity and diabetes are affecting more and more people each year – four diseases that are already shown to have a very strong nutritional basis. For the first time in recent history, Americans are living shorter lives. The entire system is in overdrive studying these diseases, millions of man hours committed, amazing treatments developed, billions of dollars poured into health sectors clogged with rich but poorly-fed casualties, and while we focus on the *symptoms*, an actual solution to the *cause* of all this dis-*ease* in our basic constitution seems as stubbornly elusive as ever.

Compare modern medicine's approach to these diseases with the notion of a hefty sugar tax that a single person could enact with the swipe of a pen. Now that, we are told, is complicated. And yet, proper taxation of terrible foods coupled with tax reductions on whole foods, ideally coupled with government initiatives encouraging home cooking, health adverts on the TV, celebrity endorsements and even mail shots of tips and tricks, would very quickly, very cheaply and very obviously reduce junk food feeding to the level of an occasional 'treat'. A truly effective tax modifies behaviour. The result would be national weight loss. We would have less disease, be more active, work harder and assumedly be happier. We would have more money for education, for the environment, for the poor and the starving. This simple approach has just one critical flaw. It profits only the people. Multinationals struggle to make insane profits on healthy humans. And that's not fair because they have rights, too, and theirs, it seems, are more important.

Health care is, in every sense of the word, vital. Good health is the glorious state most of us hope to find ourselves in for the majority of our lives. And yet, like so many good things in life, you only appreciate it when it's gone. I now think of health as a 0 to 100 scale, where 0 is top health, up to 50 is good health, 50–80 is a few creaks and a few warning lights perhaps (take it easy, a better road is needed). 80 to 99 is varying degree of sickness and 100 is death. Incredibly, few of us care about our health until 80% of it is gone. Now you need modern medicine.

Because it only kicks in when you are sick and it rarely if ever treats the cause of disease in the first place, it's fair to say modern medicine has little to do with actual *health* care today. It now concerns itself primarily, if not totally, with *sick* care. Health care, on the other hand, involves a multitude of disciplines such as, but not limited to, nutrition (including the use of food and herbs as medicine), both physical and mental health management, stress and sleep management. Sadly, modern medicine, be it of the human or every-other-animal kind, considers these disciplines add-ons to sick care and are commonly referred to today as *alternative therapies*. In fact, veterinary medicine has gone one further today and put in place legislation that ensures sick care is the first port of call for all pet owners with a health issue. Their reason, we assume, is that the true value of these other scientific disciplines wane considerably for a patient presenting with stage IV cancer. But this, while often true, is not where most of these disciplines are strongest. While eating a high sugar/carbohydrate diet during out-of-control cancer growth is sure to quicken your demise, nutrition, physical and mental health are critical to not only *avoiding* such dis-*ease* in the first place but recovering from disease should one come knocking. The very fact hospitals serve such terrible food is but one, albeit highly telling, sign of how disconnected things have become in this regard. That modern doctors feel it's OK to prescribe head pills for outwardly depressed people following a single 20-minute appointment is another. In fact, America's lethal addiction to properly prescribed tablets tells us all we need to know about dangerously broken our 'healthcare' system is today.

Accounting for an ageing population, prescription drug use in the United States is exploding. Kantor *et al.* (2015)[1] report the prevalence of prescription drug use among people aged 20 and older had risen to 59% of Americans. From 2000 to 2012, the percentage of people taking five or more prescription drugs nearly doubled (from 8–15%). The prescription drug market in America alone is today worth $450 billion per year, a market that Reuters says is growing at 6–9% per year,[2] growth they expect to continue long into the next decade. In part, this increase in demand stems from a major drive by pharmaceutical companies to focus on 'lifetime' drugs, including those for hypertension, heart failure, diabetes, cancer and other consequences of a nation eating the worst diet on the planet. But antidepressants and opioid-based drugs are gaining ground.

A 2011 report by the National Centre for Health Statistics found that 11% of Americans over the age of twelve years are on antidepressants.[3] To support this sudden and growing need for mood stabilisers is a litany of bad science that makes for depressing reading. Irving Kirsch, a lecturer in medicine at Harvard Medical School, conducted a major review of all the published data but also the unpublished data on antidepressants which were hidden by drug companies. It found that most (if not all) of the benefits were due to the placebo effect.[4] A third of meta-analyses of these antidepressant studies were written directly by pharma employees,[5] with a difficult-to-decipher amount of the rest being industry-sponsored. More worryingly, a study published in the *British Medical Journal*, looked at documents from 70 different double-blind, placebo-controlled trials for antidepressants. They found that pharmaceutical companies were not disclosing the full extent of side effects and serious harm revealed in their trials.[6]

> We found that a lot of the appendices were often only available upon request to the authorities, and the... authorities had never requested them. I'm actually kind of scared about how bad the actual situation would be... if we had the complete data.
>
> **Sharma *et al.*, (2016)**[6]

Even more worrying is the growing market for opioid-based painkillers. It is reported that pharmaceutical companies are knowingly making their prescription opioids, such as OxyContin, increasingly more powerful while sowing misinformation about their addictive properties.[7]

It all began in 1996 when American drug giant Purdue Pharma held more than 40 national 'pain management symposia' at fancy locations all around North America, inviting thousands of American doctors, nurses and pharmacists to attend. Once there, they were drilled on the firm's new star drug, OxyContin, and they were recruited as advocates. The US government publication on the whole affair, titled "The Promotion and Marketing of OxyContin: Commercial Triumph, Public Health Tragedy", makes for a sickening read.[8] This 'new' (it's a semi-synthetic version of morphine) 'wonder drug' (studies show it had no benefit over other similar drugs, Van Zee, 2009)[8] simply took best advantage of a new market that was emerging from the relaxation of laws and the general liberalisation of the use of opioids in the treatment of chronic, non-cancer pain. And they did it the tried and tested way – by influencing physicians. In fact, Van Zee (2009)[8] uses eight studies to clearly demonstrate how Purdue was able to first determine and then target the physicians who were the highest prescribers for opioids across the country and then incentivise them.

And they were very successful. Prescriptions for their drug increased 10-fold, from 670,000 to more than 6 million between 1996 and 2002. When others saw what was going on, they wanted in on the game, too, and soon the market was flooded with highly addictive painkillers. Crucial to their success, though, was hiding how addictive their drugs can be, which eventually got OxyContin in some trouble. On May 10, 2007, Purdue Frederick Company Inc., an affiliate of Purdue Pharma, along with three company executives, pleaded guilty to making false claims about OxyContin's addictiveness and was ordered to pay $634 million in fines.[8]

With no monopoly on pain, America is now consuming 80% of global opioid pills even though it has less than 5% of the world's population. This has resulted in tragic amounts of addiction and death. In 2016, two-third of the more than 63,600 drug overdose deaths in the United States involved an opioid,[9] equating to around 115 deaths a day. More than gun crime and car crashes combined. Thanks to the efforts of these charming companies, there is now a common but dangerously incorrect perception that prescription drugs are less harmful than illicit drugs.[10] Prescription drugs are killing more than 100,000 Americans a year.[11,12] To clarify, that is 100,000 people dying as a result of taking drugs that were properly prescribed by a doctor and *excluding* the 60,000 Americans who die from their opioid addiction each year, many of whom quickly turn to cheap Mexican heroin and synthetic Fentanyl as a cheaper way to fulfil their terrible, unending need. Around every single one of those poor people is a family torn apart.

And all this goes on, necessarily though somewhat unbelievably, with the full approval of the Food and Drug Authority (FDA). In 2013, with the epidemic raging, the FDA permitted the sale of a powerful opiate called Zohydro, despite the near unanimous objection of its *own review committee*.[13] It's patently clear that commercial concerns trump that of a doctor's opinion in corporate America.

The small bit of good news is that opioid deaths and misuse now appear to have peaked in the United States and, while opioid abuse continues to climb in Europe, it is nothing like the rates witnessed in America.[14]

> The medical profession is being bought by the pharmaceutical industry, not only in terms of the practice of medicine, but also in terms of teaching and research. The academic institutions of this country are allowing themselves to be the paid agents of the pharmaceutical industry. I think it's disgraceful.
>
> **Arnold Relman (1923-2014), Harvard Professor of Medicine, former Editor-in-Chief of *The New England Medical Journal***

It goes almost without saying that the root of the problem in this instance is corporate influence. When human health systems interact with big industry, it produces outcomes not in keeping with the patient's best interests. This includes influencing a doctor's behaviour, the creation of favourable results[15] from industry-sponsored research and ultimately increased product usage. Corporate-funded studies are significantly more likely to favour the sponsor's product compared to the comparator drug in head-to-head trials.[16] Colossal review studies that amalgamate all industry-funded studies produced over a lengthy period reveal they consistently favour those sponsored by the industry, beyond 96% in fact.[17,18] How do they do it? The answer is copious amounts of pseudoscience.

By definition, pseudoscience is a set of ideas, practices or claims that present themselves as science but do not meet the criteria to be properly identified as such. Pseudoscience comes in many forms but more often than not involves bias, whether deliberate or otherwise, a lack of openness to evaluation by other experts (this is where studies are first scrutinised by a board of peers prior to publication) and a general absence of systematic practices that are critical to sound scientific method. Used almost exclusively today by marketeers, pseudoscience is sadly not only a highly effective strategy but thanks to near bottomless budgets, it is practically an art form. This means that to the untrained eye, even to the trained one, it is often very difficult to separate the wheat from the chaff.

In his highly lauded follow-up to *Bad Science*, titled "Bad Pharma: How Drug Companies Mislead Doctors and Harm Patients", a highly recommended if deeply unsettling read (not one for the holiday, don't make the same mistake I did), Ben Goldacre explains many of the tricks used by the industry to produce the results they want. The British medical doctor lays out for us in forensic detail how devious, how unregulated and how morally bankrupt our drug industry has become.

In relation to the studies our drug industry produces, there are many ways to get the results you need.

First, drug companies are not required to publish the trials that didn't work or, worse still, those that found side effects. Furthermore, researchers are free to do as many trials as they wish and publish only those results where they fared positively. It's like flipping a coin 100 times and only publishing a 10-flip section where heads (good results) appeared eight times and tails (minor side effects) appeared only twice. Then there's clever sampling methods; very small sample sizes, handler bias, flexibility with design or definitions, interpretations of outcomes, ranging all the way up to the massaging and even withholding of vital data, and good old blatant lies.

As the saying goes, bad science gets results.

Behind all this terrible over-prescription, addiction and death are usually smart and almost certainly well-educated doctors prescribing what they feel is best for their patient at the time. So, simply producing bad science is not enough, you need to insert it into the medical psyche and big pharma do it by targeting health sectors and universities with their vast cash reserves. Assistant Professor Roy Moynihan spends a lot of time speaking out against the cosy financial relationships between our health systems and big pharma. In 2006, his *British Medical Journal* piece titled "Who Pays For The Pizza? Redefining The Relationships Between Doctors And Drug Companies", a reference to the fact drug reps still today use the method of buying lunch (invariably pizza, go figure) for anyone in a doctor's clinic that is willing to listen to their sales pitch, is a terrifying read.[15] From the very first line 'twisted together like the snake and the staff, doctors and drug companies have become entangled in a web of interactions as controversial as they are ubiquitous' to the last 'the flipside of this sense of entitlement is of course indebtedness, which, as Katz points out, is to be repaid by support for the patron's drugs, with a sense of obligation in direct conflict with doctors' primary obligation to their patients' – the bias and impact on patient welfare is truly terrifying.

It has to be said at this point, in Europe we are guilty of assuming this is just a US thing, that we have another level of protection from such infiltration, but nothing could be further from the truth. In Ireland, a Business Post investigation revealed big pharma is funding the positions of numerous medical and nursing positions, with one-third of our Heath Service Executive's (HSE's) most senior doctors receiving money directly from big pharma.[19]

In his piece, Moynihan draws our attention to the fact that the process of hooking doctors likely begins from the moment they step into college. The University of California, in San Francisco (UCSF) has a reputation for having one of the strictest policies in the United States on financial ties between researchers and study sponsors. While most other institutions do not feel the need to advertise a researcher's relationship with a company if it is worth less than $10,000 in any given year, UCSF researchers with any ties worth more than $250 must disclose it to the institution. Second, anyone conducting research at the college is expressly prohibited from having any other form of financial tie with that sponsor while that research is being conducted. And yet, a little digging reveals a worrying amount of undisclosed ties between academics and biotech companies, including numerous paid-speaking arrangements (ranging from $250 to $20,000 a year), paid consultancies (mostly less than $10,000 but up to $120,000 a year), paid positions on advisory boards and even equity holdings in said companies (mostly over $10,000 and ranging up to $1million).

People tend to assume that doctors are sitting at home each night, after long days in the office, reading and correctly interpreting scientific papers and drug trials for every product they recommend. However, this is an extremely daunting task. The depth of the deception coupled with the sheer volume of information now coming out means you need to be something between an academic and an investigative journalist to tease apart the nonsense around a single drug, let alone *all* the drugs they prescribe daily.

Milton Packer is an American doctor and leading cardiologist known for his clinical research concerning heart failure. In a recent piece titled *"Does Anyone Read Medical Journals Anymore?"*,[20] he notes that young physicians no longer even pretend to keep up with the medical literature. At a meeting of two hundred young physicians, Packer asked how many actually read an issue of *any* journal that was delivered to them, electronically or physically. The answer was zero. Not one. When pushed if they picked a single journal in their field of interest and try to keep up there, not a single hand went up. Packer then asked if these young physicians has read a *single paper* on *any topic* from start to finish? Silence. Stunned by the response, Packer asked why, and the answer was: 'We don't know how to read them. And most papers will subsequently get contradicted by another paper published somewhere else. So, it makes no sense to read any single paper.' He could sympathise, in part, with this response as he, an eminent and highly regarded cardiologist, must read dozens of papers every day and even then, feels he is not staying abreast of the information arising in just his field alone, something to which I can greatly sympathise.

The reason for this deluge is perhaps best highlighted by a piece in the *British Medical Journal* titled "Why Doctors Don't Read Research Papers? Scientific Papers Are Not Written To Disseminate Information." The piece explains how modern authors are eager to get their names in print less for reasons of enlightenment and more for reasons of self-interest.[21] The issue is science. Scientists and indeed universities have moved toward a 'publish or die' mentality. Frequency of publication is now the deciding factor in a university employing an academic as it is what the university in turn is judged on, something that will be reflected in the cash investments they can attract. In fact, universities are hiring new faculty members based on little more than their publications list.[22] There is now pressure to publish, the inevitable result of which is quantity over quality. One tactic adopted by 'salami slicers' is to divide decent works down into the smallest publishable unit in order to lengthen their publication list. The other, clearly, will be questionable research. The result is in 2006 alone, approximately

1.3 million peer-reviewed scientific articles were published. As of the last count, and not including the predatory or fake journals, from 2001 to 2006 the number of available scientific journals increased from 16,000 to somewhere close to 23,750.[23]

> It seems to me that we should for an experimental period of a year, declare a moratorium on the appending of authors' names and of the names of hospitals to articles in medical journals. If the dissemination of information is the reason why papers are submitted for publication, there will be no falling off in the numbers offered... But if far less material is offered to the journals, we shall have unmasked ourselves.
>
> **Healy, 1976**[24]

So expecting our young doctors to stay abreast of the 'science' is no small task, certainly not when you're studying to be a doctor. Young doctors, out of necessity, are left placing large amounts of faith in the supposition that 'good science' supports each of their lessons and thus decisions in practice. However, as the prescription drug epidemic at least in America clearly demonstrates, an environment of weak regulation and clever-but-self-serving science that is poorly understood, if read at all, by the practitioner leaves our health practitioners vulnerable and open to abuse. It is leading to bad decisions with potentially dire consequences for the patient. More simply put, in a class action lawsuit filed in Ontario, Canada alleging that Purdue was 'negligent in the development, manufacture, distribution, marketing and sale of OxyContin', Dr. David Juurlink, Associate Professor Of Medicine, Paediatrics and Health Policy, Management and Evaluation at the University of Toronto makes the following observation:

> ...doctors swallowed the firm's promotional messages 'hook, line and sinker'...

Nor is it just in the drug sector that we see a pollution of the science. America is in the grasp of an obesity (and, thus, heart disease, diabetes and cancer) epidemic. This, too, is fuelled by a lot of very bad science, albeit from a different type of drug pusher. Independently funded studies find correlations between sugary drinks and poor health, whereas those supported by the soda industry do not.[25] Marion Nestle,[26] Professor of Nutrition, Food Studies and Public Health at New York University, highlights how corporate influence is destroying the credibility of the food industry's research. She uses two examples to support their systematic abuse of the science.

First, Nestle highlighted an article by *The New York Times*,[27] which exposed a new organisation of academic researchers, the Global Energy Balance Network, who promoted physical activity as a more effective method than calorie control for preventing obesity (e.g. rather than avoiding sugary sodas). The group was supported by Coca-Cola. Nestle then introduced us to a study published in the prestigious *British Journal of Nutrition*. It concluded that cocoa flavanol compounds 'improved accredited cardiovascular surrogates of cardiovascular risk, demonstrating that dietary flavanols have the potential to maintain cardiovascular health even in low-risk subjects'.[28] The study, which followed well-established scientific protocols, was funded in part by Mars Inc. Nothing wrong so far. The problem, Nestle points out, is not the science itself, but how they used it.

On September 27, 2015, Mars took out a whole page ad in The *New York Times*. It stated 'cocoa flavanols lower blood pressure and increase blood vessel function in healthy people'. As Nestle (2015)[26] explains, what was not explained was that cocoa flavanols are largely destroyed during all but the most careful processing of chocolate. But Mars didn't mention chocolate, specifically. As Nestle states, they didn't have to.

> Multinationals use science like a drunken man uses a lamppost, for support rather than illumination.
>
> **Adapted from a quote by Andrew Lang**

Michele Simon is a public health lawyer specialising in legal strategies to counter corporate tactics that harm the public. From her platform www. EatDrinkPolitics.com, she has been researching, writing about and exposing the food industry and its politics since 1996. In her analysis of the US Academy of Nutrition and Dietetics (AND), titled "And Now a Word From our Sponsors: Are America's Nutrition Professionals in the Pocket of Big Food?[29]," Simon presents some damning findings. Besides it's growing list of food industry sponsors, including a long-term affiliation with The National Cattlemen's Beef Association and processed food giants ConAgra and General Mills, the AND allows their sponsors to give Continuing Education lectures to members. The messages taught by Coca-Cola include sugar is not harmful to children, aspartame is entirely safe – including for children of 1 year and the Institute of Medicine (IOM) is too restrictive in its school nutrition standards. At their 2012 annual meeting, of the major attendees, only two out of the 18 represented whole, nonprocessed foods.

While large review studies conclude that through the sale and promotion of ultra-processed food and drink, multinational corporations are 'major drivers of global epidemics of non-communicable diseases' and as such should play no role in any strategies laid out to combat said diseases,[30] it seems every major nutrition group in the United States is still happily supping from the corporate teat. The American Dietetic Association lists Coca-Cola, Hershey's, Kellogg's, Mars and Pepsi among its fourteen sponsors. The AND is the same. Representing over 7,000 US dietitians, their journal describes itself like this: *The Journal of the Academy of Nutrition and Dietetics* is the premier source for the practice and science of food, nutrition and dietetics. The monthly, peer-reviewed journal presents original articles prepared by scholars and practitioners and is the most widely read professional publication in the field. The American Journal of Clinical Nutrition thanks the following sponsors on its website (www.ajcn.org): Abbott Nutrition, Bush Brothers Inc., Cadbury, Campbell Soup Company, The Coca-Cola Company, ConAgra Foods Inc., The Dannon Company Inc., DSM Nutritional Products Inc., General Mills, GlaxoSmithKline, Consumer Healthcare, Kellogg Company, Kraft Foods Inc., Mars Inc., Martek Biosciences Corp., McDonald's, McNeil Nutritionals, Mead Johnson Nutrition, Metagenics Inc., Monsanto Company, National Dairy Council, Nestlé Nutrition Institute of Nestlé USA, Pepsi Co, Pfizer, Pharmanex, POM Wonderful LLC, The Procter & Gamble Company, Sara Lee Corporation, The Solae Company, The Sugar Association Inc., Tate and Lyle, Unilever North America and Welch's.

Even the US government seems to be doing its bit to ensure Big Sugar holds its lofty position in the American food pyramid. In the midst of a terrible obesity epidemic, with the average citizen consuming approximately 100 lb of sugar a year, the US Department of Agriculture decided to employ a new methodology for recording how much sugar people were eating, shaving 20 pounds of sugar off the average American's annual intake in the process. Covered by *The New York Times* (NYT), Dr. Michael Jacobson, executive director of the Center for Science in the Public Interest, worries that this new lower figure might 'take some pressure off companies that make sugary foods'.[31] The NYT dug further and revealed an e-mail from Jack Roney, the then-director of economics and policy analysis at the American Sugar Alliance, where he states 'we perceive it to be in our interest to see as low a per-capita sweetener consumption estimate as possible'.

With such powerful interests pulling the strings, obese America just can't seem to get on top of its raging diabetes crisis. According to the US Centre for Disease Control, by 2050 diabetes will affect one in three Americans. When Mayor Bloomberg proposed a soda portion size limit in New York City, the AND issued a statement declining to support the ban, saying that the education of sound nutrition should be reemphasized (as that's been working so well to this point – kids, just say no to the tasty, legal highs you can buy with your own money each day, think of your future waistlines).

> So much research is sponsored by industry that health professionals and
> the public may lose confidence in basic dietary advice.
>
> **Nestle, 2015**[26]

And as with the prescription drug epidemic, don't assume your doctor will be able to protect you from this. Nutrition does not rank highly on their agenda. Authors note doctors are grossly under-trained in nutrition in favour of time spent on medication and surgery.[32,33]

From drugs to food, from sports to politics, when it comes to decisions that affect consumption, it's difficult to think of a single example where corporate influence was for the common good. Our primary defence to the tidal wave of useless and often harmful products is *good* science but it seems, with the tide of bad science now at epidemic proportions today, that barrier is wholly ineffective. The most widely accessed article in the history of the Public Library of Science, was written by John Ioannidis, an epidemiologist and maths legend at the Stanford University School of Medicine. Titled "Why Most Published Research Findings are False", Ioannidis turned his attention to the 49 most widely cited studies found in the world's three most prestigious medical journals (*The Lancet, The New England Journal of Medicine, The Journal of the American Medical Association*) published between 1990–2003. He found that in more than 40% of them, their findings were significantly exaggerated or flat out wrong.[34]

The issue of bad science is now so endemic that Richard Horton, editor-in-chief of the world's most respected, peer-reviewed medical journal, *The Lancet*, states:

> Much of the scientific literature, perhaps half, may simply be untrue.
>
> **Horton, 2015**[35]

Horton cited small sample sizes and flagrant conflicts of interest as the chief protagonists, concluding with the remark that science 'has taken a turn towards darkness'. And he is far from alone in his sentiments among editors of top scientific journals:

It is simply no longer possible to believe much of the clinical research that is published, or to rely on the judgment of trusted physicians or authoritative medical guidelines. I take no pleasure in this conclusion, which I reached slowly and reluctantly over my two decades as an editor of *The New England Journal of Medicine.*

Dr Marcia Angell, former Editor-in-Chief of The New England Journal of Medicine

Richard Horton, now 58, has been the Editor-in-Chief of *The Lancet*, the prestigious British medical journal founded in 1823, for twenty-three years. He began working there when he was just 33 years old. He is one of the world's most eminent scientists, of that there is little doubt, but even he too is clearly fallible, leaving little hope for the rest of us. Horton will never be forgiven by many for being the editor that published the paper that forged unfounded links between the measles, mumps and rubella (MMR) vaccine and autism in children back in 1998. Concerns were first raised in 2004 and many times in the years following but it wasn't until 2010 that *The Lancet*, following the General Medical Council's decision that its lead author, Andrew Wakefield, had been dishonest (and was later censured), and the paper was retracted (essentially struck from the record). The debacle became one of the biggest and ongoing calamities for the MMR campaign and public health in general. By all accounts, Horton now deeply regrets sitting on the decision for so long.[36] Indeed, it appears a lot of what Horton has done since has been shaped significantly by the event. But it is his words to the *Guardian* newspaper in 2010 that should frighten us the most:

> Wakefield "was dishonest", said Horton. "He deceived the journal." *The Lancet* had done what it could to establish that the research was valid, by having it peer-reviewed. But there is a limit, he said, to what peer-review can ascertain.
>
> **Boseley, 2010**[36]

Peer-review are two words that are supposed to instil in us a measure of calm reassurance that 'the science' is sound. We can trust it. It has been verified typically by a group of colleagues with specialty backgrounds or an Editorial Board of Reviews. But with so much insidiously false, self-serving science appearing *daily* in a now vast array of journals that are of questionable quality themselves, it can be hard to keep up. Even if directed to the paper in question, these falsehoods are so delicately and expertly woven that it can take a team of top scientists in that very field many days to undercover where the treason had been committed.

I remember, upon submitting my doctorate, I had to go through the *viva* process. It was terrifying. In science, there is always a fear you will be found out because there are always better scientists around. Better biologists. Better behaviourists. Better statisticians. And for peer-review, you are meant to ship in a couple to critically interrogate your work, your workings and your conclusions. If you're not cheating at any point, there is nothing whatsoever to fear. Few get through unscathed. Most walk out beaming with 'minor corrections' one or two have a bit more to do in some places. I have yet to hear of a fail but no doubt they occur. The point is: they are not there to 'do' you. Your supervisor would not let your work embarrass them. Sitting in front of me I had two 'friendly' scientists, one was my supervisor and the other a professor from my own faculty that, while I would be on a first name basis in the corridors, friends we were most certainly not. The other two scientists were two heavyweights of my field. Both were flown in, put up, wined and dined but of cash payment there was none. Peer-review is a voluntary process. You don't get your name on anything. There is no formal recognition you were even there. You are expected to contribute your valuable time (there are heads of departments, extremely busy people) for nothing more than the advancement of science. Herein lies the problem. While we would like to think everyone is in it just to move our understanding forward, we have clearly seen there are too many scientists out there with more self-serving motives in mind. The chances of these types wanting to conduct peer-review is considerably less. Moreover, your team picks who sits opposite you. This opens the door to all sorts of shenanigans. And all the time the people on the other side of the table are working with the data I hand them. Little more.

This, it seems, is peer review of the highest quality. You're going for a doctorate after all. When publishing a science paper, the legitimacy of 'peer-review' goes downhill steeply from this point.

> ...some systems are very different. There may even be some journals using the following classic system. The editor looks at the title of the paper and sends it to two friends whom the editor thinks know something about the subject. If both advise publication the editor sends it to the printers. If both advise against publication the editor rejects the paper. If the reviewers disagree the editor sends it to a third reviewer and does whatever he or she advises. This pastiche—which is not far from systems I have seen used—is little better than tossing a coin, because the level of

agreement between reviewers on whether a paper should be published is little better than you'd expect by chance.

Lock, 1985[37]

Peer review, it seems, has never been a standard over which anyone can really stand. A systematic review of all the available evidence on peer review concluded that 'the practice of peer review is based on faith in its effects, rather than on facts'.[38]

Richard Smith was editor of the *BMJ* from 1991–2004. While at the *BMJ*, he used to amuse himself by inserting very major errors into papers to check how thoroughly their reviewers were going about their business.[39, 40] In his words 'nobody ever spotted all of the errors. Some reviewers did not spot any, and most reviewers spotted only about a quarter'. It's fair to say, in peer-review, he sees some room for serious improvement, but his 2006 book "The Trouble with Medical Journals" lays out just how critical the problem now is. Smith states that medical journals have become little more than 'creatures of the drug industry', riddled with fraudulent research usually conducted by the pharmaceutical companies themselves.

> This is why Robbie Fox, the great 20th century editor of the Lancet, who was no admirer of peer-review, wondered whether anybody would notice if he were to swap the piles marked 'publish' and 'reject'. He also joked that the Lancet had a system of throwing a pile of papers down the stairs and publishing those that reached the bottom. When I was editor of the British Medical Journal I was challenged by two of the cleverest researchers in Britain to publish an issue of the journal comprised only of papers that had failed peer review and see if anybody noticed. I wrote back 'How do you know I haven't already done it?'
>
> **Smith, (2006) in "Peer review: a flawed process at the heart of science and journals"**

This is why Horton and many others in his position admit perhaps half of what the top journals publish may be false. Big brother is *not* watching. When the study gets published, and it will somewhere, eventually, the paper will be either readily accepted by the wider scientific community (they cannot *prove* their conclusions false) or it will be rejected (proven false). How long that process takes will vary. But being proven false, as the Wakefield study demonstrated, does not mean the paper has been *redacted*. It takes serious malpractice for a paper to be pulled and this takes time. In this way, a misleading paper, much like a terrible fart, can hang around for too long, polluting the atmosphere for everyone but its creator.

Starting to feel a little uncomfortable? The only solace I can offer you is that when I read a study I always ask myself: can these findings be used to sell something? If not, my trust-meter happily jumps a click or two. If the study concerns an effect on a disease and the answer is negative – x *causes* y, so don't do it – I listen with an open mind. However, any positive findings in relation to disease – x *prevents* y, so take it OR x *does not cause* y, so take it – do not get my trust. That finding has to be repeated a number of times by people not profiting from the result. Of course, discerning who is funding what is the most confusing task of all. Not sure that has helped, actually.

Bad science today is clearly at epidemic proportions. We are now in a time that if we don't read the scientific evidence, we are *un*informed but if we do, we risk being *mis*informed (a line I adapted from Mark Twain, who first said this in relation to reading the newspaper). Knowing this, the irony of my using scientific references as the supportive structure for this book is not lost on me. Seeing our top journals struggling to tease the wheat from the chaff, it leaves me (your average researcher) on rockier ground when using numerous studies to support my arguments. I try to filter the best that I can but as you will soon understand, this is no small task. I primarily use studies because our vet sector need to see them to act when in actual fact a simple test using their most gut sick or itchy clients would tell them all they needed to know.

In 2019, Roy Moynihan, one of the most vocal advocates for the preservation of evidence-based medicine, was back – this time teaming up with another eighteen relative giants in the field. Published again in the BMJ, they re-highlight the issue – the commercial distortion of the scientific evidence must stop. This time they offered some immediate solutions to stem the destruction of trust in the science, including research being conducted without industry ties and government reforms to ensure both product testing and regulatory agencies are independent of industry.[41] In short, get them out of both research and regulation or full disclosure where they are in.

With all this in mind, let's take a look at the companies behind the top pet food brands, their affiliation with the veterinary industry, the science used to support their stance and the regulators in place to make sure they're all behaving themselves.

TAKE-HOME POINTS

✓ With the majority of pet food regulations and information coming from the United States, we begin with an analysis of the US human drug sector, assuming the science employed here is at least as robust as that used to buoy the pet sector.

✓ The US prescription drug market is exploding. It is currently worth half a trillion dollars a year and growing by 6–9% a year.

✓ Eleven percent of Americans over the age of twelve years are on antidepressants. The science supporting this market is highly questionable. At least a third of meta-analyses are written by pharma employees and side effects are not being disclosed.

✓ OxyContin was the first ultra-successful opiate-based pain killer. When restrictions were eased, PurduePharma was able to target the physicians who were the highest prescribers for opioids across the country and incentivised them. The market exploded.

✓ America is now consuming 80% of global opioid pills even though it has less than 5% of the world's population. In 2016, opioids were killing 115 Americans a day – more than gun crime and car crashes combined – and make addicts out of countless more.

✓ Excluding deaths from opioid addiction, prescription drugs (that is drugs properly prescribed by a doctor) are accountable for more than 100,000 American deaths per year.

✓ The problem is the influx of industry cash into the scientific process from those who wish to use it for marketing purposes.

✓ From how data are collected to how you process that information, there are many ways to get the answers you need – participant recruitment, sample sizes, massaging the data and handler bias are all commonly employed. It is not required that researchers publish the trials that showed the drug was ineffective or where side effects were seen. This is the scientific equivalent of flipping a coin 100 times and publishing only the 10-flip section where heads came up eight times in a row.

✓ Of 49 of the most widely cited studies found in the world's three most prestigious medical journals from 1990–2203, more than 40% were found to be significantly exaggerated or flat out wrong.

✓ The same corporate corruption of not only the science but also of the authorities and regulatory bodies can be seen in the food sector.

✓ Bad science in the human sector is now at epidemic proportions. Horton, editor of *The Lancet* stated, 'of the scientific literature, perhaps half, may simply be untrue'.

✓ Doctors are bamboozled by the deluge of bad science. Studies show they are no longer staying abreast of the scientific literature. Faith is placed in the regulators but, as we see with the prescription drug epidemic, the regulators are more than struggling, sometimes they are part of the problem, such as seen with the big sugar and the obesity epidemics.

Chapter Sixteen References

1   Kantor, E.D., Rehm, C.D., Haas, J.S. *et al.* (2015) Trends in Prescription Drug Use among Adults in the United States from 1999–2012. Journal of the American Medical Association, 314(17): 1818–1831

2   Berkrot, B. (2017). *U.S. prescription drug spending as high as $610 billion by 2021: report.* Reuters. Published online, Mar 3rd, www.reuters.com

3   National Centre For Health Statistics (NCHS, 2011). Data Brief No. 76

4   Kirsch, I. (2014). Antidepressants and the Placebo Effect. Zeitschrift Fur Psychologie, 222(3): 128–134

5   Ebrahim, S., Bance, S., Athale, A. *et al.* (2016). Meta-analyses with industry involvement are massively published and report no caveats for antidepressants. Journal of Clinical Epidemology, 70: 155–163

6   Sharma, T., Guski, L.S., Freund, N. *et al.* (2016). Suicidality and aggression during antidepressant treatment: systematic review and meta-analyses based on clinical study reports. British Medical Journal, 352: i65

7   Webster, P.C. (2012). Oxycodone class action lawsuit filed. Canadian Medical Association Journal, 184(7): E345–E346

8   Van Zee, A. (2009). The Promotion and Marketing of OxyContin: Commercial Triumph, Public Health Tragedy. American Journal of Public Health, 99(2): 221–227

9   US Centre for Disease Control and Prevention (2017). Understanding the Epidemic. CDC Official Publication. Published online, www.cdc.gov

10   Daniulaityte, R., Falck, R, and Carlson, R.G. (2012). "I'm not afraid of those ones just 'cause they've been prescribed": Perceptions of risk among illicit users of pharmaceutical opioids. International Journal of Drug Policy, 23(5): 374–384

11   Petersen, M. (2009). *Our Daily Meds: How the Pharmaceutical Companies Transformed Themselves into Slick Marketing Machines and Hooked the Nation on Prescription Drugs.* Ed. Picador

12   Null, G. (2011). *Death by Medicine.* Ed. Praktikos Books

13   Sullivan, L. (2014). *Critics question FDA's approval of Zohydro. Interview transcribe on National Public Radio.* National Public Radio, published online, Feb 26th, www.npr.org

14   van Amsterdam, J. and van den Brink, W. (2015). *The Misuse of Prescription Opioids: A Threat for Europe?* Current Drug Abuse Reviews, 8(1): 3–14

15   Moynihan, R. (2006). Who pays for the pizza? Redefining the relationships between doctors and drug companies. 1: Entanglement. British Medical Journal, 326(7400): 1189–1192

16   Bero, L., Oostvogel, F., Bacchetti, P. *et al.* (2007). Factors Associated with Findings of Published Trials of Drug–Drug Comparisons: Why Some Statins Appear More Efficacious than Others. PLoS Med, 4(6): e184

17   Bekelman, J.E., Li, Y. and Gross, C.P. (2003). Scope and Impact of Financial Conflicts of Interest in Biomedical Research. A Systematic Review. Journal of the American Medical Association, 289(4): 454–465

18   Bourgeois, F.T., Murthy, S. and Mandl, K.D. (2010). Outcome reporting among drug trials registered in ClinicalTrials.gov. Annals of Internal Medicine, 153(3): 158–166

19   Horgan-Jones, J. (2017). *HSE pleads ignorance on Big Pharma's payments to doctors.* Irish Business Post. Published online, Mar 12th, available from www.businesspost.ie

20   Packer, M. (2018*). Does Anyone Read Medical Journals Anymore?* Med Page Today. Published online, Mar 28th, www.medpagetoday.com

21   O'Donnell, M. (2005). Why doctors don't read research papers. Scientific papers are not written to disseminate information. British Medical Journal, 330(7485): 256

22   Rawat, S. and Meena, S. (2014). Publish or perish: Where are we heading? Journal of Research in Medical Science, 19(2): 87–89

23   Björk, B., Roos, A. and Lauri, M. (2009). Scientific journal publishing: yearly volume and open access availability. Information Research, 14(1)

24   Healy, J.B. (1976). Letter: Why do you write? Lancet, 1(7952): 204

25   Massougbodji, J., Le Bodo, Y., Fratu, R. *et al.* (2014). Reviews examining sugar-sweetened beverages and body weight: correlates of their quality and conclusions. American Journal of Clinical Nutrition, 99(5): 1096–1104

26   Nestle, M. (2015). Corporate Funding of Food and Nutrition Research Science or Marketing? Journal of American Medical Association Internal Medicine, 176(1): 13–14

27   O'Connor A. (2015). *Coca-Cola funds scientists who shift blame for obesity away from bad diets.* New York Times. Published online, Aug 9th, www.well.blogs.nytimes.com

28   Sansone, R., Rodriguez-Mateos, A., Heuel, J. *et al.* (2015). Flaviola Consortium, European Union 7th Framework Program. Cocoa flavanol intake improves endothelial function and

Framingham Risk Score in healthy men and women: a randomised, controlled, double-masked trial: the Flaviola Health Study. British Journal of Nutrition, 114(8): 1246–1255

29   Simon, M. (2013). *And Now a Word From our Sponsors: Are America's Nutrition Professionals in the Pocket of Big Food?* Eat Drink Politics. Published online, Jan 22nd, www.eatdrinkpolitics.com

30   Moodie, R., Stuckler, D., Monteiro, C. *et al.* (2013). Profits and pandemics: prevention of harmful effects of tobacco, alcohol, and ultra-processed food and drink industries. The Lancet, 381(9867): 670–679

31   Strom, S. (2012). *U.S. Cuts Estimate of Sugar Intake.* New York Times. Published online, Oct 26th, www.nytimes.com

32   Lo, C. (2000). Integrating nutrition as a theme throughout the medical school nutrition. American Journal of Clinical Nutrition, 72: 882S–889S

33   Pearson, T.A., Stone, E.J., Grundy, S..M. (2001). Translation of nutritional science into medical education: the Nutrition Academic Award Program. American Journal Clinical Nutrition 74: 164–170

34   Ioannidis, J.P.A. (2005). Why Most Published Research Findings Are False. PLoS Med, 2(8): e124

35   Horton, R. (2015). Editorial note, Apr 11th. The Lancet, 385

36   Boseley, S. (2010). *Lancet retracts 'utterly false' MMR paper.* The Guardian Newspaper. Published online, Feb 2nd, www.theguardian.com

37   Lock, S. (1985). *A difficult balance: editorial peer review in medicine.* London: Nuffield Provincials Hospital Trust, 1985

38   Jefferson, T., Alderson, P., Wager, E. *et al.* (2002). Effects of editorial peer review: a systematic review. Journal of the American Medical Association, 287: 2784–2786

39   Godlee, F., Gale, C.R. and Martyn, C.N.E. (1998). Effect on the quality of peer review of blinding reviewers and asking them to sign their reports: a randomized controlled trial. Journal of the American Medical Association, 280(3): 237–240

40   Schroter, S., Black, N., Evans, S. *et al.* (2004). Effects of training on quality of peer review: randomised controlled trial. British Medical Journal, 328(7441): 673

41   Moynihan, R., Bero, L., Hill, S. *et al.* (2019). Commercial Influence in Health: from Transparency to Independence. British Medical Journal, 367: l6576

Corporate Influence in the Veterinary Sector

He who pays the piper names the tune.

The Pied Piper of Hamelin

A substantial majority of the dry food brands we know today originate from the same four multinationals. Mars produces Pedigree, Royal Canin, Whiskas, Kitekat, Advance, Schmackos and Cesar, to name but a few. Nestlé produces Purina, Beneful, Alpo, Felix, Dog Chow and Cat Chow. Procter & Gamble manufactures Eukanuba and Iams while Colgate-Palmolive owns the veterinary-favourite, Hill's Pet Nutrition.

Today, Mars and Nestlé are the number one and three confectionery companies in the world.[1] As of 2016, their approximate wealth is $35 billion and $230 billion respectively, and it is thanks largely to their sales of sweets, processed foods, bottled sugar drinks and water. However, with sales of these products now stuttering in human markets, these companies are increasingly focusing their efforts on the pet market, which now accounts for $17.2 and $12.5 billion dollars of Mars and Nestlé's turnover each year, according to the Pet Food Industry's online database.

> Candy makers have been diversifying their business as calorie-conscious consumers... increasingly shun sugary sweets, a trend that has weighed on the $183 billion global confectionery market.
>
> **Reuters, 2017[1]**

Writing for Nestlé Purina Research, Laflamme *et al.* (2014)[2] state that veterinarians should consider the history of the company, their pattern of investment into research and their safety record when considering whether or not to recommend a product, so that is exactly what we'll do in this section with each of the major players, above beginning with Nestlé.

Makers of Purina, Friskies, Felix, Bakers and Beneful, Nestlé is one of the market leaders in 'complete' pet food. They are also the company that has perhaps spent more time, money, effort and credibility trying to develop and market the only 'complete' foodstuff available for humans than any other company in history. Let's see how that's gone for them.

In the 1950s, Nestlé had placed themselves at the forefront of post-natal nutrition with their cutting-edge breast milk replacement formula leading the charge. Unfortunately for Nestlé, Trojan work by groups such as World Health Organisation (WHO) and United Nations International Children's Emergency Fund (UNICEF) soon revealed the true powers of mother's milk with one of the key bits being colostrum. Colostrum contains high-quality protein, vitamins, minerals, digestive enzymes, hormones and, most importantly, antibodies that provide passive immunity to the baby (the baby's immune system is not fully developed at birth) and many other bits and pieces that cannot be produced in a lab. These help to develop the newborn's digestive system to grow and function properly. Countless studies now show that breast milk decreases the likelihood of contracting infections such as ear, cold and flu bugs, decreases the risk of asthma and eczema, lowers diabetes and possibly childhood leukaemia, may reduce psychological disorders and lowers the risk of sudden infant death syndrome (for a multitude of clinical evidence, please go to the WHO website or www. usbreastfeeding.org).

However, authors note that despite the science catching up by the 1970s and now clearly demonstrating that breast was indeed best, it seemed Nestlé was not going to walk away from this highly profitably market without a fight. It took years for them to admit defeat, and they only did so after one of the biggest corporate boycotts of the last century, beginning in the US in 1977 and spreading into Canada and Europe in the 1980s.[3]

With the US and European markets less open for business, Nestlé increased its promotion of their breast milk substitutes in less economically developed and thus less educated countries.[4] This move prompted Professor Derek Jelliffe and his wife Patrice to find the World Alliance for Breastfeeding Action and attempt to take them to task for such a move. They had some success and they are part of the reason baby formula ads now say '...*of course* breast feeding is best for your child, but *should you choose to move on* then new *follow-on* milk is shown to...'

Yet still, the practice goes on. A work published in the *British Medical Journal* in 2008, titled "Misperceptions and Misuse of Bear Brand Coffee Creamer as Infant Food: National Cross-Sectional Survey of Consumers and Paediatricians in Laos", makes for disturbing reading. The study was in response to reported cases of malnutrition among infants who had been fed coffee creamer. According to the authors, the product used was Nestlé's Bear Brand coffee creamer, which at the time carried a logo of a cartoon baby bear being held by its mother in what appears to be the breastfeeding position.[5] The largest ingredient in Bear Brand coffee creamer was sugar. Thanks to the study, Nestlé has since tweaked the potentially misleading logo on their creamer.

Frances Mason, senior nutrition advisor at Save the Children, is a vocal critic of Nestlé's marketing practices. In 2013, the charity funded a study called "Superfood for Babies". They found that one-fifth of health professionals surveyed in Pakistan said they had received gifts from representatives of breast milk substitute companies, with over half of these gifts reported to have been Nestlé-branded products. The same report found 40% of Chinese mothers had been contacted directly by breast milk substitute companies, with Nestlé among them, in direct contravention to the International Code of Marketing of breast milk substitutes they are supposed to be operating by.

Dr. Khaliq Zaman is a paediatrician at Sajida hospital, Bangladesh. He told a *Guardian* reporter that he receives frequent visits from baby formula manufacturers, including Nestlé, makers of Lactogen, one of the leading brands in Bangladesh. He states:

> The reps are very aggressive – there are three or four companies, and they come in every two weeks or so," he says. "Their main aim is to recommend their product. Sometimes they bring gifts – Nestlé brought me a big cake at new year. Some companies give things like pens and notebooks, with their brand name on them. They try very hard – even though they know I am not interested, that I always recommend breastfeeding, still they come.
>
> **Moorhead, 2007**[6]

When the Department of Trade and Industry in the Philippines, which publicly stated that it lobbies on behalf of the industry, expressed concern a proposed ban on advertising for milk products 'jeopardises multinationals' plan to invest $400 million', the response from Mike Brady, Campaigns and Networking Coordinator of the NGO Baby Milk Action, was as follows:

It is quite simply disgusting that Nestlé and its colleagues are using economic blackmail against the Philippines in an attempt to force members of Congress to accept a bill that the Department of Health, WHO and UNICEF have clearly stated will be damaging to Filipino society. The industry's boast of how sales of infant formula contribute to government revenues should be offset against the needless death and suffering – and cost to the economy – that occurs through infants and small children not being breastfed. The Supreme Court was very clear in 2007 that trade must be subjected to some form of regulation for the public good, but that cuts no ice with Nestlé Chairman, Peter Brabeck-Letmathé, who cares more about Nestlé profits. Nestlé only stops harmful marketing practices when forced to by law or through pressure from boycott supporters. Not for nothing is Nestlé one of the four most boycotted companies on the planet.

http://www.babymilkaction.org/archives/1073

Now Nestlé is pursuing the water market. Considered 'the most vital element in Nestlé's future growth' (quote Chairman of Nestlé, Peter Brabeck), Nestlé recently bought out a huge North American water company called Poland Springs. Documentary footage by Swiss journalist Res Gehringer in his documentary "Bottled Life: Nestlé's Business with Water" (2012) shows numerous gigantic tankers leaving the village Poland Springs every day. They can pump one million litres of water out of this town's aquifer in 24 hours. Gehringer explains that Nestlé now want to open up a second pumping station, this time in a wildlife reserve, but the town said no. Nestlé went to the county court. They said no. So, Nestlé went to the state court system. They, too, said no, so Nestlé is apparently suing them all.

We are told that a single road-tanker can hold 30,000 litres of water, for which the private landowner is given a whopping $10. Once bottled, this water is worth $50,000 when sold over the counter. With these sort of profits on the table, we begin to see what's fueling the fight in Nestlé

By the end of the documentary, we see Nestlé moving from small Californian towns into poorer regions of the globe, apparently draining aquifers and water tables beyond the reach of the local wells. Then, they sell the water back to them in bottles. In defence of their position on Larry Mantle on AirTalk, Nestlé Waters North America CEO, Tim Brown, explained that Nestlé was simply 'fulfilling a role' in this respect, that it's all driven by 'consumer demand'.

With the Poland Springs lawsuit, Nestlé's position was that nobody has any evidence to support the fact that taking more than 1 million litres of fresh water from a single spring, every single day, would have any damaging repercussions whatsoever to the surrounding environment or community. In the absence of evidence, until someone can prove otherwise, they should be free to take as much as they like.

This is a perfect example of the way of things today. Mirroring the success of big tobacco, big pharma, the chemical companies and now new food products such as baby formula, once a product makes it to market, often under a cloak of highly questionable scientific data, the onus is then shifted to *us*–the consumer – to prove what they are doing is wrong or causing harm. The analogies to the pet food market should be clear. *We* must produce the science. Until we do, the laws of capitalism state that they should be free to continue doing business.

Unfortunately, without *extremely* robust scientific evidence, taking years and costing many millions, proving something categorically wrong is a highly onerous task, certainly to a single consumer or small town like Poland Springs. You need a very strong, very driven, very skilled and very well-funded group to take the bull by the horns. In fact, anything short of a large, rich country (Nestlé has more spare cash than most), tackling corporate greed is often the typical David versus Goliath analogy, but without the fairytale ending. For the large part they do what they want until the weight of evidence builds to a critical mass where proceeding further would damage their profits.

While this sort of attitude may appal most, Maude Barlow, former Senior Advisor on Water for the United Nations, winner of the alternative Nobel Peace Prize, stated in the Gehringer documentary that hating these faceless megacorporations is a pointless exercise. They have no connection to a place or a people and consume without emotion. They don't love you. They don't hate you. All they care about is feeding a small handful of shareholders somewhere, and those shareholders are eternally hungry. Reflecting on this, I feel the word parasitic would be more suitable. These companies don't kill you outright. Where's the value in that?

As distasteful as this sounds, like it or not, we live in a capitalist society and big business is absolutely ruthless. Of course, it is. Your job as chair of one of these companies is to make money, above all else, year-on-year. If you don't, you will be fired and someone else will have taken your place before you even had a chance to ring your Mum. Your more ruthless replacement will be better versed in the basics of big business, which for established multinationals is to sell more or make it cheaper.

One way to make it cheaper is slave labour. In 2015, Nestlé admitted that it had found instances of forced labour in its seafood production supply chain in Thailand.[7] This resulted in pet food customers filing a class action lawsuit alleging Nestlé's cat food was the product of slave labour (Barber v. Nestlé USA, 27/01/2016). Barber lost.

For the moment, let's park our analysis of Nestlé as, in terms of corporate influence of our veterinary sector, there are two far bigger players that deserve our time, Colgate-Palmolive and Mars Inc.

The most powerful weapon available to the consumer is reliable information and pet food multinationals know this all too well. This is why their main goal is to thoroughly own and distribute the information that you, the consumer, receives. Their approach uses the tried and tested methods first invented by big tobacco, but perfected by the oil, drug and junk food companies. The process is as follows:

> **Step 1** Own the knowledge centres. Via cash incentives or outright buy-outs.

> **Step 2** Produce vast volumes of information, ideally in the form of 'studies' to corroborate their claims and bolster their agenda.

> **Step 3** Disseminate these agendas through both industry and cloaked mouthpieces.

> **Step 4** Deny, deny, deny until the weight of scientific and public opinion is so great it is no longer profitable to the company to hold its position.

In the late 1970s ,Colgate-Palmolive struck on marketing gold by paying dentists to recommend their toothpaste[8] something that, somewhat remarkably, hadn't been thought of until then. By the early 1980s, Colgate toothpaste had dominated the market, making them a pretty penny. Flushed with this success, Colgate-Palmolive then turned its focus on vets to recommend their pet food lines. In her article in the Wall Street Journal, titled "For You, My Pet: Why The Veterinarian Really Recommends That Designer Chow – Colgate Gives Doctors Treats For Plugging Its Brands, And Sees Sales Surge", Parker Pope documents the whole affair.

For their approach to be truly successful, Colgate-Palmolive first needed a great brand of pet food. As building one is both difficult and time expensive for multinationals, using their vast cash reserves to purchase established companies is often the quickest and easiest route to market. The Mark Morris Institute

(MMI) was a company with a long history in pet food research, development and education. The MMI also owned Hill's Science Diet, a pet food so scientific that it has the word science in the title. Now *this* was a brand vets might get behind. But MMI had more than just well branded pet food.

In 1987, the MMI published the *Small Animal Clinical Nutrition* (SACN). Now in its fifth edition,[9] the SACN is today the mainstay of small animal nutrition for the world's vets. It is edited by a plethora of highly qualified vets and is packed with thousands of references. And yet, while protein (20%) and carbohydrates (50–60%) are, by weight, the most important constituents of cereal-based pet food by a very considerable degree, the evidence used to support some of their more worrying stances is all but absent. The SACN makes statements such as 'starch levels found in commercial cat foods, up to 35% of the food's DM, are well tolerated' without using a single reference in support of such a crucial point. In their all-too-brief section on protein, the SACN makes the following unreferenced statement 'it is important to note the AAFCO recommendations should be interpreted as daily allowances, not as absolute minimum requirements'. This is despite the The Association of American Feed Control Officials (AAFCO) stating that they are in fact exactly that, *minimum* requirements (18% crude protein for an adult, 22.5% for a puppy).[10] Most worryingly, nowhere in this colossal nutritional manual (1300+ page) does the SACN discuss the importance of fresh, biologically appropriate ingredients for dogs or cats.

In 1988, Colgate-Palmolive bought the MMI and then, as Parker Pope highlights, began to focus their attentions on the veterinary departments of US universities, offering cash-starved universities generous financial donations in return for veterinary endorsements, product placement and allowing them to distribute their nutritional information, such as the SACN, to veterinary students.[8] Within one year they had made large financial contributions to all twenty-seven university veterinary departments in the United States. John Steel, a once senior vice-president of global marketing and sales for Colgate-Palmolive, said 'the bulk of our expenditure goes to the veterinary community'.[8]

It's fair to say, Hill's Science and Prescription Diets are now the dry food of choice by the vast majority of vets today in a global market of $72 billion per year. Thirty years on and it is very difficult to find a university veterinary department not promoting Hill's Pet Food in some form. Whyte and Robinson (2016)[11] reported that trainee vets in the prestigious Murdoch University in Perth, Western Australia today are now wearing Hill's branded clothing and nearly all of Murdoch's discharge letters recommend a Hill's diet for pets. In 2016, when Sydney University admitted that a Hill's Pet Food employee directly teaches nutrition to their third-year students,[11] something the department said was 'appropriate for an identified industry and academic expert to present to students as part of a professional program', a lecturer in ethics from the very same University, Anne Fawcett, admitting the potential for conflict of interest in the situation was a concern, stated:

> I think we need to be really aware of the problem. Companies wouldn't be giving freebies if they weren't getting something out of it.
>
> **Whyte and Robinson, 2016**[11]

Today, if you look closely enough, you will see a link to Hill's sponsorship on most university veterinary department website pages. Sometimes this link can be hard to find, so an easier way, is to Google your vet department of choice with the words, 'Hill's Pet Nutrition' or simply ring your university veterinary department and ask them what dry food brands they stock in their waiting room. The answer is rarely more than one.

It's not just the universities in receipt of Colgate-Palmolive's generous cash grants but also the veterinary governing bodies and journals. The American Animal Hospital Association (AAHA) is one such recipient. Among a great number of other projects, the AAHA's Weight Management Guidelines Implementation Guidelines was 'sponsored by a generous educational grant from Hill's Pet Nutrition'.[12] The AAHA, for some reason, needs a lot of money to do its job and a lot of it comes via 'sponsorship'. As of 2018, their Strategic Alliance Program says would-be donors can choose from the Diamond, Platinum, Gold, Emerald and Silver Strategic Alliance Programs. This gets you various advantages. For instance, you can get recognition on www.aaha.org, advertise in the JAAHA or even give 'scientific educational sessions', depending on your membership. The AAHA Convention in 2010 sported giant Hill's and Pfizer advertisements outside its venue. Perhaps they were welcoming their new CEO, Michael T. Cavanaugh, who was previously, from 2000–2010, the Director of Veterinary Hospital Services with Pfizer.

On the American Veterinary Medical Association (AVMA) website, another colossal veterinary governing body in the United States, on the images of their 2016 convention, there are Hill's stickers with the tagline 'one of the reasons people flock to the AVMA Annual Convention is the superb educational programming, Hill's Pet Nutrition plays a big role in supporting this'.

The Canadian Veterinary Medical Association's (CVMA) annual report for 2007 highlights a CVMA and Hill's Pet Nutrition new venture called the "Pet Health and Nutrition Tool Kit", whose purpose is to:

> ...help veterinarians facilitate an open and honest dialogue with clients about nutrition and the crucial role it plays in the overall health and wellbeing of their pets...
>
> **Hodgkins and Smart, 2008**[13]

Even the World Small Animal Veterinary Association (WSAVA), the 'association of veterinary associations' and authority for vets worldwide, has Hill's as a gold sponsor (as of February 2019), their 'longest-standing industry partner', apparently. A search of the WSAVA website reveals numerous programs involving Hill's Pet Food.

While all this was going on, the candy company and dog food manufacturer Mars Inc. was not about to sit on their hands and allow the carpet to be pulled from under them. Mars is the world leader in pet food production, holding a quarter of the $71.77 billion global pet food market as of 2015,[1] and they have taken great steps of late to establish themselves as the world's largest providers of pet health care, albeit in a slightly different manner to Colgate-Palmolive.

As with Colgate-Palmolive employees teaching nutrition directly to veterinary students, Mars too have used paid residents to access the highest levels of veterinary university education. The results of a crucial Freedom of Information Act Enquiry, published by the UK Raw Meaty Bones (UKRMB) website,[14] shows details of correspondence between the veterinary department of the University of Edinburgh (The Royal Dick School of Veterinary Studies) and Mars Pedigree Pet Foods beginning in 1993 and ending in 2003. The conversation was concerning a draft of their partnership. What it disclosed was staggering. They got straight to the point from page 1 (italics added by me for effect):

> ...This plan is a natural progression; reflecting our mutual interests in the *education of veterinary students*...

> ...Final impetus to the development of a firm partnership has been provided by the company's *wish to become... more closely associated with the education process in veterinary schools* and by the opportunity to *fund the... Clinical Nutrition Residency*...

Mars divides their demands into four sections:

Section 1 was regarding the funding of a full time 'resident' who would play 'a key role in our overall partnership'. Below are some examples, cited by Mars, of what they expect the full time resident to be responsible for.

...the teaching of Small Animal Nutrition, including Clinical Nutrition, to veterinary students...

...to disseminate this knowledge to the undergraduate students and professional colleagues by written papers, lectures and tutorials, in order to improve the awareness of the importance of nutrition...

Section two of four in the Mars contract was concerning their products. Here Mars states:

...Pedigree Pet Food products will be used exclusively in the Faculty of Veterinary Medicine...

...This will not only apply to the Pedigree & Whiskas Clinical Diets, but to the 'core' brands such as Pedigree...Chum, Chappie and Whiskas ranges...

...Pedigree Pet foods will supply the above products free of charge, which can then be used to generate further...income for the Department...

Section three of four was concerning 'commercial development'. Here Mars states:

...This partnership will offer a unique opportunity for mutual activity in the areas of waiting & reception room...merchandising, staff training in retailing skills and pet health counselling...

Section four was entitled 'contractual expectations'. Here Mars states:

...Within the undergraduate curriculum, the use of speakers, written material and promotional visits from other prepared pet food manufacturers will be discussed with the company prior to any arrangements being made...

Also released in the same FOI request were the responses by the Head of Department to Mars Pedigree Pet food as well as to Purina Pet food whom, and I'm paraphrasing, they also wanted to work with.

...We are, as I mentioned, obliged to use and recommend Pedigree diets as our first choice...but, clearly, we will be able to be of enormous help [to Purina] in the generation of publicity through lectures etc. and the… publications by the appointee…

Head of the Veterinary Department at Edinburgh University to Purina Pet Food, October 31, 1997

On January 7, 2000, the Head of Department writes to Mars (italics added by me):

…I am trying to develop a more aggressive sales pitch in respect of the Pedigree products as we have yet to…recover anything like the sales levels that existed prior to the change in agreements. My task has not been aided…by Hill's, who have developed a direct sales pitch to our students, *which we are powerless to stop.* So what I…have to do is to ensure that the students know of the superiority of the Pedigree products…

On December 18, 2003, the head of the Veterinary Department highlights just how successful their partnership has been over the last decade. Among their many successes, they cited:

…collaboration on several projects which ultimately led to the publication of one textbook on clinical nutrition…and nine scientific papers. In addition X lectured on behalf of the company in several countries including…Israel, Hungary and most recently Greece…several road shows aimed at increasing awareness of the 'Selected Protein' range of diets, which led to a significant increase in sales of the product and allowed Pedigree to…firmly stamp its authority in this area of the… market…

When we look at the studies cited, most of which published in reputable journals, we see no mention of the paid position, simply that they were produced by the Department of Veterinary Clinical Studies, Royal (Dick) School of Veterinary Studies, Summerhill, Edinburgh.

In their letter, the University gets the Mars-funded resident to say a few words. We learn that while resident, she apparently taught:

…all the small animal basic nutrition lectures to the preclinical veterinary students, as well as many of the small animal medicine classes, which include an introduction to therapeutic…diets. Teaching the use of clinical diets… has resulted in greater awareness of clinical nutrition among our students and therefore more use of special…diets in the patients…

…the final year clinical nutrition tutorials, and also taught final year seminars, practicals, and…day to day teaching at ward rounds, on the use of clinical diets and specifically Waltham-Royal Canin diets…

The Mars-funded resident summed the whole relationship perfectly:

…This means our students on clinics are predominantly exposed to Waltham-Royal Canin diets, encouraging their use later in their careers…

Emboldened by their success, the UKRMB later sent out a similar FOI request to the Royal Veterinary College (RVC), London (Sept. 1, 2005) concerning a Mrs. Hill MRCVS who recently took up a senior position there. They requested all correspondence between Mrs Hill and any processed pet food companies from 1998 to present. The RVC refused on the grounds they believed the request to be 'vexatious' as 'it does not appear to have any serious purpose or value and will therefore not disclose any information'. Countering, the UKRMB highlighted that at the time, Hill was president of the Royal College of Veterinary Surgeons (RCVS), the group responsible for regulating the veterinary profession in the United Kingdom. The UKRMB noted it was a matter of public interest that prior to these two powerful positions Mrs. Hill was previously a senior executive for a pet food company. The RVC, a public-funded body, offered no more information.

On the February 14, 2007, the UKRMB uncovered via an FOI request (again, published on their website) that Hill's Pet Nutrition sponsored a clinician in their Small Animal Practice and a veterinary nurse in their Small Animal Intensive Care and Emergency Medicine in the University of Bristol. Hill's also provided one lecture on nutrition to students. Mars Waltham were funding a postgrad student.

Nor is it simply the UKRMB having success in this area. In 2012, Australian vet, Dr Tom Lonsdale, one of the 'founding fathers' of raw (author of *Raw Meaty Bones*) published the contract between Mars Petcare and the School of Veterinary Science in Queensland University on his website (www.rawmeatybones.com/foi. php). Among free food, scrub tops and kitten packs, Mars will deliver 'nutrition lectures to the vet school as required' and 'at least one Continuing Education Workshop per year for postgraduates, students and staff'.

In 2014, Lonsdale revealed the contract between Murdoch University and Hill's Pet Food. In return for the cash sponsorship fee ($135,000) that Hill's will provide ($45,000 every year for three years) Murdoch will agree to do quite a number of things for Hill's. First, they will promote Hill's pet food in their hospital. They will also permit the sponsor to 'engage' with the veterinary profession. This apparently includes Continuing Education sessions focusing on small animal internal medicine but also:

- access in person to veterinarians interested in small animal medicine

- verbal acknowledgement of sponsorship at the beginning of each session

- opportunity for a company representative to mingle with attendees prior to the lecture

- opportunity to provide promotional material to attendees

- [their] logo on all promotional material

Finally, they want access to the students there, too. This involves:

- The sponsor's representatives will be provided the opportunity to present education nutritional sessions for students, academic and clinical staff up to four times annually and up to two product information sessions annually.

- The sponsor will be provided the opportunity to promote the online nutrition course 'Veterinary Nutrition Advocate' to students two times annually.

I don't know much about business, but I would say that's $135k well spent.

Author's note:

If you would like to know more about the relationship the veterinary department of your local university has to whatever pet food they are selling in their foyer, you will have to submit a Freedom of Information request. Write to the institution, ask them for their FOI officer and address it directly to them, ideally stating the specific FOI act that supports your request. The wording is key and often tricky. Be polite but direct and clear. For example, the UKRMB get straight into it with wording like 'In respect of all processed pet food companies with which Liverpool Veterinary School is associated whether in a scientific, social, educational or research capacity, please supply…'. They then go on to ask for current contracts and memoranda of agreements. They also regularly ask for all correspondence between the school and pet food companies in certain years, something you are entitled to know. Don't ask for a 'cash sponsor'. It's an easy out for them. The money-trail you are trying to decipher is rarely delivered in a suitcase. There are many ways to fund an institution, including providing grants, scholarships, bursaries, guest lecture appointments, equipment (new or 'loaned'), field excursions to pet food setups or even funding new building projects. Do some research on how best to phrase each question but even then, the institution is not obliged to provide you with supporting or original documentation unless their answers are deemed unsatisfactory. You might be charged for some of this information. If it looks of value, consider a GoFundMe campaign and advertise it in your favourite raw feeding Facebook groups, asking for $1 from everyone. Always thank them for engaging with you and make sure to send them what you found. If they were motivated enough to send you money, they will be the ones to spread your findings across social media.

Much like Colgate-Palmolive's MMI and their SACN manual for vets, Mars Inc. too, has, a science arm called The Waltham Centre for Pet Nutrition, which has been 'advancing research into the nutrition and health of pets for over 50 years'. Waltham is a formidable collection of veterinary heavyweights, who release enormous amounts of literature through various outlets, including their own veterinary journal *Veterinary Focus* (previously *Waltham Focus*). Much like Colgate-Palmolive with their SACN, Mars Waltham has their version of a small animal nutrition book titled "Clinical Nutrition of the Dog and Cat" (first published in 1993). Popular with vets, it does not discuss the use of fresh, biologically appropriate ingredients in pets.

The use of strings-attached residencies greatly clouds the waters when trying to decipher if a study has any conflicts of interest but, in my opinion, this stretches into everything that the resident might do in the future. Richard Hill, VetMB, PhD, MRCVS, DACVIM, DACVN, is the *Waltham* Associate Professor of Small Animal Internal Medicine and Clinical Nutrition at the University of Florida College of Veterinary Medicine (as of January 2018). He is also sits on the ad hoc committee of the national Research Council (NRC) for dog and cat nutrition. Herein lies the problem. The NRC produces possibly the most influential and referenced (by vets at least) manual on canine nutrition next to Colgate-Palmolive's *Small Animal Clinical Nutrition*.[9] It is called *Nutrient Requirements of Dogs and Cats*.[15] The NRC, it is claimed, is a governmental body whose mission statement enthuses independence (italics added by me for effect):

> ...to improve government decision making and public policy, increase public understanding, and promote the...acquisition and dissemination of knowledge in matters involving science, engineering, technology, and health... the Research Council's *independent*, expert reports and other scientific activities inform policies and actions...that have the power to improve the lives of people in the US and around the world...

While being careful not to question the role of such an esteemed scientist, it's not unfair to ask how, with a title of Mars Waltham Associate Professor, you can get on a board of *independent* experts that governs many of the rules and guidelines used in dog food production and legislation. Nor is he alone. Professor John Bauer also sits on the ad hoc committee on the NRC dog and cat nutrition. Since 1991, he has worked exclusively for Texas A&M University. On his CV it lists his position as 'Mark L. Morris Professor of Clinical Nutrition, Department of Small Animal Clinical Sciences, Texas A&M University', Mark L. Morris being the science arm of Hill's pet food. The argument here, I assume, would be that their wages are not paid by said multinationals but by the university that employs them.

At any rate, like both the SACN owned by Hill's Pet Food and Mars Waltham's *Clinical Nutrition of the Dog and Cat,* the NRC (2006) also fails to consider the need or potential benefit of fresh, species-appropriate food for dogs or cats. And again, like these aforementioned works, it makes its argument for high carbohydrate usage in dogs and cats without using a single long-term study that compared a group of dogs fed such diets to a control group of dogs fed a normal, fresh, species-appropriate meat and bone diet.

While Mars has clearly had some success with their use of residents in universities, it's fair to say Hill's Science and Prescription diets seem to dominate in the veterinary university and governing body sector, judging by the apparent domination of Hill's Pet Food in University Veterinary departments (*personal comment*). Mars needed another plan to break into the veterinary game, and since the 2000s, it seems they have been putting that plan into action.

Over the last two decades, Mars has focused their enormous cash reserves on buying up independent veterinary practices, now at a staggering rate. Among their bigger purchases, we introduced you in Section 2 to the US veterinary giant Banfield. With more than 800 hospitals in 43 US states, as well as having more than 13,000 associates, including 2,600 licensed veterinarians, Banfield has access to over two million dogs and half a million cats. It produces the State of Pet Health Report, which gives us key figures for the growth of various chronic conditions in dogs today. Mars Inc. made their first investment in 1994 buying it outright in 2007 and we lose the Banfield report as an independent source of vital information in the process. In 2015, Mars bought Blue Pearl, adding another 53 specialty veterinary hospitals in the United States to their portfolio. In 2016, they bought Pet Partners and just a year later they made their biggest buy yet, VCA, for a staggering $7.7 billion (750 animal hospitals, 4,700 vets). In June 2018, Mars acquired the European group AniCura (200 hospitals, 4,000 vets) and Linnaeus Group Ltd. in the United Kingdom (82 clinics and five specialist referral centres). The latest investment was into the new and fast-growing Chinese market where Mars is now a partner in the RingPai Pet Hospital group who have 4,000 employees. And these are just the major buyouts we hear about. A single buyout of a veterinary hospital is not worth column inches, but they are happening all the time. Like any shop, when an independent vet wants to move on, their practice and turnover is worth good money. For years, the likes of Mars Banfield have been targeting these too.[16] The net result is that by mid-2018, Mars Inc. had more than 50,000 veterinary professionals in their pocket.[17]

Nor is it just Mars. Everyone knows there is big money to be made from our pets and where that happens, you will find investors looking to turn a buck (italics added by me for effect).

> In 2014 a chain of 250 hospitals called National Veterinary Associates was purchased by Ares Management for $920 million. In 2015 the Ontario Teachers' Pension Plan spent $440 million to buy a pet hospital group. Last May, VCA spent $344 million for a group of 56 hospitals pooled together by a smaller consolidator *for the express purpose of flipping them.*
>
> **Clenfield, 2017,[16] writing for Bloomberg News**

While most of us would find it hard to swallow the notion of a global, multi-billion candy company gaining control of our hospitals, we are not suggesting there is anything inherently wrong with corporate-owned vet hospitals. We need only look at our own privately run human hospitals to see the difference in care these groups can put out (at least in terms of waiting times, possibly more modern equipment and certainly fancier surroundings with better food). However, there are many reasons why the analogy here to pet sector is a poor one.

First, in human medicine, independent doctors must refer us to private hospitals, though they too suffer industry rep influence. In the pet world, no such filter now exists. By cash-sponsoring the universities and governing bodies, sitting on boards where it counts, as well as buying up our vet hospitals and practices, corporations are buying out our one and only line of defence. We have only their employees for advice.

Second, all our private hospitals have to deal with the insurance companies directly. Insurance companies are great at keeping medical costs down by constantly querying bills and procedures, as well as investigating many of the claims that come to them. In the pet world, bills are smaller and pet owners largely pay cash. Moreover, should insurance be needed, usually the client pays first and negotiates with the insurer themselves for reimbursement, which reduces scrutiny on the hospital setting the bill.

Finally, keeping everyone on their toes, when human doctors make a mistake, the financial implications for the hospital can be dire. With pets there are no real financial consequences for vets that do wrong. Pets are still treated as property and pay-outs are thus very low, topping out at approximately $1,500 for the death of a pet. This means few, if any, court cases. Without the sword of Damocles hanging over them, it is perceivable that companies who want to boost profits, might take greater risks.

In 2017, Bloomberg[16] took a look at how the Mars Banfield group now operates. The piece centred on vet John Robb, a vet who franchised a vet practice from Banfield and had a less than positive experience. Robb became concerned about the side effects he was seeing from the over-vaccinating pets. Unbelievably, they give the same size vaccination to a Great Dane as they do a Chihuahua. Studies show this is absolutely not working out for smaller dogs.[18,19] Robb began to give half-doses of vaccine to smaller dogs. Despite pharma giants such as Boehringer Ingelheim supplying a new half-dose shot for just this reason, Banfield was not happy and ultimately took Robb's practice from him. They are still today locked in a legal battle, and it has gotten very messy. Robb began picketing his own practice and more than once has been removed and arrested, one time strapped to a stretcher.

This might seem a bit rash until you consider the difference between a family vet and a global corporation. An independent vet is surely more likely to employ restraint on a client they might meet in a supermarket. Corporations might lean toward a more maximalist approach each visit. To quote Tom Fuller, a chief financial officer for Mars, the company's business strategy is:

> ...to leverage our existing customer base by increasing the number and intensity of the services... received during each visit...
>
> **Clenfield, 2017**[16]

To facilitate this process, Mars is getting into supplying diagnostics and laboratory services. The 2017 purchase of the animal hospital behemoth VCA (Veterinary Centres of America) Inc. was, of course, a tactical one. VCA owns ANTECH, which is the biggest diagnostics laboratory in the US if not the world. ANTECH's website informs us that they service more than 19,000 animal hospitals throughout North America, operating more than 50 reference laboratories in the United States and Canada. Diagnostics actually make up 41% of VCA's operating profit.

With their dominance in vet hospital ownership and now equipped with the likes of VCA, Mars has firmly established their new approach to the pet health market.

> Banfield's Pet Ware manual makes for interesting reading. In one example, explaining how the software is used to prescribe treatment, the book shows a checklist of therapies for a dog with atopic dermatitis or itchy skin. Doctors are encouraged to recommend a biopsy, analgesics, topical medications, antibiotics, a therapeutic dietary supplement, an allergy diet, and a flea control package. They're required to recommend antihistamines, shampoos, serum allergy testing, lab work, a skin diagnostic package, and anti-inflammatories. It's a treatment course that might run $900 for symptoms that, in a best-case scenario, indicate something as prosaic as fleas. In bold print, the manual reminds doctors: "You cannot change items that were initially marked Required. They must remain required".
>
> **Clenfield, 2017**[16]

To help their vets hit their sales targets, they give them *actual targets*. Clenfield (2017)[6] cites Wendy Beers, DVM, who quit a Mars hospital in 2014. She stated that they were sent printouts of what you sold that month with suggested targets for the following month. Leticia German, DVM, chief of staff at a Banfield hospital in Colorado from 2010 to 2013, stated those who didn't meet their targets were made to attend workshops 'to school them into how to better meet their numbers... it was definitely intimidating'.

In the face of a slowdown in human drug approvals and greatly encouraged by the increased medication of our pets in the developed world,[20] the big drug companies are now turning their attentions to the pet health market with increasing vigour, pouring millions of dollars into research and development of pet medicines. And it's working for them. In just the United States alone, the pet drug market was worth $7.6 billion in 2013, up 60% from 2006. The figure at 2016 was approaching $10 billion (pet ownership during this entire period was relatively stagnant). And it's not just the US market. In 2006, Statista put the global market for animal health at $16 billion US dollars. Just 10 years later it had nearly doubled to some $30 billion with the veterinary drug market accounting for 84% of it ($25.3 billion). In just 8 years (2024) the market is expected to double again in size to nearly $50 billion. In 2015, the third-biggest initial public offering on Wall Street was the pet medicine company, Zoetis.

We need to accept that pet owners are pretty much the perfect market. Most owners love their dogs as they do their own kids and they would do anything for them. In the last global downturn, pet care, encompassing food and health, was one of the only markets not to see a dip in spending with owners stating they would cut their own food bill before their dogs.[21] The above sales figures show this market is more than susceptible to the market pressure placed on them, spending often large portions of their hard-earned money on countless products and treatments including grossly over-priced pet foods and such treatments as chemical parasite 'prevention' (like chemically de-nitting your kids *before* they go to school), annual boosters (for dogs already adequately vaccinated for viruses as a pup, and against advice from WSAVA who state every three years is adequate) and kennel cough (akin to a common cold in a dog, one still without an effective vaccine, even if you thought it was necessary).

Moreover, the pet route incurs significantly less regulatory impediments. Amazingly, in the last 10 years, while hundreds of human drugs have been removed from the market over safety concerns and billions paid out in compensation, you will struggle to find a single pet drug pulled by a governing body over safety concerns, despite pets being repeatedly maimed and dying from their consumption. In a piece titled "Tick And Flea Control Agent Bravecto Continues To Be Acceptably Safe To Use"(17/08/2017, published online, www.ema.europa.eu), the European Medicines Agency revealed that less than 1 in 10,000 dogs will have convulsions after its use and apparently less than 1 in 50,000 doses kills (kill figure based on cited figures of 18 million doses in the European Union between February 2014 and December 2016 and 342 'reported' deaths between February 2014 and August 15, 2017). Before we even consider the fact that for every side effect that is documented, nine more go unreported in humans[22] – a figure we can surely multiply in pets, and ignoring the fact that pets can receive such medicines each and every month of their life, let's quickly imagine these figures in human terms–let's take the population of the European Union as a throwaway example. With 500 million people, assuming 200 million of these are children, consider an EU wide child-vaccination program that is deemed 'acceptably safe' when it is known it will result at the *very least* in 4,000 deaths (200 million children at a rate of 1 in 50,000)?

To understand if such a potentially lethal drug was necessary to inflict on the population, you might do a quick risk/benefit analysis. Do we need to treat every single child for parasites, such as head lice, when the vast majority of healthy Western children are not only unlikely to pick them up but are highly unlikely to succumb to them should they do? For parasites, a quick, easy and noninvasive skin or stool examination would indicate their presence and then a single (safer, more natural?) treatment might be applied. Why is this not an option? Are we to believe parents can be entrusted with the health and well being of their own children in this regard but not that of their pets?

It gets even better for pet drug manufacturers. The users never complain in any meaningful way and, best of all, *should* you kill one or two and *should* the owner and vet suspect the drug (or food), and *should* the client have the means to send the dog for a thorough autopsy and *should* they have a supportive vet to take it to the next level and *should* they have the time, financial means and dogged determination to take the colossal, well-armed, multinational company on in court for years, then the maximum payout is rarely more than the cost of the animal! The drug companies literally can't lose.

And with all this extra medicine to dispense comes a need for more vets. From 1996 to 2013 the National Bureau of Economic Research states the number of veterinarians in the United States almost doubled.[23] All this despite Statista reporting US dog ownership only increased by 22.5% in approximately the same period. From 2000 to 2014 US dog ownership rose from 68 to 83.3 million dogs, with cats adding similar figures. That's a lot of extra health care (and vets) per pet. In fact, from just 2010 to 2014, in the depths of recession and with the pet population relatively stagnant, The American Pet Products Association reports that total spending on vet health care jumped by 17% from $13 billion to $15.2 billion.

Responding to the rise in costs, pet health insurance in the United States is rising quicker than even human health care,[23] which probably explains why less than 1% of American pet owners have pet health insurance (1.6 million US pets were insured in 2015; there was an estimated 160 million dogs and cats in the US in 2015).[24,25] The inevitable consequence here is sick pets are going untreated.

Whatever way you look at it, owning a dog is clearly becoming a *very* expensive thing to do, at least in the US but something we can all probably now testify to.

It's fair to say not everyone is a fan of this great corporate buyout of the vet sector. While it's thought corporations today own 15% to 20% of America's 26,000 pet hospitals,[16] the process is only really beginning in the United Kingdom and Ireland. In 2015, the UK Vet Council amended its Code of Professional Conduct to allow non-vets, including limited companies, to own veterinary practices, with Ireland following suit a year later, as she tends to do. However, speaking to a major Irish newspaper, Veterinary Ireland, a group that represents vets in Ireland said it has serious concerns with respect to the changes relating to the ownership of veterinary practices and the impact that these changes would have for both animal health and welfare and the veterinary profession as a whole.[26] It says that the changes are contrary to the Veterinary Practice Act 2005 and that 86% of its members are against the notion. They have sought clarification from the Veterinary Council of Ireland as to the meaning and implications of such a move and have not ruled out legal action to prevent the process from happening.

Nor are they entirely alone. To quote Dr Malik, one of the world's leading authorities in cats and former consultant to Zoetis, who is now petitioning his own Veterinary Council to distance itself from global pet care industry influence:

> …we're on this slippery slope of influence that pervades the things we do… it saddens me that despite…terrific developments, we have gone down this pathway of commercialism…
>
> **Whyte and Robinson, 2016[11]**

Speaking up for vets promoting the feeding of biologically appropriate food to pets, the Raw Feeding Veterinary Society, formed in 2014 in the United Kingdom now has more than 100 paid up members as of January 2020. It's fair to say these vets are still very much in the minority. It seems the vast majority of our vets remain steadfastly convinced by the science supporting their product of choice. So, let's take a look at some of the evidence used to prop up the dry pet food sector.

TAKE-HOME POINTS

✓ Mars and Nestlé, the world's biggest candy manufacturers, are also the biggest players in pet food, annually grossing $17.2b and $12.5b of turnover, respectively.

✓ Nestlé is the most boycotted company in the United Kingdom, much of it a result of their relentless pursuit of the baby formula market in the 1970s. Sadly, studies show the pursuit of young mothers and health professionals is still going on today in poorer regions.

✓ The multinational's stance was they had the right to make money. That it was up to the market to prove what they were doing was wrong or harmful. That is a very difficult, laborious, lengthy and costly thing to do.

✓ Colgate-Palmolive bought out the MMI, creators of Hill's Science Diet and publishers of the SACN, the leading canine nutrition manual for vets today.

✓ CP were the first multinational to properly pursue vets to recommend their pet food. Authors note they did it by offering generous cash donations to cash-hungry veterinary departments. It is now recommended by most veterinary departments in the Western World. CP also cash-sponsor the biggest veterinary organisations and scientific journals.

✓ Mars does their share of veterinary department sponsorship too. FOI requests reveal their desire to be 'more closely associated with the education process in veterinary schools'. In return for monies given to the University of Edinburgh, Mars Inc. was the first to teach small animal nutrition to veterinary students. Further FOI requests reveal this implantation of industry 'residents' into veterinary colleges happens the world over.

✓ Over the last three decades, Mars has been buying up independent vet practices. They also bought veterinary giants Banfield, Blue Pearl, Pet Partners, Antech Diagnostics and VCA, to name but a few. Mars now has more than 50,000 vets worldwide on the payroll.

✓ Mars also owns The Waltham Centre for Pet Nutrition, the science and marketing arm of Mars Pet Food. They publish the popular *Clinical Nutrition of the Dog and Cat*. Much like CPs' SACN, it does not discuss the potential benefits of fresh, biologically appropriate ingredients in meat-eating cats and dogs.

✓ Bloomberg highlights how companies such as Mars Banfield have provided their vets a long list of treatment recommendations for diseases such as atopy and actual sales targets to hit.

✓ The pet drug market is now exploding. In the last decade, the global pet health market has doubled in value (from $16b to $30b per year). In just 8 years, it is anticipated to double again. Vet numbers have doubled from 1996-2013. Pet ownership has been relatively stagnant during this time.

✓ Insurance costs are now spiralling. The majority of pet owners can no longer afford it. Inevitably, sick pets are going to go untreated.

Chapter Seventeen References

1   Reuters (2017). Mars to buy pet healthcare provider VCA for $7.7 billion. Published online, Jan 9th, www.reuters.com

2   Laflamme, D., Izquierdo, O., Eirmann, L. *et al.* (2014). Myths and misperceptions about ingredients used in commercial pet foods. Veterinary Clinics of North American Small Animal Practice, 44(4): 689–698

3   Deacute, B. (1985). *The evolution in Canada of the citizen's movement against Nestlé, 1978–1984: A descriptive study*. Masters thesis. Waterloo, Canada: Wilfrid Laurier University.

4   Wise, J. (1997). Baby milk companies accused of breaching marketing code. British Medical Journal, 314(7075): 167

5   Barennes, H., Andriatahina, T., Latthaphasavang, V. *et al.* (2008). Misperceptions and misuse of Bear Brand coffee creamer as infant food: national cross sectional survey of consumers and paediatricians in Laos, British Medical Journal, 337: 1379

6   Moorhead, J. (2007). *Milking it*. The Guardian. Published online, May 15th, www. theguardian.com

7   Marschkea, M. and Vandergeestb, P. (2016). Slavery scandals: Unpacking labour challenges and policy responses within the off-shore fisheries sector. Marine Policy, 68: 39–46

8   Parker-Pope, T. (1997). *For you, my pet: Why the veterinarian really recommends that designer chow – Colgate gives doctors treats for plugging its brands, and sees sales surge – Offering a fat-cat bounty*. Wall Street Journal (Eastern Edition), Nov 3rd.

9   Hand, M.S., Thatcher, C.D., Remillard, R.L. *et al.* (2010). *Small Animal Clinical Nutrition, 5th Edition.* Topeka, KS, Mark Morris Institure

10   Association of American Feed Control Officials (AAFCO, 2016). Dog and Cat Food Nutrient Profiles. Official Publication, see www.aafco.org

11   Whyte, S. and Robinson, L. (2016). *Vet industry compromised by influence of pet food and pharmaceutical companies, expert says.* ABC News Australia. Nov 12th, www.abc.net.au

12   American Animal Hospital Association (AAHA, 2014). *2014 AAHA Weight Management Guidelines for Dogs and Cats. Veterinary Practice Guidelines.* AAHA Official Publication. Published online, www.aaha.org

13   Hodgkins, E. and Smart, M. (2008). Who is responsible for the efficacy and safety of pet foods? Canadian Veterinary Journal, 49(10): 945

14   www.ukrmb.co.uk/images/RoyalDickCorres.pdf

15   National Research Council (NRC, 2006). *Nutrient requirement of dogs and cats.* Washington, DC: National Academies Press.

16   Clenfield, J. (2017). *The high-cost, high-risk world of modern pet care.* Bloomberg News. Published online, Jan 5th, www.bloomberg.com

17   Lau, E. (2018). *Mars Inc. buys British veterinary-hospital chain.* Veterinary Information Network news. Published online, Jun 8th, www.news.vin.com

18   Moore, G.E., Guptill, L.F., Ward, M.P. *et al.* (2005). Adverse events diagnosed within three days of vaccine administration in dogs. Journal of the American Veterinary Medical Association, 227: 1102–1108

19   Novak, W. (2007). *Predicting the "unpredictable" vaccine reactions.* Proceeding of the NAVC North American Veterinary Conference. Jan. 13-27, Orlando, Florida

20   Ward, A. (2015). *Pharma groups eye healthy returns from animal drugs market.* Financial Times. Published online, Jul 1st, www.ft.com

21   Sanburn, J. (2011). *12 things we buy in a bad economy.* Time Magazine. Published online, Oct 19th, www.business.time.com

22   Hohl, C.M, Small, S.S., Peddie, D. *et al.* (2018). Why Clinicians Don't Report Adverse Drug Events: Qualitative Study. JMIR Public Health Surveillance, 4(1): e21

23   Einav, L., Finkelstein, A., and Gupta, A. (2017). Is American Pet Health Care (Also) Uniquely Inefficient? American Economic Review: Papers & Proceedings, 107(5): 491–495

24   North American Pet Health Insurance Association (2015). *State of the Industry Benchmarking Report 2014.* Published online, Jul 7th, www.naphia.org

25   American Pet Products Association (2016). *Pet Industry Market Size & Ownership Statistics 2016.* Published online, www.americanpetproducts.org

26   Donnelly, M. (2017). *Vets may challenge new rules to allow non vets own practices.* Irish Independent Newspaper. Published online, Dec 28th, www.independent.ie

What Does *Scientifically Proven* Mean?

Unfalsifiable Comparisons: The Foundation of the Dry Pet Food Industry

I was recently debating the use of chemical parasite control with a small group of vets at a seminar. In short, I absolutely do not recommend chemical parasite *prevention* in pets with no parasites. Rather the critter than the chemicals used to prevent them, as they say (fleas are a non event, *if* you find them on your dog, use a bit of diatomaceous earth; for worms do a stool count where you post off a poo sample to them, and for as little as €15/$20, they will tell you if they have worms, cheap and definitive. Should an issue be identified there are a great variety of simple, natural and highly effective home-remedies to try before going nuclear. Please see www.dogsfirst.ie for more). The conversation soon turned to ticks. I hate ticks as I have seen firsthand what Lyme disease and co-infections, resulting from a tick bite, can do to someone. During the debate, a vet informed me of a study of more than 15,000 UK dogs which found 31% of them had ticks.

It has to be said, this was quite shocking news to me. Not one to normally doubt figures quoted offhand, I did think this figure might be a touch high, so I wanted to see who was behind the study. A little digging on the website responsible (www.bigtickproject.co.uk) quickly revealed it was sponsored by MSD Animal Health (Merck Sharp & Dohme Corp, aka Merck Animal Health) the makers of the chemical flea, worm and tick preventative product, Bravecto®, a company the university lists as a proud sponsor that year. While this does not invalidate the work, it does put you on alert.

The study used to support their claims, titled "Ticks Infesting Domestic Dogs in the UK: A Large-Scale Surveillance Program", was conducted by Bristol University (encouraging) under the stewardship of Professor Wall, head of Veterinary Parasitology and Ecology (very encouraging). However, it was not published in a peer-reviewed journal but in the University's own research section. This is instantly disappointing from a research and reliability point of view – why did they not publish it in a reputable journal? A second warning bell.

The clincher comes when you read how the study was conducted. In their methods, they state (italics added by me for effect):

> …The overall prevalence of tick attachment was 30% (range 28–32 %). *The relatively high prevalence recorded is likely to have been inflated by the method of participant recruitment…*

That last line stopped me in my tracks. I thought I would have to work a little harder than this. It is quite literally admitting that the high prevalence of tick infestation found was inflated by the method of sampling. As such, the study's findings are beyond useless, they risk being misleading.

Just 2 months later the BBC in the United Kingdom aired an episode of their popular *Trust me I'm a vet* program. This particular episode, titled "Raw Meat Trend", did not come down kindly on the side of feeding pets fresh, species-appropriate diets. It focused on the usual drama, in particular, microbiological concern and the as-of-yet-to-be-seen threat to you and yours, something we have adequately dissected in Section 2, with the usual lack of balance. Thankfully, the online response to this most recent effort to suppress the use of fresh food in pets was overwhelmingly negative. The show based the majority of its conclusions on research by The University of Nottingham, which was cash-sponsored by Hill's Pet Food at the time of airing. The UK Pet Food Manufacturers Association, to their credit, wanted to see the research as shown in the following:

> The PFMA and our members have serious questions over the accuracy and relevance of the research undertaken by Nottingham University and aired by the BBC. We do not believe the findings reported reflect the actual situation with products on the market. Conversations with representatives of Nottingham University have led us to question the research methodology and testing regime used in this study... we are disappointed that Nottingham University have to date failed to

provide requested details of their study and the products tested so that manufacturers can investigate this matter further.

https://www.pfma.org.uk/news/pfma-statement-on-trust-me-im-a-vet-regarding-the-nottingham-university-research

It seems that the vet departments of universities often publish terrifying studies that are contrary to what people are seeing in actual application. Martinez-Anton *et al.* (2018)[1] presented a very widely shared study that apparently highlights the danger of feeding fresh chicken to dogs. The study investigated the link between the incidence of Acute Polyradiculo-Neuritis (APN), an immune-mediated peripheral nerve disorder of dogs) and the bacterial pathogen *Campylobacter* spp., which they theorised might be a trigger. The study concludes, raw chicken in the diet is *highly likely* to increase the risk of developing APN in dogs in Australia. (Italics added by me.)

This was shocking to learn, considering I and many like me, promote raw meat and bone to tens of thousands of healthy, raw-fed dog owners, many Australians among them, so I needed to learn more quickly. The researchers found that around half of their test dogs with APN (13 of 27, 48%) had *Campylobacter* in their faeces and 98% of their dogs with APN (26 of 27) had been fed raw chicken (including such pieces as necks and wings), which is a known source of *Campylobacter*. From this and precious little else, the study rules out all fresh food for pets worldwide 'until we know more'.

However, the authors of this study made some critical flaws. We know that half of apparently healthy dogs can normally house *Campylobacter* in their guts,[2-5] and these studies were of *both* dry and raw-fed dog populations! So, it's apparently quite a normal thing for assumedly non-APN dogs to be walking around with. Still, when these authors found that half their test dogs housed *Campylobacter,* they somehow attributed this very rare disease to eating raw chicken. An extraordinary leap, particularly when you flip it and consider that more than half of their test dogs with APN did not test positive for *Campylobacter*. Not to mention 23% of their test dogs that tested positive for *Campylobacter* did not have APN.

Both the authors and the university, via its website, clearly point their finger at chicken necks to be the most likely cause – the authors note that the APN dogs were more likely to be fed chicken wings and necks and the University of Melbourne website, from where the researchers hail, recommends that "owners choose regular dog food rather than chicken necks until we know more about this debilitating condition". However, the authors failed to balance the average weight of both test groups very well. The APN group of dogs had an average body weight of 8.5 kg while the control group averaged 14 kg. When you consider that smaller dogs are more likely to be fed chicken necks and wings than medium or large dogs, this deviation could lead to bias. It seems an unusual oversight, when a veterinary department as large as this would have endless records to choose from, thus ensuring body size was not at play. What makes it all stranger is that the authors clearly stated they are aware that smaller dogs are more likely to be fed chicken necks and wings, which is absolutely the case.

Most damning is their sampling method. First, this study is talking about 27 dogs with APN, quite a small number of cases to be working with, certainly not the sort of sample population you would use to justify removing fresh food from the world's pets. Second, their test group was not selected at random. This is fatal. Martinez-Anton *et al.* (2018)[1] compared their test population of raw chicken eaters to a selection of client-owned and 'staff-owned dogs'. However, we must assume that the staff at this hospital are largely feeding dry food, considering that the reception at Melbourne University's veterinary department sells nothing but Hill's Prescription and Science Diet (as of the video tour they made available on YouTube, April 29, 2014). A randomly selected control group is crucial in trials. It's science 101. A random sample reflects a fair representation of the *normal* population, a group that you can compare your test group with, to see if there's anything going on. As these particular dogs were significantly less likely to be fed fresh meat, this immediately skews the data and when you are talking about such small sample sizes, this can have a colossal effect.

The truth is there are many potential causes of APN out there. Contrary to the findings in this study, previous authors found no such link with *Campylobacter* and APN in dogs.[6] In fact, these authors investigated the link between six microbes (*Ehrlichia canis, Borrelia burgdorferi, Toxoplasma gondii, Neospora caninum, Campylobacter and distemper*) with APN and found that *T. gondii* was the only significant culprit. In fact, APN has been linked to a great variety of maladies, including vaccinations,[7] as well as common upper respiratory and gastrointestinal infections.[8,9] Other authors have found a strong seasonal effect, where APN was more likely to strike in autumn and winter. Are the authors suggesting we don't feed chicken in spring? They also noted a breed effect, with Jack Russell terriers and West Highland white terriers most affected.[10] None of this fits in the slightest with a *Campylobacter* cause.

Two years on, and millions more dogs now converted to species-appropriate food, there has been little mention of APN in the literature and no further links to raw dog food. The issue has apparently evaporated or, in the very least, retreated back to its current position of incredibly rare in the general population with no known direct cause, as of yet.

All published papers provide a contact email for the first one or two authors on the piece so you can contact them and discuss their findings. Most authors are very obliging, as they relish the opportunity to discuss their work with any peers that may be interested (so few often are!). This sharing of information is the root of good science. I was thus a little disheartened when I contacted the authors of the APN piece with my concerns but received no response. This is disappointing; however, I am not the only researcher to struggle in this manner. When Schulof (2016)[11] tried contacting Dr. Tiffany Bierer to discuss her piece cited in Section 2 which found dogs on diets of a higher protein dry food lost *six times* the body fat of their higher-carb fed counterparts, something that fits perfectly with the ideal approach to canine obesity, he, too, was surprised when she didn't respond. But this can happen, people are busy, and emails can go into junk. After some weeks, he tried again via Twitter. No response again. Some weeks passed before he got his response, but it wasn't from Bierer. It was from a public relations representative of Mars Petcare who responded on her behalf! Their message read:

> Hi Daniel, I am writing in response to a tweet from you to Dr Tiffany Bierer regarding a request to speak to her about a pet obesity book you are writing. Would love to understand more about your project. Thanks, Angel.

Is it just me or does that strike anyone as a little chilling? From a scientific point of view, it is extremely worrying. Why can't we speak to the author? Schulof (2016)[11] sums it up best:

> …it seemed the company was – at least in my case – exerting a measure of control over the scientist who had produced it…

More worrying is when weak science is used to include some potentially toxic ingredients in pet food. We all know grapes may lead to acute renal failure in dogs.[12-15] Recently, Hill's Science Diet started using grape pomace (the dried leftovers of the wine industry) in some of their products. Leftovers of the food industry, including corn gluten pulp (the leftovers from corn processing), beet pulp (the leftovers from beet processing) and meat meal (the leftovers of the meat industry), are a lucrative option for pet food and they are used extensively in dry pet foods worldwide. But here we have a pet food manufacturer using grape pomace in their mixes – an ingredient that is not defined by the AAFCO and thus, supposedly, not permitted to be used in pet food, and it gave me cause for concern.

Originally thought to be the result of a mycotoxin that lives on the skin, the exact causative agent in grapes remains unknown, though it does appear to be in the flesh of the fruit (peeled grapes or seedless varieties don't appear to be any less toxic). Doses ranging from 3 g per kilo of body weight[14] to as little as 0.21 mg per kilo of body weight[15] can do damage, in other words, one or two grapes.

> Poisoning has occurred in dogs following ingestion of seedless or seeded grape varieties, commercial or…homegrown fruits, red or green grapes/raisins, organic or non-organic fruits, and *grape pressings from… wineries…*
>
> **Ahna Brutlag, Assoc. Director of Veterinary Services, Pet Poison Helpline,**
>
> **Mars VCA Hospital. *Grape, Raisin, and Currant Poisoning in Dogs.* Published online**
>
> **www.vcahospitals.com/know-your-pet/grape-raisin-and-currant-poisoning-in-dogs**

We contacted Hill's about the use of this ingredient. To support its inclusion, they cited a study by Martineau *et al.* (2016),[16] a study which published some 15 years after they first released Hill's Prescription Diet b/d Canine on the market. These authors evaluated the renal and hepatic safety of an "*extract* from grape and blueberry" on a group of dogs over 24 weeks. They used a range of doses, topping out at 40 mg of extract per kilo of body weight per day. In what proportion the berries were included or how the extract was prepared, remains unknown. If we assume a 50/50 inclusion rate then the dogs were consuming 20 mg per body weight of some part of the grape in some form for 24 weeks, 5% lower than the lowest dose so far found to cause harm. Perhaps they used substantially less due to risk, we don't know. They found no hepatic or renal injury for this extract and concluded that this extract can therefore be considered safe. OK, so far.

The study by Martineau *et al.* itself cited two works that suggested grape skin/grape pomace might be of no harm in dogs. The first was a test of grape skin in 7 dogs over 8days and measured only platelet activity.[17] The second study by Milgram *et al.* (2005)[18] and titled "Learning Ability in Aged Beagle Dogs is Preserved by Behavioral Enrichment and Dietary Fortification: A Two-Year

Longitudinal Study",[18] was an interesting and enlightening insight into how the *scientifically proven* pet food industry works. This 2-year study of 65 beagles, 48 of whom were middle aged and older, aimed to preserve cognitive abilities in ageing dogs using behavioural enrichment and diet supplementation. Two groups of dogs were fed 'identical diets' as a baseline (using a complete Hill's Pet Food) although the test group diet was supplemented with a mix of ingredients including alpha-tocopherol (vitamin E) and ascorbic acid (vitamin C) as well as 1% inclusions of spinach flakes, tomato pomace, carrot granules, citrus pulp and *grape pomace*. After one year, the two groups were given a size discrimination task. After 2 years they were given black and white discrimination tasks. At no point did the researchers measure or mention the hepatic or renal health of the dogs.

What they did find was that dietary fortification worked to preserve cognitive ability in the test dogs. This is a very interesting finding. For anyone interested in the *how*, one of the scientists involved in the study by Milgram *et al.* (2005)[18] investigated further and found that an antioxidant diet (Vitamins E and C, fruits and vegetables) alone improved mitochondrial function in aged dogs when environmental enrichment did not.[19] In 2012, Fahnestock *et al.*[20] demonstrated that an antioxidant diet coupled with environmental enrichment, increased levels of brain-derived neurotrophic factor (BDNF) when compared with untreated aged dogs, approaching levels measured in young animals.[20] This, the authors suggest, was the likely dominant explanation for neural improvements seen. It was the first demonstration in a higher animal that 'non-pharmacological changes in lifestyle in advanced age can up-regulate BDNF to levels approaching those in the young brain'. You would think doctors treating neurodegenerative issues in humans would insist on something so simple in the background for their patients but when you see the slop served in most hospitals, I wouldn't hold my breath.

At the bottom of the original study by Milgram *et al.* (2005)[18], we learn that one of the authors, Zicker, works for the Science and Technology Centre at Hill's Pet Nutrition. The 'conflicts of interest' statement at the bottom of the study reads:

> Steven Zicker is an employee of Hill's Pet Nutrition Inc., which has commercialized the antioxidant-fortified food used in the study.
>
> **Milgram *et al.*, (2005)**[18]

This is likely the supportive work that helped the formulation of Hill's Prescription Diet b/d Canine for 'brain aging care', a product lauded as "clinically proven nutrition to help fight age-related behaviour changes in older dogs". It lists spinach, dried tomato pomace, carrot, dried citrus pulp and grape pomace in its list of more than 30 ingredients.

First, it's a touch worrying that all of these ingredients are ordered by weight. Grape pomace is seventeenth on the list. Despite the AAFCO still not permitting it to be included in pet food as of January 2018 which Hills has chosen to ignore (and yet still boasts as of April 2018 that this very product adheres to the AAFCO's requirements, stating on its website 'balanced nutrition that exceeds the AAFCO nutrition standards'[16]), how long will it be before this *potentially*-toxic-but-now-*assumed*-safe-until-someone-proves-otherwise ingredient is seized upon by less discerning pet food manufacturers than Hill's, who will move it higher up the inclusion list to greater financial gain? If you make millions of tonnes of dog food each year and grape pomace is *possibly* safe, has been 'clinically proven' by the pet food producers to make dogs think better, and your shareholders are breathing down your neck looking for profit year-on-year, I can't imagine we'll be waiting too long to find out.

The issue of grapes aside, this study serves as the perfect example of an unfalsifiable comparison and it these is on these works the entire house of cards is built.

Unfortunately for pet owners, the term *scientifically proven* now means about as much as the word *natural*. The words have been hijacked and today are little more than marketing hyperbole. The truth is science never *proves* anything. Real science can only ever *disprove* theories. The more experiments that are conducted around a hypothesis, the more it is tested, the surer we can be that it is right, but the positive is rarely, if ever, *proven*. The same applies to *clinically proven*, which is shorthand for 'shown to be better than placebo in a statistically significant number of cases'. But *clinically proven* is certainly a lot better than *clinically tested,* which suggests it was *clinically trialled* but for all we know the results could have been really bad. However, it gets the word 'clinical' in there and that does the job for many consumers. In pet food land, *scientifically* or *clinically proven* is most commonly found on vet-prescribed products.

> OK, your product is clinically *proven* but what has been clinically *proved*?
>
> **Unknown**

The thing is, for the very large part, it's not that the cereal-based pet food sector has made up a lot of data and produced a lot of bogus studies. Far from it. They have now a vast amount of legitimate scientific studies and less useful trials built up. The problem is most of them are very largely irrelevant to the dry versus fresh debate. If a study was used to support a cereal-based dry food product, it almost always (I have never read one that doesn't) relates to a feeding trial where the manufacturers compared one group of dogs fed a commercially available dry/tinned product compared to another group of dogs fed the same dry/tinned food product but with one or two small changes. Never do they compare their product to a control group of dogs fed a biologically appropriate raw meat and bone diet.

The grape study above is the perfect example. They fed one group of dogs dry food (made by their company) and compared this to another group of dogs that were given the same dry food but with a sprinkling of natural items that have long been known to boost cognitive function, including carrot,[21] tomato,[22] spinach[23] and berries.[24] When they find that group B does a bit better than group A, then this amazing, new food has been *clinically proven* to do whatever and your now confident vet can *prescribe* this non-medicinal-regular-dry-food-with-a-smattering-of-dried-fruit-and-veg-powder to you, at a hugely inflated price.

Adding plain old fish oil is another favourite. Supplementing dry-fed dogs with omega-3 is proven to aid skin repair, enhance the development of the nervous system and overall cognition, significantly reduce steroid need, improve visual performance and fight cancer in dogs.[25-33] Ricci *et al.* (2009)[34] suggested the reason behind the partial amelioration of clinical symptoms of pruritus on commercial hypoallergenic diets could be largely down to the fact the hypoallergenic diets contain fish oil. Thus, when a group of dogs fed a poor-quality food substrate such as a cereal-based pet food are compared to another group of dogs fed the same poor substrate but with added fish oil, you can expect to find that after a year, group B might be able to see a touch better, solve problems a touch quicker, may perhaps have less dandruff. These are all things a rudimentary knowledge in nutrition will tell you to expect from having better fats in the diet. But in the hands of a marketeer, this second diet has now been *clinically proven* to be better for your dog's vision, brain or skin. Moreover, it IS actually slightly better for your dog's vision, brain or skin compared to their control group of choice!

And they can do this with virtually any condition. Despite studies in overweight dogs showing that higher protein (and lower carb) diets produce better weight loss in dogs while retaining lean body mass,[35,36,37,38,39] that they are more satiating, leading to greater compliance in weight-loss programs,[40] that they reduce problem behaviours such as begging and scavenging,[41] and that hydrated diets produce better results in pet cats,[41] and thus likely in dogs, vets continue to recommend a high-carb, low-protein, ultra-processed and rapid-to-digest diet over a fresh diet containing lots of lean animal protein, for an animal that requires zero carbohydrates in its diet. Why? Well, light food has been *clinically proven*. Yes. The manufacturers housed a small number of overweight beagles on their new light product containing 13% inedible plant fibre, comparing it to another small group of overweight beagles fed regular dry food containing less than 2% fibre. Group A lost more weight over time.

It seems we must ignore the lessons learned in Section 2, that this weight loss can come at the cost of lean muscle mass, that an owner will likely fail with such a product in real life as they increase scavenging behaviour and that these foods are shown to cause further nutritional deficiencies.[42, 43] This food has been *scientifically proven* to result in weight loss. If it doesn't work, *you* must be doing something wrong, you have been killing him with love. A grossly unfair line trotted out in veterinary clinics everywhere to countless owners of overweight pets today.

Unfalsifiable comparisons are used to promote the benefits of their products as if they were good for health when in actual fact, they are actually just slightly less bad. This was first employed by the tobacco industry when they advertised their new lower-tar cigarettes were *good* for lung health. It seems absolutely preposterous to us now, but it was more than enough to get our doctors on side. They simply were not aware of the consequences, despite the prevalence of lung disease in their practice at the time. These tactics are still used to sell poisons today. Insanely sugary and nutritionally bereft breakfast cereals are 'fortified' with vitamin B and iron, nutrients that are *scientifically proven* to be good for young minds, to inexplicably cajole uninformed parents in. It is the nutritional equivalent of me comparing two groups of children fed nothing but gobstoppers for a week. To one group I feed regular candy gobstoppers but to the other I feed gobstoppers that had been supplemented with omega-3 fatty acids and vitamin E. If, at the end of the trial, the supplemented group had slightly less skin rash, would this be enough for my doctor to recommend these 'new and improved gobstoppers' for my kids? Or perhaps the advice would be that if you *have to* eat gobstoppers, then the latter are the slightly less-worse option by a tiny fraction? And sure, when your teeth start to fall out, you can switch to our new dental-type that contains less sugar!

In fact, think about the implications of a vet selling a certain dry kibble that is supposedly better for teeth – if a new dry food is *scientifically proven* to out-perform another product in the same manufacturer's range, by extension does this imply that all of the other products made by them don't provide this benefit, and are therefore bad for my dog's teeth? Shouldn't my vet now be taking these products off their shelves?

As more and more of these inconsequential, self-serving, in-house and often self-published studies are produced, the scientific validity of the products they support gets more and more established in the general psyche. In all the noise, we lose track of the whole debate. With great stealth, these 'tried and tested', 'scientifically proven', 'vet-recommended' and now 'prescription' products begin to switch the focus of the debate. As we saw with their approach to selling baby formula, the demand for scientific evidence is shifted to the consumer. We must prove that *normal* food is better! You have to hand it to them, it's a brilliant lesson in marketing and all without the burden of having to produce a single study documenting their products outcompeting a control group of normal, healthy animals fed a biologically normal diet.

> Proponents of home-prepared or raw food diets cite various benefits, including control over...ingredients used, avoidance of artificial preservatives, and preservation of natural enzymes and... phytonutrients. However, no published data are available to support an actual health benefit to pets... fed such diets.
> **La Flamme *et al.* (2008), for Nestlé Purina Petcare Research**[44]

In fact, Laflamme *et al.* (2008)[44] draws our attention to a study whereby owners who fed one of two home-prepared diets (one with meat, one without) had a greater prevalence of health problems compared to those that fed 'nutritionally balanced, commercial diets'. The 'study', which, after an awful lot of searching, turns out to be an unpublished oral poster presentation first for Nestlé Purina (entitled 'Commercial vs Traditional Food in Canine Health' in St. Louis, Missouri, 1999) and later at the Mars Waltham International Nutritional Science Symposium (in Washington, DC, in 2005). It arose from the veterinary department of the University of Agricultural Sciences, Hebbal, Bangalore, India. Shared extensively both online and in numerous academic texts in support of cereal-based pet food, it cites the use of 1,229 dogs split into three diet groups, one of which was fed a homemade diet of some sort (we are not told). While I am unsure if it was a survey or they actually housed these dogs, and the exact content, quality and suitability of the homemade diets they used aside, their findings were startling. It turns out the incidence of gut issues, including parasitic enteritis, bacterial enteritis, nonspecific anorexia, indigestion and ascites, were all less on the commercial diet. Similarly, the incidence of dermatologic disorders such as pyoderma, dermatomycoses, atopic dermatitis, hormonal disorders, dry coat, pruritus and dandruff, not to mention parasitic infestation with ticks, fleas and sarcoptic and demodectic mites, were all less in dogs fed commercial diet. It is a remarkable and apparently highly comprehensive victory for 'complete' pet food, it seems, just not something a single author has managed to replicate since, on any point, with any dry food product – ever. You would think any one of these points would be explored more and then promoted heavily by the industry.

All Animals Are Equal, But Some Are More Equal Than Others

It's often the case that the louder someone shouts about science, the weaker their stance is in exactly that regard. The Royal College of veterinary Surgeons (RCVS) is the main governing body of vets in the United Kingdom today. It has a subsidiary called RCVS Knowledge whose mission statement assures us they wish to 'advance the use of evidence-based veterinary medicine in veterinary practice'. This is most welcomed. One of the ways they aim to do this is via their peer-reviewed veterinary journal *Veterinary Evidence*. One article in this journal, titled "In Dogs Does Feeding Raw Dietary Treats Reduce or Prevent Periodontal Disease?"[45] did not come down favourably on the side of raw meaty bones in the diet of the dog. After excluding all the aforementioned evidence highlighted in Section 2, most of which was missed, they were left analysing the strengths and weaknesses of a single study supporting the use of raw meaty bones in the dog's diet. The authors conclude that vets should *not* rely on the available published literature but instead employ their clinical *experience* until more is known (italics added by me below for effect).

> …considering the weak evidence on raw bones and lack of evidence on other types of raw treats, veterinarians and veterinary nurses should be cautious when recommending raw treats to support periodontal health in dogs. Additionally, they should advise clients accordingly by *relying on their clinical experience rather than the literature* until more and better-quality evidence is generated.

Their conclusions aside, the wording here was familiar to me, having been used in a similar extent to wrap up another paper in the same journal only 4 months previously. This time two researchers (a degree student and a masters' student) set out to highlight the inadequacies of feeding pets fresh, species-appropriate food, this time by focusing on kidney disease in pets. In their paper, titled "In Adult Dogs, Does Feeding a Raw Food Diet Increase the Risk of Urinary Calculi Formation Compared to Feeding a Complete Dry Kibble Diet?", the authors again used only a single study to make their case.[46] This study found that raw-fed dogs had higher levels of creatine in their blood when compared to levels normally seen in dogs fed a 'complete' dry food, something we know to be very normal in dogs fed a diet containing adequate amounts of protein (more in Section 4). So quick, it seems, were they to highlight their concern regarding the *possible* link between a high-protein diet and the increased risk of renal damage in dogs, they entirely neglected to mention the studies that strongly suggest dogs with chronic kidney failure, often with up to 90% loss of kidney function, seem to not only safely deal with higher protein diets but do significantly *better* when fed them.[44, 47-49]Despite this, they conclude:

> …the evidence provided by the single study identified is weak and the outcomes can neither support nor challenge the hypothesis that a raw food diet increases the risk of urinary calculi compared to a kibble diet. Therefore, professionals working within the veterinary science or nutrition field should proceed with caution when advising clients and *rely on their professional experience until more evidence is generated.*
> **Taylor and van Neggel, (2018)[50]**

Both these peer-reviewed papers published in the RCVS's Journal *Veterinary Evidence* conclude it's better for vets to rely on their professional experience and not so much the literature until *more evidence* is generated. Their use or lack thereof of the published literature aside, there's nothing too much wrong with that sentiment. We surely want our trained professionals to use their valuable 'professional experience' now and again.

Sadly, we know this scientific freedom is absolutely not extended to all vets, just the ones on their list. Not on their list is any other alternative therapy, such as homeopathy, a far older medical practice than dry feeding and with arguably more positive, peer-reviewed, clinical trials supporting its use. At least it has been compared to a suitable control and it has come out on top, something cereal-based dry food has not yet managed to do.

> Homeopathy exists without a recognised body of evidence for its use…
> in order to protect animal welfare, we regard such treatments as being
> complementary rather than alternative to treatments for which there
> is a recognised evidence base or which are based in sound scientific
> principles.
>
> **RCVS statement on homeopathy, Fearon, 2017**[51]

A 'recognised evidence base' is a tricky one. How much evidence is required? And recognised by whom? The fact remains, there is adequate evidence supporting the use of homeopathy which should at least be stimulating further scientific investigation. In 2011, an independent report commissioned by the Swiss health authorities concluded 'there is sufficient evidence for the preclinical effectiveness and the clinical efficacy of homeopathy and for its safety and economy compared with conventional treatment'.[52] In 2016, a comprehensive literature review of peer-reviewed studies into the efficacy of homeopathy in replacing the use of antibiotics in cattle, pigs and poultry, spanning four decades, was published in the Veterinary Record.[53] 48 publications produced 52 trials that were said to fulfil the necessary scientific criteria. 28 of these trials were apparently in favour of homeopathy, with 26 trials showing a significantly higher efficacy in comparison to a control group, whereas 22 showed no therapeutic effect. This is very far from zero evidence. After all, prescription drugs are notoriously hit and miss. Nobody batted an eyelid with Dr. Allen Roses, renowned vice-president of genetics at GlaxoSmithKline, Britain's largest drug company, admitted to the science editor of the Independent newspaper that most prescription medicines do not work on most people who take them.[54] It came as no great surprise, at least to anyone in the scientific community, as studies clearly show drugs for the likes of Alzheimer's disease work in fewer than one in three patients. Drugs for cancer are only effective in a quarter of patients. The problem, Dr. Roses explains, is that different people carry genes that interfere in some way with the medicine, concluding 'the vast majority of drugs – more than 90 per cent – only work in 30 or 50 per cent of the people'. This failure rate is acceptable in modern medicine, as are the side effects, apparently (properly prescribed drugs are killing more than 100,000 Americans a year). Side effects, and certainly death, are virtually unheard of in homeopathy. Sadly, this incredible flexibility is not offered to any 'alternative' medical practice.

Available, peer-reviewed evidence aside, the RCVS made their statement on homoeopathy without any prior consultation or debate with established homeopathic vets.[51] Nor did they discuss the matter with any of the various governing bodies overseeing the many hundreds of highly qualified homeopathic vets worldwide, including the British Association of Homeopathic Veterinary Surgeons (BAHVS) and the International Association for Veterinary Homeopathy. Both groups claim that 'powerful interests had determined the RCVS Council's decision'. A spokesman for the BAHVS said the RCVS had been 'seduced' into a 'precedent setting restriction on the clinical freedoms the profession has always enjoyed'.[51] And yet it remains, a statement that relegates homeopathy and a number of other effective therapies to the status of 'complementary', whereby it cannot be recommended by the vet ahead of conventional treatments, regardless of their opinion or that vet will face reprisal.

Of course, the RCVS is not alone in its repression of homeopathy. The (Australian) National Health and Medical Research Council (NHMRC) got itself in hot water recently when it was tasked with assessing the available evidence supporting the use of homeopathy. Their concluding write-up (it was not a published study as it was not submitted to peer review), was titled "Evidence on the Effectiveness of Homeopathy for Treating Health Conditions" (2015), argued against the effectiveness of homeopathy. However, discrepancies found in the work by various homeopathy research groups, including cherry-picked data from available evidence and a panel of homeopathic experts containing no actual homeopathy experts, a group that was chaired by a member of an anti-homeopathy lobby group, led to public scrutiny of the piece as a whole. It soon came to light there was an earlier work that wasn't made public. It took three years, multiple Freedom of Information requests and members of the Australian Senate to make the NHMRC admit the fact. Eventually, the original work, titled "The Effectiveness of Homeopathy: An Overview Review of Secondary Evidence" and dated 2012, was published in September 2019. In this report, it states, 'there is *encouraging evidence* for the effectiveness of homeopathy' for five health conditions.

> To see this document finally seeing the light of day is a major win for transparency and public accountability in research.
> **Rachel Roberts, Homeopathy Research Institute Chief Executive**

I know practically nothing about homeopathy, but I do have a keen interest in science and fairness as a whole. The studies I have read in animals and the fact I have seen it work in dogs and horses means the placebo line does not hold for me. One of the constant criticisms of homeopathy is that the treatments are so dilute they are in fact just *water*. They contain no active components whatsoever. However, in unpublished trials, scent detection dogs can identify a homeopathic treatment diluted down beyond Avogadro's number (0.1^{-23}), the dilution at which the molecule is said to be no longer present in the water. The dogs are detecting *something*. It might simply be that the tools science has available for investigating it are inadequate. Ask any physicist about trying to measure dark matter, something we *know* is there. It has great mass, accounting for perhaps 85% of the matter in known universe, affecting dust and universes alike and yet remains invisible to our current instruments or understanding. In this day and age, with antibiotic resistance now a very real and imminent threat to our health, an area where homeopathy has great potential, it is surely an area that warrants further research. At the very least, why would any scientific body wish to repress exploration of a new field by any of their highly trained members?

Our feelings or knowledge of homeopathy aside, the fact remains the RCVS is standing shoulder to shoulder with dry food, a product that by its own admission is based on "recent scientific publications, *practical experience* and *unpublished data*".[55] In the past, the RCVS have elected presidents who were once senior executives of dry pet food companies. Nor is this the only practice the RCVS has endorsed that lacks much by way of scientific credibility. Take, for example, the annual boosting of dogs already adequately vaccinated for at least the core viruses (distemper, parvovirus, adenovirus) as pups, something we know from Section 2 is wholly unnecessary.[56,57,58,59] In fact, even the studies produced by the vaccine manufacturers predict a duration of immunity of 3 years or longer for canine distemper and adenovirus.[58] Revaccination annually thereafter fails to stimulate a secondary response as a result of interference by existing antibodies.[58] In fact, there is evidence that it could be potentially harmful to your pet. Authors have found reactions ranging from the more common fever, stiffness, sore joints, abdominal tenderness and behavioural changes to the more serious increased susceptibility to infections, autoimmune disease, cancer, neurologic disorders, encephalitis, jaundice as well as organ failure and collapse.[60-67] It's very far from a *perfectly safe* practice, certainly in small dogs that are significantly more likely to suffer adverse reactions than larger dogs.[68,69] For all these reasons, The World Small Animal Veterinary Association now stipulate boosting dogs for most viruses no more than every three years.[70] And yet, so many UK (but also US) vets continue to recommend annual boosting with full support from the RCVS. Writing to the *Vet Times*, 21 homeopathic vets attempted to highlight this conundrum but were met with apparent indignation.

> Rather than acknowledging the fact, the council accused [its homeopathic] members of bringing the profession into disrepute. When the press

became interested the charges were dropped, and the vaccination guidelines subsequently changed.

www.bahvs.com/articles-parent/bored-to-death

How long before vet governing bodies feel free to move in a similar 'evidence-based' manner on raw feeding vets is a matter of debate; for now, it seems all animals are free, but some are freer than others.

Again, this is not to invalidate the findings of any of the above authors or the journal *Veterinary Evidence* as a whole. It's just I find it incredible that such pieces are rarely, if ever balanced, with an analysis of their own product of choice. In what context have diets high in rapidly digested carbohydrates ever outperformed diets high in protein for obese meat-eaters? Where is the evidence that dry food is better for teeth than fresh meat and bone? Has anyone *ever* shown that a *dry*, hard-to-digest, ultra-processed, high salt, chemical-laden product does *not* negatively impact kidney health over time when compared to a suitable control? How safe is dry pet food for pets in comparison to premade raw? As with the dry versus raw-fed dog population health comparisons, these sorts of works are conspicuous for their absence. In classic sleight of hand, what we get are literature reviews bemoaning the state of the science supporting the use of species-appropriate food in our pets but never the opposite. These works are then referenced tirelessly by the industry in support of whatever point they are trying to make, offering a warm blanket of scientific solace to the average vet who might not have the time or expertise to investigate further. So far, we have provided evidence that suggests a raw or homemade meat-based diet improves behaviour, benefits gut health and reduces stress metabolites, as well as greatly benefitting dogs suffering atopy and canine hip dysplasia.[71,72] However, in all the minutiae, such works are roundly ignored by the veterinary sector as readily as studies highlighting flaws in their product of choice are welcomed, should they happen to read them at all.

With little by way of real science in support, the near pious devotion of our young vets to the dry pet food sector is based on little more than faith. I don't mean to be facetious here. It's highly unlikely a recent visitor to earth, upon reviewing the available evidence, would shun a species-appropriate diet for this meat-eater in favour of a dry, high carb, low protein, high salt, chemically preserved and ultra-processed pellet made a year ago by candy companies with woeful reputations for good nutrition and health in human circles. Pose the same question to a man interested in making a profitable product and he might say the opposite. To believe him however, you're going to need a little faith.

As we saw with the poorly read doctors at the beginning of the section believing the drug reps pseudoscience 'hook, line and sinker', ferociously filling out prescriptions for highly addictive opiates and potentially useless antidepressants, the entire cereal-based pet food industry is built on little more than faith. Our young vets necessarily place their faith in the university lectures given to them and in the vet governing bodies that oversee them. Vets next have faith in their own ability to notice any side effects should problems arise from poor diet and yet we continue to watch in helpless horror as nutritional diseases such as obesity, diabetes and foul dentition continue to spiral, mirroring what we see in human populations for the same reasons. Next, and much like Packer's two hundred young physicians who had not read a single study in their field *whatsoever*, our vets are clearly placing faith in the company reps and the largely in-house science used to support their claims, because if they went looking for some evidence by themselves, if they peeked behind that curtain, they would quickly see little Oz furiously peddling the machine. Finally, faith is placed in the regulatory bodies that are meant to be patrolling the producers, ensuring some sort of quality standards are met. Unfortunately, as you are about to learn in the next chapter, this faith is perhaps the most ill-judged of all.

TAKE-HOME POINTS

✓ Bristol University self-published a work that implied 31% of UK dogs might have ticks. The work was used as the foundation to get more UK pets chemically treated for the parasite. In their methods, the authors state 'the relatively high prevalence recorded is likely to have been inflated by the method of participant recruitment…'.

✓ In 2018, using just 27 dogs, a widely shared study linked *Campylobacter,* raw dog food and APN in dogs, concluding 'raw chicken in the diet is highly likely to increase the risk of developing APN in dogs in Australia'. The widely shared work had numerous critical flaws. There has been no mention in the literature of raw chicken causing APN in dogs since.

✓ Unfalsifiable comparisons are when one group of caged dogs is fed a standard, cereal-based pet food and is compared to another group of caged dogs fed the same diet but with one small change, be it a pinch of extra ingredients known to preserve cognitive abilities in old age (senior care dry food), a spoon of fish oil that is known to reduce inflammation (dermal dry food) or added indigestible fibre to make dogs lose weight (light dry food). When an effect is noticed in the test group, this becomes *scientifically proven* pet food.

✓ These studies are replicated and cited endlessly, offering a warm blanket of scientific 'evidence' to the vet who will then sell the product to you under 'prescription', despite the fact you can buy it off the shelf, having no medicinal qualities whatsoever.

✓ The RCVS is the main governing body of vets in the United Kingdom. While standing over dry, ultra-processed, cereal-based pet foods for meat-eaters without the benefit of *a single head-to-head study* of any value in support of that stance, the RCVS hold themselves up as protectors of evidenced-based veterinary medicine. It does not support homeopathy, a field with significantly more peer-reviewed head-to-heads in support.

✓ The industry is keen to produce literature reviews highlighting potential flaws in fresh feeding, but never do they turn the looking glass on their dry product of choice.

Chapter Eighteen References

1   Martinez-Anton, L. Marenda, M., Firestone, S.M. *et al.* (2018). Investigation of the role of *Campylobacter* infection in suspected Acute Polyradiculoneuritis in Dogs. Journal of Veterinary Internal Medicine, 32(1): 352–360

2   Olson, P. and Sandstedt, K. (1987). *Campylobacter* in the dog: A clinical and experimental study. Veterinary Record, 121: 99–101

3   Baker, J, Barton, M.D. and Lanser, J. (1999). *Campylobacter* species in cats and dogs in South Australia. Australian Veterinary Journal, 77:10

4   Wieland, B., Regula, G., Danuser, J. *et al.* (2005). *Campylobacter* sp. in dogs and cats in Switzerland: Risk factor analysis and molecular characterization with AFLP. Zoonoses and Public Health, 52(4): 183–189

5   Chaban, B., Ngeleka, M. and Hill, J.E. (2010). Detection and quantification of 14 *Campylobacter* species in pet dogs reveals an increase in species richness in feces of diarrheic animals. BMC Microbiology, 10: 73

6   Holt, N., Murray, M., Cuddon, P.A. *et al.* (2011). Seroprevalence of various infectious agents in dogs with suspected acute canine polyradiculoneuritis. Journal of Veterinary Internal Medicine, 2: 261–266

7   Gehring, R. and Eggars, B. (2001). Suspected post-vaccinal acute polyradiculoneuritis in a puppy: short communication. Journal of the South African Veterinary Association, 72(2)

8   Cummings J. (1992). *Canine Inflammatory Neuropathies*. In: Current Veterinary Therapy XI. Kirk, R.W., Boagura, J.D., eds. Philadelphia, PA: WB Saunders; 1992: 1034–1037

9   Cuddon P. (2002). Acquired canine peripheral neuropathies. Veterinary Clinics of North America, 32: 207–249

10 Laws, E.J., Harcourt-Brown, T.R., Granger, N. *et al.* (2017). An exploratory study into factors influencing the development of acute canine polyradiculoneuritis in the UK. Journal of Small Animal Practice, 58(8): 437–443

11 Schulof, D. (2016). *Dogs, Dog Food and Dogma*. Present Tense Press, Salt Lake City

12 Mazzaferro, E.M., Eubig, P.A., Hackett, T.B. *et al.* (2004). Acute renal failure associated with raisin or grape ingestion in 4 dogs. Journal of Veterinary Emergency Critical Care, 14: 203–212

13 Eubig, P.A., Brady, M.S., Gwaltney-Brant, S.M. *et al.* (2005). Acute renal failure in dogs after the ingestion of grapes or raisins: a retrospective evaluation of 43 dogs (1992–2002). Journal of Veterinary Internal Medicine, 19: 663–674

14 Morrow, C.M.K., Valli, V.E., Volmer, P.A. *et al.* (2005). Canine renal pathology associated with grape or raisins ingestion: 10 cases. Journal of Veterinary Diagnostic Investigation, 17: 223–231

15 Sutton, N., Bates, M. and Campbell, A. (2009). Factors influencing outcome of *Vitis vinifera* (grapes, raisins, currants and sultanas) intoxication in dogs. Veterinary Records, 164(14): 430–431

16   Martineau, A.S., Leray, V., Lepoudere, A. *et al.* (2016). A mixed grape and blueberry extract is safe for dogs to consume. BMC Veterinary Research, 12: 162

17   Shanmuganayagam, D., Beahm, M.R., Osman, H.E. *et al.* (2002). Grape seed and grape skin extracts elicit a greater antiplatelet effect when used in combination than when used individually in dogs and humans. Journal of Nutrition, 132(12): 3592–2598

18   Milgram, N.W., Head, E., Zicker, S.C. *et al.* (2005). Learning ability in aged beagle dogs is preserved by behavioral enrichment and dietary fortification: a two-year longitudinal study. Neurobiological Aging, 26: 77–90

19   Head, E., Nukalab, V.N., Fenoglio, K.A. *et al.* (2009). Effects of age, dietary, and behavioral enrichment on brain mitochondria in a canine model of human aging. Experimental Neurology, 220(1): 171–176

20   Fahnestock, M., Marcheseae, M., Head, E. *et al.* (2012). BDNF increases with behavioral enrichment and an antioxidant diet in the aged dogNeurobiology of Aging, 33(3): 546-554

21   www.hillspet.com/dog-food/pd-bd-canine-dry

22   Nabavi, S.F., Braidy, N., Gortzi, O. *et al.* (2015). Luteolin as an anti-inflammatory and neuroprotective agent: A brief review. Brain Research Bulletin, 119(A): 1–11

23   Ferrari, C.K.B. and Torres, AC.K.B (2003). Biochemical pharmacology of functional foods and prevention of chronic diseases of aging. Biomedicine & Pharmacotherapy, 57(5–6): 251–260

24   Kiefer, I. (2007). Brain food. Scientific American Mind, 18(5): 58–63

25   Andres-Lacueva, C., Shukitt-Hale, B., Galli, R.L. *et al.* (2013). Anthocyanins in aged blueberry-fed rats are found centrally and may enhance memory. Nutritional Neuroscience, 8(2): 111–120

26   Scott, D.W., Miller, W.H., Jr, Decker, G. A. *et al.* (1992). Comparison of the clinical efficacy of two commercial fatty acid supplements (EfaVet and DVM Derm Caps), evening primrose oil, and cold water marine fish oil in the management of allergic pruritus in dogs: A double-blinded study. Cornell Veterinarian, 82(3): 319–329

27   Scott, D.W. and Miller, W.H. (1993). Nonsteroidal anti-inflammatory agents in the management of canine allergic pruritus. Journal of South African Veterinary Association, 64(1): 52–56

28   Scott, D.W., Miller, W.H., Jr, Griffin, C.E. (1995). *Structure and function of the skin.* Muller and Kirk's Small Animal Dermatology (5th ed.). Philadelphia, PA: Saunders, pp1–54

29   Scott, D.W., Miller, W.H., Reinhart, G. A. *et al.* (1997). Effect of an omega-3/omega-6 fatty acid-containing commercial lamb and rice diet on pruritus in atopic dogs: Results of a single-blinded study. Canadian Journal of Veterinary Research, 61(2): 145–153

30   Logas, D. (1995) *Systemic nonsteroidal therapy for pruritus: the North American experience.* Proceedings of 19th WALTHAM/OSU Symposium Dermatology, pp32–36

31   Sture, G.H. and Lloyd, D.H. (1995) Canine atopic disease: therapeutic use of an evening primrose oil and fish oil combination. The Veterinary Record, 137: 169–170

32   Watson, T. D. G. (1998). Diet and skin disease in dogs and cats. Journal of Nutrition, 128(12): 2783S–2789S

33   Heinemann, K.M., Waldron, M.K., Bigley, K.E. *et al.* (2005). Long-chain (n-3) polyunsaturated fatty acids are more efficient than alpha-linolenic acid in improving electroretinogram responses of puppies exposed during gestation, lactation, and weaning. Journal of Nutrition, 135: 1960–1966

34   Ricci, R., Berlanda, M., Tenti, S., *et al.* (2009): Study of the chemical and nutritional characteristics of commercial dog foods used as elimination diet for the diagnosis of canine food allergy. Italian Journal of Animal Science, 8: 328–330

35   Lenox, C.E. (2015). Timely topics in Nutrition: An overview of fatty acids in companion animal medicine. Journal of the American Veterinary Medical Association, 246(11): 1198–1202

36   Hannah, S.S. and Laflamme, D.P. (1998). Increased dietary protein spares lean body mass during weight loss in dogs. Journal of Veterinary International Medicine, 12: 224

37   Hannah, S. (1999). Role of dietary protein in weight management. Compendium on Continuing Education for the Practicing Veterinarian, 21: 32–33

38   Diez, M., Nguyen, P., Jeusette, I. *et al.* (2002). Weight loss in obese dogs: Evaluation of a high-protein, low-carbohydrate diet. Journal of Nutrition, 132: 1685S–1687S

39   Blanchard, G., Nguyen, P., Gayet, C. *et al.* (2004). Rapid weight loss with a high-protein low-energy diet allows the recovery of ideal body composition and insulin sensitivity in obese dogs. Journal of Nutrition, 134: 2148S–2150S

40   German, A. J., Holden, S.L., Bissot, T. *et al.* (2010). A high protein high fibre diet improves weight loss in obese dogs. Veterinary Journal, 183: 294–297

41   Weber, M., Bissot, T., Servet, E. *et al.* (2007). A High-Protein, High-Fiber Diet Designed for Weight Loss Improves Satiety in Dogs. Journal of Veterinary Internal Medicine, 21(6): 1203–1208

42   Cameron, K.M., Morris, P.J., Hackett, R.M. *et al.* (2011). The effects of increasing water content to reduce the energy density of the diet on body mass changes following caloric restriction in domestic cats. Journal of Animal Physiology and Animal Nutrition, 95: 399–408

43   Zentek J. (1995). Observations on the apparent digestibility of copper, iron, zinc and magnesium in dogs. Deutsche tierarztliche Wochenschrift, 102(8): 310–315

44   Laflamme, D.P., Abood, S.K., Fascetti, A.J. *et al.* (2008). Pet feeding practices of dog and cat owners in the United States and Australia. Journal of the American Veterinary Medical Association, 232(5): 687–694

45   van Veggel, N. and Oxley, J. (2018). Treats Reduce or Prevent Periodontal Disease? A Knowledge Summary. Veterinary Evidence, 3(3)

46   Dijcker, J.C., Hagen-Plantinga, E.A., Everts, H. *et al.* (2012). Dietary and animal-related factors associated with the rate of urinary oxalate and calcium excretion in dogs and cats. The Veterinary record, 171(2): 46

47   Bovée, K.C. (1991) Influence of dietary protein on renal function in dogs. Journal of Nutrition, 121(11): S128–S139.

48   Finco, D.R., Brown, S.A., Crowell, W.A. *et al.* (1994). Effects of aging and dietary protein intake on uninephrectomized geriatric dogs. American Journal of Veterinary Research, 55: 1282–1290

49   Hansen, B., DiBartola, S.P., Chew, D.J. *et al.* (1992). Clinical and metabolic findings in dogs with chronic renal failure fed two diets. American Journal of Veterinary Research, 53(3): 326–334

50   Taylor, E. and van Veggel. N. (2018). In adult dogs, does feeding a raw food diet increase the risk of urinary calculi formation compared to feeding a complete dry kibble diet? Veterinary Evidence, 3(2)

51   Fearon, R. (2017). No evidence for homeopathy, says RCVS. BMJ Vet Record, 181(19): 494–495

52   Bornhöft, G., Matthiessen, P. and Saar, M.M. (2011). *Homeopathy, in healthcare: effectiveness, appropriateness, safety, costs.* A HTA report on homeopathy as part of the Swiss Complementary Medicine Evaluation Programme. Springer, Bornhöft, G. and Matthiessen, P.F. (eds)

53   Doehring, C. and Sundrum, A. (2016). Efficacy of homeopathy in livestock according to peer-reviewed publications from 1981 to 2014, Veterinary Record, 179(24): 628

54   Connor, S. (2003). *Glaxo chief: Our drugs do not work on most patients.* The Independent UK. Published online, Dec 8th, www.independent.co.uk

55   Association of American Feed Control Officials (AAFCO, 2016). Dog and Cat Food Nutrient Profiles. Official Publication, ww.aafco.org

56   Carmichael, L.E. (1999). Canine viral vaccines at a turning point - a personal perspective. Advances in Veterinary Medicine, 41: 289–307

57   Mouzin, D.E., Lorenzen, M.J., Haworth, J.D. *et al.* (2004). Duration of serologic response to five viral antigens in dogs. Journal of the American Veterinary Medical Association, 224(1): 55–60

58   Schultz, R.D. (2006). Duration of immunity for canine and feline vaccines: A review. Veterinary Microbiology, 117(1): 75–79

59   Bonagura, J.D. and Twedt, D.C. (2008). *Kirk's current veterinary therapy XIV.* Philadelphia, PA: Saunders

60   Phillips, T.R., Jensen, J.L., Rubino, M.J. *et al.* (1989). Effects of vaccines on the canine immune system. Canadian Journal of Veterinary Research, 53: 154– 160

61   Tizard, I. (1990). *Risks associated with use of live vaccines.* Journal of the American Veterinary Medical Association, 196(11): 1851–1858

62   Duval, D. and Giger, U. (1996). Vaccine associated immune-mediated hemolytic anemia in the dog. Journal of the Veterinary Internal Medicine, 10: 290–295

63   Dodds, W.J. (1999). More bumps on the vaccine road. Advances in Veterinary Medicine; 41: 715–732

64   Dodds, W.J. (2001). Vaccination protocols for dogs predisposed to vaccine reactions. Journal of the American Animal Hospital Association, 37(3): 211–214

65   Hogenesch, H., Azcona-Olivera, J., Scott-Moncrieff, C. *et al.* (1999). Vaccine-induced autoimmunity in the dog. Advances in Veterinary Medicine, 41: 733–747

66   Scott-Moncrieff, J.C., Azcona-Olivera, J., Glickman, N.W. *et al.* (2002) Evaluation of antithyroglobulin antibodies after routine vaccination in pet and research dogs. J Am Vet Med Assoc, 221: 515–521

67   Horzinek, M.C. (2006). Vaccine use and disease prevalence in dogs and cats. Veterinary Microbiology, 117(1): 2

68   Moore, G.E., Guptill, L.F., Ward, M.P. *et al.* (2005). Adverse events diagnosed within three days of vaccine administration in dogs. Journal of the American Veterinary Medical Association, 227: 1102–1108

69   Novak, W. (2007). Predicting the "unpredictable" vaccine reactions. Proceeding of the NAVC North American Veterinary Conference. Jan. 13-27, Orlando, Florida

70   Day, M.J., Horzinek, M.C., Schultz, R.D. *et al.* (2016). Guidelines for the vaccination of dogs and cats. Journal of Small Animal Practice, 57: E1–45 f

71   Grundström, S. (2013). *Influence of nutrition at young age on canine hip dysplasia in German Shepherd dogs.* The WALTHAM International Nutritional Sciences Symposium (WINSS) 2013, Oct. 1-4, Oregon, USA

72   Roine, J., Roine, M., Velagapudi, V. and Hielm-Björkman, A. (2015). *Metabolomics from a Diet Intervention in Atopic Dogs, a Model for Human Research?* 12th European Nutrition Conference (FENS), Berlin, Germany

CHAPTER 19

Where Are the Pet Food Police?

1. AAFCO: An Advisory Body and Nutritional Protocol Grossly Unfit for Purpose

In Section 2, we learned Hills Pet Nutrition underwent the largest, single brand pet food recall in history. Driven by consumer complaint, Hills ended up voluntarily recalling a huge portion of their range when it was discovered they were potentially including a toxic amount of vitamin D in every line. As an American company, the Food and Drug Administration investigated Hill for their fatal lapse and found that the vitamin premix Hill's was buying in had not been analysed by Hills themselves before usage. OK, we could probably forgive that. However, the FDA also noted that at no point were any of the products ever tested by them prior to leaving the factory (FDA Warning Letter to Hill's MARCS-CMS 576564), despite each product having a 'guaranteed analysis' above the ingredients on the side of each packet. That's 22 *million* cans of highly scientific and 'complete' pet food emanating from the world leader in pet food for an undetermined amount of time going out entirely *unchecked*, resulting in untold death and suffering. Their punishment? The FDA said, 'It will verify *Hills proposed voluntary corrective actions*—submitted in March, May and August *last year*—during a future inspection.'!

A number of things should be leaping out of that paragraph, such as: How did this happen? Who can we blame? Might this be happening in every pet food factory? Who is supposed to be keeping an eye on these guys? And then, *voluntary corrective actions*? Proposed by the offending company themselves?! That doesn't sound like much of a punishment. And to be investigated at a *later* stage?! In any other food industry, you would expect a lethal lapse might, if not instantly, close the factory until their systems are thoroughly verified externally, put it under very strict, very immediate surveillance from the powers that be.

Who's supposed to be overseeing these guys?

You may have noticed on the front of your dry food of choice that most, if not all, now proudly boast something like 'Complete for lifetime feeding as per AAFCO standards' on the front. But what does the term 'complete' pet food mean? Afterall, bar breast milk (made by Mother Nature Incorporated), we still do not have a *complete* food for humans. The closest they came to that was baby formula – and look how well that worked out for Nestlé.

And yet, there it is in black and white, giving both the vet and customer great solace that the product in question is sure to contain everything your pet needs to be in peak physical condition. So, now's a good time to take a look at the AAFCO, see exactly who they are and what their standards entail.

In human health and nutrition, the burden of ensuring a product's safety, efficacy and any claims of benefit is on governmental organisations that independently test drug and food product manufacturers. In dog health and nutrition, this filter is virtually nonexistent. There are no governmental organisations supervising the nutritional content of pet food anywhere in the world, that I am aware of. They are concerned only for the layout, operations and cleanliness of the premises and microbiology content of the finished product.

Today, pet food in the United States is overseen at different levels by a mishmash of numerous groups. At the federal level, under the Federal Food, Drug and Cosmetic Act, the industry is regulated by the FDA. Think of them as the police. Once alerted to an issue, they have been known to inspect a manufacturing premise (such as the melamine scandal in 2007). The FDA does not require preapproval of new foods, whether intended for humans or animals. Rather, they simply ask that foods not be 'adulterated' or 'misbranded' with false or misleading information. The adulterated food bit is interesting. They define it as 'food packaged or held under unsanitary conditions, food or ingredients that are filthy or decomposed, and food that contains any poisonous or deleterious substance'.[1] They also state that a food may be deemed adulterated if it contains 'any part or product of a diseased animal'.[2] Not quite sure how most pet food ingredients, particularly meat meal, get the green light with this in place.

The problem that the FDA has is resources. In that, they don't have a whole lot. Unfortunately for them, the FDA/Centre for Veterinary Medicine have a mandate from Congress that requires them to regulate the pet food sector. To fulfil this requirement, they used a branch of the FDA called the National Research Council (NRC). Then it was decided to form cooperative partnerships with other groups who might do it for them. Enter the AAFCO. In the mid-1980s, the US Government shut down the NRC's Subcommittee on Dog Nutrition, dissociated its regulatory agencies and turned the entire pet food industry entirely over to AAFCO.[3]

> …continued partnership with AAFCO is vital to the continued regulation of pet food products… because FDA has limited enforcement resources that are focused on human food safety… issues.
> **S. Benz, *FDA's Regulation of Pet Food*, FDA Veterinarian, Vol. XVI,**
> ***supra* note 23**

The AAFCO (the Association of Animal Feed Control Officials) is now the biggest player in terms of pet food policy worldwide. It's safe to say their recommendations are seen by the industry as the gold standard. Everybody copies them. For example, the European Pet Food Industry Federation (FEDIAF), oversees what goes on in pet food this side of the pond. Unlike the AAFCO, however, the FEDIAF freely admits they concern themselves with 'promoting the views and interests of around 650 European pet food producing companies'. In the line underneath, they then assure us that FEDIAF is also very concerned for 'quality and safety, nutritional balance and palatability, variety and value for money, pet owner demands and convenience'. While their goals may be admirable, it is clearly impossible to safeguard the interests of both sides of the debate, particularly when one side is making money while the other is parting with it. While the FEDIAF have released their own nutritional guidelines for European pet food manufacturers (see www.Fediaf.org), their guidelines are, to all extents and purposes, very similar to those produced by the AAFCO, one of the standout differences being that FEDIAF do allow young pups and some adults an extra four percentage points of protein (22% versus 25%, and 18% versus 18-21%, AAFCO and FEDIAF respectively).

> …The industry uses as a basis and is a contributor to the research studies published by the internationally recognised authorities, the American Association of Food Control Officers and the National Research Council (NRC) of the National Academy of Sciences in the USA…
> **http://www.fediaf.org/self-regulation/nutrition.html**

So, who exactly are the AAFCO? AAFCO Official Publication (2016)[4] tells us that the AAFCO first met as an organised grouping around 1909. Their mandate was to prepare a uniform bill of feeding, formulate regulations and definitions regarding what was or wasn't permitted and establish some labelling requirements. We are assured that protecting the consumer remains the AAFCO's primary goal.

Unfortunately, as reported by *The New York Times*,[5] by the 1970s the US Government and the pet food business had grown particularly close. Earl L. Butz, chair of the Ralston Purina board (an American animal feed company, bought out by Nestlé in 2001) and Clifford M. Hardin, Secretary of Agriculture, effectively swapped jobs. The first national guidelines for nutrition originated from a Ralston Purina research team. Right from the start, nobody seemed to mind that the industry was beginning to self-regulate.

Today the AAFCO sets the guidelines to which pet food manufacturers should adhere, including the nutritional standards, feeding trial protocols and label requirements for pet foods. I say 'should' as AAFCO is a nongovernmental organisation. They have absolutely no statutory or regulatory powers whatsoever. The AAFCO has neither the capability to approve nor the power to ban pet foods. It has no labs, no investigators, no laws, makes little to no checks on the industry and has absolutely no teeth in a court of law.[6] Its role is purely advisory (although I hear changes are currently afoot where AAFCO, an Non-Governmental Organisation (NGO), are now straying into making actual policy). Currently, pet food manufacturers are free to follow their recommendations or not.

To make matters considerably worse, its board has a history of being populated with dry food reps. In his piece for the Harvard Law School titled "Deconstructing the Regulatory Facade: Why Confused Consumers Feed their Pets Ring Dings and Krispy Kremessit either as AAFCO committee members or AAFCO "industry advisors", Patrick (2006)[7] notes an AAFCO Official Publication from 1994 which lists a group of members charged with developing and reviewing standards for terms found on pet food labels. Of the group's six members, four were pet food company employees (Ken Johannes, Hill's Pet Products Inc.; Dan Chauslow, Westreco, Inc.; Dave Bebiak, Ralston Purina Co.; and Mark Finke, Alpo pet foods, Inc.). There is similar infiltration of many other sections of the AAFCO, including the Inspection and Sampling Committee, the Feed Manufacturing Committee and the Feed Labeling Committee.[7] Extensively researched by Martin (2007), the AAFCO holds a convention once a year to discuss and vote on issues relating to the pet food industry. Apparently, it's not uncommon to see more lobbyists from the pet food industry in attendance at these conventions than AAFCO members.[6] To quote Douglas Knueven, DVM, 'talk about the fox guarding the henhouse'.[8]

> Today, representatives from Cargill, ADM, Purina, the Pet Food Institute (the primary lobby group for Big Kibble), and both the American Feed Industry Association and the National Grain and Feed Association (two other carbohydrate lobby groups) all sit either as AAFCO committee members or AAFCO "industry advisors".
>
> **Schulof, 2016**[9]

And yet, with no other players offering anything by way of a suitable alternative, the AAFCO appear to be the only group setting the standards for pet food worldwide. So, let's take a look at the AAFCO protocol, the standards to which pet food manufacturers must adhere if they are to state 'complete for lifetime feeding' on the front of their packets.

Glaring Issues With the AAFCO Feed Trials

There are three ways a pet food producer can demonstrate their product is 'complete' in the eyes of the AAFCO and producers are free to pick whichever method suits them the best. The first option is that they establish that their product's formula meets AAFCO's *minimum* nutrient requirement profile. This profile is beset with an incredible array of issues. First, certain nutrient groups are absent from the profile, such as carbohydrates, one of the reasons you will not see the carbohydrate content mentioned on your dry pet food of choice. Unlike human nutrition, it's not a requirement. No mention of sugar. As we stated previously, you can work it out by adding up all the bits that are mentioned (protein, fat, ash) and take this total figure from 90 (assuming 10% of the dry food is water). Fibre doesn't get a mention either. As with the obesity foods, manufacturers can and do use as much as they like, regardless of the issues this may be causing digestively for the dog. Unbelievably, it wasn't until 2014 when public backlash had built to a sufficient level, that calories were required to be stated. This all seems a little odd from a group whose primary goal, apparently, is to protect the consumer!

But focusing on what *is* actually mentioned, according to the AAFCO manual, their nutrient profile is based on a previous profile established by the NRC's Committee on Animal Nutrition. However, at some point, the AAFCO took it upon themselves to tweak some values, stating 'values for specific nutrient requirements were added or modified…supported by recent scientific publications, practical experience, and unpublished data'. One of the ingredients they felt was a touch excessive was – you guessed it, protein, so they dropped it from 22% to 18% of dry matter for adult maintenance in dogs. It's crucial to note here that AAFCO (2016)[4] explicitly states this is a list of *minimum* nutrient requirements should normal function be desired in the dog (over 6 months). At no point do the AAFCO discuss the *optimum* requirements of dogs. Thus, 18% crude protein figure is the *minimum* amount of protein permitted in products seeking to state, 'complete as per the AAFCO guidelines' (in puppy food it is 22.5% protein) on their label. Sadly, these minimums now appear to be targets of the industry with few cereal-based dry foods now offering more than 1% or 2% points of protein more than this. In this way, any vets recommending such products are endorsing the use of the minimum amount of protein for your dog for life, not the optimum.

As discussed in our chapter on Vitamins and Minerals, the AAFCO concerns itself only with synthetic nutrition. At no point is fresh or optimum nutrition ever-considered. While they continue to obsess on the minimum required, and considering the danger of too much supplementary nutrients, there is a worrying lack of maximums in place. Of the 12 minerals listed, there are maximums in place for only four. Of the 11 vitamins listed we have maximums for only two. Using figures from swine, huge quantities of cheap iron and zinc oxide are permitted for use to replace the lack of these nutrients in the premix. Gross excesses of calcium carbonate, copper sulfate and various salts are undoubtedly posing a health risk to pets today.

At no point is fresh food, normal vitamin and mineral absorption or optimum nutrient requirements considered by this industry. Worse, as they busy themselves with minimum nutrient requirements and often using figures from swine, the inherent dangers posed by excessive supplementary nutrients in ultra-processed pet food have fallen by the wayside. There is a worrying lack of nutrient maximums in place. Remember, of the 12 minerals listed, there are maximums in place for only four. Of the 11 vitamins listed we have maximums for just two. With the breaks off, great quantities of cheap mineral oxides and sulfates are used to replace the lack of these nutrients in the premix coupled with terrible quantities of salt to make sure the pet eats it.

We know the body does not treat inorganic, supplemented forms of calcium or phosphorus the same as minerals found in nature chelated to a protein. Women on calcium supplements, despite consuming more calcium per meal, have lower bone density in their hips and spines. Phosphorus occurring naturally in the diet appears to have little or no effect on postprandial plasma phosphorus in cats. In fact, being harder to absorb, mineral supplements will result in more useless by-products which will increase the strain on the body's filtration system. This is the route to toxicity. In this way, maximums for supplements will very surely differ from nutrients in their natural form.

While the AAFCO's minimum nutritional guidelines were surely a God-send to dry pet food sector when they were devised in the 1970s when thousands of pets were going blind and dying for the want of taurine (the second most abundant amino acid in meat), undoubtedly pulling some atrociously inadequate products off the floor, the fact remains they are only truly relevant to dry food producers interested in making this quality of product. Worse, over time, these standards seem to have had the inadvertent effect of establishing a new low for the market. There was no longer any incentive for some dry food manufacturers to be a little better, use a little more animal protein or choose a better meat meal with less dogs in it. They certainly will not be rewarded by the consumer who, given adequate exposure to salt to hunger, will eat it regardless. Today, all that matters to the vet and owner is that the product has attained the AAFCO standard. More is not required. Better will not be rewarded. A rush to the bottom to remain competitive inevitably ensues.

It is disgraceful that the processed version of food and the synthetic version of nutrients have become the nutritional standard by which we must all now go by and it is clearly absurd. Currently any nutritionists trying to formulate AAFCO-compliant, species-appropriate raw dog food products must run around looking for ingredients that are high in items such as zinc and vitamin E (usually plant sourced, such as seeds; I like hemp seeds in this regard as they don't contain phytic acid which we know can cause its own problems) or risk their products not being deemed 'complete' by the dry food industry. I'm not quite sure what the plan is for obligate carnivores such as cats in this regard. It is for these reasons I say the AAFCO *minimum* nutritional profile requires very urgent revision if it is to play any role whatsoever in the fresh/raw sector and their lofty ideals of *optimum* nutrition for pets.

The Problems with AAFCO's Feed Trials

From here, somewhat unbelievably, things get worse with the AAFCO protocol. The second way of showing your product meets the AAFCO's 'complete for lifetime feeding' claims is to demonstrate that your product is practically identical to another product that has already been deemed 'complete' as per AAFCO standards. This apparently is the favoured route for dry pet food manufacturers today, in large part as their products *are* practically identical to others on the market.

But it is the third and final method of demonstrating your product is adequate for 'lifetime feeding' (an AAFCO feed trials using live dogs) that is the most inept – in-house food trials. The criteria for these trials are as follows:

- All food trials can be conducted in-house. (by the pet food companies themselves…).

- Manufacturers should conduct feeding trials on eight caged dogs for six months to check if the food is appropriate to sustain life.

- Growth food testing is similar to maintenance food testing, except that growth food testing need only run for 10 weeks despite being fed for 6–12months in most cases.

- Six of eight caged dogs must not show signs of nutritional deficiency or excess.

- Two dogs are allowed to be removed from the trial; the data recorded from the dispatched animals does not have to be included in the final reports.

- No animal is allowed to lose more than 15% of its starting weight although weight gain is not considered.

- At the end of this trial, four blood values should be taken – haemoglobin, packed cell volume (amount of red blood cells, a measure of fitness in sporting circles), serum alkaline phosphates (monitoring the kidneys) and serum albumin (monitoring the liver); levels must fall between accepted high and low values.

Once those criteria are satisfied and the in-house trial results are submitted, large-scale production may begin. If we are to ignore the fact that AAFCO is happy to bestow the lofty claim of 'complete for lifetime feeding' on a product that has been tested for six months, so many issues leap off the page at this point. The first is sample size. The AAFCO recommends a test of just eight caged dogs. Tiny sample sizes are the *modus operandi* of marketeers as it hides effects that would be seen when a greater number of test subjects are included. Small sample sizes mask issues, and these small sample sizes can get even smaller. Manufacturers are permitted to remove dogs for 'non-nutritional' reasons in case these dogs fudge their results. These reasons include skin or coat conditions, dental disease, gastric dilation, torsion, anal glands and a great deal of other 'non-nutritional' issues. Similarly, should one of the numerous food additives or their combination have a negative effect on their behaviour, it will not be measured. Not that laboratories would be equipped to assess problem behaviour in caged dogs – I defy anyone to spot *normal* behaviour in a beagle kennelled for 6 months in a laboratory.

From this point, manufacturers are free to repeat these trials as often as they like. This is crucial. Should they find side effects in their trials, manufacturers are not required to report or retain this information. Thus, they are free to repeat their tiny trials until one group of six dogs gets over the 6-month line and publish the results of that trial only. This is akin to rolling a dice eight times but repeating this feat ten times in a row. You then select the effort where it happened to land on heads six of eight times. Do it enough times and you will get eight in a row. It took the magician Derren Brown nine excruciating hours of coin-tossing to flip 10 heads in a row, check it out on YouTube, *Derren Brown, Ten Heads in a Row*.

The next issue is time. Nutritional deficiencies can take many months and even years to have a noticeable effect. Remember John Crandon from Section 2, who entirely deprived himself of vitamin C for 18 weeks before symptoms started popping up, symptoms that nearly killed him. How long before symptoms would pop up on a diet containing 50% of his Recommended Daily Allowance of vitamin C? Thirty-six weeks? A year? And would we be able to filter out all the noise at this point in order to quantify it in any meaningful way? Very likely not. While the ability of six of eight caged dogs to survive for six months on a commercial diet has been amply demonstrated by these manufacturers, to date a solid body of studies examining the health implications of these high-carb, ultra-processed, pelleted diets over years is missing from the literature. It is up to us the consumer to provide the link, should it exist.

The only requirement prior to the start of an AAFCO feeding trial is an initial physical examination, then after 26 weeks of eating the food being trialled, four blood parameters are measured, none of which directly correlates to nutrient levels in the body (haemoglobin, packed cell volume, serum alkaline phosphatase and albumin).

What is actually measured is also of huge concern. Only four blood values are taken. Measures must fall between predetermined minimal and maximal values. Thus, should the minimum be 1, the maximum be 10 and the ideal be 5, a reading of 9 in a pup consuming the food for 10 weeks is acceptable. Also not measured is the animal's nutrient levels before or after the trial! There is no measurement of vitamin levels, no measure of zinc, calcium, phosphorus, magnesium, iron, copper or manganese, which is all the more breathtaking an oversight when you consider this is a product based almost entirely on difficult-to-digest vitamin and mineral supplements.

As if it were possible, it gets worse. The AAFCO does not carry out checks or regulate these trials. The less-than-stringent, *in-house* tests are conducted by the manufacturers themselves and the results submitted on faith. Oversight is not the role of the AAFCO (or its equivalent in Europe, FEDIAF). In the United States, that is left to the FDA. However, the FDA only responds to issues if and when they arise, usually lead by consumer complaint or pet death. As in Europe, random investigations of pet food manufacturing premises are conducted by the relevant Department of Agriculture, where the condition of the premises and exact processes is their primary concern. Products are not spot checked although in Ireland and the United Kingdom they *ask* the manufacturer for their microbiology readings. To clarify, in no country that I am aware of is there an official body that randomly samples pet food or treats for their nutrient quality or content

This is the current state of pet food regulation in both the US and the EU (the latter uses FEDIAF nutritional and operational guidelines which, as a body of pet food producers, are virtually identical to that of AAFCO). But for all their woes, concerns and irregularities, at least the AAFCO / FEDIAF pretend to offer some form of control in the US and EU. Countries such as Canada have not even the pretence. The sector there is entirely unregulated. It's based on trust. No inspection. No verification. Nothing but the word of the producer!

> As a former CFIA veterinarian, it concerns me that, to date, there are still no federal regulations…governing the production of pet food in Canada…
> **Dr. Harper, retired from the Canadian Food Inspection Agency (CFIA), Jan 13, 2017**
> **https://truthaboutpetfood.com/the-failed-trust-of-the-canadian-pet-food-regulatory-system/**

This in part explains how, when the US FDA ordered a pet food company to recall a product that claimed, 'may help reduce feline urological syndrome', the company could keep on selling it with these claims in Canada.[6]

Unchecked Label Claims

It follows that you can write what you want on the label and put what you want in the product and, should nothing go wrong, be relatively free of persecution. With nobody keeping tabs, studies show ingredients in dry pet foods can vary widely from one sampling period to the next, even between foods that were the same flavour and brand.[10] Single-protein diets commonly used for dogs with atopy are routinely adulterated with potentially allergenic proteins or fats not listed on their labels, even when the label specifically states otherwise.[11-14] The inevitable result, we now know, is that a shocking amount of 'complete' dry, canned and indeed raw pet foods fail to achieve even the minimum benchmark set out by the AAFCO.[15-18]

If the market should learn how truly awful a certain ingredient is, manufacturers are free to simply change its name. In response to the public's growing recognition and repulsion of meat and bone meal as their sole 'meat' ingredient, the minutes of one AAFCO meeting is particularly revealing (January 23, 2018). At this gathering of minds, 'villain ingredients' were discussed. These are, the pet food producers explain, 'ingredients of confusion', a result of internet forums 'misleading consumers' – one of them being that recycled meat waste is in the form of meat meal. It is their belief that meal is actually a fantastic food source, so they wanted to change the names of ingredients to protect the consumers. It's all for you, you see! The result of such casual discussion is why you will now see the term 'dehydrated' or 'dried' meat on many pet food products. To most, the terms dehydration or dried calls forth desirable images of slow and gentle water removal, an excellent way of preserving meat integrity, although a time and cost expensive way of doing so. It most certainly does not call forth images of a giant pressure cooker in Asia stewing up often hazardous mystery meat waste, emerging from the cooker as grey gloop, arriving to the factory as a twice-cooked, nutrient bereft and likely antigenic powder.

The UK's Number 1 pet food (in terms of sales) is Bakers. On the back of their 'meaty chunks' product, the ingredients simply state it contains 15% 'meat and animal derivatives'. Normally, this would imply the meat ingredient went in fresh, which is better than meal form as they must be non-hazardous (fit for human consumption) when they arrive at the factory. But then, underneath the ingredients, we see mentioned that when these ingredients are 'rehydrated' they are actually 30% of the mixture. This is confusing. If you have to rehydrate, that means it has been somehow *de*hydrated first, implying the possible use of meat meal. When I emailed the manufacturer on their use of 'dehydrated meat', asking specifically if it was meal they were using, they responded that it was meat "in its concentrated form". I pushed again with the same question – does this mean it was meat meal? The answer was yes.

Buzz words such as 'natural' or 'super premium' are not defined or regulated by the AAFCO, FEDIAF or any government body. They mean absolutely nothing in the pet food world. Manufacturers use them with reckless abandon. The very fact these products state they are *prescribed* is indicative of the state of things. In December 2016 and using the Illinois Consumer Fraud and Deceptive Business Practices Act, two cat owners filed a putative class action lawsuit against Mars Pet Care, Purina Pet Care, Blue Pearl Vet Hospital and the multichain pet store Pet Smart, Hill's Pet Nutrition and Phoenix-based pet shop PetSmart.[19] The complainants alleged that these companies were colluding to charge consumers more than was justified for regular pet foods simply by making them available under the 'prescription' title, despite the fact these foods are comparable to their less expensive ranges, contain no drug or active medical ingredients that are not found in conventional foods and not to mention they are sold in regular stores by non-health professionals (Case No. 3:16-cv-7001). The US District Court in Chicago dismissed the case. Persisting, the defendants alleged that it was entirely outside the remit of the FDA to permit such a practice as it does not establish industry-wide standards for the labelling and marketing of pet food intended to treat or prevent disease. In 2019, a federal three-judge appeals court panel overturned the ruling and reinstated the putative class action lawsuit against Hill's Pet Nutrition and PetSmart (*Holly B. Vanzant and Dana Land, on behalf of themselves and all others similarly situated v. Hill's Pet Nutrition Inc. and PetSmart Inc.*).

Lacking the oversight, all too rarely are the fantastical claims of manufacturers called into question in this regard. In 2016, the Federal Trade Commission (Docket Number 152-3229) forced Mars Eukanuba to backtrack on its huge advertising campaign after they stated:

> …10 years ago, we launched a long life study. What we observed was astonishing. With Eukanuba and proper care, dogs in the study were able to live beyond their typical lifespan…by 30%…

The advertising campaign consistently implied that Eukanuba pet food plays a key role in dog longevity, only they didn't have any data to back up that claim. The truth was their product was used in a lifestyle study examining the effect of 25% food intake and better exercise. These leaner, healthier dogs lived longer. Mars was found to be too selective about these other details, however. You can't help but worry how many such claims get through, and onto walls of veterinary clinics the world over, if just for a short amount of time. If they are forced to take it down years later, the message is surely still implanted.

The longevity claim is a popular one in vet circles. In the opening paragraph of their study investigating the importance of manufactured dog food to health in older dogs, Pugliese *et al.* (2005)[20] make the following, perpetually unreferenced statement:

> …recent advances in the nutrition of companion animals has resulted in a longer possible lifespan for dogs and cats and an improvement in their quality of life…

I strongly disagree with this typically unsupported comment. Dogs are enjoying an ever-increasing social status in our lives today. More and more dogs sleep inside, and owners are increasingly ready to empty their bank accounts to get them fixed up when things go wrong. Dog laws are up, free-roaming and traffic accidents down. Most importantly, however are the advances in science and medicine. We know this from the increase in longevity of human populations with terrible diets. Take the United

States for example. The average American is living longer than they were 50 years ago, but today, few would dare to argue it is thanks to their diet choices. They are living longer *despite* their diets. We have to assume things would be even better if their diet was free of processed food, in line with advice following colossal global initiatives examining the dangers of ultra-processed food in humans highlighted in Section 2. But this advice we are all ignoring, which is likely at the centre of the sad fact that the average American's longevity is now decreasing for the second year running.[21]

And it seems we humans are not alone in this downward trend. In 2004, one of the largest health surveys of a canine population was undertaken by the UK Kennel Club and the British Small Animal Veterinary Association Scientific Committee.[22] The median age of death of 15,881 dogs representing 165 breeds was 11 years 3 months. Ten years later, the UK Kennel Club again reached out, this time receiving detailed information on 5,684 deceased dogs representing 191 breeds.[23] This time, while a very small number of breeds appeared to be living a touch longer (six at my last count), the overall resounding trend for longevity was highly negative. The overall median age at death was now 10 years 4 months, equating to an 11% fall in longevity, on average.

It is very strongly suspected poor diet, too, is implicit to this falling figure. A report for the Prince Laurent Foundation Price, a Belgian NGO set up in 1996 for the advancement of welfare in domestic and wild animals, titled "Relation Between The Domestic Dogs Wellbeing And Life Expectancy", indicates a similar slippery slope for our dogs too. Lippert and Sapy (2003)[24] surveyed 500 dog owners and found:

> …Animals fed with homemade food (based on similar food as the family) reach an average of 13.1 years… the animals fed with canned industrial food reach an average of 10.4 years. The animals fed with mixed food… (homemade plus canned food) reach an average of 11.4 years… Giving it homemade food is a guarantee for… better protection, wellbeing and longer life expectancy…

Not only did they find a close to 30% greater longevity in dogs fed home-cooked food but adding commercial food actually appeared to shorten their life expectancy. Sadly, this report was not peer reviewed but we already suspect raw-fed dogs are costing less at the vets (as per Brisbane Guide Dogs and Wylie Vets the latter we will learn about later) so it stands to reason that they are healthier and thus, assumedly, living longer. Using veterinary records, this will be easy enough to determine in the coming years. Rumour has it this process has already begun and the answers are very much as expected.

I think it's fair to say that the AAFCO is only considered the industry watchdog by the industry itself, a dog that is not on the company payroll but is toothless, de-balled and sound asleep. Today their *minimum*, unenforced criteria are at risk of cajoling both vet and consumer alike into believing their product of choice has obtained a gold star of nutritional completeness, something even members of their own panel of experts admit to:

> Although the AAFCO profiles are better than nothing, they provide false securities. I don't…know of any studies showing their adequacies or inadequacies.
>
> **Rogers Quinton DVM, PhD, one of the AAFCO panel experts,**
> **cited in Butterwick *et al.* (2011)[25]**

2. The Worrying, Willing Participation of Governments in the Pet Food Scandal

To coin Leonard Cohen – you want it darker?

So far, we have just been focusing on the corporate links to our veterinary sector and regulators. However, in a way, we expect multi-billion-dollar companies to run riot in such sectors when and where they can. That's what they do. From tobacco to oil to pet food, the same old tricks. It's more worrying when government departments get involved. And they do, repeatedly. The following is an outstanding example.

While working in the United States, Ilze Matīse-Vanhoutana, a Latvian veterinary pathologist and researcher, was pulled away from her microscope by a phone call from a colleague which changed the course of both her professional and personal life for the next few years. Below I paraphrase from her TedX talk on October 26, 2017, titled "I Did My Research, Blew The Whistle And Found Myself At War", which you can find on YouTube.

Ilze's friend asked whether she noticed the increased amount of megaoesophagus in dogs recently. Moreover, did she know they had all been eating the same food?

ME is a terrible condition in mostly dogs which involves an unusual enlargement of the oesophagus, the muscular tube connecting the throat to the stomach, that ultimately results in significantly decreased to absent motility. In other words, the dog can no longer swallow. It is extremely distressing and often results in the dog slowly starving and very often being put to sleep. Those that make it have owners who are prepared to administer many small meals to their dog while they are in an upright position, for the rest of their lives. And it requires constant surveillance as even a small treat off the ground will surely choke them. Up until this phone call for Ilze, and indeed this TedX talk for the rest of us, it was assumed to be the result of a genetic defect only.

Slow to jump the gun, Ilze was hesitant to accept her friend's observation as it was. There must be something more to it than simply the wrong food. But being the scientist she is, Ilze was keen to understand more. Within 2 years they had produced three studies on the matter. To summarise the findings, the average number of ME cases in Latvia from 2011–2013 was approximately ten cases per year, a rare enough disease in the grand scheme of things. However, 2014–2016 saw a 10-fold increase in cases, to approximately 104 cases per year (a quarter of them each year succumbing to the disease).

Ilze and her team determined that the problem was in the nerves, that it is was most likely caused by a toxin and that a common factor in the cases they were seeing was the food they were eating, a pet food made in Latvia. Armed with their findings, they felt obliged to inform the authorities of the outbreak they had identified and approached the chair of the board of the pet food manufacturer in question. Their response, perhaps unsurprisingly, was immediate denial.

> Your data must be wrong…those dog owners are probably lying about the dog food they feed…
>
> **Matīse-Vanhoutana, 2017**[26]

The Latvian Ministry of Agriculture agreed to fund a further study and Ilze was tasked to find the toxin in question. By the time the six months was up, as the ME cases continued to roll in, her team had eliminated more than half of the potential culprits. But more work needed to be done. At this point, the authorities said to stop, that there was 'no evidence of an outbreak'. They said that *not enough* dogs were affected and that too much money had already been spent (so far, her investigation has cost the state a mere €35,000 over 6 months).

> …we also learned that the chairman of the board had made a donation to the political party that the minister of Agriculture belonged to…
>
> **Matīse-Vanhoutana, 2017**

This brought with it more problems as, now without backing from her government, Ilze and her team could not get access to the list of ingredients used in the pet food in question.

Thankfully however, the media soon got hold of the story and following interviews with various TV and media outlets, now Ilze's investigation found itself under the microscope. On the plus side, this led to crowdfunding and they very quickly secured the monies needed to continue the research her own government 'found too sensitive to fund'. They conducted a case-controlled study which found a correlation coefficient of more than 100 (anything over four is considered strong). The higher the figure, the more likely the correlation is to the actual cause. In this case, the risk of a dog getting ME upon eating the pet food in question is 100 times higher than for a dog eating another kind of food. In short, very concrete proof. Ilze felt she had to warn the public and 2 years later she is still suffering the repercussions of that selfless action. In her words: (italics added by me for effect)

> ...this investigation has been a heavy burden on my shoulders for the past two years...I'm sure we were heard by those people in power, but politics turned out to be more powerful than science, the price of life and common sense...the peak of absurdity came when I heard the news that me, several other veterinarians and their clinics had been sued by the dog food company...if we lose we have to pay €500,000. But if you think that was the peak, it wasn't, because *the dog food company also sued the owners of the sick dogs for sharing their stories on social media...*
>
> **Matīse-Vanhoutana, 2017**

The net result of this team's actions resulted in a dramatic decrease (from 100 cases per year in 2014–2016, to just 18 cases mid-June 2016 to mid-June 2017) of ME in the Latvian dog population; Ilze states there was a four-fold decrease in the sales of the product in question (the name of which she does not mention in the entire piece).

Two years later, in a piece entitled *Pet food Advance Dermocare linked to megaoesophagus outbreak, research shows,*[27] ABC News Australia was reporting on 100 cases of ME in Australian dogs from 2017–2018. This included nine Victoria police dogs. It was perhaps the inclusion of these highly prized dogs which arguably brought the media's attention back to this scandal. In their piece, Scopelianos and Donnellan quote Caroline Mansfield, U-Vet Hospital director who looked at a sub-set of dogs with ME 'and found the odds of them being fed Advance Dermocare in the six months prior to diagnosis were 437 times greater for cases compared to the control group'.

> This is an extremely strong association, there is about a one in a million probability that this occurred by chance, supporting the hypothesis that Advance Dermocare was associated with this outbreak of idiopathic megaesophagus in dogs.
>
> **Caroline Mansfield, ABC News, cited in Scopelianos and Donnellan (2018)**[27]

Following this very public outbreak, Mars voluntarily recalled the product in question in Australia in March 2018.[28]

In terms of government's stepping in to affect the pet food sector for the bad, it's fair to say the US FDA takes the cereal-based biscuit.

Dr. Victoria Hampshire's job in 2004 was to keep count of side effects from animal drugs for the FDA. Proheart 6, a 3-year-old injectable drug to prevent heartworm made by Wyeth, came up on her radar. With over 500 deaths officially recorded from autoimmune, allergic, liver and other reactions, Proheart 6 for heart worm was killing more dogs than all its competitors combined. As adverse events coordinator, Hampshire alerted her peers to the issue she was seeing but in trying to do her job, she ended up losing it. The NBC news covered the story in detail[30] and I recount it in part as follows:

> What happened next — and the price she paid for speaking up — have spurred a US Senate inquiry and shined a spotlight on the complex topography of drug safety, where interests collide like tectonic plates and squeeze decisions from all sides.

Proheart 6 was very successful for the company, but for vets, too. Injectable drugs such as Proheart 6 are favoured by vets as it means the client must come into the clinic twice a year for a shot. Donn (2007)[29] highlights how one vet with ties to Wyeth, lectured his colleagues about 'seizing on Proheart 6 as a hook to pull in healthy pets for profitable regular exams'. It wasn't going away without a fight, and Hampshire was ready to give it to them. She was initially successful. Wyeth recalled all Proheart 6 products from vets in the United States, perhaps the largest (and possibly only) major pet drug recall in the 2000s (though it continued selling Proheart 6 in Canada, Europe and elsewhere).

However, just 2 months later, things went south for the whistle-blower. Following a meeting with Wyeth's Chief Executive, the then FDA Commissioner, Lester Crawford called Hampshire into her office. The FDA had detected financial irregularities in Hampshire's records which might be construed as a conflict of interests when evaluating the safety of Proheart 6. In particular, it was Hampshire's use of a certain website for prescribing drugs for her patients, a practice that grossed her $160 over two and a half years. Crawford, who would suddenly quit the FDA only a year later, admitting he was hiding stocks in medical and food companies the FDA regulated and was fined about $90,000, thought it best 'to protect Tory [Victoria Hampshire] to get her out of it completely'.[29] Just a few months later, Hampshire was called into the office of Dr. Linda Tollefson, then deputy head of the FDA's CVM. She was being moved out of her current job and into a desk job significantly beneath her abilities.

> "Wyeth has pulled all the plugs at the level of commissioner," Tollefson told a stunned Hampshire. They were transferring her to the vaccines building to care for the rats and monkeys.

The FDA later detected some residual solvents used in the manufacturing of Proheart 6 were allergenic, prompting Wyeth to change how the drug was manufactured. Adverse reactions declined and the product was relaunched in 2008 to the US veterinary market but with restrictions such as vets were required to attend in-depth training, restrict treatment to 'healthy' dogs aged 6 months to 7 years of age and obtain a signed consent form from the owner. Zoetis purchased Wyeth soon after and after a 4-year internal safety review had the FDA lift the restrictions on Proheart 6.

Just a year after her ordeal, in 2006, the US Public Health Service awarded Hampshire its vet of the year award.

> [Wyeth] tried to destroy a reputation...her own agency sold her down the river.
> **Senator Chuck Grassley, Donn, 2007**[29]

Switching our focus to pet food, we have already covered some of the more questionable practices of the FDA in Section 2. These include policy 690.300 which permits the use of material from diseased animals for animal consumption and their worryingly slow response to protect consumers by naming the affected pet food products during the melamine scandal in 2007, something Susan Thixton pursued with interest.

Thixton's site TruthAboutPetfood.com is the primary source for pet food recalls, manufacturer indiscretions and labelling irregularities. As much as she is a champion of pet owners, she is a thorn in the side of the AAFCO and the FDA, standing practically alone in holding pet food manufacturers to account for their indiscretions. Her fully referenced articles keep tabs on the AAFCO, often comparing industry-proposed changes to the legislation already in place that is supposed to be governing the process in the first place. I urge you to keep tabs on her website. She was the first to sit in on AAFCO meetings and report back to consumers what was happening. She lasted six months in this regard. When she was eventually turfed out of these *public* meetings, she received these words in an email from Mr. Stan Cook, AAFCO's President-Elect and Chair of the AAFCO Pet Food Committee:

> Any of the people providing input to the group and thus to AAFCO as a whole, serve at AAFCO's discretion. It's AAFCO's party, we can invite who we want to the party...
>
> **Email to Susan Thixton, published online (https://truthaboutpet food.com/its-aafcos-party/)**

One of Susan's articles, titled "A Pet Food Betrayal Like None Other", followed the 2007 melamine scandal that killed and maimed tens of thousands of pets. Dead pets aside, this was a full force storm for the industry. It serves as an excellent example of how exposed you guys truly are. Following the scandal, pet owners were given promises by Congress that the Food and Drug Administration Amendments Act (FDAAA) will 'ensure the safety of pet food'. They passed the *Ensuring the Safety of Pet Food Law* and handed it to the FDA to implement...which it decided not to do. In 2018, after the FDA had entirely ignored their mandate for more than a decade, the *Pet Food Industry Magazine*[30] discovered the law was apparently no longer on the table. Gone. The piece goes on to quote Dr. Steven M. Solomon, director of the FDA's CVM, who made a surprising announcement during a presentation at the Ninth Annual Feed and Pet Food Joint Conference, a meeting of minds between the National Grain and Feed Association and the Pet Food Institute. It came in his final slide, which mentioned *the deletion* of the ingredient standards and definitions provision in the FDAAA. He commented that the FDA 'will continue working with AAFCO for that'.[31]

> In fairness, even the editor and chief of the Pet Food Industry Magazine was surprised. And that was it! Solomon offered no further explanation, and there was no opportunity to question him later about this potentially significant development with pet food ingredients...
>
> **Phillips-Donaldson, 2018**[31]

It's fair to say the FDA appears overly distracted by the raw dog food sector. In 2015, they announced that they would be doubling down on hazardous microbiology in raw dog food.[34] The announcement stated that, despite permitting large amounts of *Salmonella* in the human food chain, any positive readings for *Salmonella, Listeria* or *E. coli O157:H7* in a sample of raw dog foods 'may result in a Class I recall, press release, and Reportable Food Registry (RFR) submission'. Zero *Salmonella* is a tough ask for raw dog food manufacturers that employ none of the chemical nor processing techniques commonly used in kibble production. Despite this, after a period of intense scrutiny, what did the FDA find? They found that the volume of dry food recalled for *Salmonella* from 2012–2019 positively dwarfed that of raw dog food. Using official recall records free to view on the FDA website, Thixton (2019)[32] collated dry and raw pet food recalls by volume over the previous 8 years. She found that 150 million pounds (68,000 tonnes) of kibble were recalled for pathogenic bacteria from 2012 to early 2019 compared to just 2 million pounds (900 tonnes) of raw dog food. What makes this difference even more dramatic is that those figures for *Salmonella* in dry food came from just the 2012–2015 period! Once the FDA decided to focus its might on the raw sector, all announced recalls for *Salmonella* in dry pet food mysteriously stopped. This is pretty astounding, considering Section 2 showed us that in the five years previously there was a constant stream of enormous recalls for exactly this issue (19 from just 2010 to 2015, involving multiple big-name companies, hundreds of products and millions of tonnes of product, each and every year). They all just somehow…stopped! Every dry and canned pet food manufacturer suddenly got its act together…for a 4-year run. You would forgive the numerous US raw dog food manufacturers for crying foul at the time.

And yet, despite all the evidence to the contrary, the FDA posted a warning on their website February 22, 2018 that instructed America to 'Avoid the dangers of raw pet food'.[32] It has since been taken down.

More recently, the FDA has shifted its attention to grain-free pet food. The US pet food market is now being driven by more natural products for their pets. More natural types of pet food are beginning to take over in the United States (next section) with grain-free pet food accounting for the largest proportion of that market. In 2018, the FDA announced it was investigating the link between some 600 cases of dilated cardiomyopathy (DCM), which is a heart condition in dogs, and grain-free pet food (FDA 2018).[33] Nothing wrong so far. Considering what we now know about DCM, it is entirely plausible that the dry, grain-free pet food sector would suffer many of the same nutritional and safety woes of the cereal-based pet food sector.

What was unusual about this case was that the FDA quickly went on to name the companies involved and the number of 'suspected' cases attributed to each of them, something that was not afforded pet owners 10 years previously during the melamine scandal when tens of thousands of pets were actually dying. Fears were adequately stoked in the general population. Soon papers such as The *New York Times* and the *Washington Post* (Furby 2018)[34] picked up on the 'link' and spread the concern to dog owners throughout the nation. Very quickly, a newly created Facebook group 'Taurine Deficient (Nutritional) Dilated Cardiomyopathy' had more than 60,000 members for 600 apparent cases.

In fact, for that number of cases to spook the FDA in this manner is highly unusual. First, we are talking about 600 potential cases in a grain-fed pet population of approximately 90 million US dogs and 60 million cats; so this is still a very, very rare issue. Then you compare it to cereal-based pet food, and it looks pretty phenomenal. DCM is historically a cereal-based dry food issue, killing many thousands of pets in the last few decades of the 20th century. Before the melamine scandal in 2007 really ignited the natural pet food sector in the US, the cereal-based pet food sector was at its zenith. It happens that Sanderson, in 2006, estimated the overall prevalence of DCM in the overall dog population at the time to be somewhere between 0.5% to 1.1%. This means you would expect somewhere between 500,000 and a million cases of DCM in the US dog population!

Moreover, no more issues have been identified since the FDA made their announcement, nor has the issue seemed to have materialised in the EU. Furthermore, as of October 2019, none of the manufacturers has yet identified an issue with their products nor conducted a recall. Finally, nearly a full year after their announcement and heightened public awareness, no more than 500 cases of DCM have been reported, in a nation of more than 90 million pet dogs.

Mansilla *et al.* (2019)[35] explain that DCM in dogs is most likely the result of insufficient circulating taurine in the body which can arise for a number of reasons. Taurine, an amino acid commonly found in meat, is a non-essential amino acid to the dog meaning, should they not consume a lot of it, they can synthesise their own from the dietary precursor amino acids methionine and cysteine, which are essential. Thus, a diet low in meat and/or low in methionine and/or cysteine may be a risk factor for DCM. There are other suspected dietary causes of DCM too, including anything that perturbs the metabolism of methionine by the body, a lack of carnitine (another amino acid found in meat, involved in energy production) and the role of too much plant fibre which may interfere with how well the animal reabsorbs bile (and thus taurine) in their small intestines. In this case, a high consumption of fermentable fibres may increase the abundance of microbial populations that degrade taurine in the small intestines. There is also a strong breed effect, not to mention the effect of age, sex, size and physiological status.

Of all dietary causes, Mansilla *et al.* (2019)[35] point the finger at a lack of methionine in the diet. Methionine is, according to the NRC (2006)[36], one of the most limiting amino acids in pet foods formulated using soy or rendered meats. As Section 2 showed us, it is highly heat sensitive and is readily broken down by the heat used in pet food processing, resulting in constant pet food recall and indeed pet deaths.

There is another suspected but hotly debated cause of DCM in dogs and that is the use of ingredients such as potatoes and pulses (peas, lentils, chickpeas and beans such as soy), now common fillers in grain-free pet food. It is these ingredients causing the FDA the most concern as they were apparently 'frequently listed' in the recent cases presented to them. Mansilla *et al.* (2019)[35] do a very comprehensive job detailing how these ingredients as a whole are yet to be correlated with DCM in dogs. They highlight that previous works that did make such an association,[37,38] involving less than 100 DCM cases between them, did not adequately address the fibre, taurine, methionine nor cysteine contents of the foods they were examining and thus provided no such proof whatsoever. In fact, the Kaplan study actually supplemented their test dogs with taurine. But in terms of worrying conclusions, the Adin work stands out as the most erroneous and I credit Daniel Schulof for pointing the issues out to me.

The FDA's concern for the apparent 'spike' of DCM cases was prompted by a group of American veterinary specialists from major research universities, most notably Dr Lisa Freeman, Dr Josh Stern and Dr Darcy Adin. Their piece,[39] titled "Diet-Associated Dilated Cardiomyopathy in Dogs: What Do We Know?" appears to be the seminal work linking DCM in dogs to grain-free pet food, in that it is certainly the most popular. Published in the *Journal of American Veterinary Medical Association*, it has been downloaded more than fifty times more often than the Mansilla *et al.* (2019)[35] piece above. With more than 80,000 downloads in just six months (Dec 2018 to July 2019), it had three times that of any article published around the same time in that journal. In fact, with those sort of numbers, it is likely the most widely read canine nutritional science article *ever written*, which is quite a remarkable feat for Freeman who also authored JAVMA's other most popularly downloaded articles, this time a piece on raw dog food in 2013, titled "Current Knowledge About The Risks And Benefits Of Raw Meat-Based Diets For Dogs And Cats."

In relation to this DCM article, all these authors openly declared financial interests with the world's biggest cereal-based pet food producers Hill's Pet Nutrition, Nestlé Purina Petcare and Mars Petcare are three of the world's largest cereal-based pet food companies. Dr. Adin declared financial interests to Purina Pet Care, Dr. Stern to Royal Canin and Purina and Dr. Lisa Freeman to all three.

Unfortunately, the piece is replete with errors and conjecture, most of which were revealed to me upon reading the 50-page redaction demands submitted to the *Journal of American Veterinary Medical Association* in July 2019 by Daniel Schulof, CEO of KetoNatural Pet Food. It was co-signed by more than 200 veterinarians, research scientists, medical professionals and representatives of the pet food industry (published online, see veterinaryintegrity.org). For instance, Freeman *et al.* (2018)[39] stated 'over the past few years, an increasing number of DCM cases involving dogs appear to have been related to diet' although they provide no evidence of this. Not a single reference. They repeatedly associate 'BEG diets' (essentially grain-free pet foods) with DCM in dogs. But again, they have no evidence to support this point. In their piece, Freeman *et al.* refer to the only two diet-associated DCM works in recent years – the aforementioned studies by Adin *et al.* 2019[37] and Kaplan *et al.* 2018[38] (the latter of which was co-authored by Stern). Neither of which were published at the time the Freeman article went to press. Furthermore, neither of these works manages to make any association between grain-free pet foods and DCM as both fail to adequately address the fibre, taurine, methionine or cysteine contents of the foods they were testing. To test the methionine issue, and submitted as part of his redaction request, Schulof sent the foods used by Kaplan *et al.* (2018)[38] off for independent testing and discovered that "the vast majority of the DCM-positive dogs in the study do indeed appear to have been consuming less than the NRCs recommended daily allowance for one or both of these DCM-linked amino acids – a fact which might well explain their DCM diagnoses".

But it gets worse. The DCM cases discussed in the study by Dr. Adin *et al.* (2019)[37] were reported in a poster presentation titled "Echocardiographic Phenotype of Canine Dilated Cardiomyopathy Differs Based on Diet" presented in the same year at the American College of Veterinary Internal Medicine Specialty Symposium, June 14–16, 2018. In this piece, Adin, a vet specialised in cardiology, discusses 49 cases of DCM in dogs, of which 22 (~45%) were consuming grain-free diets while 27 (~55%) were eating grain-based diets, which is almost exactly as you would expect considering the spread of these products in the market. However, by the time Adin submitted her work for actual publication in the *Journal of Veterinary Cardiology*, the number of DCM-positive dogs consuming grain-based diets had dropped from 27 to 12, increasing the prevalence of those consuming grain-free diets from 45% to 75%. Schulof contacted Adin about this anomaly and she claims 15 of the grain-consuming dogs were dropped from the final study due to not having 'airtight diet histories'. In comparison, only one dog consuming a grain-free diet at the time of diagnosis was dropped for the same reason.

It is because they have no evidence that the article by Freeman wanders so repeatedly into open conjecture, such as the following statement (italics added by me for effect):

> The *apparent link* between BEG diets and DCM *may* be due to the grain-free nature of these diets…possible nutritional imbalances or inadvertent inclusion of toxic dietary components. *Or, the apparent association may be spurious.*
>
> **Freeman *et al.* 2018**[39]

How can such vagary get through onto a scientific publication? Well, Freeman's piece wasn't peer reviewed. The article was labelled as an 'op-ed', an opinion piece. This is the one area of which *JAVMA* does not require peer review for. However, in reality, as the title clearly states (bold added by me for effect) *Diet-Associated Dilated Cardiomyopathy in Dogs: What Do We **Know**?*, thereby removing, the notion of opinion and leads the readers, via copious use of the literature, down the road of a factually-focused literature review, a work demanding peer review before publication so as not to possibly mislead consumers.

So erroneous and potentially damaging was the piece that Schulof, a lawyer by trade, has filed a federal lawsuit against the FDA for their part in the debacle. As part of his investigation, Schulof asked the FDA to disclose records concerning its relationship with the *JAVMA* article's authors as well as the three pet food companies to which several of the authors have financial ties.

> Because it was never peer-reviewed, the article is rife with the kinds of false and misleading statements that reviewers surely would have caught if given the chance. It grossly mischaracterizes the evidence surrounding its subject, it relies on anecdotes and conjectures instead of evidence for its most basic assumptions, it misrepresents studies that were unpublished at the time it went to print, it overlooks suspicious methodological irregularities in recent DCM studies published elsewhere by its own authors, and its authors have financial ties (including undisclosed ones)

to "Big Kibble" pet food companies with clear incentives to promote a link between "BEG diets" and canine DCM, even if one doesn't really exist.

Daniel Schulof, owner of Keto Pet Grain-Free Pet Food, leading the charge in redacting Freeman's 2018 *JAVMA* article, stated on www. veterinaryintegrity.org/

Just before this book went to print, there was one more effort by the industry, again by Stern at UC Davis, to drum home the apparent dangers of DCM from 'non-traditional' diets, meaning those higher in legumes but low in grains.[40] This work resulted in the online publishing platform PLOS ONE issuing the authors with an 'Expression of Concern' concerning its content (https://doi.org/10.1371/journal.pone.0233206). The issues included questions regarding the criteria used to categorise diets, the fact the authors focused on the dangers of legumes in the 'non-traditional' diets whilse apparently ignoring the fact soybeans are also in the legume family and that diet history prior to a subject's current diet and indeed the varying lengths of time each group spent on their diet might impact the study's outcomes. There were questions regarding the statistical analyses reported in the article and regarding their concluding statement which read 'Grain free diets, produced by small companies, including legumes within the top five ingredients, represent a risk for the development of taurine deficiency and echocardiographic abnormalities consistent with DCM in the golden retriever.'

But of all the concerns highlighted by PLOS ONE, it was the issue with their undeclared competing interests that stood out. The initial declaration read:

> A.J. Fascetti [Andrea Fascetti, one of the corresponding authors] is the Scientific Director of and J. Yu is employed by the Amino Acid Laboratory at the University of California, Davis that provides amino acid analysis on a fee for service basis. This did not influence the collection or interpretation of results in this study. This does not alter our adherence to PLOS ONE policies on sharing data and materials.

In response to the concerns raised by PLOS, the authors changed the statement to the following:

> AJF is the Scientific Director and JY is the Technical Director of the Amino Acid Laboratory at the University of California, Davis (UCD) that provides amino acid analysis on a fee for service basis. AJF received remuneration for

lectures or as an advisor on behalf of Nestlé Purina PetCare, Mars Petcare, Synergy Food Ingredients, the Mark Morris and Pet Food Institutes. AJF received funding from Nutro for graduate student training. A resident on the Nutrition Service, mentored in part by AJF, received funds from the Hill's Pet Nutrition Resident Clinical Study Grants program, matched by the Center for Companion Animal Health, School of Veterinary Medicine at UCD. The Veterinary Medical Teaching Hospital at UCD received funding from Royal Canin to support a resident, and from Nestlé Purina PetCare to partially support a nutrition technician. AJF has a contract with the FDA on unrelated research. Since the time of article submission, JAS [Stern] has received research support from Nature's Variety Inc. Collectively, this did not influence the collection or interpretation of results in this study. There are no patents, products in development or marketed products to declare. This does not alter our adherence to PLOS ONE policies on sharing data and materials.

In 2019, Statista confirmed Schulof's fears regarding the impact of the FDA getting involved in the debate. Reports show a significant drop in sales of grain-free pet food in the United States in 2019. Where previous years, it had enjoyed year-on-year growth of nearly 10%, in 2019 sales had fallen by 0.3%"[41]

If by this stage you are wondering why the US government appears so willing to step in and assist the plight of the poor, suffering cereal-based pet food sector, then consider the fact that the cereal-based pet food is a profitable end point for the waste of the human food industry. It is an outlet for poor-quality grain, as well as indigestible leftovers from the likes of the beet, corn and grape industries. Most importantly, it is the dumping ground for the meat industry.

The meat lobby is immensely powerful, particularly so in the US. Their rapid adoption of incredibly inhumane Concentrated Animal Feed Operations (CAFO's), which now account for the vast majority of the meat consumed by Americans, is but one indicator of the sector's power to grow questionable businesses behind closed doors. Today Americans are eating a LOT of animal protein in the form of meat, eggs, cheese and milk. The problem is this sector produces a lot of hazardous waste. Typically, less than half of a slaughtered cow is consumed by humans. The rest, much of the head, brain, carcass, much of the organs, innards, feet and tail, is waste, as far as the human market is concerned. The producers have two options available to them at this point – sell it direct to the pet food companies or sell it to the rendering plants (which will stew it with all other meat waste) and inevitably send it on to pet food companies, among other animal feed groups.

There is a third option and that is to send their more hazardous waste (nonedible parts such as brains and guts but also meat from dead, diseased, dying, disabled) for incineration. While this latter step is a requirement for hazardous waste in the European Union, in the United States this material is permitted to be handled by the renderers and sold on for animal feed; so there's little point paying to dump what the renderers will pay you to send them or in the very least take for free. In this way, pet food provides a valuable outlet for meat waste, if just in the United States. Here are some throw away figures to give us some context: the US produces more than 50 million tonnes of meat each year (beef, chicken, turkey and pork, combined, United States Department of Agriculture (USDA) figures). That is potentially 25 million tonnes of animal waste each year (or 25 billion kilos). If we estimate that the producer asks for just $0.10 per kilo of their product (in Ireland, chicken and duck carcass is worth €0.30/kg when bought by the tonne, beef organs €0.70/kg), that's a market value of $250 billion.

This shifts our focus immediately. No longer are we talking about a $30 billion US pet food market. Now we are talking figures of a quarter of a trillion. In fact, we could easily double that figure, considering now we are asking the meat industry to adapt its supply lines and storage facilities and start *paying to dump* what was once a profitable commodity. At least half a trillion dollars, or 1.5 times the size of the US entire prescription drug market. Either the producers pay or the home of capitalism, currently $20 trillion in debt as a result, will be picking up the tab to manage it for them. This is something the FDA is currently completely unable to do, financially or otherwise. They could insist meat prices increase significantly but this would result in less US meat being consumed, which is equally bad news for the economy, big pharma and heavily lobbied governments as a whole. There is simply no profitable way out of this, so they dig in and continue to relentlessly drive consumption by any means necessary.

Lacking any form of appropriate, independent regulation, power is going to be abused. That is the way we work. From governments to churches to banks to big pharma and now with multibillion dog-food-making candy manufacturers, once they get into a position of real power, self-preservation quickly overrides any concern for the safety and well-being of the masses. All that matters is the preservation and growth of the company and for that job they will always find the right person.

> All governments suffer a recurring problem: Power attracts pathological personalities. It is not that power corrupts but that it is magnetic to the corruptible.
>
> **Frank Herbert, Author of Dune**

Unfortunately for us, there is no pet food police. Today our top veterinary governing bodies, including the RCVS, the American College of Veterinary Nutrition (ACVN), the AVMA, the AAHA and even WSAVA, and now even governments themselves, are all 100% behind cereal-based pet food for dogs and cats. Whatever defences we had are completely overrun. It seems that *nobody* is protecting our pets from what are some truly awful food products. With little by way of a filter on the nonsense they speak, science has been reduced to little more than a marketing tool and it used with great abandon. So we get what we have today – increasingly scientific and difficult to interpret labels that leave the poorly versed vet and pet owner alike utterly bamboozled. Hard-to-pronounce protein names and complex molecular structures are used on the front of nutrient-defunct, ultra-processed, junk food products, giving a rubbish food product an air of scientific prowess which comforts and cajoles the consumer into parting with their cash.

> It's funny, all you have to do is say something nobody understands and they'll do practically anything you want them to.
>
> *The Catcher in the Rye*, **J.D. Salinger**

Today pet owners are walking into a vet's office looking for a specific diet for a specific illness in a specific breed of dog of a specific age in a particular moment in time. We are forced to decide between a product that boasts better cognitive function in our ageing dog or the dental variety for his kibble-rotted teeth. What to do?! Next month, are they to trade a healthy gut with nice, firm stools for a sleeker coat? Maybe focus on his stiffening joints over winter and then slim him down in the summer in time for the beach! Does it seem right that you have to choose?

The good news is, there is another way. Imagine for a second a diet that accommodates *all* of the body's needs throughout the year. One that you can tweak as you see fit, as life throws out its stumbling blocks, one that is not only beautifully simple, fresh and nutrient dense but also, enjoyable to prepare and so extremely palatable for your best friend that he risks dislocating his butt from excessive tail wagging. A diet free of nasty chemical adulterants and made from local ingredients, maybe even, dare we hope, from more ethically treated animals? A diet that offers *real* value for money that will save you on vet visits and that is absolutely expected to add many healthy years to the already too-short lives of your pets?

Doesn't this sound like something you should at least *try* for a few weeks before making up your own mind? You certainly can't do much worse.

TAKE-HOME POINTS

✓ The largest recall ever of a single brand of pet food occurred last year. Hill's Science Diet distributed more than 22 million cans of pet food with potentially toxic amounts of Vitamin D without nutritionally checking a single one. The FDA said it would 'verify Hill's proposed voluntary correction actions'. Who is supposed to be supervising the manufacturers?

✓ There are no governmental organisations supervising the nutritional content of pet food. They are merely concerned only for the layout and cleanliness of the premises and microbiology content of the product.

✓ In the 1980s the American FDA handed over the regulation of the pet food industry to the American Association of Feed Control Officials (AAFCO). The AAFCO sets the guidelines for what 'complete' pet food means but they do not enforce it. They have many established ties to the pet food industry.

✓ FEDIAF in Europe effectively copies the AAFCO feed guidelines and does not enforce either. That is left up to each individual country. Unlike the AAFCO, the FEDIAF admits it concerns itself with 'promoting the views and interests of around 650 European pet food producing companies'.

✓ The AAFCO minimum nutritional profile is a list of amino acids, vitamins and minerals that is supposed to determine what is 'complete' food for dogs. While useful in the first few years, it is in urgent need of review, certainly for the raw food industry.

✓ As the industry bases its recommendations on poorly absorbed nutritional supplements, the minimum requirement for zinc and vitamin E is absurdly high (it has little likeness to their availability in nature).

✓ Vitamin C is not required by the AAFCO, despite sick dogs benefitting from its addition.

✓ The AAFCO allows just 18% and 22.5% protein for adults and pups, respectively.

✓ There is no labelling requirement for carbohydrates and no maximums in place for sugar, salt or fibre. In fact, there are maximums in place for only four of 12 minerals and two of 11 vitamins.

- ✓ The AAFCO's *minimum* guidelines have slowly but surely become the *optimum* for manufacturers.

- ✓ Due to how differently the body treats synthetic supplements and nutrients in their natural form, the AAFCO's guidelines are of very little value to anyone formulating a fresh diet for a dog using real ingredients.

- ✓ Another way to verify that your dog food is 'complete' is to conduct an AAFCO food trial. The requirements here have major concerns – the trials are short (6 months), involve a handful of dogs (eight dogs start but two can be removed for 'non-nutritional reasons') and only four blood values are measured at the end. The trials are conducted in-house. The manufacturer can repeat the trial as many times as they like and publish only the most satisfactory results.

- ✓ The AAFCO does not supervise these food trials or the manufacturers themselves. That is left up to the US FDA which tends to respond to issues when they arise. As we see in each European country, the USDA does conduct some random site visits but never checks the nutritional quality or safety of the products being pumped out.

- ✓ Buzzwords such as 'natural', 'super premium' or 'prescription' are not regulated by the AAFCO, so they mean nothing. Further, manufacturers are free to change the name of less desirable ingredients such as meat meal.

- ✓ The recent ME and melamine scandals told us that governments of the world seem worryingly ready to step in and assist ultra-processed pet food manufacturers, often to the detriment of pet and pet owner alike.

- ✓ Unlike its own meat chain for humans, where *Salmonella* is permitted, the US FDA insists on zero *Salmonella* of any kind in US raw dog food.

- ✓ In 2015, the US FDA appears highly concerned about the raw sector. So much so that, in the face of an avalanche of dry food recalls for *Salmonella*, the FDA ceased recalling dry food products and dedicated all its energies to the raw dog food sector. Despite their best efforts, the net result was that by 2019, still 76 times more kibble was recalled for *Salmonella* (from 2012–2015) than raw dog food (from 2012–2019).

✓ With grain-free pet food sales beginning to dominate in the US market, accounting for approximately 50% of dry pet food sales there, in 2018 the US FDA turned its focus on the grain-free pet food sector. The FDA announced it was investigating a possible link between some 600 cases of dilated cardiomyopathy (DCM) in dogs, a long-standing issue in the cereal-based pet food sector. Unlike the melamine scandal, the FDA chose to name the 'suspected' companies involved.

✓ All the authors involved in the piece that alerted the FDA were affiliated to the world's biggest cereal-based pet food producers. The article, which bypassed peer review, is replete with errors including crucial statements going unreferenced, questions over sampling methods and the two most critical works propping up their hypothesis did not support their claims (both unpublished at the time of printing).

✓ The grain-free pet food products were never found at fault for causing DCM in dogs. Grain free pet food did not appear to be linked to DCM in any other country at the time and since the article was published seems to have stopped causing the issue in the United States. Regardless, grain-free pet food sales fell significantly in 2019.

✓ Why do governments get involved? Because pet food offers a profitable end point for much of the meat and cereal industries spewing out of the human food industries.

Chapter Nineteen References

1   Federal Food, Drug, and Cosmetic Act (FD&C Act). Published online, www.fda.gov/animal-veterinary/animal-food-feeds/product-regulation

2   USC 342: Adulterated food. United States Code 342(a)(5) 2006, Published online www.uscode.house.gov

3   Brown, A. (2006). *The whole pet diet*. New York: Celestial Arts

4   AAFCO (Association of American Feed Control Officials). Dog and Cat Food Nutrient Profiles 2016. Official Publication, available from www.aafco.org

5   Cunningham, L. (1981). *Pet food esthetics: A human concern*. New York Times. Published online, Dec 16th, www.nytimes.com

6   Martin, A.M. (2007). *Food pets die for: Shocking facts about pet food*. Troutdale, OR: Newsage Press

7   Patrick, J. (2006). *Deconstructing the Regulatory Facade: Why Confused Consumers Feed their Pets Ring Dings and Krispy Kremes*. Dissertation thesis, available online www. harvard.edu

8   Knueven, D. (2005). *The Five Supplements Every Dog Needs*. Clean Run Magazine, 11(12).

9   Schulof, D. (2016). *Dogs, Dog Food and Dogma*. Present Tense Press, Salt Lake City

10 McDonald, B.W., Perkins, T., Dunn, R.R. *et al.* (2020). High variability within pet foods prevents the identification of native species in pet cats' diets using isotopic evaluation. PeerJ: 8: e8337

11 Raditic, D.M., Remillard, R.L. and Tater, K.C. (2011). ELISA testing for common food antigens in four dry dog foods used in dietary elimination trials. Journal of Animal Physiology and Animal Nutrition (Berlin), 95(1): 90–97

12 Ricci, R., Granato, A., Vascellari, M. *et al.* (2013). Identification of undeclared sources of animal origin in canine dry foods used in dietary elimination trials. Journal of Animal Physiology and Animal Nutrition, 97: 32–38

13 Willis-Mahn, C., Remillard, R. and Tater, K. (2014). ELISA testing for soy antigens in dry dog foods used in dietary elimination trials. Journal of American Animal Hospital Association, 50(6): 383–389

14 Horvath-Ungerboeck, C., Widmann, K. and Handl, S. (2017). Detection of DNA from undeclared animal species in commercial elimination diets for dogs using PCR. Veterinary Dermatology, 28(4): 373–386

15 Hodgkinson, S., Rosales, C.E., Alomar, D. *et al.* (2004). Chemical nutritional evaluation of dry foods commercially available in Chile for adult dogs at maintenance. Archivos de Medicina Veterinaria, 36(2): 173–181

16 Gosper, E.C., Raubenheimer, D., Machovsky-Capuska, G.E. *et al.* (2016). Discrepancy between the composition of some commercial cat foods and their package labelling and suitability for meeting nutritional requirements. Australian Veterinary Journal, 94(1-2): 12–17

17 Hendriks, W.H. and Tarttelin, M.F. (1997). Nutrient composition of moist cat foods sold in New Zealand. Proceedings of the Nutrition Society of New Zealand, 22: 202–207

18 Davies, M., Alborough, R., Jones, L. *et al.* (2017). Mineral analysis of complete dog and cat foods in the UK and compliance with European guidelines. Science Reports, 7: 17107

19 Wall, T., (2016). FDA update: Jerky treats sickened 6,200 dogs, killed 1,140. Pet Food Industry Magazine. Published online, May 6th, www.petfoodindustry.com

20 Pugliese, A., Gruppillo, A. and Pietro, S. (2005). Clinical nutrition in gerontology: Chronic renal disorders of the dog and cat. Veterinary Research Communications, 29(2): 57–63

21 Kochanek, K.D., Sherry, M.A., Murphy, L. *et al.* (2017). Mortality in the United States, 2016. NCHS Data Brief No. 293. Published online, www.cdc.gov

22 UK Kennel Club (2004). The Purebred Dog Health Survey. A report from the Kennel Club / British Small Animal Veterinary Association Scientific Committee. Published online www. thekennelclub.org.uk

23   UK Kennel Club (2014). The Purebred Dog Health Survey. A report from the Kennel Club / British Small Animal Veterinary Association Scientific Committee. Published online, www. thekennelclub.org.uk

24   Lippert, G. and Sapy, B. (2003). The relation between the domestic dogs' well-being and life expectancy statistical essay. Essay for the Prince Laurent Foundation Price

25   Butterwick, R.F., Erdman Jr., J.W., Hill, R.C. *et al.* (2011). Challenges in developing nutrient guidelines for companion animals. British Journal of Nutrition. 106, S24–S31

26   Matīse-Vanhoutana,I. (2017). TedX Talk "I did my research, blew the whistle and found myself at war". Published online, Oct 26th, www.youtube.com

27   Scopelianos, A. and Donnellan, A. (2018). Pet food Advance Dermocare linked to megaesophagus outbreak, research shows. ABC News Australia. Publised online, Dec 13th, www.abc.net.au

28   Wall, T. (2018). Mars Australia recalls dog food after megaesophagus. Pet Food Industry Magazine. Published online, Mar 27th, www.petfoodindustry.com

29   Donn, J. (2007). Watchdog risked career over pet drug warning. Associated Press. Published online, Apr 22nd, www.nbcnews.com

30   Phillips-Donaldson, D. (2018b). FDA's big (yet sly) pet food ingredient announcement. Pet Food Industry Magazine. Published online, Oct 1st, www.petfoodindustry.com

31   Phillips-Donaldson, D. (2018a). FDA's fixation on raw pet food ratchets up again. Pet Food Industry Magazine. Published online, Mar 12th, www.petfoodindustry.com

32   Thixton, S. (2019). When second place is very bad. Truth About Pet Food website. Published online, Mar 14th, www.truthaboutpetfood.com

33   FDA 2018. FDA investigating potential connection between diet and cases of canine heart disease. US FDA Official Publication. Published online, July 12th, www.fda.gov

34   Furby, K. (2018). Grain-free, exotic dog food linked to heart disease. Washington Post Newspaper. Published online, Aug 29th, www.washingtonpost.com

35   Mansilla, W.D., Marinangeli, C.P.F., Ekenstedt, K.J. *et al.* (2019). Special topic: The association between pulse ingredients and canine dilated cardiomyopathy: addressing the knowledge gaps before establishing causation. Journal of Animal Science, 97(3): 983–997

36   Freeman, L.M., Stern, J.A., Fries, R. *et al.* (2018). Diet-associated dilated cardiomyopathy in dogs: what do we know? Journal of the American Veterinary Medical Association, 253(11): 1390–1394

39   Freeman, L.M., Stern, J.A., Fries, R. *et al.* (2018). Diet-associated dilated cardiomyopathy in dogs: what do we know? Journal of the American Veterinary Medical Association, 253(11): 1390–1394

40   Adin, D., DeFrancesco, T.C, Keene, B. *et al.* (2019). Echocardiographic phenotype of canine dilated cardiomyopathy differs based on diet type. Journal of Veterinary Cardiology, 21:1–9

41   Kaplan J.L., Stern, J.A., Fascetti, A.J. *et al.* (2018). Taurine deficiency and dilated cardiomyopathy in golden retrievers fed commercial diets. PLoS One 13(12): e0209112

42   Ontiveros, E.S., Whelchel, B.D., Yu, J. *et al.* (2020). Development of plasma and whole blood taurine reference ranges and identification of dietary features associated with taurine deficiency and dilated cardiomyopathy in golden retrievers: A prospective, observational study. Published May 15, 2020, https://doi.org/10.1371/journal.pone.0233206]

43   Phillips-Donaldson, D. (2019). Pet food brands named by FDA in DCM alert see sales loss. Pet Food Industry Magazine. Published online, Oct 16th, www.petfoodindustry.com

Feeding Species Appropriately

CHAPTER 20

The Raw Market

The pet market is moving toward more natural and raw products for their pets, something that is reflected by falling sales of dry pet food worldwide. In 2010, in the face of rising pet ownership, the quantity of dry food sold worldwide fell for the first time in 50 years.[1] Despite this fall in *quantity*, for the next few years, dry food sales still managed to rise in cash money due to the expansion of ever more expensive veterinary recommended specialty diets, although this trend has slowed and begun to reverse. By 2015, worldwide sales value of pet food had peaked at $77.7 billion. Since then, it has fallen year-on-year, to where it is today at approximately $75 billion,[2] despite rising pet ownership in that time.

While dry food sales fell, the Euromonitor International (2010)[3] report found that sales in the fresh/frozen pet food market jumped by more than 13% during the same period. In fact, the 'natural' pet food segment of the market is today seeing the fastest growth among pet owners. In the United States this market doubled from $2.0 billion in 2008 to $3.9 billion in 2012,[4] and this trend is expected to continue. In their 2016 review of the current pet food sector,[5] *Packaged Facts* notes the natural segment of the pet food market will increase by 15% each year at least until 2019. As of 2017, data released by Growth From Knowledge (GFK) data analysts in the United Kingdom show natural pet food now makes up more than a third of the UK's total £940 million spent within the pet specialty market, with grain-free food accounting for 15%. And all this growth in the natural market is coming at the cost of the cereal-based pet food market, still pushed by our vets today. In a piece titled "The Rise of Niche Pet Food Brands in the UK", a Euro-monitor report notes that the top dry food manufacturers are losing market share to more natural, meat-based products such as Lily's Kitchen, many of which cost significantly less than super premium dry food.

> …Leading brands such as Mars Petcare and Nestlé Purina are losing share to smaller niche players like Lily's Kitchen, which is going from strength to strength recording double-digit growth in 2017.

> **Shah, 2018**[6]

Companies like Nestlé are slowly trying to adapt. Recently, they brought out a 'gourmet' range of products called *Chef Michael's* range which comes in flavours like 'Sirloin Steak with Rice and Pea Garnishes' or 'Pork Tenderloin with Carrot and Barley Garnishes'.[7] But then in 2020, it simply used its vast cash reserves and bought out the popular grain-free pet food company Lily's Kitchen.[8] Watch this space: with Colgate-Palmolive spending so heavily in the veterinary universities and governing bodies and Mars busy buying up veterinary practices, it is my belief that Nestlé is going to start going after the natural market in earnest in the coming years. By the time Mars and Colgate-Palmolive change tact, they may find themselves struggling to catch up.

Authors note the sales of raw dog foods are rising rapidly.[9,10] In 2008, 16.2% of dog owners in the United States and Australia were providing bones or raw meat as a part of the main meal.[11,12] Australia was the first to adopt the idea, in earnest, thanks largely to the pioneering work of Australian vets, Lonsdale and Billinghurst, who for the last four decades have never relented in the fight to remove junk food from veterinary surgeries. By all accounts, they were vilified and ostracised for their efforts. But in the last 10 years we are beginning to see the fruits of their labour. According to the Australian Companion Animal Council's *Contribution of the Pet Care Industry to the Australian Economy*, 7th Edition (2010), in 2010 36% of Aussies owned a dog, equating to roughly 3.41 million dogs and bringing in some $3.5 billion a year in revenue. In terms of average diet, it states:

> …the significance of non-prepared food fed to pets needs to be recognised as a substantial… ontributor to total dog food consumption. While a dollar value is difficult to estimate, over half (53%) of all dog food consumed in Australia is made in the home…consisting of leftovers, table scraps and homemade food…

More recently, a survey of some 3,673 English-speaking dog and cat owners, published in the *Veterinary Record*, suggests that raw foods were fed to two-third of the dogs surveyed and more than half of cats. While bearing in mind raw feeders are more active online than dry-feeders, these findings hold added weight as the work was sponsored by Pet Curean, a UK-based, grain-free pet food company. They are selflessly advertising the competition with their findings.

> Only 13% (381) dogs and around a third (32%; 488) of cats were exclusively fed a conventional diet for their main meals. Many respondents said they fed their animals a diet that included home-made foods (63.5% of dogs; 45.5% of cats), although few were fed this diet exclusively (7% of dogs;

3.5% of cats). Raw animal foods were fed to over half of all the animals represented in the survey: two thirds of dogs (66%) and 53% of cats.

Dodd *et al.* **,2020**[13]

A 2014 survey of more than 2,000 breeders in the United States and Canada revealed one in seven were preparing food for their pets themselves.[7] In the same year, raw frozen pet food sales in the United States jumped 32%.[14] An interesting report by GFK summarised at the Pet Food Industry Leadership Conference by Lange (2017) shows huge growth in the US raw dog food sector. From 2011 to 2015 sales of raw dog food increased year-on-year by approximately 33%, totalling $120 million in 2015. By anyone's estimation, this annual double-digit growth of the natural and raw pet food market is not about to ease, any time soon.

Other studies have UK pet owners feeding the least amount of dry food.[15] While reliable figures for the UK raw market are still unavailable, in 2017 company reports from just the top 10 retailers indicate that together they are moving over £90 million ($100 million) of material; approximately 10% of the UK dog food market (the latest figures from the UK Pet Food Manufacturers Association reveal that less than 2% of raw pet food sales in the United Kingdom in 2018 was for cats). When you add in the companies we do not have figures for (many raw dog food companies are privately owned and thus their incomes are not published) and the pet owners who are not using actual dog food products but meats from the human food chain, I believe the raw feeding figure to be closer to 20% of the UK dog food market in 2019.

The domination of dry, ultra-processed, high-carb foodstuffs is most certainly over and the future is clearly bright for natural and raw feeding. As the human market tries to turn its back on processed foods in favour of fresh fruits, vegetables and whole grains,[16] we are turning our attentions toward what we are putting in their bowl. Spurred on by social media, the logic leap is not difficult for pet owners. They are now flocking to fresher, lower carbohydrate, more natural pet foods for the nutritional benefits they are assumed to convey.[17-26] These include,but are not limited to, the following:

- the resolution of recurring skin and gut conditions (thanks to a removal of wheat gluten, cooked meat protein and chemicals, the top food antigens in pet food today).

- better control, and possible resolution of kidney and pancreatic issues.

- better condition of their dogs (whereby higher protein diets fuel better weight control and muscle growth).

- better coat condition (as higher protein diets mean more protein for skin and hair maintenance).

- better dental hygiene (kibble offers no abrasion, ground raw meat and bone diets don't either, but proponents tend to enforce the necessity of raw meaty bones, which do).

- resolution of hyperactive behaviour (possibly).

- value for money (many pet owners are currently wasting at least €5/kg on what is largely cheap cereal with a token meat meal addition, when the same money can buy a kilo of high-quality meat-based raw dog food delivered to their door).

Often motivated by one of these health issues above, it is the quick turnaround in their pets following a simple 2-week trial of species-appropriate food, that makes very vocal advocates out of these owners, at least online. This sort of growth becomes self-perpetuating and exponential.

I remember I was giving a seminar in London one day and an elderly couple were sitting right up front, listening intently. After my talk, the man's wife turned to him and said, 'Show him your business cards.' A little bashful, the gentleman eventually showed me a bunch of simple cards with my name, number and website on them. Apparently, after my advice returned his beloved Westie, Tom, back to good health, he took it upon himself to make up these cards so he could hand them out to any dog owners he met in the park.

In this way, as with all good revolutions, this *rawvolution* is happening from the ground up. It is your lack of participation in their market that forces change. To quote Jim Morrison, '*They got the guns but we got the numbers*' (although Morrison likely nabbed it from Stalin who stated ,'*There is a quality in quantity*'. The comment was made in reference to his massive, but very poorly equipped, standing army of farmer peasants whom he threw at German machine guns to essentially exhaust their ammunition).

As Section 3 alluded to, any vets now stubbornly holding the line risk losing the trust of their client base. Customers will find vets to support them. Conversations with vets who do recognise the importance of species-appropriate nutrition reveal they are positively thriving, sucking in clients from a very large radius. In the increasingly competitive environment vets now find themselves in, it may soon become a case of adapt or starve for anyone pushing alternative facts located close by. Luckily, the process is not without incentive for vets, too:

> In our practice, we support owners who feed bones and raw food (BARF) and other raw meat diets. We formulate the diet specifically for each pet's health status, so that the diet is complete, balanced, medically

appropriate, and of high-quality. In addition, we educate owners as to food preparation, food handling safety, and feeding practices during a 30 to 40-minute consultation with our nutritional consultant. They are given typed instructions for the diet, food handling safety and preparation, and a shopping list. We charge $45 for this service.

Stogdale and Diehl, (2003)[18]

I have, up until this point, painted quite a bleak picture of veterinary medicine, but as always, there are very encouraging stories out there, too. I see the future in Wylie Vets, of Essex, United Kingdom. Wylie's consists of two practices: one a formal hospital, and as it is staffed by more than 20 raw-promoting vets, it is possibly one of the largest independent vet hospitals in the country. If you do not support fresh, species-appropriate nutrition for pets, you won't get a job with them. By focusing on *health*care (they call it *wellness*) instead of *sick* care, they have flipped the modern veterinary approach on its head, bringing medicine back to its roots. That is, you used to pay a doctor to keep you healthy, otherwise you risk encouraging the system we have today.

Morkel and Richard's practice offers a plan whereby the client pays a baseline annual fee, much like insurance, and *all* health care is provided for their pet for nothing from that point to the day they die. This means, rather beautifully, the practice makes the most money keeping your dog free from illness as it will cost them in resources to resolve any maladies that do arise. They employ a variety of measures to ensure this happens, like all visits are free, as often as you like, 24/7, so they can keep an eye on them. With so many vets at their disposal, they have most areas covered.

All vaccinations and parasite control are free (they check for parasites rather than blindly using chemicals, which not only saves your pet's health but saves Wylie's money on treatments). But most importantly for Wylie's, your dog *must be* raw-fed. According to their director, Morkel Piennaar, this is *the most important factor* in their client's health and longevity. Dry-fed dogs are not welcome on their plan – they are simply too costly to maintain to old age. To encourage this approach in their clients, they offer 10% off raw dog food purchased from them which they sell many tonnes of each week. They are so confident in this approach that the price you pay yearly for a pup is the same as a geriatric dog. No hidden increases for any reason. In this way, Wylie's is now notorious for keeping your dog healthy. As such, they are sucking in clients within a 100-mile radius. Any conventionally trained vets pushing contrary messages close by risk being starved of business.

I mean, it's quite simple: we shift them to raw food, they get better.

Morkel Piennaar, Director of Wylie Vets, *personal correspondence*, **2018**

TAKE-HOME POINTS

✓ The natural pet food market is growing by around 15% year on year. In 2017, it accounted for ⅓ of the UK's £940m market.

✓ Nestlé bought Lily's Kitchen in 2020 - the beginning of multinationals buying top natural pet food labels.

✓ In 2014, one in seven breeders in the United States were raw feeding. From 2010–2015, raw pet food sales jumped 33% per year. Australia was the leader, the United Kingdom leads in raw dog food sales, with at least 10% of the pet food market I estimate this figure could be as high as 20%.

✓ Pet owners are mainly jumping to raw in the hope of resolving stubborn health issues including those of the skin and gut but also for better muscle and coat condition, better dental hygiene, resolution of poor behaviour, as well as a better value-for-money proposition.

✓ Vets are changing. Many vets promote only raw. While still too few, they are increasing in numbers.

Chapter Twenty References

1   Euromonitor International Pet Food Report (2010). Available online www.euromonitor.com

2   Lange, M. (2017). *Pet Food Trends Shaping the World.* Pet Food Industry Leadership Conference, 2017. Available online www.pida.memberclicks.net

3   Euromonitor International's Pet Care 2010-20111 Report. Available online www. euromonitor.com

4   Lummis, D. (2012). *Natural, organic and eco-friendly pet products in the U.S.* Packaged Facts, Rockville, MD.

5   *Pet Food in the U.S., 12th Edition.* Available online www.prnewswire.com

6   Shah, T. (2018). *The Rise of Niche Pet Food Brands in the UK.* Euromonitor International. Published online Mar 22nd, available from www.blog.euromonitor.com

7   Tarkan, L. (2015). Raw pet food sales are booming, but are the products safe? Fortune Magazine. Published online, Aug 6th, www.fortune.come

8   Koltrowitz,S. (2020). Nestle buys Lily's Kitchen pet food, sees some coronavirus stockpiling. Reuters. Published online, Apr 1st, www.reuters.com

9   Wall, T. (2017). *Raw pet food growth continues despite concerns.* Pet Food Industry Magazine. Published online, Apr 27th, www.petfoodindustry.com

10 Connolly, K.M., Heinze, C.R. and Freeman, L.M. (2014). Feeding practices of dog breeders in the United States and Canada. Journal of the American Veterinary Medical Association, 245(6): 669-676

11 Laflamme, D.P. (2008). Pet food safety: Dietary protein. Topics in Companion Animal Medicine, 23(3): 154–157

12 Laflamme, D.P., Abood, S.K., Fascetti, A.J. *et al.* (2008). Pet feeding practices of dog and cat owners in the United States and Australia. Journal of the American Veterinary Medical Association, 232(5): 687–694

13 Dodd, S., Cave, N., Abood, S., *et al.* (2020). An observational study of pet feeding practices and how these have changed between 2008 and 2018. Veterinary Record BMJ, 186(19): 643

14 Lange, M. (2016). *Pet Food Trends Shaping the World.* Pet Food Industry Leadership Conference, 2016

15 Lonsdale, T. (2001). *Raw meaty bones promote health.* Wenatchee, WA: Dogwise Publishing

16 Berschneider, H.M. (2002). Alternative diets. Clinical Techniques in Small Animal Practice, 17(1): 1–5

17 Joffe, D.J. and Schlesinger, D.P. (2002). Preliminary assessment of the risk of *Salmonella* infection in dogs fed raw chicken diets. Canadian Veterinary Journal, 43: 441–442

18 Stogdale, L. and Diehl, G. (2003). In support of bones and raw food diets. Canadian Veterinary Journal, 44(10): 783

19 Hill, D.A. (2004). *Alternative proteins in companion animal nutrition.* Presented at the Pet Food Association of Canada Fall Conference, Toronto, 27th Oct

20 Weese, J.S., Rousseau, J. and Arroyo, L. (2005). Bacteriological evaluation of commercial canine and feline raw diets. Canadian Veterinary Journal, 46: 513–516

21 Finley, R., Reid-Smith, R. and Weese, J.S. (2006). Human health implications of *Salmonella*-contaminated natural pet treats and raw pet food. Clinical Infectious Diseases, 42: 686–691

22 Morley, P.S., Strohmeyer, R.A., Tankson, J.D. *et al.* (2006). Evaluation of the association between feeding raw meat and *Salmonella enterica* infections at a greyhound breeding facility. Journal of the American Veterinary Medical Association, 228: 1524–1532

23 Strohmeyer, R.A., Morley, P.S., Hyatt, D.R. *et al.* (2006). Evaluation of bacterial and protozoal contamination of commercially available raw meat diets for dogs. Journal of American Veterinary Medical Association, 228: 532–542

24 Remillard, R.L. (2008). Homemade diets: Attributes, pitfalls, and a call for action. Topical Companion Animal Medicine, 23(3): 137–142

25 Schlesinger, D.P. and Joffe, D.J. (2011). Raw food diets in companion animals: A critical review. Canadian Veterinary Journal, 52(1): 50–54

26 Buff, P.R., Carter, R.A., Bauer, J.E. *et al.* (2014). Natural pet food: A review of natural diets and their impact on canine and feline physiology. Journal of Animal Science, 92: 3781–3791

CHAPTER 21

Will A Meat Diet Provide *Everything* They Need?

It is now accepted, at least for humans, that the diet of our Palaeolithic hunter–gatherer ancestors would better fit modern man than our current nutrition. Put simply, eat the stuff you evolved on and you'll likely be healthier. The discordance hypothesis, originally proposed by Eaton *et al.* (1988),[1] states that the change from Palaeolithic to current nutrition occurred too rapidly for adequate genetic adaptation. It also states the resulting mismatch fuels many 'diseases of civilisation', such as diabetes mellitus, obesity and dental disease. We have spent millions of years adapting to our feeding niche. Dogs and cats are no different.

Having no requirements for plant carbohydrates, we know a meat-based diet must meet all the dog's nutrient requirements. Dierenfield *et al.* (2002)[2] analysed the total nutrient composition of various whole vertebrate prey species and found that a whole prey diet, as long as the soft tissues and some bones are consumed, is more than adequate to meet the needs of the meat-eater. Whole prey species exceed the minimum recommended macronutrient concentration for both cats and dogs,[3,4] and meet or exceed essential fatty acid requirements.[2,4]

The key here is *whole* prey, ideally using *all* the bits (or as many as you can find). This is why the statement by the Mars Waltham scientist Richard Hill, a member of the subcommittee on dog and cat nutrition for the National Research Council (NRC), is absolutely correct, if entirely redundant (italics added by me for effect).

> …meat is not a *balanced* food and is *deficient* in essential vitamins and minerals…a dog cannot live on meat muscle alone…
>
> **Hill, (1998)**[5]

Of course, no single animal protein source supplies everything the dog needs, surely now in this century that is a moot point. As many thousands of sailors have already amply demonstrated for humanity at the cost of their lives that you cannot eat the same thing for *too long* without nutritional inadequacies popping up. In fact, even feeding dogs just one type of whole animal every day for long periods of time is not advisable, as we saw in Section 2, where the cats living on whole rabbit for months, sadly, became taurine deficient.[2]

It begs the question: what ingredient does Hill think might be a balanced and complete for dogs? His counterparts in Hill's Science Diet seem to believe it's corn. The following quote (italics added by me for effect) is taken from the Hill's website, dated October 30, 2019:

> Corn is a *well-rounded* nutritional package and an *ideal* choice as a cat food ingredient. No other ingredient is as versatile as this golden grain. That's why you'll find corn in most Hill's Science Diet brand cat foods.
>
> **www.hillspet.com/pet-care/nutrition-feeding/**
> **benefits-of-corn-in-pet-foods**

So, according to the industry, meat is not a balanced ingredient for a meat-eater, but ultra-processed corn is not only well rounded but *ideal*.

This industry nonsense aside, a lot of people and most vets come to the raw table with an ingrained fear of imbalance, deeply concerned they might get it wrong and their dog's butt will fall off. It costs a lot of money to make you feel that helpless, a helplessness that keeps you and your vet reaching for those grossly overpriced bags of ultra-processed, nutritionally bereft crackers.

> Dog food companies make a point of emphasizing that canine nutrition is a science best left to qualified experts – namely them (or research projects sponsored by them). Ads for 'super premium' and 'prescription' dog foods now incorporate actors or models wearing goggles and white lab coats, shown holding clipboards as they measure out healthy looking ingredients amid a clinical forest of test tubes, computers, and diagnostic equipment…Terms such as 'chelated minerals', 'ME', and 'amino acid profile' combine to both intrigue and confuse even the most savvy consumers…
>
> **Thurston, 1996,p.244**[6]

Allow me to alleviate some of that concern with the following story. A few years ago, I joined an online veterinary seminar that promised to give us the pros and cons to feeding pets fresh food. Considering the platform is owned by a dry food company, we suspected to hear far more cons than pros, and we weren't disappointed. We listened to a highly qualified vet, top of her field, specialised in (dry) canine nutrition and gastrointestinal diseases. We'll call her M. Near the end of the hour, after all the usual hoo-hah about inadequacies and dangers of fresh food for dogs, we were given the chance to ask questions. I asked, 'Hey M, I see you're married, I'm going to hazard that you have kids. Can you tell me what a child's RDA for calcium is?' Her answer, much to the attendee's approval, was that 'She only does dogs' and on they went to the next question, entirely missing my point. Nobody thought she was either a terrible parent, or that her child was at risk of immediate death, and not a soul recommended she run along to the nearest vending machine for an immediate nutrient boost from her favourite candy company. This vet, with an apparent deep understanding of the pharmacological concepts of nutrition and disease, has no idea what her kids' recommended daily allowance (RDA) of calcium is, how much she gave them last week nor how much they actually absorbed.

Instead of considering exact nutrient quantities, if the average Joe was asked what a 'complete' human diet might look like the best most could come up with would probably be lots of whole, fresh, organic plant ingredients, be it vegetables, grains, fruits, a bit of organic meat or fish, maybe a bit of dairy and as little processed food as possible. Essentially, *whole* foods. Every health, nutrition and dieting book written in the last three decades confirms this fact as they can all be summed up in three simple words – eat whole food. There's nothing more to it than that. Study after study shows that if everyone followed this basic advice there would be significantly less obesity, less diabetes, significantly less cancer, less chronic disease, better skin, better teeth, better behaviour, better everything. We would be more energetic, live longer, healthier lives and we would save billions on health care. And it's the very same for our dogs, only with a meatier food pyramid. If you stick to the game plan, they'll be more than fine.

Take further solace from the fact lots of us are getting it a bit wrong. The latest World Health Organisation reports show that only 11% of Americans consumed their RDA of fibre, only 5% consumed enough potassium and most fall short in vitamins A, C and D as well as calcium and iron. Essentially, all the stuff you get from fresh fruit and vegetables. At the same time, they were overeating in saturated fat and salt (guess where that's coming from). And still, no multinational has thought to produce a nutritious 'complete' food for us? I think I've spotted a gap in the market!

I say the following without an ounce of satisfaction – console yourself that most cereal-based pet food is so far off the mark nutritionally for a dog, so deficient in all the little life-affirming bits and so dangerous to your pet, that even your most casual effort after reading this book is likely to have them in better shape than the very vast majority of Western vets could ever hope to achieve on their fanciest bag of crackers.

No single meat ingredient or single prey animal is adequate for the lifetime feeding of a dog or cat as all animal parts are thought to convey some unique nutritional advantage (or potential deficiency) to the meat-eater. It is for this reason, using their incredible senses of smell, that wild predators seek to achieve balance by selectively feeding on body parts according to their macronutrient composition and personal need at that moment in time.[7] Meat muscle meets all the dog's and cat's protein requirements but if they need some taurine, they are expected to seek out those animals, or at least those parts of animals, that provide more of it. Cartilage supplies them with glucosamine, chondroitin, vitamin C and all the other bits and pieces they need to build their joints. If they need Vitamin A, they might eat more liver. Fresh bone provides all their calcium but also a whole swathe of minerals that are harder to find when you're a meat-eater, including zinc, copper, selenium, etc. Even poorly digested items such as hair, hide, skin, nails and bone are thought to play a role. Depauw *et al.* (1998)[8] highlight its potential importance by showing how animal tissues (such as chicken cartilage, collagen, glucosamine-chondroitin, glucosamine, rabbit bone, rabbit hair and rabbit skin) influenced large intestinal fermentation in cheetah, indicating indigestible prey material in meat eaters likely acts the same way as indigestible plant fibre for humans.

What many people are missing, most certainly the Association of American Feed Control Officials (AAFCO)/The European Pet Food Industry Federation (FEDIAF nutritional guidelines, is that food goes far beyond these more commonly discussed nutritional elements such as protein, fat, vitamins, minerals and fibre. There is a whole range of bioactive compounds out there that we need to consume daily to keep us healthy, many of which you've already heard of.

Plants provide for us an incredible array of life-bestowing phytonutrients that, when consumed and digested, have a marked effect on us, something the drug industry knows only too well. Willow bark, used by ancient Egyptians, contains salicylic acid, which we now know as aspirin. Penicillin arose from a humble fungus growing on bread. Morphine, an opiate, comes from the poppy. They put plant stanol esters in heart-stopping margarine as, when ingested, they're clinically proven to reduce the level of low-density lipoprotein (LDL) cholesterol in the blood. Lycopene in tomatoes and lutein in spinach are not only great for hearts but are proving successful in the fight against cancer. Curcumin, the active ingredient in turmeric, is a highly potent natural anti-inflammatory, supported by literally hundreds of high-quality randomised controlled studies. Milk thistle restores our liver functions. Cannabidiol from the cannabis plant can be used for a great variety of issues, many of them neural, from issues ranging from anxiety to epilepsy to autoimmune disease. Slippery elm works on our digestive tract, as will a nice peppermint tea. Echinacea is good when you're run down, lavender makes us calm. The list is endless: Pick any part of your body, pretty much any malady and you will find numerous naturally occurring phytochemicals that can assist it in some form. In fact, there are more than 4,000 phytochemicals documented thus far. Some of the more commonly known include the alkaloids (the famous codeine is one but alkaloids are also used to improve heart function, suppress coughs, repel insects), terpenoids (used to prevent metabolic disorders, fight cancer, exert anti-ageing benefits), polysaccharides, such as inulin, lignin and pectin (gut flora love them and they produce a nice poo), as well as the highly potent and anti-oxidative phenolic compounds (improve immune, heart and cognitive function and fight cancer) which include flavanols (blood vessel function) and anthocyanins, (found in colourful fruit and veggies, these are potent antioxidants).

But did you know that meat, too, contains its share of bioactive compounds, many of which you already know from the land of plants? These include:

- Tocopherols (a form of vitamin E).

- Carotenoids: an anti-oxidative tetraterpenoid.

- Ascorbic acid: vitamin C.

- Glutathione: found in both plants and animals, glutathione has a range of benefits. As well as providing cellular defence against toxicological and pathological processes, it is involved in making DNA, supporting immune function, forming sperm cells, regenerating vitamins C and E, helping the liver and gallbladder deal with fats and assisting in apoptosis or 'cell death'.

- Lipoic acid: a wonderfully beneficial organic compound made inside mitochondria of both plants and animals. It is both water- and fat-soluble, allowing it to work in every cell or tissue in the body.

- L-carnitine: while found in some plants, L-carnitine is largely obtained from animal sources. It assists the body in producing energy, lowers the levels of cholesterol and helps the body to absorb calcium to improve skeletal strength. As it plays a crucial role in preventing skeletal muscle myopathy associated with heart failure.

- Ubiquinone: aka co-enzyme Q10, is a vitamin-like compound ubiquitous to animals and bacteria. While it is found in some plant sources, meat is by far the best source, with liver and kidney being top of the list. CoQ10 is involved in the production of cellular energy and is used as a popular antioxidant in the prevention and treatment of some chronic diseases.

Meat is also host to a wide range of bioactive compounds found *only* in meat, again some of which you may already have heard of. These include the following:

- Conjugated linoleic acid (CLA): An omega-6 fatty acid, commonly found in meat and dairy. While essentially a trans fat, it is a naturally occurring form that is actually beneficial to the body, including boosting heart health and aiding with weight loss.

- Taurine: An amino acid found only in meat, commonly the brain, eyes, heart and muscle. It has been shown to have several health benefits, such as a lower risk of disease and improved sports performance. It is the lack of taurine from a lack of meat in pet food that results in much-repeated pet illnesses and death from DCM.

- Creatine: An organic compound found in the muscles of cells where it plays a critical role in muscle energy metabolism. Creatine is now famous for its use by gym enthusiasts. Studies show it can increase muscle mass, strength and exercise performance as well as potentially provide a number of other health benefits, including protecting against neurological disease.

- Anserine and carnosine: Protein building blocks that are naturally produced in the muscles and bones of animals, these two compounds have risen to stardom of late as they have such a diverse range of beneficial impact, including boosting muscle strength and performance but also potentially treating nerve damage, eye disorders, diabetes and kidney problems, wound healing, fatigue and stress-related diseases.

- Spermine: Found in many tissues, it's essentially a bacteria growth factor; hence, it's concentrated around the gut.

In addition to these bioactive compounds, meat-protein-derived peptides are another promising group of bioactive components.[9] These are the by-products of the enzymatic digestion of meat and the ageing of meat (and God knows dogs like eating aged meat!). Digestive enzymes, (pepsin, trypsin and α-chymotrypsin) in the gastrointestinal tracts generated angiotensin-converting enzyme (ACE) inhibitory activity from porcine skeletal muscle proteins.[10,11]ACE inhibitory peptides such as myosin, actin, tropomyosin and troponin, linked to the reduction of blood pressure, are generated from meat digestion.[12] Furthermore, several anti-oxidative peptides are generated from meat proteins by enzymatic digestion. The protease digestion of pork meat has been reported to exhibit high levels of antioxidant activity in the linoleic acid peroxidation system.[13,14]

Haemoglobin, the red protein in blood, contains biologically active peptides with an affinity for opioid receptors.[15,16] These opioid peptides, such as endorphins, encephalin and prodynorphin (opioid polypeptide hormone involved in cell communication), can induce opiate-like effects in animals, affecting the nervous system as well as gastrointestinal functions.[17]

> …bioactive peptide generation from meat and meat products, and their functionality and application as functional ingredients, have proven effects on consumer health. Animal food proteins are currently the main source of a range of biologically active peptides which have gained special interest because they may also influence numerous physiological responses in the organism…
>
> **Albenzio et al., (2017)**[18]

And then we come to the organs. We know phytochemicals can bioaccumulate in various parts of the prey animal, depending on the food they are eating [19,20]. In this way, each prey organ is potentially host to a cacophony of vital chemical compounds, many unique to that organ itself. The eye is a great example. Lutein and zeaxanthin are essential to eye function. Lutein is only synthesised by plants while zeaxanthin is best sourced from plants although some micro-organisms do produce it, too. You have two options at this point. Make it yourself (mammals can't), eat something containing it (unlikely for true carnivores) or eat *someone* who has some. As they are stored in the retina, the occasional eyeball might save a carnivore a trip to the opticians.

But with organs, it goes deeper than this. In the early 20th century scientists examined a pig's pancreas to find out how to help a human being with diabetes. They discovered insulin and started injecting insulin into patients with diabetes, saving many lives, certainly of late. However, insulin is but one of the pancreas's amazing compounds. The pancreas also produces glucagon which assists in blood glucose levels, amylin which controls how fast the gut empties and ultimately the food intake, as well as pancreatic and vasoactive polypeptides which function in various gut contractions, among other functions. Of course, not all the hormones present in an organ will escape the digestive process. Some, notably the protein-based ones, are susceptible to the stomach acids. Sadly, for dogs with diabetes, this includes insulin. But many do make it through digestion, including all the steroid ones. As do the enzymes, present in the organ. All these together are useful to an animal with a struggling pancreas. In fact, authors discovered that the addition of raw pancreas to de-pancreatised dogs fed a meat and sugar diet greatly increases their longevity compared to dogs that are not fed it, even though these dogs were on insulin therapy.[21]

This is surely the case with each and every secreting organ of the body, none of which limits themselves to the production of a single, life-affirming compound. The thyroid gland produces triiodothyronine and thyroxine (often known as simply T3 and T4, respectively), which regulate many aspects of your metabolism. It also produces calcitonin, which helps construct bone. The adrenal gland produces cortisol (the 'stress hormone'), epinephrine (aka adrenalin) and aldosterone. The anterior pituitary gland produces seven hormones. These are the growth hormone (GH), thyroid-stimulating hormone (TSH), adrenocorticotropic hormone (ACTH), follicle-stimulating hormone (FSH), luteinising hormone (LH), beta-endorphin and prolactin. The gut produces cholecystokinin (controls release of enzymes and bile) and ghrelin (regulates the appetite). Your liver produces angiotensinogen, thrombopoietin, hepcidin and insulin-like growth factor, among a number of others. The heart produces atrial-natriuretic peptide and brain natriuretic peptide. The pineal gland on your brain produces melatonin, which controls your circadian rhythm. Blood platelets produce thromboxane. Your skin produces prostacyclin and fat produce adiponectin. The sex organs (testes and ovaries) contain all the sex hormones, including testosterone, progesterone and oestrogen, among many others. If your dog is neutered or spayed, there is a very good argument for supplementing their diet with these meats as a form of natural hormone replacement therapy, if you can find them (raw testes are now readily available). The placenta, the brain, the nervous system, each one produces lots of different fantastically useful chemical compounds, many of which we are yet to even discover. It's a fascinating, poorly understood and almost entirely unexplored facet of carnivore nutrition today.

It is for this reason we say organs are to the dog what green vegetables are to humans.

And these are just the compounds *in* the meat parts themselves. We haven't even begun to discuss the advantages of the stuff that might be found *on* the meat itself! It is thought that a significant quantity of the rising allergy and asthma cases we are experiencing today may be explained by living *too clean*, that it is our routine and harmless exposure to every day microorganisms in the environment that trains our immune systems to ignore the more benign stuff such as pollen or doggie dandruff. There is a common phrase used in most societies that goes something like 'farmers are healthier as they live with a pinch of dirt'. There is likely an enormous amount of truth to this. In Chapter 4, we saw how Irish soils contains microbes with strong antibacterial properties, effective against four of our top six antibiotic-resistant superbugs, including Methicillin Resistant *Staphylococcus Aureus*.[22] Gabrielová *et al.* (2018)[23] found the single celled oomycete *Pythium oligandrum* can suppress and kill the causative agents of dermatophytosis. This fascinating little fungus-like eukaryotic microorganism is a parasite of fungi. It lives symbiotically in and around the roots of many plants. The roots likely feed them in return for their protection. It is now used very successfully for treating stubborn dermatophytosis, such as yeast infections of the skin and ears (common in dogs fed high-carb diets). But did you know that there's potentially a natural antidepressant in there too? It's true. Seized upon by gardeners the world over as proof that gardening, makes you happy, it appears that a simple concoction derived from the non-pathogenic (do not cause disease), saprophytic (lives on dead stuff), bacterium *Mycobacterium vaccae*, commonly found in soil, can improve the lives of patients with inflammatory disorders and even cancer. Incredibly, patients with lung cancer who were injected with heat-killed *M. vaccae* reported better quality of life, less nausea and less pain.[24] Lowry *et al.* (2007)[25] later found that it targets the same nerves as Prozac, stimulating serotonin production in mice. So, how much *M. vaccae* would you like on your Weetabix on a cold, wet winter morning?! Two heaped spoons, please.

People supporting the use of heavily processed food stuffs replete with anti-life chemicals over real ingredients are making the same mistake that those who supported bottled milk over breast milk made back in the 1970s and that is the total disregard for the plethora of bioactive compounds in fresh food. We have spent millions of years evolving around these naturally occurring dietary chemicals. Which of them is truly essential to our optimum health and in what quantity is still virtually unknown. Moreover, the complex interactions of all these compounds are all but impossible to replicate in the lab. The few that can now be synthesised are characteristically less effective in isolation, harder to absorb by the body and suffer degradation during the harsh cooking temperatures and long storage times that occur in pet food production.

If you require more solace than that, there are always blood tests. Never a bad idea. With all this in mind, we raw feeders include a range of fresh meat pieces in a proportion that might reflect how our pets would find them in the wild. We then ensure we vary the meat sources (not daily or even weekly necessarily) in proportions we deem necessary and from there hope for the best, because making a truly 'complete' or 'balanced' meal for an animal, which it will consume day in day out, is as impossible a concept as it is unnecessary.

Many authors still miss this crucial concept when analysing raw recipes for 'completeness'. A survey of recipes being used by German home-feeders revealed as many as 60% of the rations had some form of imbalance.[26] Of the 200 from texts, books and web articles (64% written by vets), only five recipes met the AAFCO or NRC minimum requirements.[27] Interestingly, while some nutritional discrepancies existed in the homemade food, no clinical deficiencies were observed.[28] This may be that the authors were using for their nutrient comparisons facts and figures from the dry food industry (they used for comparison data from the NRC 2006)[29,30] or potentially just a matter of time and sample size (nutrient deficiencies are hard to spot). At any rate, much, if not all, of this potential risk will be offset by raw feeders knowing variation is crucial to the whole process. It's how we humans manage it, after all.

The notion of a single meal providing everything at once is pure marketing hyperbole, and it is irresponsible, bordering dangerous, to suggest otherwise. That said, should the AAFCO/FEDIAF minimum requirement guidelines be your benchmark of choice, Honey's Pet Food adequately demonstrated that a raw diet can most certainly tick all the boxes. At great financial cost, the study (Raw Proof, free to view online from the Honeys website) involved twenty-six adult dogs in an extended version of the AAFCO food trial protocol. No dogs experienced any adverse health effects or significant loss of weight. The authors concluded the range of raw diets they formulated (based on raw meat, raw bone and raw vegetable) were all "wholly adequate...when fed in conjunction with each other", easily meeting the European Pet Food Industry Federation's nutritional guidelines without the need for additional, synthetic supplementation.

But in terms of a single diet long-term, the 'perfect' canine diet remains as elusive as our own, with leading specialists all coming up with slightly different variations of what they deem to be the ideal for the dog, day-to-day. If ever the phrase applied, it seems like the more you know about this subject, the more you realise you don't know. Or, the ignorant are full of conviction, the learned full of doubt.

I hope this provides newbies with a little solace. We're all a little unsure. Like a form of rebirth, we are emerging from the dark, blinking. There is so much to learn. So much to gain. Don't let the fear of the unknown stop you from taking those first few steps. Sometimes in science, certainly in life, you have to make the leap.

TAKE-HOME POINTS

✓ A whole-prey diet (all the parts, less the gut contents) fulfils all the dog's nutrient requirements.

✓ A dog or cat cannot live on one meat (or animal) alone for too long.

✓ You need to know the dog's RDA for calcium about as much as you need to know your own.

✓ Each part of the animal offers a different array of nutrients to the carnivore.

✓ Hard-to-digest items (hair and hide and feathers) offer roughage to the carnivore, likely stimulating large intestinal fermentation and also contain manganese.

✓ A dizzying array of plant-based bioactive compounds exist in nature and we exploit many of them for our own health. Studies show they can accumulate in various parts of herbivorous prey. For example, lutein is essential to eye function. It exists only in the plant kingdom and the eyes of herbivores.

✓ Meat contains a range of bioactive compounds that are much harder to source in the plant kingdom, including gluthionone, L-carnitine, co-enzyme Q10. But meat also contains compounds that do not exist in plants, such as CLA, taurine, creatine, anserine, carnosine and spermine. Meat is a source of meat-protein peptides, as is blood, and the latter are known to induce an opiate-like effect in animals. Also, the by-products from the digestion of meat, such as angiotensin–converting enzyme, have known health benefits. Bar taurine, none of these compounds are even on the AAFCO nutritional profile. We have no idea how vital any of these are to the carnivorous dog.

✓ Organ meats contain a huge array of compounds that are known to have major health benefits when ingested, the most famous being insulin but that is just one hormone from one organ. There are many.

✓ Even the microorganisms in the dirt on their food are potentially vital. We have literally no idea.

✓ Raw feeders are recommended to feed a variety to touch all these bases, achieving balance over time.

Chapter Twenty One References

1   Eaton, S.B., Konner, M. and Shostak, M. (1988). Stone agers in the fast lane: chronic degenerative diseases in evolutionary perspective. American Journal of Medicine, 84: 739 – 749.

2   Dierenfeld, E.S., Alcorn, H.L. and Jacobsen, K.L. (2002). *Nutrient composition of whole vertebrate prey (excluding fish) fed in zoos*. U.S. Department of Agriculture. Published online, www.researchgate.net

3   Butterwick, R.F., Erdman Jr., J.W., Hill, *et al.* (2011). Challenges in developing nutrient guidelines for companion animals. British Journal of Nutrition, 106: S24 – S31

4   Kerr, K.R., Kappen, K.L., Garner, L.M., *et al.* (2014). Commercially available avian and mammalian whole prey diet items targeted for consumption by managed exotic and domestic pet felines: Macronutrient, mineral, and long-chain fatty acid. Zoo Biology, 33: 327–335

5   Hill, R.C. (1998). The nutritional requirements of exercising dogs. Journal of Nutrition, 128(12): 2686S–2690S.

6   Thurston, M.E. (1996). *The lost history of the canine race*. Kansas City, MI: Andrews McMeel.

7   Kohl, K.D., Coogan, S.C.P. and Raubenheimer, D. (2015). Do wild carnivores forage for prey or for nutrients? Evidence for nutrient-specific foraging in vertebrate predators. Bioessays, 37(6): 701–709

8   Depauw, S., Hesta, M., Whitehouse-Tedd, K. *et al.* (1998). Animal fibre: The forgotten nutrient in strict carnivores? First insights in the cheetah. Journal of Animal Physiology and Animal Nutrition, 97(1): 146–154

9   Glasgow, A.G., Cave, N.J., Marks, S.L. *et al.* (2002). *Role of diet in the health of the feline intestinal tract and in inflammatory bowel disease*. Center for Companion Animal Health, School of Veterinary Medicine, University of California, Davis, California

10 Arihara, K. (2006a). Strategies for designing novel functional meat products. Meat Science, 74, 219–229

11 Arihara, K. (2006b). *Functional properties of bioactive peptides derived from meat proteins*. In Advanced Technologies for Meat Processing, Publisher: CRC Press (Boca Raton), pp245–273

12 Arihara, K., Nakashima, Y., Mukai, T. *et al.* (2001). Peptide inhibitors for angiotensin I-converting enzyme from enzymatic hydrolysates of porcine skeletal muscle proteins. Meat Science, 57: 319–324

13 Katayama, K., Fuchu, H., Sakata, A. *et al.* (2003a). Angiotensin I-converting enzyme inhibitory activities of porcine skeletal muscle proteins following enzyme digestion. Asian-Australian Journal of Animal Science, 16, 417–424. 11 Bioactive Compounds in Meat 247.

14 Katayama, K., Tomatsu, M., Fuchu, H. *et al.* (2003b). Purification and characterization of an angiotensin I-converting enzyme inhibitory peptide derived from porcine troponin C. Animal Science Journal, 74: 53–58

15   Saiga, A., Tanabe, S. and Nishimura, T. (2003). Antioxidant activity of peptides obtained from porcine myofibrillar proteins by protease treatment. Journal of Agricultural and Food Chemistry, 51: 3661–3667

16   Nyberg, F., Sanderson, K. and Glamsta, E.L. (1997). The hemorphins: A new class of opioid peptides derived from the blood protein hemoglobin. Biopolymers, 43, 147–156

17   Zhao, Q., Garreau, I., Sannier, F. *et al.* (1997). Opioid peptides derived from hemoglobin: Hemorphins. Biopolymers, 43, 75–98

18   Albenzio, M., Santillo, A., Caroprese, M. *et al.* (2017). Bioactive Peptides in Animal Food Products. Foods, 6: 35

19   Pihlanto, A. and Korhonen, H. (2003). Bioactive peptides and proteins. Advances in Food and Nutrition Research, 47, 175–276

20   Hershey, J.M. and Soskin, J.M. (1931). Substituion of leicithin for raw pancreas in the diet of the depancreatised dogs. American Journal of Physiology, 98: 74–85

21   Krajcovicova-Kudlackova, M., Simoncic, R., Bederova, A. *et al.* (2000). Correlation of carnitine levels to methionine and lysine intake. Physiological Research, 49:399–402

22   Terra, L., Dyson, P.J., Hitchings, M.D. *et al.* (2018). A novel alkaliphilic streptomyces inhibits ESKAPE pathogens. Frontiers in Microbiology, 9: 2458

23   Gabrielová, A., Mencl, K., Suchánek, M. *et al.* (2018). The oomycete *Pythium oligandrum* can suppress and kill the causative agents of dermatophytosis. Mycopathologia, 183(5): 751–764

24   Assersohn, L., Souberbielle, B.E., O'Brien, M.E. *et al.* (2002). A randomized pilot study of SRL172 (*Mycobacterium vaccae*) in patients with small cell lung cancer (SCLC) treated with chemotherapy. Clinical Oncology, 14(1): 23-27

25   Lowry, C.A., Hollis, J.H. and S.L. Lightman (2007). Identification of an immune-responsive mesolimbocortical serotonergic system: Potential role in regulation of emotional behaviour. Neuroscience, 146(2-5): 756–772

26   Mir, P.S., McAllister, T.A., Scott, S. *et al.* (2004). Conjugated linoleic acid-enriched beef production. American Journal of Clinical Nutrition, 79(6): 1207S–1211S

27   Dillitzer, N., Becker, N. and Kienzle, E. (2011). Intake of minerals, trace elements and vitamins in bone and raw food rations in adult dogs. British Journal of Nutrition, 106 Suppl 1: S53-56

28   Stockman, J., Fascetti, A.J., Kass, P.H. *et al.* (2013). Evaluation of recipes of home-prepared maintenance diets for dogs. Journal of the American Veterinary Medical Association, 242(11): 1500–1505

29   National Research Council (NRC, 2006). *Your dog's nutritional needs*. A Science-Based Guide For Pet Owners. National Academy of Sciences.

30   National Research Council, NRC, (2006). *Nutrient requirement of dogs and cats*. Washington, DC: National Academies Press.

What Might the *Ideal* Raw Dog Food Diet Look Like?

There are essentially two feeding styles employed by raw feeders today. The first is the Prey Model. This feeding style is based on the desire of the owner to feed the dog as close as they can to whole prey. It is based around a ratio of 8:1:1, that is eight-parts raw meat to one-part secreting organ (later) and one-part raw bone, that being the very approximate amount of those bits you would find in the dog's typical prey such as a rat.

Most Prey Modelers clobber their meals together from bits and pieces they find online, using their local butcher and rummaging through the half-priced aisle of supermarkets. Others buy in premade, preground raw dog foods made to the 8:1:1 formula, which is most of them. The most extreme followers use actual whole prey–whole baby chickens, rabbits, rats, frogs. The dog tucks in as they would in nature. Taking what they want, leaving what they want. I know of a guy who lives in the hills. He leaves out whole deer carcass in his back garden, when he can shoot one. The dogs eat it for a few days. The birds finish it off. Not sure how this would go down in my housing estate.

While there are different methods, all followers of this strategy do unite over one concept though, and that is, asides medicinal plant inclusions such as herbs and berries, their dogs do not receive plant matter as nutrition. Vegetables are not part of the Prey Model. They are steadfast in their belief the dog is a carnivore, not an omnivore.

Nutritionally, this diet makes sense in that the dog is certainly a whole prey eater, when that animal is small enough. Everything is in there and undeniably in the correct proportions. However, as it excludes plant matter, I personally do not recommend it long term for a number of reasons. We can't trust a domestic meat sector, with animals reared on poor quality forage, to supply all the nutrients wild prey are assumed to contain. Furthermore, we have shown the dog has taken some minor evolutionary steps toward plant matter consumption. Why exclude it now? Finally, wild prey is not only hard to find but I fear it's cost prohibitive to many, particularly when you're looking at a hungry Shepherd...or two! It is perhaps for these reasons, this particular method is not followed diligently by most of the top canine nutritionists.

The other method doesn't have a fancy name or even an exact ratio. For now, we'll have to call it Prey & Plant model. This provides flexibility to the people who wish to include some plant matter. How much is a hotly debated subject that has many people barking ferociously at each other online. Some use 5%. Some 10%. Some more. It is because we vary that an exact ratio is hard to give but if you were to twist my arm then I would recommend something around 7:1:1:1, giving us around 10% plant ingredients.

For now, please don't get hung up over the ratios or percentages here. While they are best practice, leave the nailing of your ingredient ratios to the raw dog food manufacturers. For you, these figures are a ball park. When you are making DIY raw dog food, it's very difficult to work out how much bone you're feeding them, for example. It's usually hidden inside the meat! We don't want folk running around with charts and calculators (a hangover of the exacting dry pet food industry)!

Over the course of the next few pages we will be breaking down each category – meat, organ, bone and vegetables- hopefully leaving you best placed to make the most ideal raw dog food you can.

Meat

Any meat you might usually find in a supermarket is fine for your dog – chicken, turkey, duck, pork, lamb, beef, rabbit, venison, fish... anything. The only meat I wouldn't feed to dogs would be that sourced from other carnivores (which usually arises from roadkill). There is a saying that dates back to ancient Rome, 'dog does not eat dog'. There is a lot of truth to this. For reasons of parasites, carnivores tend to avoid the carcasses of other carnivores.[1]

And they want any part of the animal – fillets, offcuts, cheek, gizzards, skirt, tail, brisket, necks, head mince (yes, this is a thing and it's what most of your burgers are made out of!), to name but a few, even heads themselves. Everything is on the menu to them and the bigger a variety of meats and indeed meat parts you feed them, the better off they will be.

Some meats are fattier than others and this should be watched. While larger animals are often fattier, as we discussed in Section 2, dogs are now more likely to hunt smaller prey with protein to fat ratios of at most four-parts protein to one-part fat, with most wild prey animals far leaner than this. We can, thus, assume a lean diet is what the average adult dog is best off fed. You will find most meats in the supermarket, certainly mince meats, are significantly higher in fat than we would hope in this regard (intensively reared, certain pieces are notoriously fatty) but raw dog food manufacturers themselves serve up some of the fattiest products out there, often containing equal parts protein to fat. There are a few reasons for this, with most stemming from the fact meat protein is expensive and most of the lean stuff makes its way to the human market for much higher financial yield.

It is tempting for manufacturers to simply grind up carcass, which is fat and bone, resulting in a much lower protein to fat ratio. Others use fattier cuts such as very low-grade beef or pork mince. Not that this is always admitted on the label (remember the lessons from the dry food sector, nobody is checking the nutrient contents of pet food, dry or raw). Diets perpetually high in fatty meat inclusions should be avoided in anything but a dog with cancer. If the evolutionary *ideal* was a concept you cared for, then leaner may be healthier for the average dog longterm. In general, white meats (chicken, turkey, fish) are generally leaner than the red ones, so they're better for fatties (although oily fish, particularly the farmed stuff, can be quite fatty). The red meats (beef, pork, lamb, duck) tend to be higher in fat, which would be better for the more active types. And usually, the wilder and more free-to-run the animals, the leaner the meat.

Fish is great but it is the only meat you might freeze first for a couple of days (there is a potential for worms from wild varieties and freezing will kill them). Also, take note that many fish species contain thiaminase, which breaks down thiamine (vitamin B_1) in the dog, so it can't be a regularly large component of their diet. Fish that contain thiaminase include (but are not limited to) herring, chub mackerel, whitefish, scaled sardines, and skip-jack tuna. Fish that do not contain thiaminase and may thus be used more readily in premades include cod, hake, Atlantic mackerel, halibut, hake, trout and haddock.

Salmon doesn't have thiaminase, although I wouldn't feed too much farmed salmon either. Huge nutritional differences and seriously high drug use aside, fish farms are highly detrimental for the environment, but then show me a mass-produced meat that isn't. Your fishmonger can provide you with cheap fish in the form of fish heads. These are great, lots of meat with the added benefit of giving your dogs' access to some eye and brain nutrition, which is often absent in the average raw dog food mix. Best to feed the fresh heads outside, mind. Ideally, in someone else's garden. It's not an easy watch!

Tins of fish are ok, but know they are cooked. Aim for the oily fish varieties like sardine, herring or mackerel and avoid the ones in sunflower oil. First off, it is high in omega-6, which negates the benefit you are trying to get from the fish oil. Second, it is cooked at high temperature. This means you can expect the oil to be *inflammatory*. Like putting sugar in little yoghurt drinks meant to help your gut, the industry is rarely thinking about your health when they sell these products. Choose tins in fresh water, tomato or brine (which you pour off).

Choose Organic and As-Ethical-As-Possible Meat Over Intensively Reared

But more important than which exact parts is the quality of the meat you are feeding. I very strongly subscribe to Pitcairn's view that animals providing the meat should be raised outside with organic farming practices and using the most humane treatment possible.[2] I just can't see how our vets balance their oath of 'do no harm', with the promotion of products containing meat from countries with terrible reputations for animal welfare, or even meats emerging from meat factories that kill without prior stun. Sadly, it's something many meat factories in Ireland and the United Kingdom are more than happy to do on a grand scale, contrary to the pleas of vet councils and animal rights organisations the world over. As a vegetarian myself, I struggle daily with the dilemma that a Labrador will eat approximately 2,000 chickens in 10 years. Who are we to condemn so many lives, in favour of a single companion animal at home? Surely the very least we can do is ensure, for the sake of an extra few pennies, the animals lived as well as possible?

Welfare aside, there are a few less talked about issues with your dog living on intensively reared meat. First, from a microbiological viewpoint, grass-fed cows have about 1/300th the chance of harbouring *E. coli* as opposed to grain-fed cows.[3]

Furthermore, intensively reared meat, such as beef and chicken, contains an unnatural amount of Omega-6, a result of the poor-quality grain they are fed,[4] with chicken being the worst offender by far. A large analysis of more than 200 studies revealed that organic meat (and dairy) is higher in omega-3[5] a result of the animals eating fresh forage. It is my opinion, if formulating raw diets on intensively reared meat, omega-3 supplementation should be considered.

Finally, over the past few decades, there has been a dramatic increase of skin and gastrointestinal diseases in both dogs and cats.[6] Section 2 showed us that today recurring skin and gut conditions are among the top three reasons for dog owners to visit their vet. Adverse food reactions are a very common explanation for these issues. Besides wheat, sensitivities to chicken or beef are very common culprits which, when you think about it, should be as strange as a cow being allergic to grass. We have already alluded to two theories for this.

The first being the harsh processing conditions used in pet food that is shown to denature protein, and as a result, making it more antigenic to the body, and the role of over-vaccination by our vets. The second theory points the finger directly at antibiotic residues in the meat chain, most importantly in intensively reared chicken. In their review of the subject, Di Cerbo *et al.* (2017)[7] highlight how a specific compound, oxytetracycline (OTC), may be the possible underlying cause of many of these inflammatory pathologies. OTC is a common component of the most widely used antibiotics in intensive farming. Unfortunately, OTC has a high affinity for calcium-rich tissues such as bone and teeth where it can accumulate and reside, even when animals are no longer subjected to it. Di Cerbo *et al.*[7] highlight, using their previous research, that chicken bones can contain a toxic amount of OTC and the chronic consumption of such bones and poultry meat derivatives (via meat meal) by pets, may result in the enhancement of the inflammatory processes, materialising in skin and gastrointestinal diseases.

The importance of organic meat is even more relevant for those meat shopping in America. As well as the liberal use of antibiotics above, a number of worrying chemicals are permitted for use in the United States. This is why the European Union can't import their meat. These include ractopamine (from Europe to China to Russia, ractopamine is banned in 160 countries. It is a repartitioning agent that increases protein synthesis, essentially making meat leaner), recombinant bovine growth hormone (rBGH is the largest selling dairy animal drug in America. Developed by Monsanto and sold under the name Posilac, it arises from the contents of genetically engineered *E. coli* bacteria. It's injected into cows to increase milk production, but it is banned in at least thirty other nations including the European Union, Canada and Australia because of potential risk to human health) and not to mention a few arsenic-based drugs that are approved for use in animal feed in the United States (they make animals grow quicker and make the meat appear pinker and thus 'fresher'. Banned in the European Union, the Food and Drug Administration believes organic arsenic is less toxic than the other in organic form, which is a known carcinogen).

Thus, organic meat is certainly recommended over intensively reared meat. But please check your sources. Organic animals can be just as intensively reared as factory-farmed animals. There are a number of clever ways to charge you more for what is essentially the same intensively reared stuff that you were trying to avoid.

Sourcing Meats

The most likely source of meat for pet owners is raw dog food manufacturers. In this instance, please do not forget the lessons learned from the pet food industry. Just because raw producers are on the right side of the argument does not necessarily make them the good guys. You need to use your eyes, nose and head when shopping for anything with a picture of a dog on the front of it. If you are buying whole pieces from them, it's easier to see what you're getting but still the most popular product on the market for pet owners is ground meat and bone. In this case, I only trust mixes that are coarse ground, I want to see the meat and bone. I do not trust finely ground minces.

While there are some very good producers out there, the sad truth of it is many raw dog food producers are simply taking advantage of a growing market with no more knowledge of or passion for ideal canine nutrition than you had when you first set out on this road. The same basic laws of business will be applied here and that is that the less actual meat muscle they include in their mixes, the nicer the car they will be driving at the end of the year. Thus, while it is hoped premade raw dog foods contain approximately 10% bone, they may contain far more bone than this as they are using little more than ground up meaty bone (necks and carcass) in their mixes. When this stuff is ground into a homogenised fine mush, even the most experienced raw feeders would struggle to tell by looking at it how much meat was actually in there. The first you will know of it is when your dog's stool will be rock hard and dry and whiter in colour. This isn't good. While a firm poo is great for expressing those anal glands, we don't want them straining or getting bunged up. Adding plant fibre (blended raw broccoli or cooked sweet potato with the skin on) will alleviate the issue temporarily until a better supplier is found. The other basic protection you have is your nose. Meat should smell OK, never bad. There is no excuse for that. Finally, use your head, check out your supplier.

Call them. Ask them about their suppliers. Are they registered with the relevant authorities? What is everyone saying online?

Raw dog food producers should not be your only source of meat. Start hanging around the half-priced aisles of supermarkets. Remember he's a dog. He buries meaty bones and digs them up a week later for a chew! It's best-before-but-not-bad-after for him. Ask someone working there when they get their beef or chicken delivery and go in the evening before when those shelves are full.

You should also make friends with your local butcher. They have stuff in their bins that they will be happy to give you, especially if you shop with them, which you should do, keeping your money in the community. But beware, butchers too often sell 'mince for dogs' but, much like the less scrupulous raw dog food manufacturers, these guys do not make money throwing meat muscle out. A mix of fat and blood can look deceptively meaty. Or they might include a lot of beef liver they couldn't sell. If you're buying this sort of product, tell him you want it whole or at least to chop it chunky, so you can see what's in there!

Organs

Raw feeders need to shop a bit smarter and not limit themselves to the stuff commonly fed to humans. This is where organ meats come in. In raw feeding, there are two types of organs, one we deem to be just meat and can thus use liberally in our mixes while the others are termed 'secreting organs'. This latter group is considered as important to dogs as green vegetables to humans, but we only include so much of them as they can pack a punch. The 'meat' organs include heart, tongue, green tripe (cow/sheep stomach), lung, diaphragm, gizzard and penis. Of all the meat organs, tripe and heart are the most popularly used. Both excellent cuts of meat, they're also cheap to source as humans are less inclined to eat them; thus most raw manufacturers bulk their products with them.

The allegiance to tripe is a funny one though. While it's a cheap source of meat protein, many raw feeders swear it is an elixir for dogs, bestowing marvellous health benefits. I struggle to see this and suspect it might stem back to breeders of old who would go to the slaughterhouse door and ask for the cheapest bit of the cow they could get their hands on. The belly of the cow or *tripe*, practically useless to the human market, was it. These breeders would go home and feed it with a cheap 'biscuit' (which wasn't even 'complete' food but simply a dried cereal filler for dogs) and their dogs would bloom. However, any meat at this point would have that effect and a chicken thigh offers far more nutritional prowess than its weight in tripe. Some say tripe is a pre- or probiotic for dogs. However, the life in the belly of the cow surely bears little resemblance to the life in the belly of the dog.

They say that as it is green, unwashed tripe is apparently best, it's an excellent source of chlorophyll. Perhaps it is. However, I prefer to let the dog choose how much of that sort of stuff he wants to eat while out on a walk. I find it hard to ignore that, as Section 1 showed us, carnivores such as wolves do not regularly consume the belly of their prey. They may tease the fatty adipose tissue from the outside for sure, and perhaps some of the intestines are eaten but the acidic stomach contents are less likely to be on the menu. I've watched dogs eating larger prey; they never, ever touch the belly of the cow, let alone the contents, although perhaps this would be different if they were reared on it. If it was in any way vital, they'd surely be at it. But whatever works for you. It's fine stuff and a cheap source of good quality meat protein regardless.

A final note on tripe, people are concerned for 'washed tripe' largely as butchers often call it 'bleached tripe'. People misconstrue this as using actual bleach, but it is usually done with warm water or harmless hydrogen peroxide to make it more attractive and less odourless to humans.

The secreting organs include liver, kidney, spleen, testicles, pancreas and brain. While nice and meaty in their own right, they also function as a sink for vitamins and minerals as well as producing a variety of hormones and bioactive compounds. The liver for example stores vitamin A, D, E, K and B_{12} and is chock full of minerals such as iron and copper. It is an elixir for dogs. However, it must be fed in moderation or they can get diarrhoea or even become dangerously ill if fed on these excessively over time. Most raw feeders not using premade foods will couple the use of storage organ meat, such as liver, with a bony addition, such as carcass, to thin it out a bit. Vital to their overall diet, it's agreed that raw liver should comprise perhaps 5% of their weekly diet, and all storage organs added up together should comprise approximately 10–15% of their diet in total, with as broad a variation as possible.

Brains are incredibly nutritious. However, they are tough to source since feed companies thought it was OK to feed cow brains to cattle resulting in the Bovine Spongiform Encephalopathy crisis (with this in mind, you can't help worry about the number of dogs still going into dry food in the United States and beyond). However, as a whole animal eater, I do believe organs in the head including brains and eyes, like every other piece, are important for dogs. In this respect, in Europe, your options include sheep or lamb heads under 1 year of age, whole rodents that you can find in the frozen section of pet shops and fish heads! They offer fantastic nutrition and cost you little to nothing as they are another waste product of the human meat industry.

Testicles are another organ of note, in that with their high sex hormone content, including testosterone, they are surely a great food item for neutered dogs. However, I am unsure how many testicles a bitch would choose to eat. Perhaps some ovary would be a better choice for the spayed female, should you be able to find them!

Meaty Bone

Section 2 showed us that you absolutely need to feed raw, meaty bones (RMBs) to your dogs in order to clean their teeth. Eight of ten dogs are dry-fed and eight of ten have gum disease by three years of age. This is no coincidence. However, it goes beyond simple abrasion and teeth cleaning. RMBs provide vital nutrition to the dog. They are the primary source of calcium to the dog, as well as offering large amounts of zinc and iron and micro-minerals such as selenium, copper and magnesium. They provide lysine, which is vital for bone growth as well as good fats, chondroitin and vitamin C, which are crucial to joints. In this way raw meaty bones are practically essential eating for young pups and brood bitches that are trying to build strong teeth, joints and bones. RMBs also provide some much-needed roughage in their diet. It has a cleansing/scouring effect on the dog's digestive tract, possibly removing parasites and encouraging healthy faecal motions that stimulate the anal glands.

Let's begin with the latter first.

Unfortunately, people are often fearful of giving their dog a bone. There are a number of reasons for this. The first is that accidents can happen, as vets will tell you. Teeth breaking, impaction (undigested bone building up in the gut like a dam) and gut punctures, when undigested bone splinters and punctures the soft intestines. However, these accidents have some common factors. Most importantly, the vast majority are occurring with cooked bones and in dry-fed dogs (with less processing abilities due to weaker stomach acids). Remember, Brown and Park (1968)[8] observed no harmful effects after feeding oxtails to 2 hundred dogs for over six years. The secret was that the bones were raw, not too tough and surrounded by meat. The rest of the accidents occur from the use of inappropriate types of raw bones.

Some more bone dos and donts

- **No cooked bones:** The worst bone out there is a cooked bone. It is these that might send your dog to the vet for an obstruction. Cooking results in Maillard reactions where the ultimate result is a piece of bone far more resilient to digestion. What was once, in fresh form, a springy bendy bone becomes a very hard, brittle mass that splinters on breaking. These splinters may pass into their intestines, potentially leading to impaction or laceration. So, please, do not feed the leftover lamb bone or chicken carcass from a Sunday roast and certainly do not feed those cooked bones in pet shops wrapped in plastic. These are twice cooked pig femurs and are likely the most dangerous food item out there sold in pet shops today. Only feed fresh bones, the meatier the better (assists in lubrication).

- **The best bones:** include necks, wings, carcass, ribs and ox tail.

- **Feed right for the size:** A simple rule is the bigger the dog, the bigger the bone, it stops them gulping it down. So, you might use chicken necks and wings for a yorkie. A duck neck for a cocker. A turkey neck, chicken carcass or oxtail for Labrador. Also, avoid small bones such as chicken necks for Labradors, they tend to swallow them like a seagull with a fish.

- **No large femurs (leg bones):** These are supporting bones and are therefore the strongest in the body. Reinforced with iron and zinc, they often have a triangular shape, which gives them added strength. However, it is this shape that can result in dogs employing huge amounts of downward pressure only for one of two things happen: either the bone breaks or their teeth lose purchase and skid off. The result is the same – a vicious clash of teeth which can result in fractures

- **Feed once or twice a week:** Opinions vary on how much recreational bone you should feed to your dog. The current consensus is at least one a week to keep those teeth and gums healthy.

- **Avoid feeding before or after dinner:** Their stomachs are only so big and an RMB needs it all to itself for adequate digestion. If you feed too much bone at once, it may not digest properly and the dog risks passing splinters into the intestines.

- **Choking is unlikely BUT accidents *might* happen:** While I have personally yet to see it, I have heard of a dog choking on a bone where the owner had to take action. Choking kills thousands of Americans every year, more than road traffic accidents. The three main culprits being hot dogs, chewing gum and raw vegetables, but would anyone use an example of someone choking on a raw sprout as a reason to ban all veg from the human diet? Of course not. Dogs in general have extra wide, hardened oesophagi to enable the eating of bones. However, flat-faced breeds with missing teeth are expected to have a harder time. They should be watched. If concerned, smash the bones with a mallet while the dog gets used to his new lifestyle. Also, go to YouTube and learn how to do the Heimlich Manoeuvre on your size dog.

- **Bones do not make them aggressive:** First, dogs are extremely passive creatures, more so than humans, and for the most part avoid confrontation at all costs. But it is possible that a dog will protect a bone, the same way they might protect a nice piece of meat or even their favourite toy. It's my experience that this occurs more often in a dry-fed dog, however. I assume they place more value on them. If a dog is not giving up their bone, then they need to be trained to do so. Start with an old dry bone of little value and offer them a sausage to drop the bone with the words 'leave it'. Then, over time, reduce the quality of the treat and increase the quality of the bone, until they get the game.

How much raw bone does a dog need in his diet?

The vast number of raw feeders and even raw dog food manufacturers allow for a specific 10% bone content in raw dog food. This is likely based on the fact the average skeletal weight of a rabbit is 8%[9], a figure that would rise slightly for leaner varieties in the wild. Skeletal weight scales with body size[2], meaning the bigger the animal the more bone they contain. Mice have a skeletal weight comprising 6% of their total body weight while almost 50% of the body weight of giant animals such as blue whales consists of bone. However, not many of us are feeding a whole lot of rabbits to dogs. We are feeding farm-reared cows, pigs, sheep and poultry.

Section 2 showed us that the calcium:phosphorus ratios of common prey of the dog seem to be dangerously out of whack with what the AAFCO recommend. This is because calcium in its natural form is handled differently than the calcium found in ultra-processed pet food. Still, if raw manufacturers want to say 'complete' on their labels then they are bound to the AAFCO/FEDIAF nutritional guidelines. This means a maximum of 2% calcium is permitted in raw mixes for adults while a maximum of 1.6% calcium is permitted for the early growth phase of pups.

What is not accounted for by prey model feeders and raw manufacturers alike is that different bones from different animals vary in their calcium offerings. The type of bone used, the age of the animal at slaughter, what that animal was fed and if that animal is free to roam will all affect how much calcium is in your mix.

For instance, pork bones are notoriously hard, considering the weight they must bear, it's not surprising. A pig bone might be 63% ash (in organic mineral content, all the stuff that is left after they incinerate the material in a lab) and 32% of that is calcium.[10] At a 10% inclusion rate, this would equate to a dry matter content of 2% calcium (where 10g of fresh bone yields 6.3 g of ash, 32% of this equates to 2 g of calcium), far too high for a growing pup, according to the AAFCO.

Then we must factor in age. As bones mature much of their moisture content is replaced by an increased mineral content, giving the bone increased density and mass over time to allow for the increasing body weight. Field *et al.* (1974)[11] analysed the ash and calcium contents of various farm animal bones as the animal ages. In pigs, they found that the dry matter (DM) content of pig bones increased with age, from 63% DM at 6–8 months to 75% in animals aged 24–48 months. Percentage ash content increased from 53% to 57%, leading to a calcium from 19% to 22%. At a 10% inclusion rate in the dog's food, this is the difference between a calcium content of **1.2% Ca/DM** (19% of 6.3 g DM equates to 12 g of calcium per 10 g of fresh pig bone, if the animal is age 6-8 months at slaughter) and a calcium content of **1.65% Ca/DM** (22% of 7.55g DM equates to 16.5g of calcium per 10 g of fresh pig bone, if the animal is age 24–48 months at slaughter), the latter being an unacceptable figure for the early growth phase of dogs.

While it is accepted that the vast majority of farmed pigs are sent for slaughter at 6 months of age, it is not always the case. More ethically produced pig meat is often given longer to live. However, the situation is certainly more complicated with cattle. Most 'beef' cattle are slaughtered at 18 months old (with young male calves, known as veal, killed days after birth). But dairy cows too make up a large part of the meat chain. They exist for 4–7 years before they are dispatched to the slaughterhouse (for use largely in the burger industry). The by-products of all these animals are all used as one by the pet food industry, both dry and raw.

Field *et al.* (1974)[11] also studied the varying ash and calcium contents of cattle bones at different ages of slaughter. The DM content of bones from 'beef' cattle (12-24 months) and 'dairy' cattle (48 months+) ranges from 68% to 73% while calcium content is 21% and 24%, respectively. The result is the difference of a calcium content approximating **1.4% Ca/DM** using 10% of bone from younger animals (21% of 6.8 g DM equates to 14.3g of calcium per 10 g of fresh bone, if the animal is 12–24 months old at slaughter) and a calcium content of **1.75% Ca/ DM** (24% of 7.3 g DM equates to 17.5 g of calcium per 10 g of fresh bone, if the animal is 4+ years at slaughter), which is excessive for the growing dog. They also analysed the bones of a 2-to 3-month old calf and found they contain a lot of water, having a DM content of just 45%. This ultimately equates to the ideal **0.8% Ca/DM** of calcium for the dog consuming a raw mix containing 10% bone from these animals.

It is the very same with the difference between sheep and lamb bones. Field *et al.* (1974)[11] found that the DM content in the bones of a 6 month old lamb is around 61%, rising to 77% in a 4 year old ewe. The ash content rose from 54% to 63%, and the calcium content rose from 20% to 24%, respectively. The bottom line for the dog is **1.1% Ca/DM** using 10% fresh lamb bone (20% of 5.4 g DM equates to 10.8 g of calcium per 10 g of fresh bone, if the animal is 5–6 months old at slaughter) and a calcium content of **1.5% Ca/DM** of calcium per 100 g of mix using 10% sheep bone (24% of 6.3 g DM equates to 15.1 g of calcium per 10 g of fresh bone, if the animal is 4+ years at slaughter).

And it is the same for chickens. Most chickens are killed very young, at just eleven weeks old and as you would expect, their bones at this age not only contain more water but are significantly less dense than those chickens that lay eggs for a year before slaughter. Field *et al.* (1974)[11] compared the two groups and found that DM content rose (and thus water content fell) from 50% to 61%, the ash content rose from 47% to 55% and the calcium content rose from 18% to 21%, in chickens of 2 to 3month old and chickens 12 months old, respectively. The result for the dog consuming a raw mix containing 10% of these bones is a calcium content of **0.9% Ca/DM** per 100 g of mix made from the bones of a young chicken, to **1.3% Ca/DM** of calcium should the mix be based on older animals (it is something similar for turkeys, too).

From this point, we must remember that both diet and physical activity can greatly affect bone mass, strength and density.[12] While the figures are not yet available, we could expect animals reared outdoors, free-to-roam on a more, natural nutritious diet than, say, the intensively reared cattle in CAFO's fed wheat and corn that make up most of the US meat offerings, highlighted in Section 2.

And yet, as the body appears to handle natural forms of calcium and phosphorus differently from the kinds found in ultra-processed pet food, supported raw meat and bone diets, even though raw dog foods have a borderline-high calcium content

Section 3 showed us they still manage to have a protective effect against canine hip dysplasia in German Shepherds.

And this is **if** the manufacturers include just 10% bone. We know this is not always the case. Carcass and necks are the most common filler used by raw dog foods as meat protein is significantly more expensive. There is a temptation to use a little more of this bony material than stated to save a little money. Just like dry food, nobody is formally verifying the nutritional status of these products. You will know you have one of these products when your dog passes a much firmer, drier, paler-bordering-yellowy-white stool, a sure sign you need a new supplier. If you want to formally check up on a competitor's product, send it to a lab and check for calcium. You can infer the bone content from the figures I have given you. It's time we start holding these people accountable, dry or raw. For now, raw food producers/manufacturers need to keep these figures in mind when formulating their mixes to the AAFCO criteria.

> ***Author's note:***
>
> If, for whatever reason, your dog cannot eat raw bone, for instance those on broth for gut issues or those suffering kidney disease where best advice stipulates to keep the phosphorus content of the food low, meaning little to no bones in the mix as they are so high in phosphorus, in both these cases, the dog still needs the calcium the bones would have provided. The temporary solution here would be to include some ground up eggshell (be wary buying this in bulk online – they often bake them dry, which is not a good idea on the calcium front) with their meat dinners, at an inclusion rate of roughly one level teaspoon per 10 kg of dog (one teaspoon of eggshell powder contains approximately 1.8 g of calcium).

Now, very clearly and very sensibly, few people put as much thought into their calcium contents as this, but one thing that can upset newbies to raw feeding is when they are instructed to feed '10% bone'. How are we going to work out how much bone is going into the mix?! Are we to get out a spreadsheet every time they make up their pet's food – how much neck did I use, what are their bone contents, how much boneless mince have I got in there? This would be an unnecessary impediment. It is for this reason I prefer the broader 'meat on the bone' term in the prey and vegetables model. This includes whole (with bone) pieces such as turkey necks, oxtail and chicken legs, pieces that contain far more bone than the coveted 10% figure stated above. But this category can also contain 'meat' items, including off-cuts, brisket, skirt, cheek and head mince, as well as the meat organs such as tripe and heart. These meat pieces 'beef' up the muscle content a bit.

If you were aiming for the 'ideal' bone content of around 10% in your mix, the throw-away maths is one part meat-with-bone to one part boneless meat (1:1). I say 'throwaway' as each piece of meat-with-bone will differ in its bone content. Take chicken for example. Information from the US department of Agriculture National Nutrient Database (handy online tool for anyone looking for the possible nutrient contents of some typical food ingredients) informs us that the average bone content of a whole, raw, broiler chicken off the shelf (thus, not including innards or organs) is around 32%. As for various chicken parts (with skin), their bone contents vary as follows: wing 46%, back 44%, neck 36%, leg 27%, and thigh 21%. Obviously outdoor-reared animals will differ, as will the bone content in other bird species. It's only a rough guide. Surely, as raw continues its advance on the pet market, more accurate information will be made available online for your pieces of choice. For now, let's imagine the meat pieces we have chosen average approximately 30% bone content. If such meat-with-bone pieces make up 4 kg of a 10 kg mix, that mix will contain around 12% bone. To this we add 4 kg of boneless meat options to get near the 80% 'ideal' meat and bone inclusion ratio, the rest being made up with our secreting organ and vegetables. But again, this will vary with the pieces used. Don't overthink it. You need to spend as much time wondering if the dog had 8% or 15% fresh bone matter over the week as you do for your kids! Take solace in the fact most raw manufacturers are not getting it right either, until we know more, the dogs are more than fine.

Exact bone contents aside, meat on the bone is almost certainly the best way to feed a meat-eater. It satisfies the dog's deep-set physical and possibly emotional need for chewing, crunching and swallowing food in this manner. The increased hassle factor cleans their teeth, massages their gums and scours their insides. But also, we know meat on the bone is likely 'safer' from a microbiological point of view. Baddies can only grow on the outside of meat. When you grind that product, you mix it into the food. Hence, you can eat very raw steaks (flash-cooking each side eliminates the bacterial content) while minced meat products tend to be far higher in pathogenic bacteria.[13] This would be of no great concern if we were thoroughly cooking it for the dog but instead, we are relying on the dog's digestive juices to do the work here, which they do. But, while we are without guiding studies here, we assume that job will be made all the easier if lumps of meat on the bone hit this small pool of acid, lumps that require some time to break down, as opposed to mouthfuls of ground mince which is rapidly digested and passed through.

That said, meat on the bone is not for everyone. It can be harder to source, harder to handle, harder to store, harder to defrost. If you have a large pack, it can be harder again. Grounding up meat and bone products from raw dog food producers are a perfectly acceptable and necessary alternative. Don't be worrying. The occasional raw meaty bone will replace the need for chewing and a good supplier will ensure their hazardous microbiology is minimal.

Plant Matter

I believe some plant material can and should be used in the dog's diet, and this sentiment appears to be echoed by most of the world's leading authorities in raw canine nutrition (Billinghurst, Browne, Lonsdale, Pitcairn, Dodds, Thompson, Becker). While it is accepted that the dog's biology, and indeed the available diet studies point toward a diet high in meat when left to their own devices, we must not ignore the lessons learned in Sections 1 and 2 which indicate plant matter must have been on the menu for dogs to some degree throughout their recent evolution. The list of reasons include the following:

- Dogs have between three and thirty-two more copies of a gene that is crucial for carbohydrate digestion than wolves.

- The liver and pancreas of the dog produce hepatic glucokinase (GCK), an enzyme used to digest sugar. True, obligate carnivores such as domestic cats, owls, dolphins and trout, do not.

- Dogs have nearly twice the capacity to assimilate glucose as cats.

- Dogs can perform various metabolic tricks (such as converting carotene to vitamin A, tryptophan to niacin, cysteine to taurine and linoleate to arachidonate) that obligate carnivores cannot.

We know dogs can digest some plant material when it is presented correctly to them, that is when it is blended or pulverised or even cooked so that the tough plant cell walls are broken down for the dog allowing them access to the goodies inside. And once inside, these bioactive compounds are shown to benefit dogs immensely. With this in mind, here are my top five reasons why you might include some vegetable material in their diet:

1. A source of harder to find vitamins and minerals

While a well-varied meat, organ and bone diet may contain enough nutrients, it's a fact that some plant ingredients can provide some harder to find vitamins and minerals such as manganese, magnesium, iodine, folic acid and vitamin K. Becker and Brown conducted an anecdotal experiment where they compared the nutritional content of two seemingly well-rounded raw dog food diets, one with vegetables and one without. The latter was low in potassium, manganese, folic acid and vitamin K. I think prey model feeders are underestimating just how nutritionally poor some farmed meats now are. Soil erosion, coupled with poor farming practices such as cheap, unnatural food substrates like cereal is producing a very different meat quality to what the dog evolved on. The value of the prey species is dependent on what the prey species consumes. Wild sourced prey is likely to be more nutrient dense than farmed prey.[14] One answer, of course, is to feed only wild meats but another answer is the occasional bit of spinach for B vitamins or a pinch of kelp for iodine, etc.

2. Studies show there are major health benefits to be had (at least when adding them to a bowl of kibble)

To shun plant ingredients is to shun the science that proves their phytochemicals offer enormous benefit to dogs, at least to dry-fed dogs, as there are no studies yet in raw-fed populations. Milgram *et al.* (2005)[15] preserved the cognitive function of dry-fed Beagles by adding simple plant additions at 1% inclusion rate, including spinach flakes, tomato pomace, carrot granules, citrus pulp and grape pomace. Dunlap *et al.* (2006)[16] boosted antioxidant levels in part dry, part raw-fed sled dogs by supplementing their diet with blueberries, thereby preventing exercise-induced oxidative damage in their dogs, undoubtedly increasing performance and recovery times, although this is yet to be measured. And these are just the studies of whole plant ingredients. The inclusion of leafy green and yellow-orange vegetables three times a week reduced the incidence of bladder cancer in dry-fed dogs.[17]

Similarly, broccoli sprouts are effective against breast cancer in mice and dogs.[18] Multiple studies amply demonstrate that bioactive plant compounds such as sulforaphane, isolated from cruciferous vegetables and lycopene, isolated from tomatoes and watermelon, are effective at fighting various canine cancers.[19-21] Isolates of grape juice are effective at reducing platelet aggregation in dogs, which may be useful for treatments of both dogs and humans with heart issues.[22] Not that you should feed grapes to dogs! Adding plant starch polysaccharides, such as inulin and yeast cell wall extract, to raw diets can increase the production of faecal short-chain fatty acids, which may be beneficial for canine health.[23]

3. Fibre

We have already touched on the importance of fibre in Section 2 but there we were focused only on plant fibre as it is the type most commonly used by pet food producers. Despite being largely meat-eaters, dogs left to their own devices surely ingest a small amount of plant fibre along the way, including any minor plant items taken for sustenance, the medicinal consumption of plant material such as grass, the stomach contents of prey too small to shake free and their penchant for poo eating. We have already shown that this fibrous plant material will affect the flow of digesta through their intestines, as it does in humans.[24,25] Soluble plant fibre is effective in the reduction of diarrhoea in dry-fed dogs,[26] preserving gut membrane health when they are sick.[27] For these reasons, pet food producers can and do use plant fibre to regulate stool quality in dogs. However, as most plant fibre additions are in fact leftovers of the human food processing (beet pulp, soybean meal, corn gluten), they are also excellent for boosting your bottom line, particularly as they can contribute protein to the mix, even if the majority of it is indigestible to the dog. As carbohydrates and fibre are not a label requirement for pet food manufacturers, it is suspected that cheap plant fibre additions are very often used to excess in dry pet food.

It is strongly suspected too much plant fibre will disrupt the normal flow of digesta in dogs eating such products, ultimately resulting in digestive issues. Authors note a decrease in nutrient digestibility in dogs with increasing levels of fibre in the diet,[28,29] likely a result of the reduction of contact between the meal and both enzymes and absorptive surfaces in the water-bulked stool.[30] Of greater concern is the alteration of the gut biome by plant fibre[31,32] which has implications for both dilated cardiomyopathy and also gas production, a particular concern for deep-chested dogs at risk of bloat and torsion. In cats, increased levels of crude fibre not only alters fermentation patterns and increased faecal output but also alters glucose absorption, insulin secretion, colonic microflora and, at higher levels, can depress diet digestibility.[33]

All this considered, the small amounts of plant fibre arising from the 5–10% less fibrous fresh plant ingredients that we might blitz in the blender (or even lightly cooked cubes of sweet potato with the skin on, should you have a dog prone to constipation) are expected to be not only well tolerated but potentially beneficial to dogs, certainly those fed a dry diet that itself is not already too high in fibre.

It is increasingly likely that the gut flora of meat-eaters would benefit greatly from more animal-sourced prebiotics. These include the indigestible parts of their prey, including hair, nails, feathers and hide[34] but also a great variety of meat protein peptides that are seen to act as a prebiotic in human infants, stimulating the growth of *Bifidobacteria* species.[35,36]

Encouraged by the fact feeding whole prey (with hide) has a protective effect against diarrhoea in captive cheetahs, Sarah Depauw investigated the importance of animal sources of fibre to the cheetah (an obligate carnivore) for her doctorate. She compared cheetahs fed whole prey (rabbit) to cheetahs fed a supplemented-beef diet. The cheetahs fed whole prey had a higher faecal output and that faeces was firmer, somewhat as predicted for a diet now higher in indigestible fibre. It was also noted some of the cheetahs eating just the beef had intermittent diarrhoea. But it was her work on putrefactive compounds that was most surprising. By-products of protein fermentation, putrefactive compounds such as ammonia, phenols, aliphatic amines and volatile sulphur-containing compounds are produced by certain bacterial groups that can make their way into the blood where they are linked to chronic intestinal inflammatory diseases in humans. In particular, these toxic metabolites can be uremic toxins resulting in kidney inflammation and chronic kidney disease, a top killer of cheetahs (and dogs and cats). In this way, the wrong prebiotics can not only alter the gut ecosystem but also influence the general metabolism of the host. The feeding of whole prey to cheetahs significantly reduced the number of putrefaction compounds in comparison to a supplemented beef diet. This author concluded by stressing the importance of promoting beneficial fermentation patterns for the overall health of carnivores such as the cheetah. But there is no reason why we would not expect such benefits in the whole prey eating dog. Unfortunately, outside of prey model supporters, hair, feathers and hide are not an attractive or desired component of raw diets. People might view it as something of a poor quality filler. I expect these attitudes to change in the future as attentions shift all too slowly toward *optimal* canine nutrition.

4. Some dogs (and owners?) *might* benefit from a carbohydrate addition

Unlike most dogs that are long-distance running machines, sighthounds such as greyhounds and lurchers have been engineered to sprint. As a result, greyhound muscle is heterogeneous and comprised of a large percentage of fast-twitch oxidative fibres,[37] and these muscles use a lot of glycogen (a.k.a. sugar). It's theorised by some that such dogs pre-race may benefit from the strategic inclusion of carbohydrates in the diet. However, the jury is most certainly out on this one, and I would venture it appears to be becoming less popular to do so.

Until recently it was believed that as muscles run on glycogen, then the more glycogen you stored before a race, the greater the battery time on the track, so to speak. Makes sense and it has been the foundation diet of marathon runners since. However, as Section 2 alluded to, some of the earlier proponents of carbohydrate loading pre-race are now questioning this theory, and that it's possibly more about fat-loading than carb-loading. More and more athletes, from running to cycling and certainly long-distance swimmers, are shunning the carbohydrates for fat in this regard. It seems the chances of carb-loading applying in an animal with no requirement for plant carbohydrate are becoming slimmer by the day.

The only time I would use carbohydrates in my dog is simply in the form of scraps. It's a sin to waste food and it's wholly unnecessary with a dog around, once fed in moderation. In fact, being a great use of leftovers is becoming an increasingly important concept these days. After being criminalised by the pet food industry in the 1970s, leftovers are now making a comeback. Dogs evolved to hang out with us for a reason! It's an environmentally sound way of getting rid of leftovers so long as they have no harmful ingredients in there (such as onion or xylitol etc). So, if I have a bit of porridge left over in the morning, I might add a big dollop into his food. I can't help but think he appreciates a nice warm meal on a brisk, Irish, winter morning. I don't overthink it.

5. Reducing cost?

There is another reason you might include carbohydrates in their diet and that is cost. Plant carbohydrates are very cheap compared to meat. While clearly some people are not going to like this, the fact remains that cost is a very real concern for many pet owners. Suddenly understanding your dog is a meat-eater, particularly if you have a giant breed and certainly if you own more than one, can pose some serious financial concerns for the owner. A Labrador can eat 1kg of meat per day. While there are many workarounds, whatever way you look at it, meat-eaters can be expensive animals to feed. Euromonitor reports tell us the pet food market is split right down the middle, with half choosing the best food for their dog and the rest choosing what they can afford. The latter love their dogs as much as the former and obviously want what is best for them, but not everyone can afford that.

If we give these people no option, they will stay with a cheap, cereal-based pet food, to the great detriment of the pet in their care. We must be careful not to put people off from the outset. Baby steps. I believe this is an important point for vets to have in the back of their minds.

I would happily stand over a homemade diet based on 75% meat, organ and bone but which incorporates some cheap plant filler if this meant the dog remained on a home-prepared diet and not shifted to a cheap, ultra-processed diet obscenely high in rapidly digested carbohydrates. While not ideal, dogs will most certainly do fine on such diets, certainly if enough of the good stuff is going in there. In terms of filler, a cheap, non-grain plant addition such as 25% amaranth would be what I would use first. It looks like a grain, but it is in fact a tiny perennial plant. As it is higher in protein, lower in carbohydrates and slower to digest than grain, it is far more suitable for carnivores, but it does contain phytic acid which is not ideal long-term as it can bind calcium and zinc from the diet. The only actual grain I would use is a porridge made from soaked/boiled oats. Slower to digest and with a lower Glycaemic Load than most grains, they are more suitable for meat-eaters than rapidly digested carbohydrates such as wheat, corn, rice (white or brown) or potato.

But again, while I can't say we're seeing much flatulence on a diet of 25% cooked porridge, we must remember oats come with soluble fibre, which puts me on alert for potential gas production and potentially gastric dilation with volvus in deep chested breeds. See? It's a tricky business not feeding them normal food!

Recommended vegetable additions include but are not limited to leafy greens, carrots, green beans, broccoli, seaweed, herbs and maybe some fruit – the latter of which I would go easy on. Dogs do not need the sugar. Studies show simple sugars promote oxidative stress and low-grade inflammation in dogs[30] though, in fairness, they do the same in humans. My favourites are a handful of dark berries (blue and blackberries), but also the occasional slice of apple or melon, which I'd probably feed separate to the main meat and bone meal. Anything really, but watch those pits/stones, no whole peaches, etc., they are a commonly choked on item.

Of all plant additions, I am fascinated with seaweed. The only supplements I sell from my site www.dogsfirst.ie are mostly seaweed-based. When people think of seaweed, they automatically think 'kelp', which forms the underwater forests you see seals swimming through. However, true kelp (*Laminaria digitata*) is but one type of seaweed. There are more than 10,000 different kinds! In fact, there are more seaweeds below the waves than herbs above them. Seaweeds are simply unbelievable from a vitamin and mineral perspective, so I use them like a multivitamin for my dog. It is notoriously a great source of iodine which is crucial to your pet's health and well being, but something the pet food sector can provide very little of. Ultra-processed pet foods vary wildly in their iodine content with many containing none at all.[38, 39] In fact, studies in cats reveal they were more than four times as likely to develop hyperthyroidism compared to cats that ate iodine-supplemented foods.[40]

Raw dog food is not off the hook in this regard either. Unnatural feed stuffs coupled with soil depletion ensures our meat chain is now very deficient in iodine. The main animal sink for iodine is the thyroid gland. However, thyroid, by and large, is not included in raw dog food for a very good reason as the only thyroid glands you can easily isolate are that of the cow and these are far too high in thyroxine and would sicken your pet when fed them. A Food and Drug Administration alert in March 2017 highlighted exactly this, where two lines of canned dog food, along with a type of pet treat, were flagged for being too high in thyroid hormones that may result in hyperthyroidism in pets consuming those products. The use of thyroid, certainly beef, in pet food is not the norm for this very reason. While chicken and duck necks are quite a common item used by raw pet food manufacturers, the actual thyroid of poultry usually resides further down the neck inside the carcass, and is often removed in the processing of the bird. It is rare to find a thyroid on a chicken neck for this reason.

The only other animal sinks for iodine are the ovaries, salivary glands and brain – all items that are regularly excluded from pet food. It my opinion, all raw-fed dogs should get some seaweed in their diet. Dogs require 1 mg of iodine per kilo of dry dog food (DM) they eat.[41] If you are using true kelp as described, know that it is the seaweed highest in iodine, twice as much as the next nearest in fact, containing approximately (there is huge seasonal variation) 1.3 mg of iodine per gram of dried seaweed. Thus, 1 g of dried *Laminaria* would be enough for two kilos of wet (with water) mix as an average dose.

More than simply iodine however, it contains a great range of antioxidative and anti-inflammatory properties, largely as it lives in such a hostile environment with twice daily changes of temperature, salinity and often air exposure. Many of these bioactive compounds are only found beneath the waves too, including fucoidans and fucoxanthin. In their review, Cornish and David, (2010)[42] cited numerous articles amply demonstrating just how anti-cancer seaweeds can be. Ensure your seaweed is sustainably harvested in clean waters and air-dried if possible; the bioactive sugars hate high temperatures. Plug coming up – we have teamed up with a seaweed scientist to bring out a range of high-quality, seaweed-based supplements using sea weeds and mosses sourced sustainably off the West Coast of Ireland. The range includes single species such as *Laminaria* but also many targeted at specific conditions such as weepy eyes (Oculus Prime), anal glands (StoolRite) or gut health (BioFunction8). You can find them at www.dogsfirst.ie and we ship worldwide.

I also love a little raw garlic. Now, at this point, some people can baulk, believing raw garlic to be dangerous due to it being in the onion family. However, it's not that simple. While raw garlic contains thiosulphate, which is responsible for causing Heinz factor anaemia in dogs and cats, the amount of thiosulphate in garlic is negligible. The only study I can find (and is actually referenced by people as a reason not to use it) is by Lee *et al.* (2000).[43] This was a pretty terrible overdose study where they used the equivalent of 5 g of raw garlic per kilo of body weight of dog and found after a week their blood results were wrong. To give the figure some context, if they were using 20-kg dogs, that would be 100 g of raw garlic per day, or 20 whole cloves. Few people are thinking about such doses in an elephant, let alone a dog.

Studies show garlic is packed full of vitamins and minerals but is also anti-cancer. It boosts liver, kidney and heart function, helps strengthen the body's defences and acts as a natural wormer. Half a raw clove per 15 kg of dog per day is fine. And don't mix it into their food. Garlic is medicinal and, as with all medicinal additions such as herbs and homemade remedies, should therefore be offered separate to the meal. The dog will take it if they want/need it, in accordance with the best principles of animal zoopharmacognosy. Never use dried garlic and avoid using garlic in pups under six months or dogs on blood thinners.

There are a variety of ground seeds out there that I often use, too (dogs can't digest them in whole form). Seeds are choc-full of all sorts but particularly vitamin E and zinc. Mentioned previously, in my opinion, the AAFCO require unnaturally high amount of these two nutrients in dog food mixes. I use some ground hemp seeds (as they don't contain phytic acid) to keep everyone happy. The other seed I love is pumpkin seeds as they have the added benefit of containing both cucurbitin and kainic acid, meaning they're anti-helminthic.[44] The oils of these two can be used but you leave a lot of the good stuff behind when you do.

TAKE-HOME POINTS

✓ Prey model is a feeding style aiming to provide the dog as close as possible to a whole prey diet. It generally involves a ratio of 8:1:1 comprising 8-parts meat, 1-part secreting organ, 1-part bone.

✓ Prey and Plant model is probably more popular. Rather than simply prey alone, it allows for some plant material. Around 10% is common.

✓ If not feeding whole, gutted prey (with breast meat) you can 'beef' up your mixes with a mix of boneless meat additions including breast meat and any meat off-cuts commonly consumed by humans such as skirt, chuck and brisket, as well as heart, tripe, cheek and tongue meat, gizzards, it's all excellent protein for your dog.

✓ Any animal is fine to feed but no roadkill and only typical prey. Freeze fish first and avoid those with thiaminase long term. Avoid tinned fish in oil.

✓ Keep it lean: 4-parts protein to 1-part fat is a good average.

✓ Premade raw can be high in fat as many grind simply carcass which is fat and bone (remember, nobody is checking the nutritional content of these foods either – they can state what they like on the label).

✓ If buying meat from pet food suppliers, avoid finely ground minces, use coarse ground at a minimum. Establish relationships with butchers and use half-priced aisles of supermarkets.

✓ Choose organic and as ethically as possible. Non-organic is higher in omega-6 and the bones may store oxytetracycline which is linked to inflammatory pathways. In the United States, meat may also contain ractopamine, recombinant bovine growth hormone and some arsenic-based drugs, all of which are not approved in the European Union.

✓ There are two types of organ meats. One type is considered 'meat' (e.g. heart, tongue, green tripe, lung, diaphragm, gizzard, penis), the other as 'secreting organs' (liver, kidney, spleen, testicles, pancreas, brain). When we say '1-part organ' we mean secreting organs.

✓ Working out exactly how much bone is in your DIY mix is difficult and not absolutely necessary. Add 1-part boneless meat to 2-parts meat on the bone to achieve a more balanced bone content.

✓ Meaty bones are vital to dental health. They are also highly nutritious and provide roughage to the dog. They need to be raw. No cooked bones or large leg bones. The best bones include necks (chicken, duck, turkey, lamb), wings, carcass, smaller beef bones. If feeding meat on the bone, you don't need to feed meaty bones on their own but it won't upset things if you do occasionally.

✓ The vast majority of raw feeders assume 10% is the ideal bone content of raw dog food. This is based on a rough average of the skeletal weight of typical prey of the dog. This means IF raw manufacturers are including just 10% beef, pork or lamb bones, they are already at their maximum for 'calcium' permitted by the AAFCO for growing pups. And still raw dog food has a protective effect against canine hip dysplasia compared to ultra-processed dry food as the body handles natural calcium differently to the likes of calcium carbonate.

✓ Raw manufacturers may include more bone than is indicated on the label. If your dog struggles to poop or passes white bullets, you need to change supplier.

✓ If you can't feed bone for whatever reason, it's possible (although not ideal) to use one level teaspoon of eggshell powder per 10 kg of dog per day. Feed a meaty bone at least once a week in a grassy patch to keep his teeth clean.

✓ There is a great debate on the use of plant matter in the dog's diet. We know it must have been a regular feature of the dog's diet to some degree as the dog has evolved extra copies of the AMY2B gene for amylase production. Other adaptations include the presence of hepatic GCK in the liver and pancreas for digesting sugar resulting in twice the capacity to assimilate glucose than cats.

✓ Reasons for including plant matter are as follows:

- a source of harder to find vitamins and minerals

- major benefits from plant-based bioactive compounds

- a source of fibre

- if necessary, a minor carb addiction for reducing cost

✓ Favourite plant additions include leafy greens, seaweed, carrots, herbs and occasionally some fruit with dark berries. Seaweed offers not only a sustainable source of nutrients including vitamins and minerals but also a range of highly beneficial, anti-inflammatory compounds not found above the waves.

✓ A little raw garlic is beneficial. It boosts immunity and protects from parasites. Half a ground clove per 15 kg of dog per day is fine but leave to the side of the bowl. It's medicinal. If they need it, they'll take it.

✓ Ground seeds are great too, full of vitamin E and zinc. Pumpkin seeds are excellent as they are also anti-helminthic. However, as a general addition to a mix, hemp seeds might be best as they contain no phytic acid.

Chapter Twenty Two References

1   Moleón, M., Martínez-Carrasco, C., Muellerklein,O.C. *et al.* (2017). Carnivore carcasses are avoided by carnivores. Journal of Animal Ecology, 86(5): 1179–1191

2   Reynolds, W.W. and Karlotski, W.J. (1977). The Allometric Relationship of Skeleton Weight to Body Weight in Teleost Fishes: A Preliminary Comparison with Birds and Mammals. Copeia, 1: 160–163

3   Russell, J.B., Diez-Gonzalez, F. and Jarvis, G.N. (2000). Potential effect of cattle diets on the transmission of pathogenic Escherichia coli to humans. Microbes and Infection, 2(1): 45–50

4   Simopoulos, A.P. (2016). An Increase in the Omega-6/Omega-3 Fatty Acid Ratio Increases the Risk for Obesity. Nutrients, 8(3): 128

5   Średnicka-Tober, D., Barański, M., Seal, C.J. *et al.* (2016). Higher PUFA and n-3 PUFA, conjugated linoleic acid, α-tocopherol and iron, but lower iodine and selenium concentrations in Organic milk: a systematic literature review and meta- and redundancy analyses. British Journal of Nutrition, 115(6): 1043–1060

6   Watson, T.D.G. (1998). Diet and skin disease in dogs and cats. Journal of Nutrition, 128(12): 2783S–2789S

7   Di Cerbo, A., Pezzuto, F., Guidetti, G. *et al.* (2017). *Functional Pet Foods*. Published in Superfood and Functional Food: An Overview of Their Processing and Utilization. Eds. Waisundara, V. and Shiomi, N.

8   Brown, E.N. and Park, J.F. (1968). Control of dental calculus in experimental beagles. Laboratory Animal Care, 18: 527–535

9   Brewer, N.R. and Cruise, I.J. (1994). The Biology of the Laboratory Rabbit. 2nd Ed. Manning, P.J., Ringler, D.H., Newcomer, C.E. Eds. San Diego Academic Press. pp63–70

10 Prikoszovits, A. and Schuh, M. (1995). The mineral content of calcium, phosphorus and magnesium in the serum and bones and the serum activity of alkaline phosphatase in slaughtered fattening pigs [Article in German]. Dtsch Tierarztl Wochenschr, 102(1): 53–57

11 Field, R.A., Riley, M.L., Mello, F.C. *et al.* (1974). Bone composition in cattle, pigs, sheep and poultry. Journal of Animal Science, 39(3)

12 Office of the Surgeon General (2004). Bone health and osteoporosis: A report of the surgeon general. PMID: 20945569

13 Tassew, H., Abdissa, A., Beyene, G. *et al.* (2010). Microbial flora and food borne pathogens on minced Meat and their susceptibility to antimicrobial agents. Ethiopian Journal of Health Science, 20(3): 137–143

14 Dierenfeld, E.S., Alcorn, H.L. and Jacobsen, K.L. (2002). *Nutrient Composition of Whole Vertebrate Prey (Excluding Fish) Fed in Zoos*. U.S. Department of Agriculture. Published online, www.researchgate.net

15 Milgram, N.W., Head, E., Zicker, S.C. *et al.* (2005). Learning ability in aged beagle dogs is preserved by behavioral enrichment and dietary fortification: a two-year longitudinal study. Neurobiological Aging, 26: 77–90

16 Dunlap, K.L., Reynolds, A.J. and Duffy, L.K. (2006). Total antioxidant power in sled dogs supplemented with blueberries and the comparison of blood parameters associated with exercise. Comparative Biochemistry and Physiology Part A: Molecular & Integrative Physiology, 143(4): 429–434

17 Knapp, D.W., Ramos-Vara, J.A., Moore, G.E. *et al.* (2014). Urinary bladder cancer in dogs, a naturally occurring model for cancer biology and drug development. Institute for Laboratory Animal Research, 55(1): 100–118

18 Curran, K.M., Bracha, S., Wong, C.P. *et al.* (2018). Sulforaphane absorption and histone deacetylase activity following single dosing of broccoli sprout supplement in normal dogs. Veterinary Medical Science, 4(4): 357–363

19 Shieh, P., Tsai, M.L., Chiu, M.H. *et al.* (2010). Independent effects of the broccoli-derived compound sulforaphane on Ca^{2+} influx and apoptosis in Madin-Darby canine renal tubular cells. Chinese Journal of Physiology, 53(4): 215–222

20 Wakshlag, J.J. and Balkman, C.E. (2010). Effects of lycopene on proliferation and death of canine osteosarcoma cells. American Journal of Veterinary Research, 71(11): 1362–1370

21 Rizzo, V.L., Levine, C.B. and Wakshlag, J.J. (2017). The effects of sulforaphane on canine osteosarcoma proliferation and invasion. Veterinary and Comparative Oncology, 15(3): 718–730

22 Osman, H.E., Maalej, N., Shanmuganayagam, D. *et al.* (1998). Grape juice but not orange or grapefruit juice inhibits platelet activity in dogs and monkeys. Journal of Nutrition, 128: 2307–2312

23 Beloshapka, A.N., Duclos, L.M., Vester Boler, B.M. *et al.* (2012). Effects of inulin or yeast cell-wall extract on nutrient digestibility, fecal fermentative end-product concentrations, and blood metabolite concentrations in adult dogs fed raw meat-based diets. American Journal of Veterinary Research, 73(7): 1016–1023

24 Burrows, C.F., Kronfeld, D.S., Banta, C.A. *et al.* (1982). Effects of fiber on digestibility and transit time in dogs. Journal of Nutrition, 112: 1726–1732

25 Lewis, L.D., Magerkurth, J.H., Roudebush, P. *et al.* (1994). Stool characteristics, gastrointestinal transit time and nutrient digestibility in dogs fed different fiber sources. Journal of Nutrition, 124: 2716S–2718S

26 Gagné, J.W., Wakshlag, J.J., Simpson, K.W. *et al.* (2013). Effects of a synbiotic on fecal quality, shortchain fatty acid concentrations, and the microbiome of healthy sled dogs. BMC Veterinary Research, 9:246

27 Apanavicius, C.J., Powell, K.L., Vester, B.M. *et al.* (2007). Fructan supplementation and infection affect food intake, fever, and epithelial sloughing from *Salmonella* challenge in weanling puppies. Journal of Nutrition, 137(8): 1923–1930

28 Earle, K.E., Kienzle, E., Optiz, B. *et al.* (1988). Fiber affects digestibility of Organic matter and energy in pet foods. Journal of Nutrition, 128: 2798S–2800S

29 Castrillo, C., Vicente, F. and Guada, J.A. (2001). The effect of crude fibre on apparent digestibility and digestible energy content of extruded dog foods. Journal of Animal Physiology and Animal Nutrition, 85: 231–236

30 De Haer, L.C.M. and De Vries, A.G. (1993). Feed intake patterns and feed digestibility in growing pigs housed individually or in groups. Livestock Production Science, 33: 277–292

31 Russell, T.J. (1998). The Effect of Natural Sources of Non-Digestible Oligosaccharides on the Fecal Microflora of the Dog and Effects on Digestion. Missouri: Friskies R&D centre, Friskies-Europe

32 Hooda, S., Minamoto, Y., Suchodolski, J.S. *et al.* (2012). Current state of knowledge: the canine gastrointestinal microbiome. Animal Health Research Reviews, 13(1): 78–88

33 Kienzle, E. (1994). Effect of Carbohydrates on Digestion in the Cat. The Journal of Nutrition, 124: 2568S–2571S

34 Depauw, S., Bosch, G., Hesta, M. *et al.* (2012) Fermentation of animal components in strict carnivores: A comparative study with cheetah fecal inoculum. Journal of Animal Science, 90: 2540–2548

35 Lieple, C., Adermann, K., Raida, M. *et al.* (2002). Human milk provides peptides highly stimulating the growth of bifidobacteria. European Journal of Biochemistry, 269: 712–718

36 Arihara, K. (2006b). Functional properties of bioactive peptides derived from meat proteins. *In Advanced Technologies for Meat Processing,* Publisher: Boca Raton, CRC Press pp.245–273

37   Dobson, G.P., Parkhouse, W.S., Weber, J.M. *et al.* (1988). Metabolic changes in skeletal muscle and blood of greyhounds during 800-m track sprint. American Journal of Physiology, 255(3): R513–R519

38   Ranz, D., Tetrick, M., Opitz, B. *et al.* (2002). Estimation of iodine status in cats. The Journal of Nutrition, 132(6): 1751S–1753S

39   Hodgkinson, S., Rosales, C.E., Alomar, D. *et al.* (2004). Chemical nutritional evaluation of dry foods commercially available in Chile for adult dogs at maintenance. Archivos de Medicina Veterinaria, 36(2): 173–181

40   Edinboro, C.H., Scott-Moncrieff, C., Janovitz, E. (2004). Epidemiologic study of relationships between consumption of commercial canned food and risk of hyperthyroidism in cats. Journal of the American Veterinary Medical Association, 224(6): 879–886

41   Association of American Feed Control Officials (AAFCO, 2016). *Dog and Cat Food Nutrient Profiles*. Official Publication, see www.aafco.org

42   Cornish, M.L. and David, D.J. (2010). Antioxidants from macroalgae: Potential applications in human health and nutrition. Algae, 25: 155–171

43   Lee, K.W., Yamato, O., Tajima, M., *et al.* (2000). Hematologic changes associated with the appearance of eccentrocytes after intragastric administration of garlic extract to dogs. American Journal of Veterinary Research, 61(11): 1446–1450

44   Amin, T. and Thakur, M. (2013). *Cucurbita mixta* (pumpkin) seeds – a general overview of their health benefits. International Journal of Recent Scientific Research, 4(6): 846–854

CHAPTER 23

DIY Raw Dog Food

To get you started, here are some simple recipe ideas. You can use any and all of the meats and pieces above. Please remember, we are not putting this forth as a 'complete' meal to be used for months but it is close to spot on as your dog is going to get. For more recipes for particular types and health conditions, go to www.dogsfirst.ie.

Standard Raw Dog Food Recipe

10 kg of Organic Chicken, Beef and Vegetables

No one recipe can ever seriously be held up as 'complete' as we do not know what a 'complete' diet for a dog is but the suggested recipe would make approximately 10 k g of the Rolls Royce of dog food. Don't worry if you don't have all the ingredients at once, you'll get there next time. I'm just showing you what FABULOUS looks like. This mix would be enough for the average 15-kg dog for 23 days at a 2.5% of body weight inclusion rate. It would be a medium calorific value and suitable for average adults and senior dogs of all sizes and breeds (for pups I would increase the calorie content slightly).

<u>Ingredients</u>

8 kg of Organic Meat and Bone:

5.5 kg fresh poultry on the bone (e.g. chicken legs or thighs or back or simply in mince with bone from a provider)

1 kg green beef tripe

1 kg raw, whole sardines (from frozen).

500 g beef heart

1 kg of Secreting Organ:

500 g beef liver

500 g beef kidney (alternate with spleen when you can find it)

1 kg of blended plant additions:

300 g broccoli

300 g kale

200 g of carrot

200 g of blueberries or blackberries

Excellent Extras:

Two tablespoons of good quality seaweed

1 tablespoon of ground hemp seed/pumpkin seed

A handful of mussels (from frozen, for the manganese, if not offering hair and feather in some form, see below)

3-4 raw eggs

Method

Implements you will need:

A very large tub for mixing the ingredients (I do it in the basin, easier to clean)

A rubber glove (easier to mix with a hand than a large ladle)

Large clip-close lunchboxes to store your mix (easier than bags, recyclable, take up less space in freezer)

Antibacterial spray, for wiping everything down afterward

Some space, time and music

What to do:

1. Chop meat and organ meat pieces.

2. Either blend or par-cook plant ingredients (if using).

3. Add power additions and mix all your ingredients together.

4. Work out what your dog needs each day (see below) and store 3 days' worth in each tub (so you're not taking them out every day).

5. Keep one tub of mix in the fridge and freeze the rest.

6. Wipe down all surfaces and tools with hot water and antibacterial cleaning product.

DIY tips

- Avoid nutrient excesses/deficiencies by varying the choice of meats and organs used each time.

- If feeding ground minced meat and bone mixes, remember to feed fresh, raw meaty bones once or twice a week for their teeth.

- If you have a big dog(s), then you may need to get yourself a chest freezer. This allows you to buy in bulk to save money and better exploit deals when they pop up.

Handling Tips:

i. We know the meat chain can contain potentially harmful bacteria, so treat it with care. Wash hands and surfaces in antibacterial after handling your meat mixes. Your meat mixes should live on the very bottom shelf of the fridge so they can't drip on your food.

ii. When thawing meat, it is best to do it in the fridge below 4° Celsius as pathogens struggle to grow below 6° Celsius. The mistake many people make is leaving the product out on the drainer overnight. This means the outside of the product can get to room temperature as it thaws. Baddies then have all night to grow in numbers.

iii. Defrosted meat lasts for 4 days in the fridge before it starts to go off... for humans. While an extra few days at this point will be no trouble to your dog, if you feed them pathogenic bacteria you can expect them to pass it in their faeces, which is to be avoided, particularly if kids are around.

Have an active dog that needs more calories? (Also suitable for pups)

Working dogs such as sled dogs burn fat. Drop the chicken content above (as it's leaner) from 5 kg to say 2.5 kg. Replace with 2.5 kg of fatty mince, such as beef or pork. More again if working hard. And/or increase the amount fed. For more information go to my feed calculator on www.dogsfirst.ie.

Have an overweight dog that needs less calories?

The ideal weight loss diet for your dog is lower in calories, high in protein, lower in fat and zero carbohydrates. This will result in gradual weight loss but will retain lean body mass, crucial to the whole process. In the standard mix above remove the red meats as they are fattier. Only use white meats such as chicken, turkey or fish mince as they're much lower in calories. Pull off the skin where you can see it to lower the fat content further. You can also increase the vegetable addition from 1 kg to 3 kg, for example (as it is so low in calories), but leaner meat is preferred. And watch the treats for at least a month! Make your own treats, based on lean meats such as chicken/turkey fillet or hearts (oven dry on low heat). Measure their tummy each week to hold yourself to account. For more information go to www. dogsfirst.ie.

TAKE-HOME POINTS

✓ No one recipe can ever seriously be held up as 'complete' as we do not know what a 'complete' diet for a dog is. But a GREAT recipe for around 10 kg of standard raw dog food might be:

❖ 8 kg of organic meat and bone (5.5 kg fresh, organic poultry on the bone, 1 kg green beef tripe, 1kg of raw whole sardines from frozen, 500 g beef heart).

❖ 1 kg of secreting organ (500 g liver and 500 g of kidney/spleen).

❖ 1 kg of plant additions.

❖ Power additions include seaweed, hemp/pumpkin seed powder, mussels, eggs.

Mix in sink, wash down with antibacterial after. Store in lunchboxes in freezer. Thaw on the bottom shelf of the fridge, not on a kitchen surface.

✓ To avoid nutritional discrepancies, vary the meats used each time and make sure to get the best spread of organs that you can.

✓ Active dogs need higher fat mixes.

✓ Overweight dogs need leaner mixes, not necessarily less food, and strict portion control.

CHAPTER 24

Raw FAQs

How much raw dog food do they need?

The average *adult* dog on an average-calorie, fresh meat diet will eat 2–2.5% of their body weight per day in fresh food. I tend to go with the latter figure intially, 2.5%. For example, an 8 kg adult Westie, might require 200 g of fresh dog food per day (1% of 8 kg is 80 g multiplied by 2.5). Of course, every dog is different so you need to keep an eye. If your dog is a little heavy or a bit lazy then you can either feed him a touch less (or choose leaner meal options). Well-exercised? Then, feed him a little more, but also increase the calorie content of the meal by including fattier cuts (dogs burn fat for energy). Working dogs can eat 3–5% of their body weight per day, depending on what you have them doing.

Pups differ greatly. The rule of thumb is that an 8-week-old pup will be eating up to 10% of his body weight per day, of a suitable puppy mix (a pup's food differs slightly to an adult's in that they need more fat). By the time they reach 50% of their adult body weight, they will be down to eating 5% of their body weight. By the time they reach full body size, they will be down to 3% of their body weight per day.

These sorts of percentages are general guides that will get you or your clients started and on which the dog won't go hungry. However, the exact results depend greatly on the type of food you are feeding. Obviously a lean mix offers less calories per kilo than a higher fat mix. For this reason, when assessing what a particular dogs energy needs it is better to talk on a calorie or resting energy requirement. The formula for your dog's Resting Energy Requirement (RER) is 70 x (your dog's body weight in kg) ^ 0.75. Once you have worked out your dog's RER, you can use the following multipliers depending on his physiological state (but know that two dogs of the same sex from the same litter with the same lifestyle can still differ in their ME requirements by up to 20%):

Average neutered adult	1.6
Average intact adult	1.8
Weight loss	1.2
Light work	2
Moderate work	3
Heavy work	5–6
Growth (<4 months old)	3
Growth (>4 months old)	2

For a more accurate assessment of a dog's needs, particularly puppies, please check out our free online calorie/food weight calculator on www.dogsfirst.ie.

How Do I Introduce Raw Food To A Dry-Fed Dog?

1. Introducing raw to a healthy dog

If this dog has been eating a dry diet for a long time, his stomach may now be somewhat conditioned to it. All that gurgling and squirting you hear before dinner is all their acids and enzymes being released into the gut in preparation for the largely plant-based meal. If you then lump a whole heap of raw dog food in there, you might get problems. Also, as we discussed in Section 1, dogs learn what foods are 'safe' from very early on in life. If they've never been offered fresh meat before, they might find it a bit unusual, certainly the texture but also the smell and could turn their nose away. We want to avoid this. As I like to say, the first time you have calamari, you don't want to see the squid. For both these reasons, I usually advise to introduce raw dog food (a meat you know they like) gradually, over the course of days, 5% raw mixed well into their usual fare one day, 10% the next, etc. Once they're doing the meat-boogie when the fridge opens, you know you have them. I would then starve them for a day and introduce their new raw dog food diet. I prefer this method, as it works for even the most cautionary of dogs.

At this point, the canine nutrition world is split down the middle as to what exactly is the best method of moving the average, healthy, robust dog over to fully raw. One option is the gradual approach. The other is to go cold turkey. Simply cut out their dry one day and getting straight into the raw the next.

However, this seemingly innocuous decision seems to have divided families and split nations. The concern is over the mixing of cereal-based dry food and raw meat. Here's the hypothesis – we have known for some time that the enzymes required to digest a raw meat and bone work better in an acidic environment. Saint-Hilaire et al. (1960)[1] found different foods stimulated a different amount of acid secretion in the gut of the dog. Meat, fish and dairy products stimulated the greatest secretion of acid (and hence resulted in the lowest pH) while fruits and cereals the least (and thus higher pH). Of all factors, protein was the most important acid-stimulating constituent in the foods tested. Numerous authors since have verified in dogs, that meat protein consumption stimulates the acid-secreting cells of the stomach to produce hydrochloric acid, which results in a noticeable drop in the stomach pH of the dog.[2-4] When the acidic chyme (food mixed with gastric juices) leaves the stomach and enters the small intestine, its acidity triggers the digestive process whereby bile is released from the liver and the correct digestive enzymes from the pancreas (those necessary for protein digestion).

Similarly, should a dog consume a cereal-based pet food, which is high in carbohydrates with some plant protein and little to no meat protein, the lack of protein would not induce such a concentration of gut acid, the pH does not drop as low and the higher pH of the acid chyme will trigger a different cascade of pancreatic enzymes less suitable to the digestion of any raw meat protein within.

The hypothesis goes, if fed together, the cereal-based kibble will slightly increase the pH of the dog's gut (likely) and this will negatively impact on the digestion of the meat protein present down the line (possible, though unproven). Partially digested protein may be passed into the intestines and disrupt the gut microflora balance, as we see in dogs with irritable bowel syndrome.

Incorrect digestion of protein aside, the concern is more for the potential partial digestion of any bone present, not to mention the fact pathogens may be lurking in the meat, pathogens that would have been destroyed in a lower acidity.

Numerous authors point to the protective effect of the low gut acidity in meat-eaters, acting as a barrier to a multitude of food-borne baddies.[5-9] That said, it seems many meat-borne pathogens that cause us concern, including *Salmonella, E. coli* and *Helicobacter pylori,* can circumvent the highly acidic conditions of a stomach. They have developed adaptive mechanisms that allow these bacteria to survive in acid environments and pass into the intestinal tract.[7] This explains why the more of these pathogens you feed to a raw-fed dog, the more they tend to excrete in the days afterwards as highlighted in Section 2.

On the differing digestion rates debate, little more is known. There are x-rays of the gut tract of dogs following a recent raw meat and bone meal (in this case, chicken leg) mixed with dry kibble that show the kibble passes through first (being carbohydrate based) with the meat portion of the chicken leg not far behind. The bone fragment is retained by the gut for hours after, as you would expect.

I have not encountered first-hand healthy dogs eating kibble with meat (introduced slowly) suffering as a result differing digestive rates, any more than I have seen or heard of such an issue in a human eating food of differing digestive rates, and we know dogs have far greater processing abilities. I'm sure someone will look into this shortly but until then, the matter remains an interesting hypothesis in dogs, not a theory and most certainly not a fact.

Still, as the hypothesis appears sound and as each dog is different, it would be remiss of us not to give it some consideration. Thus, for those doing the gradual introduction approach in a healthy, robust dog, it's best to use a minced, boneless raw meat product such as beef or turkey mince. Feel free to cook it as an extra precautionary step from a microbiological concern point of view. From then on, if you would like to mix dry with raw feeding, certainly if feeding meat on the bone, it would be best to do it in separate meals. If you detect digestive issues, you have a likely culprit.

2. Introducing raw to a picky dog

If you know you have a healthy but picky dog, you can slow it down even further by putting half a teaspoon of raw mince into a mug of hot water and using it like a light gravy over their normal food. Over time, you make your gravy meatier and meatier.

Despite your best efforts, in rare cases, you can have a dog that is hesitant (cats are notorious, they get hooked on the salt in dry food). One sure way to aid the transition is to employ a little cooking. Make a small patty out of their raw mix and cook it on the pan for a short amount of time, let's say 2 minutes each side. They will love this, as they have no doubt had cooked meat in the form of scraps and treats sometime in the past. Next time you cook it for 1 minute 50 seconds, cooking it less and less over time. To jazz this up even further, you can sprinkle a little salt on both sides, using less salt over time. Bold but so what, it's just a short transitional period. And dogs love it!

If you find yourself having to feed him from your hand, you know you've gone wrong somewhere. Dogs do not need this. It's incredible how well they can train us. You're moving into more of a behavioural issue at this point and less of a diet thing. To alter this behaviour, you need to change what you're giving them, change who feeds them, change where they're fed, put them in a room on their own or even move them to a friend's house for a few days (someone who doesn't fall for all their little cues).

3. Introducing raw to an unhealthy or gut-sick dog

If your previously dry-fed dog is suffering recurring gut issues (IBS/colitis type issues, recurring diarrhoea etc.), most likely from a food sensitivity, we take a little extra care moving them over to their new diet, in particular, if we suspect the gut is malfunctioning, perhaps in a state of 'leaky gut', where the gut has deteriorated to the point that little gaps have developed in the gut lining. This is dangerous as it may grant passage to not only partially digested food proteins, but also a myriad of bad bacteria that can be present in food. The body will thus elicit an appropriate immune response, which in itself can be quite detrimental to the animal in question.

To avoid this happening, we begin the gut-issue dog on bone broth made from a single animal protein (ideally one that has been determined to be safe by the owner or a food sensitivity test). The process of stewing bones in this manner extracts vital nutrients from bone and cartilage, notably collagen, proline, glycine, arginine and glutamine, which boost the immune system, reduce inflammation and are central to repair of the damaged gut lining. They also ensure a relatively inert food is being used, eliminating any threat of harmful bacteria.

To make your broth, simply pick up all the ingredients of one of the diets mentioned previously (the diet you will be using for the next few weeks). You need to use meat on the bone, so the likes of beef knuckles and pork trotters are excellent. If using poultry, it's best to buy a whole, organic turkey or duck and chop into lumps. However, I never start with chicken in a gut-sick dog as they can often be intolerant of it. So, try other meats first.

Put the meat and bone mix into a very large pot and cover with water. Add a dash of apple cider vinegar (helps leach the goodies from the bones) and leave on a low heat for 24 hours. Over time the fat will float to the top and the meat and bone will likely separate on the bottom. When cool, simply dump the cooked bones and the rest is your dog's dinner.

How much do you feed? Well, let him guide you. Start with the juice to ease him into it. He'll adore it. You'll have an idea of how much mix you used at the start. Let's say, 3 kg of meat and bone and vegetables. Assume 15% of it was bone, which you binned. So, you have around 2.5 kg of food there (exclude the water from your calculations).

To this diet I would always add canine probiotics to help restore their gut flora. Also, for bad cases, consider goat colostrum, the growth factors therein are excellent for ruined guts

After 4–8 weeks of broth, though many natural vets push bad cases up to 12 weeks, we begin to gradually move them onto raw by cooking the meat and bone soup less and less over time.

While this method is excellent for your gut-sick dog, many people use this method to move your average healthy or picky dog over, too. Whatever works for you!

For more on moving over gut-sick dogs or those suffering food intolerances please see www.dogsfirst.ie.

Do I Need to Supplement Their Fresh Mixes with Anything?

There are a couple of harder to find nutritional elements you might keep in mind. The National Research Council (NRC) tells us that dogs need a surprising amount of manganese, around 2.3 mg of manganese daily for every pound of dog food they eat (on a dry matter basis, NRC requirements). If we divide this figure by three (as fresh food contains say 65–80% water), that's still 0.7 mg of manganese per pound (454 g) of fresh raw dog food. However, meat, fat and bones do not offer anywhere near the degree of manganese that the dog requires. The highest amount of manganese in a meat source I could find was liver, where raw liver contains 0.35 mg of manganese per 100 g. Everything else paled in comparison, but this would mean you would have to feed 50% of raw liver to your dog each day, which would sicken him very quickly (the liver is a storage organ, avitaminosis is possible if you feed too much of it).

And yet, Dierenfeld *et al.* (2002)[10] showed us that the manganese needs of dogs and cats would likely be met by most *whole* prey. The problem is most of the manganese your dog or cat needs is in the hair, hide and feathers of the prey they consume. Hair is an excellent source of manganese, however indigestible it may be.[11] It is carnivore fibre and expected to help maintain the flow of digesta in intestines and may scour their intestinal tracts free of parasites. The problem is raw dog food manufacturers do not include this material in their mixes, whether out of ignorance of the issue at hand or the fact the market might view the sight of such material as penny pinching by the manufacturer.

For this reason, many premade raw mixes will be found very wanting for manganese. By far the best animal source of manganese I can see is mussels, which contain around 43 mg of manganese per 1,000 kcal. Best if you pick them up frozen in the supermarket, raw if you can though most are cooked. But don't worry manganese is fairly resistant to cooking. A mussel a day will supply him with not only enough manganese but some excellent quality fats, too. The second-best option is to pick up some mussels in a tin (best find the ones packed in freshwater or brine and pour off the excess juice. Though vegetable oil will do if there's no alternative, we just want to feed as little cooked vegetable oil as possible to dogs).

Other than that, raw spinach is just as good. However, spinach is also quite high in oxalic acid which, if used too much, can sort of cancel out the good effects. Sweet potato is another good plant source of manganese (with skin on, boil up some cubes and feed – great for fibre, too) although not everyone wants to give their dogs carbohydrates. Finally, I love pumpkin seeds as they're also anthelminthic, which means it keeps the worms away (blitz in a food processor).

Iodine is commonly low in raw dog food, which we have already dealt with in our piece on seaweed.

Another important ingredient mentioned above is CLA conjugated linoleic acid, which is commonly found in unpasteurised raw dairy (harder to find) but also grass-fed beef. Here in Ireland and the United Kingdom, grass-fed beef is the norm. However, in the United States the very large majority of beef is reared in concentrated animal feeding operations (CAFO's). These poor animals live a life on nutrient-poor grain and their meat will be lower in CLA as a result. If your dog is living on meat from these animals, you may need to go looking for some raw dairy or a decent CLA supplement. Most are made by chemically altering vegetable oils.

Finally, raw dog food is naturally low in salt, so an occasional pinch of good quality salt offers a great nutritional boost to the raw-fed dog. Also, don't forget my salt therapy tip in Section 2. Now and again, offer your dog a range of waters with some good quality salt in there. See what he selects.

Choosing a good premade raw food

The only thing dry has over raw is convenience. The number of meals being made in the US home today is steadily decreasing,[12] so you can see why dry food has gotten so popular. We are getting busier or food-lazy, most likely a bit of both. So premade raw products will play a large role in the feeding of dogs in the future. However, I will repeat the caveat – after years inside the industry, I can say with some authority that just because a raw dog food manufacturer is on the right side of the argument does not make them the good guys. Or even the knowledgeable guys, nutritionally speaking. There are plenty of bad products out there, with studies showing they, too, suffer nutrient imbalances.[13] That said, unlike dry pet food, premade raw have none of the body count. So, if using these products, always add in your own bits, and always vary your products of choice as often as possible to avoid the pitfalls.

The fact remains, like dry food companies, I have yet to meet a raw manufacturer using sirloin steak as the beef in their products. If they did, it would be five times the price. From that, the question becomes what bits *do* they use? In the poultry products – chicken, duck, turkey and wild game, the filler is always neck and carcass. These items cost the manufacturer around 30 cents per kilo when bought by the tonne. If they use largely this meat bone material, they will grind their product very finely, so you won't know by looking at it. Unfortunately, the producer is free to state 'duck' or 'chicken' on the label and not specify which part they use. This means you might be paying upward of €4 per kilo for a product worth a tenth of that, money that would have been far better spent, value-wise, on meat on the bone from the supermarket.

Dogs need that meat muscle. Unfortunately, there is nothing in place to prevent this. In the same way, some producers might state 'chicken legs and carcass' as their main ingredient. Again, they could buy a single tonne of legs a year to fulfil this promise. It wouldn't make much market sense for them to include a piece that is four times more expensive than the other if their clients won't know the difference. While most dogs do fine on such high-bone mixes, the risk is their clients might give the game away by pooing very firm, white bullets.

So, while I know lots of great raw dog food producers, I do want to instil caution. Trust nobody with the health of your pet. Here are some checks that can help you build trust with your producer and product of choice:

- Never buy a finely ground product. Ideally, it will be chunky so you can see the meat to fat to bone ratio with your own eyes. I trust what I see and *smell*.

- Fatty mixes are oily to the touch. To get an idea of the fat content of your meat mixes, take 100 g of their mix and place it in boiling water for 15 minutes (you're effectively rendering it). The fat will float to the top. Allow the mix to cool, scrape the fat off the top and weigh. It should correspond very roughly to what is written on the packet.

- Do the mixes contain everything in the right proportion? A good spread of organ meats? How much bone do they use? If they only use 10%, your dog is unlikely to become constipated. If they use vegetables, how much are they using?

- Find out who's behind your company. Do they look the part? Sound the part? Anyone with real dog experience there? Is there anyone credible associated with the company?

- Contact them. Are they open and friendly? You can get a great feel for a product just by getting them on the phone for 5 minutes.

- Google your company of choice. See who the directors are, try to find out a little info on them, they might be owned by a dry food company with a bad reputation.

- Ask them what meat pieces they use and who their suppliers are, then contact the supplier and ask where *their* meat comes from. Foreign meat can be run through two or three companies to cover its tracks. Neither is obliged to supply you with this information, but it says a bit if they don't.

Freezing Meat to Control Meat-Borne Parasites

Freezing first kills some parasites common in our meat chain, but not others. A common concern for new raw feeders is the consumption of raw pork by dogs, largely a result of the great fear we have of raw pork in the human food chain. However, pork is as clean as our other meats. Always has been, at least in Europe. In the United States they had an outbreak of *Trichinella spiralis,* a round worm that can cause all sorts of trouble in a human if ingested, and your dog, too, albeit examples are hard to find here. I can't find one example in a domestic dog. In their *Trichinellosis Fact Sheet* (CDC 2012) the US Centres for Disease Control and

Prevention report that this disease is now almost fully under control, with only twenty cases per year reported in Americans, and they eat a *lot* of pork. It's almost entirely absent in European meat.

Another concern with pork is the occurrence of toxoplasmosis.[14] Although this again is largely in American and Asian pork, significantly less so in European pork. It accounts for nearly a quarter of all US deaths from food-borne pathogens, sending 4,428 Americans to the hospital in 2017 and killing 327 of them.[15] A simple, single celled organism, it is an extremely successful parasite. While its primary host (the host in which the parasite matures and reproduces) is the cat, toxoplasmosis is known to thrive in numerous warm-blooded animals. Unfortunately, humans are a common secondary host (holding the parasite for a short, transitional period). Incredibly, 30–50% of the world's human population, largely in poorer regions, is estimated to carry a toxoplasma infection.[16] Infection is acquired by ingestion of viable tissue cysts in undercooked meat, poorly cured meats, contaminated water or oocytes excreted by cats that contaminate the environment. Initially, signs of infection are mild, perhaps some flu-like symptoms or, more often than not, no illness as all. Thereafter, the parasite rarely causes any symptoms in otherwise healthy adults. Unhealthy, immune-compromised individuals, however, such as those with AIDS or pregnant women, can suffer issues of the brain including encephalitis (swelling of the brain) and brain cancer, as well as causing numerous neurological illnesses such as depression, anxiety and schizophrenia. The brain is a popular organ for the parasite to set up home, although it can also affect most of the other organs too. A key part of the parasite's success is how it can affect the behaviour of its intermediate hosts, among which are rodents. Infected rats and mice are less fearful of cats, with some infected rats even seeking out cat-urine-marked areas,[17] which of course is advantageous to the parasite, as it can then fulfil its lifecycle.

A parasite very similar to *Toxoplasmosis gondii* is *Neospora caninum*, in that they share a similar form and, indeed, disease symptoms. In fact, until 1988, the two were assumed to be the same thing. However, an *N. caninum* infection can have a more severe impact on the dog's neurological and muscular system. A common parasite of wild canids (wolves and coyotes), *Neospora* can use cattle, sheep, goats, horses and deer as the intermediate host. Rarely will cattle exhibit issues, though abortion of the foetus is one symptom of a large infestation. Where dogs and cattle cohabit, transmission is possible through the contamination of infected meat. Mum can pass *Neospora* to her pups via the placenta.

If concerned about these potential meat baddies, the good news is that freezing meat first, from 2–3 days, depending on the bug, is highly likely to kill off all of the above parasites (Trichinella, Toxoplasmosis, Neospora) and it will also kill any worms present. Worms are common in fish and wild prey, but extremely rare in farmed land animals. Hence, anyone feeding US or Asian pork raw or raw fish, might consider this preventative step to sterilise their meat products.

However, please note that freezing is less effective on pathogenic bacteria. While it can reduce the numbers of *Campylobacter* over time, it will not safely eradicate them.[18] Freezing has no effect on pathogenic bacteria such as *E. coli*, *Salmonella* and *Listeria*, beyond putting them into stasis. Once that meat gets above 5° Celsius, they will happily bloom again. Only heat above 70°C for a set period of time or chemicals will kill these baddies.

Nor will freezing kill *Brucella suis*. Two years ago, a Dutch dog of unknown health status was infected with *Brucella suis*.[19] While this was not the first time this parasite had been detected in a dog,[20,21] it is the first time the issue was attributed to a meat source (in this case, the dog was fed *Brucella*-infected raw heads of Argentinian hares). The dog was first castrated (that's where the infection resided) but was euthanised two weeks later when he did not make a recovery. *Brucella suis*, particularly the biovars 1 and 3, are a relatively common zoonotic (will transfer from animal to human) species in the Americas. It can populate most livestock, usually swine and many wild animals, including rabbits, hare and deer. Europe has the biovar 2, which is considerably less pathogenic.[14]

Can you feed cooked home-prepared food?

Yes, absolutely. In fact, a recent, award-winning study found that some gut-sensitive dogs do better on a cooked meat diet than a raw. It's surely not as good nutritionally and a life of cooked meat is far from ideal but a diet using the ingredients above cooked at the lowest temperature possible, is very vastly superior to any dry, processed food pretending to use the same ingredients. In fact, as long as you don't overprocess it, very lightly cooked meat can be easier to digest as some of the bonds holding it together have been broken down pre-digestion. Pythons experience 13% lower costs of digestion when fed on lightly cooked meat instead of raw,[22] so the same should apply to dogs. So, don't be so hard on yourself. There is a lot of fear at the start, so do whatever makes you feel comfortable. When you're comfortable, you can start cooking it less and less. But remember don't give them cooked bone! If making home-prepared food and cooking it, you can only use boneless meats and add in eggshell, as mentioned previously.

What Should I Not Feed?

The following alphabetical list consists of things that REALLY should not be given to a dog. Their metabolism is a little different and this needs to be considered. Excluded from this list are coffee, alcohol, cigarettes and marijuana. While they may be bad (but fun) for humans, they are positively toxic to pets.

Chocolate: Unfortunately, chocolate is a definite no. This is due to theobromine and theophylline, which can be toxic to dogs, particularly dark chocolate. It can cause panting, vomiting and diarrhoea, as well as damage to a dog's heart and nervous system. Of course, we have all heard of a dog eating a whole box of chocolates and getting away with it, but the same box of chocs could kill another.

Cooked Bones: These are really bad for dogs. They can cause the cracking of teeth, perforated throats and intestines, as well as resulting in impaction.

Corn on the Cob: Cob pieces do not break down. If swallowed, they can easily get lodged in the small intestine causing issues.

Dental Sticks: Brought to you by the same companies that gave your dog the gum disease in the first place, the majority of these 'treats' have wheat gluten (or milk casein) as their number one ingredient, the most antigenic protein on earth for dogs. The third ingredient is sugar, the fourth salt, and the fifth is sugar again. For teeth! I strongly recommend removing these from the diet. Replace with fresh meaty bones. They're free and infinitely more nutritious.

Fat (too much of): Dogs can have the scraps of fat from the dinner table, that's fine, certainly for a raw-fed dog. Dry-fed dogs are a little different, however. As Section 1 showed us, we expect their pancreas to be under enormous pressure from trying to digest a diet of 50–60% carbohydrates every single meal and then produce enough insulin to balance the soaring blood sugars. With a dry-fed dog, the fat trimming from one steak can be enough to push this struggling pancreas over the edge.

Fresh Fish: Plenty of people feed their dogs fresh fish but it's probably not great practice. At least, the best advice is to freeze the fish first for a few days. Freezing kills any worms that can be present.

Grapes and Raisins: Grapes contain a toxin that can cause severe liver damage and kidney failure in dogs.

Human Multi-Vitamins: Often too high in the wrong things, do not give these to your dog. At any rate, fresh fed dogs don't need them. Dry-fed dogs might, but it would be far better to use something like kelp.

Macadamia Nuts: These contain a toxin that can inhibit locomotory activities in dogs resulting in weakness, panting, swollen limbs and tremors, as well as possible damage to the dog's digestive, nervous and muscle systems. Not good.

Milk from cows: Like 75% of humans on the planet after 2 years of age, dogs are intolerant to the lactose in milk. They simply don't retain the enzymes for milk digestion. It's not going to kill him as such, just block absorption of vital nutrients and minerals in him, and subject you to some smelly farts with the occasional bouts of diarrhoea.

Onions and Chives: No matter what form they're in (dry, raw, cooked, powder, within other foods), onions contain disulphides and sulfoxides (thiosulphate), both of which can cause anaemia and damage red blood cells in dogs.

Peaches and Plums (whole): Indigestible peach and plum pits often cause intestinal obstruction and enteritis in dogs. Avoid at all costs.

Pigs' ears & Raw Hide bones: As with many other cheap 'all-meat' pet treats, most notably raw hide chews (something akin to leather), most are imported from India and China where chemical use is highly questionable. These are meat-based pieces that are many months old, which have been sitting in a sweaty Perspex box in the pet shop for weeks, yet they don't decay… Since 2007, the Food and Drug Administration reports indicate imported pet treats (chicken, duck and sweet potato) from China have sickened many thousands of pets and in the decade from 2007 to 2016 killed 1,140 pets,[23] possibly as a result of antimicrobial and antiviral residues. The issue is still on-going.

Sweets: The real problem here is xylitol. While we are told it causes no apparent harm to humans, it is extremely toxic to dogs. Even small amounts can cause low blood sugar, seizures, liver failure or even a pup's death.

Raw-fed dogs will have different blood readings

Dogs consuming higher protein diets have elevated plasma urea nitrogen levels.[24] ANTECH Diagnostics® is the largest veterinary analytics company in the world, servicing more than 19,000 animal hospitals throughout North America, operates more than 50 reference laboratories in the United States and Canada and processes more than 45,000 samples a day. In 2003, ANTECH conducted a 'raw food diet study' where they compared 227 raw-fed dogs to 75 healthy adult dogs fed a commercial cereal-based diet. The raw-fed dogs exhibited statistically higher packed cell volume (haematocrit, i.e. the amount of red blood cells in the blood), higher blood urea nitrogen (BUN), (19.9 versus 15.5 mg/dL) and higher serum creatinine in some (1.20 versus 1.07 mg/dL). They conclude that dogs (with whom they call 'natural carnivores') fed raw meats have higher red blood cell and BUN levels than dogs fed cereal-based food. Thus, the normal reference values for dogs fed raw food diets should probably be revised.

Jean Dodds is a world-leading veterinary haematologist and immunologist. In 2005, she and Susan Wynn examined blood reference range differences between raw (n=227) and dry-fed (n=75) dogs over 9 months.[25] They found that raw-fed dogs had higher haematocrit (the measurement of the percentage of red blood cells in whole blood) than dry-fed dogs (51-53.5% versus 47.6%, in raw and dry-fed dogs, respectively). The accepted 'normal' haematocrit levels being 37-55%, though these figures arise from the study of dogs fed a low-protein, cereal-based dry food.

They further found that BUN, (a waste product derived from protein breakdown in the liver) was also higher in the raw-fed dogs (18.8-22.0 mg/dL versus 15.5 mg/dL, in raw and dry-fed dogs, respectively) with accepted norms (again for dry-fed dogs) being 6–24 mg/dL.

Finally, most raw-fed dogs had higher blood creatinine (also the result of protein deamination) than dry-fed dogs (1.20 mg/dL versus 1.07 mg/dL, for raw and dry-fed dogs, respectively) with accepted normal values in dry-fed dogs being 0.4–1.4 mg/dL.

BUN and creatinine are often expressed as a ratio of BUN/creatinine ratio, whereby an increasing ratio suggests protein building the blood. It is the primary test used to check how well the kidneys are functioning. When either or both levels are low, it can indicate inadequate protein intake or something more sinister such as liver damage. Increased levels can result from kidney issues, but also low water intake, poor digestion, intestinal bleeding, even heart failure and drug issues. This can indicate proteinuria (protein in the urine) and worsening kidney function. Or it may be simply that the animal is eating more protein so that the body is excreting more. In this case, raw-fed dogs typically had higher BUN because they were consuming more protein.

In the wrong hands, this blood work could be misinterpreted. A conventional vet might compare your raw-fed dog's blood results to the to accepted norms for dry-fed dogs consuming a diet low in protein and conclude that the higher blood protein is something more sinister.

Fasting dogs

Digesting food is hard work. It takes a lot of energy. This is why you want to fall asleep after you stuff your face at Christmas. All spare resources are directed to the gut to get the meal digested and absorbed. It's thought that if you don't eat for a prolonged period, the body will have more energy available to do other things such as repair, toxin removal and regeneration. Basic housekeeping really, that's the crux of it. Plus, the science is strongly in support.

While we are still only guessing at the exact processes involved, it is thought that during times of calorie restriction, the body goes through a detox program, killing off older or malfunctioning cells. This process of cellular cleansing is known as autophagy and stems from the Greek *auto* (self) and *phagein* (to eat). In 2016, Yoshinori Ohsumi won the Nobel Prize in medicine for discovering autophagy is switched on via nutrient deprivation. During this time, macrophage activity increases. Macrophages engulf and destroy bacteria, viruses and other foreign substances but they also ingest worn-out or abnormal body cells.

This process of housecleaning has enormous benefits for the body. A fascinating study in mice revealed that if you starve mice every other day but allow them to feed *ad lib* in the days in between, they are not only healthier but live longer. [26] In fact, when mice are starved for 48 hours before receiving a high dose of chemotherapy drugs, they are far more protected from harm.[27] Just one death occurred among 28 mice that had food withheld for 48 hours prior to receiving the drugs. The other 27 mice not only regained the weight they lost but showed no signs of any other side effects. In the control group that were not starved prior, only 17 of 37 survived the drug administration. These are startling results that have been replicated many times since.[28]

It's the reason you and almost every other animal on the planet is averse to eating when you're sick, your body is switching off hunger to divert its attentions to the front lines. A group of researchers set out to investigate the saying 'feed a cold, starve a fever'. Turns out it's spot on. The difference is down to whether you have a virus (cold) or a bacterial infection (fever). It seems in humans, while we stop eating when infected with either, we get back to eating quicker if it's a virus. To investigate this perspective, he injected mice with either a bacterial or viral infection and divided the mice into eating or fasting groups. Mice that ate with viral infections recovered faster. The mice that ate with a bacterial infection all died.[29]

Fasting may also boost recovery after acute spinal cord injury. Compared to controls, fasting rats with damaged spinal cords showed they recovered better, had smaller injury-site lesions, and increased neuronal regeneration over rats fed more liberally.[30]

Long-term diet restriction, where calorie consumption is slashed by 20–40%, has been shown to reduce cancer and cardiovascular disease in monkeys. In fact, the literature is rife with studies clearly indicating diet restriction and fasting is effective at preventing obesity, type-2 diabetes, inflammation, hypertension and atherosclerosis, as well as improving mental clarity and concentration in humans.

> …starvation for 48 hours or longer protects normal yeast and mammalian cells but not cancer cells from chemotherapy, an effect we termed Differential Stress Resistance (DSR). In a recent article, ten [human] patients who fasted in combination with chemotherapy, reported that fasting was not only feasible and safe but caused a reduction in a wide range of side effects accompanied by an apparently normal and possibly augmented chemotherapy efficacy…
>
> **Raffaghello et al., 2010**[31]

It's safe to say it's likely something you might consider in your dogs, too.

There are two ways to fast (you or them). One is the old-school whole day fast (two days in humans is even better. I did it a few times and you can taste the fruity ketones after 24 hours. Burn, baby burn!). In this case, quite simply, your dog won't get fed one day in a week, although he has full access to limitless fresh water. But he doesn't lose this food entirely. If your dog currently eats 1 kg of fresh, biologically appropriate raw dog food each day, then you would simply up their daily feed to 1.1 kg for 5 days, and then perhaps give them 1.25 kg either side of the fasting day. In this way, your dog is still getting everything he needs, you just displaced it a little to allow the fast to do its thing. And no, it doesn't matter the size or breed of dog, they're all the same on the inside.

The other way is even easier! A study in mice reveals that feeding them simply in line with their diurnal rhythm has positive net effects on their general health.[32] This, too, makes sense. Over the millennia, your internal computer has adapted to a morning and evening feeding pattern, typical of most group-living animals, and has developed mechanisms to switch off the apps it's not using during the day, diverting power to system maintenance, so to speak. Called intermittent fasting, the key, apparently, is to consume the two meals within 6–8 hours of each other. This gives the system 16–18 hours without food, which is the magic number for the body to go into ketosis (fat burning, which is good, but also that's where a lot of your toxins are stored).

In this way, the current trend is to move back from two meals per day (which I currently do) to one meal per day – evening is best (your liver works best at night, apparently). Of course, it's hard to enjoy your brekkie looking at his little face, so you won't be able to just cut his food out suddenly, one day. The trick is to reduce the size of the morning meal over time. In my head I have been mentally calculating how much longer Dudley might last on the planet and balancing it with not giving him his brekkie. I think if he could vote, he'd happily trade the few weeks or months.

It's important to note here that we are not talking about starvation. In fact, dogs are remarkably capable at going very, very long times without food. Back in the day when they could do horrific tests on dogs for the fun of it, scientists have on record dogs going more than 100 days without food, given adequate access to water, etc. So, don't worry, neither you nor your healthy adult dog will die for want of food over the course of the day. That said, please don't fast pups, dogs with diabetes, bitches in whelp or overweight cats (which can get fatty liver disease as a result).

Can my child get infected if my raw-fed dog licks them?

As Section 2 laid out, it seems today you and yours are statistically safer feeding your dog raw food than dry food. Perhaps owners who raw feed are, by necessity, better educated in canine nutrition having tended to do their own research online. In this manner they will have learned not just the benefits of fresh food but also its dangers, and will take appropriate steps to prevent contamination. Ensure hands, surfaces, bowls, feeding and toileting areas are regularly cleaned and sterilised. Make sure food is stored correctly and always, always pick up their poop. Daily.

Another feared, often cited but less likely, vector for infection is a dog licking his bottom and transmitting any germs there to his mouth, ready to lick your face and hands. However, Section 2 showed us the dog has an oral disinfectant built-in where a number of antibacterial factors ensure their mouths, outside of meal times, are significantly cleaner than yours. Throughout history, this has been taken advantage of, for instance, for cleaning wounds on battle fields. This implies that the dog's mouth is less likely to be a vector of disease. That said, 'don't snog the dog'. But then, you mightn't snog humans either! With nowhere near that level of protection in our oral cavity, many of our mouths are total jungles. It's estimated that there are over 100 million germs in every millilitre of saliva from more than 600 different species! Granted most are harmless, like the many sub-species of *Streptococcus* but in the right circumstances, we've all had throats infected by them. Then there's *Porphyromonas gingivalis* from periodontal (gum) diseases, as well as *Staphylococcus epidermidis* and a few *Lactobacillus*, depending on the individual and their oral hygiene. That's not to mention viruses like good old herpes simplex (cold sore) and his pal the human papillomavirus, as well as a few endearing fungal infections such as oral thrush (*Candida albicans*). So yeah, keep that in mind next time you meet your partner at the airport. Go for the hi-five maybe…Actually, don't get me started on fingers…

Raw feeding puppies

Correct puppy nutrition actually begins when they are developing in the womb. Mum and pups have never needed fresh ingredients more. A suggested pup diet is noted previously, but I wouldn't begin on this diet. Puppies should be moved to real food from weaning, which is at 3–4 weeks of age. For the first few days of the transition, it's thought the best meats to start with are plain, raw, boneless, white minces such as chicken, fish or turkey. Feel free to leave out a large meaty beef bone for them to gnaw on but make sure it is not small enough to chew. This will help grind down those jagged little puppy teeth that are hurting their jaw and ultimately destroying the furniture. After a couple of days of white meats, you're ready to move on to red minces (duck, beef, pork, organ meats) and these can contain ground bone, just like Mum would regurgitate. Of course, if you've got a teacup breed, you, may need to select a product where the bone content has been ground fine into a homogeneous mix. Most breeds will be eating meat on the bone by 6 weeks and onward.

How Much Raw Dog Food Do Puppies Need?

An 8-week-old puppy will eat 10% of his body weight per day in fresh food! When they reach 50% of their adult body weight, this drops to around 5% of their body weight per day and 3% by the time they reach full size. However, all dogs will differ depending on their expected adult size and growth rate. For a more accurate figure, see my online dog food calculator (www.dogsfirst.ie).

How often should pups be fed?

Most young pups are fed three to four times a day (I prefer the latter). Drop to three meals a day by 3 months. Aim to be feeding them two meals by 5–6 months. However, your breed can go through quite predictable growth spurts (ask your breeder or research your breed online) as hormones kick in at various ages. During this period, your pup will need extra feeding so don't be afraid to give them the odd extra meal here and there if you think they need it. After 6 months, many stay at two meals or drop to one meal a day, whatever works for you. They'll be happy with either, although there are the possible health benefits of occasional fasting linked to the longer periods of abstinence from food when only feeding once per day.

Feed puppies fresh bones for their teeth

Puppies will cut their baby teeth between 4 and 8 weeks old. They will cut lots of sharp little teeth poking out through their gums. It's sore. They need to chew things to relieve the pain. The best things for dogs to chew are fresh raw meaty bones (RMBs). Puppies will chew and get a bit of meat, but crucially bits of cartilage and bone with which they will build their own joints.

Perhaps the best bones for little puppies are big bones, so they can't really try and swallow them, just sort of gnaw at them. At 4–6 months, they will start teething their adult teeth. Very sore, and you will see a little red line above their teeth on the gum line indicating that. RMBs are even more important now, as the baby teeth need to be massaged out.

What about the calcium/phosphorus ratio?

Remember the line – how much calcium did you give your child growing up? They will get what they need from their diet. We don't recommend supplementing with calcium. It's a dark art, particularly in pregnant and nursing bitches. It can all be done with the diet but please get the hand of a good vet for your first rodeo.

Fortified milk mix for young pups

For the unfortunate situation where it is necessary to substitute the mother's milk, try the following. It's rocket fuel and they will LOVE it.

- One cup (250 ml) of goat's milk (never feed cow's milk)

- One can of evaporated milk (for energy)

- Tablespoon of probiotic yoghurt (for the gut)

- Two raw eggs

- Tablespoon of kelp (natural multivitamin and antioxidant)

- Optional: One or two teaspoons of coconut or almond oil

Raw feeding pregnant bitches

There is nothing overly complicated about raw feeding a pregnant bitch. Remember, what diet advice do pregnant human females receive? Little to none. Nonetheless, we naturally worry, so here are some tips to guide you through.

A well-balanced raw meal made with good, fresh, organic ingredients has everything she needs to build mini copies of herself; she will simply need more of it. A variety of ingredients is crucial during pregnancy to avoid nutritional discrepancies. Each meat offers a different amino acid profile, each organ a unique array of nutrient and bioactive compounds. Ingredients differ on where they grow, season, age at inclusion. Trust no single product or recipe to provide everything she needs, particularly as during pregnancy her nutrient needs fluctuate on a nearly daily basis. Variety, such as changing up your recipes each week, leads to balance over time (and has the added benefit of reducing future pickiness in pups!).

For the first half of the pregnancy, nothing much will change for Mum and she will eat as normal. Many breeders like to use a touch more heart muscle which can be higher in folic acid, but I suspect this is a human concern pushed on dogs. It's no harm, anyway. I would turbocharge my recipes with all the usuals, including some raw eggs, some good seaweed, some fish oil (with no added vitamin A), some frozen mussels (for manganese) and a handful of blueberries here and there (antioxidants).

As always, she needs access to fresh, chlorine-free water. Also, don't forget the "salt therapy" tip we spoke of in Section 2. Raw dog food is naturally low in salt.

A little good quality salt (anything with a name, not the refined stuff) dissolved in a separate water bowl offers harder to find minerals such as potassium and magnesium. Let her take what electrolytes she needs.

By week 5, start to increase the quantity fed to her. The general rule is that by week 6 food will have increased by 5–10%, by week 7 it will have increased by another 5–10%, by week eight it will have increased by another 5–10%, depending on what you think she needs.

By week 6, I would start to accommodate the lessening space by feeding her smaller meals more often. She can move from two to three and even up to five meals a day, whatever works.

I would also be moving to slightly higher-fat mixes (simply swapping out some of her usual diet for high-fat beef mince is an easy way to do it), certainly in the latter stages: less space, more oomf per gram.

Online you will see mentioned the importance of dropping the bone content, beginning around week 6 and dropping to nil in the week before the pups are born. There are two reasons cited for this. The first is we don't want her constipated. This is understandable although well-made raw diets shouldn't constipate. The second is a fear that too much calcium can negatively affect her pregnancy. Calcium is stored in the bones. Before birth, the parathyroid pulls calcium from the bones to help form the skeletons of the new pups but also to increase the contractibility of heart and uterine walls. The concern, it seems, is that feeding too much calcium now can play havoc with this system. However, support from the literature here is sadly lacking, certainly in dogs provided real food consuming calcium in its natural state. As we showed in Section 2, the body does not metabolise natural and supplemented calcium the same way.

However, as a non-vet, I cannot advise in such matters. Personally, I aim for a happy medium until more is known in raw fed dogs. In the latter half of pregnancy, I feed ground, premades to reduce the workload on the stomach. I reduce the bone content down to around 5% by adding boneless meats to her regular food in week 7 and 8, and by week nine, she is eating nearly bone free. Crucially, post-birth, you ramp back up the calcium fed via her meals but also by offering extra RMBs. Milk production is a significant draw on calcium stores, so let her take what she needs. A lack of calcium in the brood bitch can result in eclampsia (seizures), something you don't want to experience.

What we do absolutely know is to never ever feed calcium supplements to your pregnant bitch unless under the guidance of a good vet.

By week 8, she may be consuming up to 50% more food than she was pre-pregnancy. By week 9, she will begin to eat less, so gradually reduce the amount of food offered. A day or two before birth, some bitches will stop eating altogether. Don't worry, you have given them lots of reserves to draw upon.

Just before birth, Dr Ian Billinghurst, author of *Give Your Dog a Bone*, recommends increasing the amount of cooked vegetable matter offered. This has a laxative effect on the dog, allowing her to more fully vacate her bowels, facilitating more space for the pups and contributing toward a more comfortable birth. This can be achieved with cooked and mashed greens or sweet potato with the skin on.

Post birth, she should be fed ad-lib, as much as she needs over the next 3–4 weeks until the puppies are weaned, at which point you begin to reduce the amount of food offered which will, in turn begin to turn off the milk. Dr Billinghurst further recommends a great smoothie for Mums in the week or two post-birth. I have tweaked it below:

- 1 cup of whole goat milk

- 1 teaspoon of raw honey

- 2 teaspoons of fish oil (containing no added vitamins!)

- 1 raw egg

- Half a teaspoon of seaweed (if not in her food!)

- A little pinch of fenugreek and milk thistle (stimulates milk production)

Can I feed my dog a vegetarian/vegan diet?

This is an interesting and hotly debated topic. First, it is entirely possible to formulate a vegan or vegetarian kibbled diet for dogs and cats without using meat, just another one of the many issues with the The Association of American Feed Control Officials (AAFCO) nutritional profile.

> …Canine vegetarian dry and wet diets are formulated to meet the nutritional levels established by the AAFCO Dog Food Nutrient Profiles for maintenance…
>
> **Royal Canin in email correspondence to Knight and Leitsberger,**
> **2016**

...The nutritional adequacy of our [vegetarian] products is fundamental. We ensure this through formulation, feeding trials, and strict manufacturing processes. We meet or exceed every major food quality and safety standard, including those issued by the FDA, USDA, AAFCO and FEDIAF...

Nestlé Purina in email correspondence to Knight and Leitsberger, 2016

Knight and Leitsberger (2016)[32] note that it was not clear from these statements if the manufacturers actually conducted the AAFCO feed trials with their products. V-Dog in the US admitted to not doing so, instead citing they've 'been in business eleven years and have *seen* thousands of dogs thrive into their golden years'. Another vegan pet food company apparently conducted 'home-feeding studies' which involved surveys of customers and aimed to assess the performance of their products in an 'actual home environment'. The participants were given free samples of their products in return for taking part.

We also know that many of these diets will suffer the same nutritional concerns as their cereal-and-meat-based counterparts. Kienzle and Engelhard (2001)[33] studied 86 vegetarian dogs and eight vegetarian cats in Germany, Switzerland and Belgium. The authors, using the AAFCO feed guidelines, were only able to recommend two without reservation. Gray *et al.* (2004)[34] analysed Evolution canned complete diet for adult cats and found it to be deficient in taurine, methionine and arachidonic acid as well as deficient in several B vitamins, retinol, calcium, phosphorus and overall protein. Kanakubo *et al.* (2015)[35] examined 13 dry and 11 canned vegetarian diets for dogs and cats. They found 25% did not meet all AA minimum requirements for the animal in question.

That said, Section 2 showed us that cereal-based pet food fails just as much, if not more so, to meet the minimum targets they set for themselves (94% of the 'complete' canned food and 62% of the 'complete' dry foods sold in the UK were not compliant with European Pet Food Industry Federation/ AAFCO guidelines). In this way, studies suggest that vegetarian pet foods can certainly compete well enough with cereal-based pet foods containing a token amount of meat meal. Semp (2014)[36] followed 20 dogs and 15 indoor cats fed a vegan diet. Participating dogs had eaten vegan diets from 6 months to 7 years, with a mean of 2.83 years. Animals were subject to clinical examination (including general appearance, body condition, skin and coat, lymph nodes, defecation and vital signs including cardiovascular, respiratory and digestive systems) and no abnormalities were detected.

Blood trials were also conducted by Semp, including measures of the liver, kidney and pancreas and evaluation of magnesium, calcium, iron, total protein, folic acid, vitamin B_{12} and L-carnitine levels. The 20 vegetarian dogs compared favourably to 20 'healthy' dogs fed a conventional, dry, cereal-based pet food. They found the following:

- 5/20 (25%) vegan-fed dogs were outside the reference range (RR) for vitamin B_{12}, compared to 7/20 (35%) of conventionally fed dogs.

- 2/19 (11%) vegan-fed dogs were outside the RR for iron, compared to 5/20 (25%) of conventionally fed dogs.

- All vegan-fed dogs had adequate protein, 2/20 (10%) of conventionally fed dogs did not.

- 5/17 (30%) vegan-fed dogs were outside the RR for folic acid, compared to 5/20 (25%) of conventionally fed dogs.

- 3/7 (43%) were outside the RR for L-carnitine, compared to 12/20 of conventionally fed dogs (60%).

Interestingly, when vegan-fed cats were compared to cats fed conventional dry food, only 1/15 cats were outside the RR for vitamin B_{12}, compared to just 10/20 (50%) of conventionally fed cats and only 1/15 vegan cats were outside the RR for iron, compared to a whopping 13/30 (65%) of conventionally fed cats, although the dry-fed cats did do better on folic acid (the only statistically relevant finding $p<0.001$).

All these numbers were too small to attach any real statistical value but the findings are interesting inso far as both products were equally poor at providing the pet with what it needs each day from conventional diets, outside of folic acid in cats appearing consistently, but not significantly, worse in terms of bloodwork. Indeed, this finding has been echoed by other authors comparing the bloodwork of populations of cats fed conventional or vegetarian/vegan dry food.[41]

Brown *et al.* (2009)[37] did an interesting, albeit small, study of 12 racing Siberian Huskies fed either a commercial diet (containing 43% poultry meal, recommended for active dogs, n = 6) or a meat-free diet (where the meal was replaced with maize gluten and soybean meal, n = 6). All dogs were kept on these diets for 16 weeks, which included 10 weeks of competitive racing, with intermittent health checks and bloodwork, all of which were conducted by a veterinarian blind to the dietary regimens. Haematology results for all dogs, irrespective of diet, were within normal range throughout the study and the consulting veterinarian assessed all dogs to be in 'excellent physical condition'.

Thus, depending on your opinion of the AAFCO feed guidelines, your need for evidence and indeed approach to pet nutrition as a whole, it seems vegetarian/ vegan pet foods, formulated on the best plant ingredients, can at least compete with cereal-based food containing some meat meal. But surely this should be no surprise. Often with no more than 4–10% meat meal, the latter are actually as close to being vegetarian as you're likely to get. In fact, it could be argued your dog would be better off not getting that antigenic powder in there in the first place.

On this I can say little more, except that I'm a vegetarian and would dearly love to read a study, conducted over years, that compares a large group of dogs fed a vegetarian diet to a large group fed a fresh meat-based diet. A study that covers the effects of such diets on pregnant bitches, pup growth, joint soundness, body mass index, behaviour, gut flora, general health and, crucially, longevity. This however is unlikely to materialise, considering the resources necessary for such a trial. Until then, it is our obligation to ensure the animals in our charge are cared for adequately. It is my opinion, considering the vast importance of meat that goes far beyond the nutrients considered in the AAFCO feed profile, it is currently neither possible nor advisable to feed a meat-eating animal a vegetarian/vegan product to dogs long term. For maximum health benefit, we must them the food they evolved upon. For dogs, this means fresh meat and bone. If this jars with your principles, please reconsider the pet you share your home with in the future.

The future of dogs, pet food and our planet

As the market continues to move toward fresh ingredients, there will come a tipping point when multinationals will weigh up the financial cost of putting out the wrong message and not being involved in the right side of the argument. At this point, inevitably, they will use their endless resources and start buying out small fresh food brands, obtaining not only their product but also the hard-earned customer's trust and loyalty. Initially, you may not even notice the change.

For a while, this move will be good news for dogs. Colossal advertising budgets will result in ads reading, '…after many years of (marketing) research, we at X have uncovered the fact that cats and dogs *may* actually benefit from eating fresh ingredients…'. Millions of dogs will be converted to a fresh diet. The business will boom, and millions of dogs will be better off.

That's the good news. The bad news is that these companies must return a profit year-on-year. One way to do this is to sell more. Once the initial surge to fresh is over you, can expect these companies to begin to make cost savings. The quality of the ingredients will be the first to fall. As most of these products will be meat, that means cleverer and cleverer ways to use poor-quality meat in their mixes. Using carcass would be one familiar way. Although I fear another would be to exploit the cheaper meat from countries with less stringent animal welfare laws. This is as sad as it is unavoidable in a capitalist world.

But millions of dogs converting to their appropriate diet calls forth a bigger problem and that is, the more we feed dogs biologically appropriate food, the greater our impact on global warming.

As stated earlier, I don't eat meat. It's not right to pen up a beautiful, smart, sentient animal in deplorable conditions for the entirety of its all-too-short life and then kill him, often barbarically, so you can spend 30 seconds eating a cheap beef burger, tasty as they are.

But let's park the welfare debate for a moment. They tried that. It's now so safely tucked behind closed doors that that message clearly does not work on the masses. Another great reason for humans not to eat meat is health, certainly red meat, cooked meat and processed meat.

Yet another reason rising to prominence above the other two is that meat is not working out for us on a global warming front. Not unlike bacteria in a jar, the human population continues to grow, consuming everything in its path and spewing out waste behind it. We simply cannot continue on the mindless consumption track we are currently pursuing. And of all sectors, meat is possibly the worst offender in terms of carbon output.

The beef sector alone produces more harmful gases than the ENTIRE transport industry, cars, planes, trains, etc.,[38] which surprises many. As Asia slowly turns to the Western diet, there isn't enough agricultural land space available to produce the cereal the cattle would need to be fed on. Not even today, let alone in 30 years when the human population is set to increase by 30%.

Now, a bit of math to put it all in context...

Dogs are predators, top of the pyramid. As such, there wouldn't normally be a lot of them around, as they are energetically very expensive animals to feed, compared to say herbivores. It's how a feeding niche works. As there's only so much meat to go around, to compensate, carnivores always have large home ranges. Take little old Ireland, an island of only 84,000km^2. Given free run of the place and considering all our other little predators need to get fed also, we'd normally be able to accommodate little more than 3,000 wild dogs (based on the very approximate figures that a 10–30 strong pack of African wild dogs on the Serengeti requires 1,500km^2, this equates to Ireland housing 56 packs of 20 dogs). Instead, we are home to 300,000 dogs.

Dudley, my cocker spaniel, weighs 12.5 kg and eats 400 g of meat per day. If he lives for 15 years, he is going to be responsible for the deaths of more than 1,100 chickens. The average weight of a live chicken at 47 days is 2.6 kg, the dressed weight being around 2 kg and your dog can eat all of it. The average Labrador will need close to 3,000 chickens in their lifetime.

Now let's scale it up a bit. On top of the 300,000 dogs in Ireland, there are 8 million in the United Kingdom and 70 million pet dogs in the United States. If we add in the rest of the countries we have information on, including Australia (4 million), Colombia (5 million), Canada (6 million), Argentina (7 million), Japan (10 million), Brazil (30 million), mainland Europe (35 million), China (110 million) and Africa (140 million, half of which are strays), it adds up to more than 500,000,000 – half a billion dogs on the planet. And all these dogs need meat.

If the average weight of a dog from these three countries is 16.5 kg (average based on the top 50 breeds) and that average dog requires 663 g of meat and bone per day, then that's 330 million tonnes of meat needed per day to feed them, close to 120 billion tonnes per year. In chickens alone, it equates to 60 billion chickens. And in 2002, The Food and Agriculture Organisation of the United Nations estimated we had 15.8 billion chickens on the planet.

So, there's that.

Of course, not all dogs will get this diet, which is sad but also inevitable. You could also say that they are eating the scraps of the industry but…(1) that's no longer really true, certainly with the advent of decent raw dog foods, and (2) even if they did, they are simply providing a valuable outlet for this material. This will, in fact, cheapen the rest of the carcass. Farmers only need so much for the animal to be competitive, meaning meat prices will fall, and the human market will consume more.

Now let's talk about meat choices. Of all meats, beef is the worst, by a significant degree. As mentioned earlier, it produces more harmful gases than the ENTIRE transport industry. In their review of the available literature on the subject,

Desjardins *et al.* (2012)[39] found that the total carbon footprint for the average cow, including cow farts, the cost of their feeding, housing and slaughtering is between 8 kg and 22 kg CO_2 per kg of live weight, depending on how and where the animal was reared. The average live weight of a cow is 600 kg. So, the average cow, from birth to supermarket shelf, will put out between 4.8 tonnes (8 x 600 kg) and 13.2 tonnes of CO_2 in her lifetime, give or take.

To give this figure some context, compare it to the average family saloon car, which puts out 1.56 tonnes of CO_2 per year (a new car today of average efficiency is putting out around 130 g of CO_2 per kilometre and the average car in the European Union does around 12,000 km per year).

While 2010 was the year that we surpassed one billion cars on the road,[30] at the same time we had 1.4 billion cows on the planet,[31] equating to somewhere between 6.7 billion and 18.5 billion tonnes of CO_2 from the beef sector alone.

> …Livestock-based food production…causes about one-fifth of global greenhouse gas emissions, is the key land user and source of water pollution by nutrient overabundance…
>
> **Eshel *et al.*, (2014)[36]**

And so far, we've just been talking beef and we've only mentioned carbon dioxide. We're not even going to touch upon methane and nitrous oxide, which, while making up a lesser quantity, cause significantly greater damage. Nor discuss the effects of the vast quantities of pesticides and chemical fertilisers used to grow the corn we feed the livestock on.

Then there's the untreated waste. Pound for pound, a pig produces four times the waste of a human. And we don't flush it through our sewerage system.

> Depending on the type and number of animals in the farm, manure production can range between 2,800 tons and 1.6 million tons a year (Government Accountability Office [GAO], 2008). Large farms can produce more waste than some US cities—a feeding operation with 800,000 pigs could produce over 1.6 million tons of waste a year. That amount is one and a half times more than the annual sanitary waste produced by the city of Philadelphia, Pennsylvania (GAO, 2008). Annually, it is estimated that livestock animals in the US produce each year somewhere between 3 and 20 times more manure than people in the US produce, or as much as 1.2–1.37 billion tons of waste (EPA, 2005).

Though sewage treatment plants are required for human waste, no such treatment facility exists for livestock waste.

CDC, 2010[41]

Their untreated effluent leaks out of the deplorable concentrated animal feeding operation (CAFO's) where 90% of American beef and pork comes from) in which they are reared and into our ground water, causing dead zones in our oceans.

…Somewhere in Iowa, a pig is being raised in a confined pen, packed in so tightly with other swine that their curly tails have been chopped off so they won't bite one another. To prevent him from getting sick in such close quarters, he is dosed with antibiotics. The waste produced by the pig and his thousands of pen mates on the factory farm where they live goes into manure lagoons that blanket neighbouring communities with air pollution and a stomach-churning stench. Fed on American corn that was grown with the help of government subsidies and millions of tonnes of chemical fertiliser, when the pig is slaughtered, at about 5 months of age, he'll become sausage or bacon that will sell cheap, feeding an American addiction to meat that has contributed to an obesity epidemic currently afflicting more than two-thirds of the population. And when the rains come, the excess fertiliser that coaxed so much corn from the ground will be washed into the Mississippi River and down into the Gulf of Mexico, where it will help kill fish for miles and miles around. That's the state of your bacon circa 2009…

Getting Real About the High Price of Cheap Food **Time Magazine, Friday, August 21, 2009**

Intensively farmed meat is an environmental catastrophe on many levels, but for now let's come back to the CO_2 cost of our dogs. My cocker Dudley eats 400 g of fresh food a day, most of which is meat. His current diet is approximately half chicken, one-quarter duck and one-quarter beef. At the finished product level, wrapped and on the shelf, the best per kilo CO_2 cost estimates for 1 kg of EU beef is around 21–28 kg of CO_2, 19-28 kg per 1 kg of EU sheep and goat, with non-ruminants like pork (7–10 kg) and poultry meat (5–7 kg) much lower, though they are higher in other things. This equates to an average of 13 kg of CO_2 per kilo of Duds' diet. Or in essence Duds diet is costing the planet 5.2 kg of CO_2 per day or 1.9 tonnes of CO_2 per year. Remember the family car is putting out 1.56 tonnes of CO_2 per year. Thus, if you own a medium sized dog of 16.5 kg then they are the equivalent of almost two saloon cars on the road per year. Own a 40-kg Shepherd? It's the equivalent of three extra cars on the road…

As of 2012, the total world energy related CO_2 emissions from the total burning of gas, petrol and coal were 32.3 billion tonnes of CO_2 per year.[41] If the half a billion dogs were all lucky enough to eat like Dudley, that would equate to perhaps 1.56 trillion tonnes of CO_2 per year, or forty-eight times the TOTAL CO_2 emissions from electricity and heat production for the entire planet.

If we cautiously assume that we as a race cannot regress further and keep animals in any worse conditions than they are currently suffering, then I think it's pretty clear that something has to give.

One thing might be to eliminate red meat, particularly beef, from their diet (and indeed, ours). More than any other meat, beef has a colossal carbon footprint. As we highlighted previously, one cow is a saloon car on the road for four years. Everyone is focusing on the one billion cars on our roads and yet we have 1.4 billion cows walking the planet. Simply stopping eating beef will decrease your carbon footprint in the quickest, easiest and most earth friendly way possible.

> …the environmental costs per calorie consumed of dairy, poultry, pork, and eggs are mutually comparable (to within a factor of 2), but strikingly lower than the impacts of beef. Beef production requires 28, 11 and 5 times more land, irrigation and water, respectively, than the average of the other livestock categories…
>
> **Eshel *et al.,* (2014)**[40]

Thus, not feeding them beef is one very likely option. Another is that we do not feed dogs as carnivores at all and incorporate some more plant additions. Studies show that greenhouse gas emissions (measured in kilos of carbon dioxide per day) for meat-eating humans are approximately twice those for vegetarians.

5.63 for medium meat-eaters (50–99 g/d)

4.67 for low meat-eaters (< 50 g/d)

3.91 for fish-eaters

3.81 for vegetarians and

2.89 for vegans.

Scarborough *et al.,* (2014)[42]

If it was an immediate solution we needed, slightly increasing plant material and removing beef dog food is certainly a more likely option than trying to tell a dog owner to stop owning dogs, which I imagine might be as calm and productive as debating the need for automatic rifles with the American National Rifles Association. The problem is, even at 50% plant material and 50% carbon-cost in meat choices, half a billion dogs still increase the earth's total output of CO_2 by multiples.

Starting to feel depressed? Me, too.

Two bits of good-ish news. Firstly, ruminants are actually a very necessary part of the environment. Their grazing and manure enrich environments and organic farms absolutely need them around–just not in the numbers we are currently cramming into filthy, hot, infected barns worldwide. So, there will always be some meat available.

Another option I can see is the advancements in lab-grown meat, a process that has already begun. There exists today, chicken nuggets from chickens that are still walking around, healthy as ever. This is not GMO meat. It is the same meat you would find in that chicken, only the cells are replicated in a nutrient-dense, plant-based liquid, as opposed to a nutrient dense animal body. The growing cells know no different. Nutritionally, we would expect this meat to be identical. While still cost prohibitive, in the near future the need for meat substitutes will drive this industry forward at a rapid rate. If this is what the market needs to wean themselves off meat, then I'm all for it.

Until then, my prediction for dog food and, indeed, dog ownership is the following:

For reasons of welfare, health and now global warming, and driven by online influencers, it seems meat consumption has now hopefully peaked in the West. Vegetarianism and veganism are now advancing rapidly, at least across Europe and North America and these areas still tend to set global trends. For instance, by 2016 Britain's vegan population had increased from 150,000 to 542,000 in the space of a decade (alongside a vegetarian population of 1.14 million) and that figure is increasing rapidly.[43] Canada is eating significantly less red meat, replacing it with chicken. Over the last three decades, beef and pork consumption by Canadians has been consistently steadily declining, from 39 kg and 32 kg per year respectively, to 27 kg and 22 kg by 2013. Demoskop in Sweden randomly polled 1,000 Swedes and found 1-in-10 are vegetarian or vegan. Hence, it was the country of choice for McDonald's to trial their new vegan burger patty.

Sales of meat and dairy alternatives are exploding. This effect will be magnified when carbon tax eventually comes in and they penalise industry and consumers for poor carbon choices. At this point, meat consumption by humans is undoubtedly going to go the way of cereal-based pet food. This is good news, as up and coming mega-societies in Asia, where the great majority of the world's population lives, generally copy what the richest societies are doing, at least diet wise. Just as we see now, with Asia, sadly, copying American diets. Pet owners who wish to feed their pets appropriately will be faced with a big cost-based, financial and now environmental dilemma. For these reasons, we can expect dog size and, indeed, numbers to decrease in the future. It's likely that having a large group of six German Shepherds walking around your house *just because you can* might become a luxury of only the super-rich and the occasional drug dealer, putting it on par socially with someone burning trash in their back garden.

But don't worry, on a slightly more positive note, the good news is we're always likely to have them around. We are learning that food waste adds a great deal to our carbon footprint, not only in food wasted by processors/manufacturers (They only send the perfect looking fruits and vegetables to be sold!), supermarkets and restaurants but in our own homes. We have until recently been putting our food waste in the garbage. This goes to landfill where it decomposes, adding more harmful greenhouse gases to the atmosphere. We must dispose of our food waste correctly, which means using a compost bin where it can go to become energy for fertiliser. We can also put some of it – any of our unused meat (the industry is not going away from a very long time, if at all as ruminants play a role in organic farming) and most of our vegetables ingredients left over from dinner (please do not use decomposing vegetables in dogs) in the dog. We know they love our scraps and if it remains only a small portion of an overall good diet, it's yet another reason to have them around.

We are now all beginning in earnest to assess our own impacts on the planet. In this way, I urge raw-fed dog owners to become as environmentally friendly as possible. Buy the most ethically sourced meat you can afford. Buy organic and address your own meat consumption. Support pet food companies trying to make a difference. Wash plastic wrappers and bring them to your local recycling depot. Force companies to use compostable packaging by shunning those that make no effort. Stop buying one-use plastic food items and pick plastic up from the beach. Shop locally and grow your own food. We raw feeders must make something good of this situation we find ourselves in.

In the meantime, I am kept awake at night. I love animals and worry incessantly about the general decline of their welfare and, indeed, their decreasing numbers in the wild, in the path of the relentless juggernaut of human progress. But of all of species on earth, I love dogs the most. When I started out, I meant for this book to help as many of them as possible. But 10 years on, when I sit back and reflect, here I am, a vegetarian who is inadvertently but significantly increasing the amount of meat consumed by both dogs and humans worldwide, to the great detriment of the animals supplying it, the humans eating it and the planet that produced it.

Much like the slight unease I now feel on a nice, warm day, I often find myself looking at my beloved Dudley, wondering if my kids will experience the utter joy of sharing a home with another dog after he's gone.

TAKE-HOME POINTS

✓ On average, dogs need 2–2.5% of their body weight per day in raw dog food.

✓ Pups need much more. An 8-week-old pup will be consuming 10% of his body weight per day of raw dog food over four meals, 5% of his body weight by 6-months and 3% of his body weight by 12-months, although this varies greatly with the size of the dog. Check with the calculator on dogsfirst.ie.

✓ There are two ways to introduce raw dog food – quickly (skip a meal or two for an adult dog and move him straight over) or gradually (slowly decrease the amount of dry and increase the amount of raw over the course of days). The latter should help picky eaters, but some hypothesise it might result in an increase in gut acid pH, potentially resulting in indigested protein or, worse still, bone entering the intestines. While the hypothesis appears sound, in thousands of dogs I have yet to hear of such an issue. But how well have I been looking?!

✓ For picky dogs make a raw meat gravy and pour some on their favourite food. Increase the meat dosage each time. Or make a burger, cook each side and sprinkle with salt. Decrease cooking time and salt over days.

✓ If moving gut-sick dogs to raw, always begin with broth. Don't forget to remove the cooked bones. Add probiotics and colostrum for bad cases.

✓ Any raw mixes without hair or feathers, etc., needs manganese supplementation. A bag of frozen mussels is great here, a pinch of good-quality seaweed for iodine. Finally, dogs need the fatty acid CLA in their diet. Lastly, consider a pinch of good quality salt.

✓ Like the changing of the tides, you can count on the fact there will be bad raw manufacturers. Many grind carcasses and sell this to you as chicken or turkey, etc. It's likely to be ground finely, so you can't see what you are getting. Another issue is very high fat mixes (typical with the red meats such as beef, pork and lamb where the meat muscle is sold to humans for higher prices).

✓ Tips for picking a good supplier include the following: Who are they? Can you talk to them? Where do they get their meats? What does the meat smell like? How is your dog's stool?

✓ Freezing for 2–3 days kills some parasites, certainly worms and their eggs but also single celled organisms such as toxoplasma. However, it's less effective for pathogenic bacteria. It will reduce *Campylobacter* but will have no effect on *E. coli*, *Salmonella* and *Listeria*.

✓ It is ok to feed a lightly cooked home-prepared diet.

✓ Don't feed dogs chocolate, cooked bones, corn on the cob, dental sticks, fresh fish, grapes or raisins, macadamia nuts, milk from cows, onions, peaches and plums with stones, pigs ears, raw-hide from pet shops.

✓ Raw-fed dogs have elevated plasma urea nitrogen, haematocrit and creatinine levels than dogs fed cereal-based pet food, as they are receiving more protein in their diet. Make sure your vet understands this when reading your dog's blood levels.

✓ Studies show fasting now and again has major health benefits, many stemming from the fact your body goes into autophagy once it is no longer assimilating food. Your body likely knows this and turns off your hunger during sicknesses, such as infections. Fasting also boosts recovery from injury, and is beneficial for cancer, obesity, diabetes and hypertension.

✓ Intermittent fasting, is when your days meals are all consumed within 6–8 hours. Hence one meal a day for the average adult dog might be best. If your dog receives two meals and you wish to change to one meal a day, simply reduce the size of one meal (the morning one, preferably) and increase the evening feed over time.

✓ Poo is the most likely vector of disease, so please pick it up regularly. Thanks to a range of built-in oral disinfectants, a dog's lick is less of a concern. It's certainly cleaner than yours. Do not allow your dog to lick you or your children soon after a raw meat meal.

✓ Pups can be weaned to raw meat from week 3. Begin with plain, boneless white meats and leave a large beef bone out for them to explore and chew. By week 4 they can be moved on to bone-containing pre-made raw dog foods (and maybe begin with the more finely ground products first).

✓ Feed pups as you would adults, although maybe increase the fat content a little. An 8-week-old puppy will eat 10% of his body weight per day in fresh food (over four meals). When they reach 50% of their adult body weight, this drops to around 5% of their body weight per day (over two meals) and 3% by the time they reach full size. These figures vary with dog size. Give them regular RMBs.

✓ Pregnant bitches should be fed as normal until week 5 when you increase the amount offered by 20–30%. Week 6 start upping the fat content as available space decreases. Start reducing the bone content in week 8, she may be eating 50% more, spread over more meals. Bone content should be close to nil. In week 9, she will start eating less. Some stop eating. Before birth, increase the fibre content to make sure she gets empties her bowels. After birth, increase the bone content offered once again.

✓ Can you feed a vegetarian diet to a carnivore? No, you are advised not to until we know more. Studies suggest that a dry, ultra-processed vegetarian diet might compare favourably.

✓ The good news is raw is taking over. The bad news is as we increase the value of their meat waste products (carcass, necks, organs), meat will become even cheaper for humans, resulting in more meat being consumed. It is unsustainable to feed every dog on the planet the species-appropriate diet they deserve. The meat industry is a top polluter and extremely carbon expensive. Soon we will be forced to make more sustainable food choices, likely via a carbon tax. If climate change is a concern of yours, feed them white meat over red. It is predicted that dogs will then decrease in size, if not in numbers.

Chapter Twenty Four References

1 Saint-Hilaire, S., Lavers, M.K., Kennedy, J. *et al.* (1960). Gastric acid secretory value of different foods. Gastroenterology, 39(1): 1–11

2 Banta, C.A., Clemens, E.T., Krinsky, M.M. *et al.* (1979). Sites of organic acid production and patterns of digesta movement in the gastrointestinal tract of dogs. Journal of Nutrition, 109(9): 1592–1600

3 Carpentier, Y., Woussen-Colle, M.C. & de Graef, J. (1977). Gastric secretion from denervated pouches and serum gastrin levels after meals of different sizes and meat concentrations in dogs. Gastroenterology of Clinical Biology, 1: 29–37

4 Carrière, F., Laugier, R., Barrowman, J.A. *et al.* (1993). Gastric and pancreatic lipase levels during a test meal in dogs. Scandinavian Journal of Gastroenterology, 28: 443–454

5 Cook, G.C. (1985). Infective gastroenteritis and its relationship to reduced gastric acidity. Scandinavian Journal of Gastroenterology, 111: 17–23

6 Hunt, R.H. (1988). The protective role of gastric acid. Scandinavian Journal of Gastroenterology, 23(146): 34–39

7 Smith, J.L. (2003). The role of gastric acid in preventing foodborne disease and how bacteria over some acid conditions. Journal of Food Protection, 66(7):1292–1303

8 Martinsen, T.C., Bergh, K. and Waldum, H.L. (2005). Gastric juice: a barrier against infectious diseases. Basic and Clinical Pharmacology and Toxicology, 96(2): 94–102

9 Callaway, E. (2014). *Microbes help vultures eat rotting meat*. Nature. Published online, Nov 26th, www.nature.com

10 Dierenfeld, E.S., Alcorn, H.L. and Jacobsen, K.L. (2002). Nutrient Composition of Whole Vertebrate Prey (Excluding Fish) Fed in Zoos. U.S. Department of Agriculture. Published online, www.researchgate.net

11 Combs, D.K., Goodrich, R.D. and Meiske, J.C. (1982). Mineral concentrations in hair as indicators of mineral status: a review. Journal of Animal Science, 54(2): 391–398

12 Kant, A.K. and Graubard, B.I. (2004). Eating out in America, 1987-2000: trends and nutritional correlates. Preventative Medicine, 38: 243–249

13 Freeman, L.M. and Michel, K.E. (2001). Evaluation of raw food diet for dogs. Journal of the American Veterinary Medical Association, 218: 705–709

14 Dubey, J.P., Hill, D.E., Jones, J.L., *et al.* (2005). Prevalence of viable Toxoplasma gondii in beef, chicken, and pork from retail meat stores in the United States: Risk assessment to consumers. Journal of Parasitology, 91(5): 1082–1093

15 Centre for Disease Control and Prevention (CDC, 2017). *Estimates of Foodborne Illness in the United States*. Official Publication. Available on www.cdc.gov

16 Flegr, J., Prandota, J., Sovičková, M., *et al.* (2014). Toxoplasmosis – A Global Threat. Correlation of Latent Toxoplasmosis with Specific Disease Burden in a Set of 88 Countries. PLoS One. 2014; 9(3): e90203

17 Berdoy, M., Webster, J.P. and Macdonald, D.W. (2000). Fatal attraction in rats infected with *Toxoplasma gondii*. Proceedings of Biological Science, 267(1452): 1591–1594

18   Bhaduri, S. and Cottrell, B. (2004). Survival of cold-stressed *Campylobacter jejuni* on ground chicken and chicken skin during frozen storage. Applied Environmental Microbiology, 70(12): 7103–7109

19   van Dijk, M.A.M., Engelsma, M.Y., Visser, V.X.N. *et al.* (2018). *Brucella suis* infection in dog fed raw meat in the Netherlands. Emerging Infectious Diseases, 24(6): 1127–1129

20   Lucero, N.E., Ayala, S.M., Escobar, G.I. *et al.* (2008). *Brucella* isolated in humans and animals in Latin America from 1968 to 2006. Epidemiology and Infection, 136: 496–503

21   Mor, S.M., Wiethoelter, A.K., Lee, A. *et al.* (2016). Emergence of *Brucella suis* in dogs in New South Wales, Australia: clinical findings and implications for zoonotic transmission. BMC Veterinary Research, 12(199)

22   Boback, S.M., Cox, C.L., Ott, B.D.*et al.* (2007). Cooking and grinding reduces the cost of meat digestion. Comparative Biochemical Physiology, 148: 651–656

23   Wall, T., (2016). FDA update: Jerky treats sickened 6,200 dogs, killed 1,140. Pet Food Industry Magazine. Published online, May 16th, www.petfoodindustry.com

24   ANTECH Diagnostics (2003). *ANTECH News*. ANTECH Online Journal, June issue, see www.antechdiagnostics.come

25   Dodds, J. (2015). Raw Diets and Bloodwork results: should you be concerned? Published online, 6th Dec 2015, www.drjeandoddspethealthresource.tumblr.come

26   Mitchell, S.J., Bernier, M., Mattison, J.A. *et al.* (2019). Daily fasting improves health and survival in male mice independent of diet composition and calories. Cell Metabolism, 29(1): 221–228

27   Lee, J.H., Verma, N., Thakkar, N. *et al.* (2020). Intermittent Fasting: Physiological Implications on Outcomes in Mice and Men. Physiology, 35(3): 185–195

28   Raffaghello, L., Lee, C., Safdie, F.M. *et al.* (2008). Starvation-dependent differential stress resistance protects normal but not cancer cells against high-dose chemotherapy. PNAS, 105(24): 8215–8220

29   Wang, A., Huen, S.C., Luan, H.H. *et al.* (2016). Opposing effects of fasting metabolism on tissue tolerance in bacterial and viral inflammation. Cell, 166(6): 1512–1525

30   Jeong, M., Plunet, W., Streijger, F. *et al.* (2011). Intermittent fasting improves functional ecovery after rat thoracic contusion spinal cord injury. Journal of Neurotrauma, 28(3): 479–492

31   Raffaghello, L., Safdie, F., Bianchi, G. *et al.* (2010). Fasting and differential chemotherapy protection in patients. Cell Cycle, 9(22): 4474–4476

32   Knight, A. and Leitsberger, M. (2016). Vegetarian versus Meat-Based Diets for Companion Animals. Animals, 6(9): 57

33   Kienzle, E. and Engelhard, R.A. (2001). Field study on the nutrition of vegetarian dogs and cats in Europe. Compendium Continuing Education for Practicing Veterinarian, 23: 81

34   Gray,C.M., Sellon, K., Freeman, L.M., (2004). Nutritional adequacy of two vegan diets for cats. Journal of the American Veterinary Medical Association 225:1670–1675

35   Kanakubo, K., Fascetti, A.J. and Larsen, J.A. (2015). Assessment of protein and amino acid concentrations and labelling adequacy of commercial vegetarian diets formulated for dogs and cats. Journal of the American Veterinary Medical Association, 247: 385–392

36   Semp, P.G. (2014). *Vegan nutrition of dogs and cats*. Master's Thesis, Veterinary University of Vienna, Vienna, Austria

37   Brown, W.Y., Vanselow, B.A., Redman, A.J. *et al*. (2009). An experimental meat-free diet maintained haematological characteristics in sprint-racing sled dogs. British Journal of Nutrition, 102: 1318–1323

38   Matthews, C. (2006). Livestock a major threat to environment. Food and Agriculture Organisation of the United Nations. Published online, see www.fao.org

39   Desjardins, R.L., Worth, D.E., Vergé, X.P.C. *et al*. (2012). Carbon Footprint of Beef Cattle. Sustainability, 4(12): 3279–3301

40   Eshel, G., Shepon, A., Makov, T. *et al*. (2014). Land, irrigation water, greenhouse gas, and reactive nitrogen burdens of meat, eggs, and dairy production in the United States. PNAS, 111(33): 11996–12001

41   Hribar, C. (2010). Understanding concentrated animal feeding operations and their impact on communities. Official Publication of the Centres for Disease Control and Prevention (CDC). Available online www.cdc.gov

42   Scarborough, P., Appleby, P.N., Mizdrak, A. *et al*. (2014). Dietary greenhouse gas emissions of meat-eaters, fish-eaters, vegetarians and vegans in the UK. Climatic Change, 125(2): 179–192

43   Hancox, D. (2018). The unstoppable rise of veganism: how a fringe movement went mainstream. The Guardian Newspaper. Published online, Apr 1st, www.theguardian. com

Abbreviations

AAFCO	Association of American Feed Control Officials
AAHA	American Animal Hospital Association
AAI	Animal Assisted Intervention
AAVLD	American Association of Veterinary Laboratory Diagnosticians
ACE	Angiotensin–converting enzyme
ACTH	Adrenocorticotropic Hormone
AGE's	Advanced glycation end products
AJCN	American Journal of Clinical Nutrition
ALA	Alpha-linolenic acid
AND	Academy of Nutrition and Dietetics
APN	Acute polyradiculoneuritis
ATP	Adenosine tri-phosphate
ATPF	Association for Truth in Pet food
AVMA	American Veterinary Medical Association
BAHVS	British Association of Homeopathic Veterinary Surgeons
BARF	Bones and raw food OR Biologically-appropriate raw food
BDNF	Brain-derived neurotrophic factor
BHA	Butylated hydroxyanisole
BHT	Butylated hydroxytoluene
BMI	Body mass index
BMJ	*British Medical Journal*
BPA	Bisphenol A
BSE	Bovine spongiform encephalopathy
BUN	Blood urea nitrogen
BW	Body weight
CAFO	Concentrate Animal Feed Operations

ABBREVIATIONS

CD	Coeliac disease
CDC	Centres for Disease Control
CDV	Canine Distemper Virus
CFIA	Canadian Food Inspection Agency
CHD	Canine hip dysplasia
CKF	Chronic Kidney Failure
CLA	Conjugated linoleic acid
CO	Cardiac output
CP	Colgate-Palmolive
CPV	Canine parvovirus
CVM	Center for Veterinary Medicine
CVMA	Canadian Veterinary Medical Association
DCM	Dilated cardiomyopathy
DCPAH	Diagnostic Center for Population and Animal Health
DEHP	Diethylhexyl phthalate
DHA	Docosahexaenoic acid
DM	Dry matter
DSR	Differential stress resistance
DTI	Department of Trade and Industry
DVM	Doctor Veterinariae Medicinae
EAA	Essential amino acids
EMA	European Medicines Agency
EPA	Environmental Protection Agency
EPI	Exocrine Pancreatitic Insufficiency
FDA	Food and Drug Administration
FDAAA	Food and Drug Administration Amendments Act
FEDIAF	The European Pet Food Industry Federation
FFDCA	Federal Food, Drug, and Cosmetic Act
FOI	Freedom of Information
FSH	Follicle-stimulating hormone
GALT	Gut Associated Lymphoid Tissue
GCK	Hepatic glucokinase

GH	Growth hormone
GI	Glycaemic index
GL	Glycaemic load
GMO	Genetically modified organism
GSD	German Shepherd dogs
HCA	Heterocyclic amines
HDL	High-density lipoprotein
HPCSA	Health Professions Council of South Africa
IAVH	International Association for Veterinary Homeopathy
IBD	Irritable Bowel Disorder
IgA	Immunoglobulin A
IgE	Immunoglobulin E
IgG	Immunoglobulin G
IOM	Institute of Medicine
JAVMA	*Journal of the American Veterinary Medicine Association*
LA	Linoleic acid
LCHF	Low-carbohydrate-high-fat
LDL	Low-density lipoprotein
LH	Luteinizing hormone
LHL	Low, then high, then low
MBM	Meat and bone meal
ME	Metabolisable energy
MMI	Mark Morris Institute
MRCVS	Member of the Royal College of Veterinary Surgeons
MRP	Maillard reaction products
MRSA	Methicillin-resistant *Staphylococcus aureus*
MSD	Merck, Sharp & Dohme
NBC	National Broadcasting Company
NGO	Non-Governmental Organisation
NHMRC	National Health and Medical Research Council
NRC	National Research Council
NSAID	Nonsteroidal anti-inflammatory

ABBREVIATIONS

OSHA	Occupational Safety and Health Administration
OTC	Oxytetracycline
PAHO	Pan American Health Organisation
PET	Positron emission tomography
PFMA	Pet Food Manufacturers Association
PLoS	Public Library of Science
PMS	Premenstrual syndrome
PR	Public relations
PTH	Parathyroid hormone
RCVS	Royal College of Veterinary Surgeons
RDA	Recommended daily allowance
RFD	Raw food diet
RFR	Reportable Food Registry
RMB	Raw meaty bones
RMBD	Raw meat and bone diets
RR	Reference range
RVC	Royal Veterinary College
SACN	Small Animal Clinical Nutrition
SPB	Sodium pentobarbital
TB	Tuberculosis
TPR	Total peripheral resistance
TSH	Thyroid-stimulating hormone
UCSF	University of California San Francisco
UKRMB	UK Raw Meaty Bones
UNICEF	The United Nations Children's Fund
USDA	US Department of Agriculture
VCA	Veterinary Centres of America
VNA	Veterinary Nutrition Advocate
VPI	Veterinary Pet Insurance
WABA	World Alliance for Breastfeeding Action
WHO	World Health Organisation
WSAVA	World Small Animal Veterinary Association

Index

INDEX

Acknowledgements

I first and foremost would like to thank my friends and family for keeping me sane during this project. I fully realise I have been nothing short of a burden for much of the last ten years as I obsessed over this manuscript. I especially want to thank my wife, Elaine. On every level, you have been the difference in getting this book done and not even beginning it in the first place. I sincerely appreciate your patience and support. I want to thank all my proofreaders (too numerous to mention) and my publisher Orla Kelly. I'm positive this has been one of the worst experiences of her life. Your patience in the face of my constant tweaking has made for a far more robust manuscript. Thanks for all your work. I want to thank my parents – my father for instilling a love of nature and the outdoors and my mother for fueling my love of dogs by driving me out weekly to those animal shelters (a 90-minute round trip...every week) and ingraining in me a strong work ethic throughout the years. I need to thank Dr Hubert Fuller. My mentor in college, Hubert talked me down from a proverbial ledge following some poor exam results one year. My best friend passed away some months before and I had neither the heart nor head to focus on my work. I was encouraged to try again and, undoubtedly with his help behind the scenes, I limped through that year second time around. From there, things improved for me and my focus returned. I wouldn't be doing this without him.

Finally, I need to thank a few vets. I have been neck-deep in research and it's fair to say, a lot of it was quite negative. It's hard to go down a rabbit hole and not realise how dark things have become. That can take its toll. The more I learned of the corruption in science, the more I feared the subject was becoming sullied beyond repair, reduced the realms of a marketing gimmick. It was meeting people like Dr Nick Thompson that returned my faith in science and discovery to full strength. Nick is a brilliant vet and formidable mind. Far longer at this game than me, I bounce all my ideas off him and the content of this book is stronger for his input. Dr Brendan Clarke the same. A formidable intellect. I love debating various scientific topics with you and one day, God willing, I will win one. Thanks to Dr Anna Hielm-Bjorkman and her crew at Dog Risk, Helsinki University, Finland, for all that you do. Still, one of the few if not only university groups that actively compare fresh and dry fed dogs. They need our support. And thanks to all the members of the Raw Feeding Vet Society whom I bother constantly. Wonderful, wonderful vets and vet nurses, one and all. Thank you for reminding me what a vital profession it is you guys practice and how crucial it is that we preserve its integrity well into the future.

Made in the USA
Coppell, TX
30 June 2021